Leisure, Pleasure and Healing

Supplements

to the

Journal for the Study of Judaism

Editor

John J. Collins

The Divinity School, Yale University

Associate Editor

Florentino García Martínez

Qumran Institute, University of Groningen

Advisory Board

J. DUHAIME − A. HILHORST − P.W. VAN DER HORST

A. KLOSTERGAARD PETERSEN − M.A. KNIBB − H. NAJMAN

J.T.A.G.M. VAN RUITEN − J. SIEVERS − G. STEMBERGER

E.J.C. TIGCHELAAR − J. TROMP

VOLUME 116

Leisure, Pleasure and Healing

Spa Culture and Medicine

in Ancient Eastern Mediterranean

by

Estēe Dvorjetski

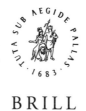

BRILL

LEIDEN • BOSTON
2007

This book is printed on acid-free paper.

Library of Congress Cataloging-in-Publication data

Dvorjetski, Estee.
  Leisure, pleasure, and healing : spa culture and medicine in ancient eastern
  Mediterranean / by Estee Dvorjetski.
    p. cm. — (Supplements to the Journal for the study of Judaism ; v. 116)
  Includes bibliographical references and index.
  ISBN-13: 978-90-04-15681-4
  ISBN-10: 90-04-15681-X (alk. paper)
    1. Health resorts—Middle East—History. 2. Mineral waters—Therapeutic
  use—Middle East—History. 3. Balneology—Middle East—History. 4. Hot
  springs—Middle East—History. 5. Baths, Hot—Middle East—History.
  6. Medicine—Middle East—History. 7. Medicine, Ancient. I. Title.

RA934.M628D86 2007
613'.1220956—dc22
                                                                    2007060882

ISSN 1384-2161
ISBN-13: 978 90 04 15681 4

PRINTED IN THE NETHERLANDS

This book is lovingly dedicated
to my husband and friend
Dubi Dvorjetski

CONTENTS

LIST OF ABBREVIATIONS

A	*Arabic*
AASOR	*Annual of the American Schools of Oriental Research*
ADAJ	*Annual of the Department of Antiquities of Jordan*
AÉ	*L'Année Épigraphique*
AIM	*Annals of Internal Medicine*
AJA	*American Journal of Archaeology*
AJN	*American Journal of Nephrology*
AJSLL	*American Journal of Semitic Languages and Literatures*
AK	*Archaeologisches Korrespondenzblatt*
AMIF	*Journal de l'Association des medecins Israelites de France*
AMO	*Acta Medica Orientalia*
AJN	*American Journal of Nephrology*
ANRW	*Aufstieg und Niedergang der römischen Welt: Geschiche und Kultur Roms im Spiegel Neueren Forschung*
ANS	*American Numismatic Society (Numismatic Studies)*
ANSM	*American Numismatic Society Museum Notes*
AR	*Archiv für Religionswissenschaft*
ARAM	*ARAM Periodical*
Archeologia	*Archeologia, Rome, Italy*
Archaeology	*Magazine dealing with the Antiquity of the World*
ARID	*Analecta Romana Instituti Danici*
Ariel	*Periodical for the Geography Eretz-Israel*
ArO	*Archiv für Orientforschung*
ArRh	*Arthritis and Rheumatism*
Art Bulletin	*The Bulletin of the College Art Association of America*
Atidot	*Scientific Literary Collection for Youth, The Zionist Organization*
'Atiqot	*Journal of the Israel Department of Antiquities, Hebrew Series*
'Atiqot EgS	*Journal of the Israel Department of Antiquities, English Series*
Ausonia	*Rivista della Società italiana di archeologia e storia dell'arte*
AUSS	*Andrews University Seminary Studies*
BA	*Biblical Archaeologist*
BAIAS	*Bulletin of the Anglo-Israel Archaeological Society*
BAMAH	*Drama Quarterly*
BAR	*Biblical Archaeology Review*
BASOR	*Bulletin of the American Schools of Oriental Research*

Behinot	*Review in Literature Criticism, Jerusalem*
Beth Mikra	*Quarterly of the Israel Society for Biblical Research*
BGA	*Bibliotheca Geographorum Arabicorum*
BGSI	*Bulletin of Geological Survey of Israel*
Biblica	*Journal, Commentarii editi a Pontificio Instituto biblico*
BHM	*Bulletin of the History of Medicine*
BIES	*Bulletin of the Israel Exploration Society*
BIHPS	*Bulletin of the Institute for Hebrew Poetry Research*
BINS	*Bulletin of the Israel Numismatic Society*
BJb	*Bonner Jahrbücher*
BJPES	*Bulletin of the Jewish Palestine Exploration Society*
Bodl. MS Heb.	*Bodleian Collection, Oxford*
BPSHE	*Bulletin of the Palestine Society for History and Ethnography*
Brit.	*Britannia, A Journal of Romano-British and Kindred Studies*
BRCI	*Bulletin of the Research Council of Israel*
BRCI	*Bulletin of the Research Council of Israel*
BSOAS	*Bulletin of the School of Oriental and African Studies*
BSSA	*Bulletin of the Seismological Society of America*
ByZ	*Byzantinische Zeitschrift*
Byzantion	*Revue internationale des études Byzantines*
BZ	*Biblische Zeitschrift*
CAC	*Commentationes de Antiquitate Classica*
Cathedra	*Cathedra for the History of Eretz-Israel and Its Yishuv*
CCSL	*Corpus Christianorum. Series Latina*
CG	*Chemical Geology*
ChE	*Chronique d'Egypte*
CI	*Classics Ireland*
CIL	*Corpus Inscriptionum Latinarum*
CJHSP	*Canadian Journal of the History of Sport and Physical Education*
Cl. Med.	*Clio Medica, Acta Academiae Internationalis Historiae Medicinae*
CM	*Classica et Mediaevalia*
CMG	*Corpus Medicorum Graecorum*
CNI	*Christian News from Israel*
CPh	*Classical Philology*
CQ	*The Classical Quarterly*
CSEL	*Corpus Scriptorum Ecclesiasticorum Latinorum*
CSHB	*Corpus Scriptorum Historiae Byzantinae*
DAH	*Das Heilige Land*

DaM	*Damaszener Mitteilungen*
EB	*Encyclopaedia Biblica*
EH	*Encyclopaedia Hebraica*
EI	*Eretz-Israel: Archaeological, Historical and Geographical Studies*
Eitaniim	*Bi-Monthly Journal for Health Affairs and Public Medicine*
EJ	*Encyclopedia Judaica*
Eretz-HaGolan	*Journal of the Golan Settlements*
Eshel Beer-Sheva	*Annual, Studies in Bible, Ancient Israel and the Ancient Near East*
Eshkolot NS	*Eshkolot, New Series: Collection Devoted to the Study of Classical Culture and Its Interpretation*
ESI	*Excavations and Surveys in Israel*
ÉT	*Études et Travaux*
Et-Mol	*Journal for the History of the Land of Israel and the Jewish People Tel-Aviv University*
Expedition	*University of Pennsylvania Museum Magazine of Archaeology and Anthropology*
FPMJ	*The Family Physician, Medical Journal*
GBS	*Greek and Byzantine Studies*
GCS	*Die griechischen christlichen Schriftsteller der ersten drei Jahrhunderte*
Geology	*A Journal of the Geological Society of America*
Germania	*Anzeiger der Römisch-Germanischen Kommission des deutschen archaologischen Instituts*
GRC	*Geothermal Resources Council*
GJ	*Geology Jahrbücher*
GSI	*Geological Survey of Israel Report*
GVJ	*Gesellschaft pro Vindonissa, Jahresbericht*
H	*Hebrew*
HA	*Hadashot Archiologiot*
HaH	*HaHinuh HaGufani*
HaKedem	*Vierteljahrschrift die Kunde des alten Orients und die Wissenschaft Des Judentums*
HaMayan	*Judaism Periodical*
HaRefuah	*Journal of the Israel Medical Association*
Harofé Haivri	*The Hebrew Medical Journal*
HaTekufah	*Annual for Literature and Meditation*
Hebrew Studies	*A Journal devoted to Hebrew Language and Literature*
Hellenica	*Recueil d'épigraphie de numismatique et d'antiquités grecques*

Hermes	*Zeitschrift für klassische Philologie*
Historia	*Journal of the Historical Society of Israel*
Historia Judaica	*A Journal of Studies in Jewish History*
HP	*The Hebrew Physician*
HTR	*Harvard Theological Review*
HUCA	*Hebrew Union College Annual*
ICS	*Illinois Classical Studies*
ICST	*Institute of Classical Studies*
IEJ	*Israel Exploration Journal*
IG	*Inscriptiones Graecae*
IGA	*International Geothermal Association*
IJES	*Israel Journal of Earth Sciences*
ILS	*Inscriptiones Latinae Selectae*
IMZ	*Internationale Mineralquellen Zeitung*
IMJ	*Israel Museum Journal*
IMN	*The Israel Museum News*
INJ	*Israel Numismatic Journal*
JAOS	*Journal of the American Oriental Society*
JAS	*Journal of Archaeological Science*
JASTR	*Journal of the American Society for Theatre Research*
JBL	*Journal of Biblical Literature*
JCE	*Journal of Chemical Education*
JESHO	*Journal of the Economic and Social History of the Orient*
JGE	*Journal of Geochemical Exploration*
JGS	*Journal of Glass Studies*
JH	*Journal of Hydrology*
JHM	*Journal of the History of Medicine and Allied Sciences*
JHS	*The Journal of Hellenistic Studies*
JHSI	*Historia: Journal of the Historical Society of Israel*
JIH	*Journal of Interdisciplinary History*
JJS	*Journal of Jewish Studies*
JÖAI	*Jahrshefte des Österreichischen archäologishen Institutes in Wien*
JÖB	*Jahrbuch der Österreichischen Byzantinistik*
JPOS	*Journal of the Palestine Oriental Society*
JQR	*Jewish Quarterly Review*
JR	*Journal of Religion*
JRA	*Journal of Roman Archaeology*
JRS	*Journal of Roman Studies*
JRSM	*Journal of the Royal Society of Medicine*

JSJ	*Journal for the Study of Judaism in the Persian, Hellenistic and Roman Periods*
JSHL	*Jerusalem Studies in Hebrew Literature*
JSJF	*Jerusalem Studies in Jewish Folklore*
Kardom	*Bi-monthly Journal for the Geography of Eretz-Israel*
KBS	*Kolner Beiträge zur Sportwissenschaft*
LA	*Liber Annus, Journal of Studium Biblicum Franciscanum, Jerusalem*
Kerem Hemed	*Periodical for Belief and Wisdom, Prague*
Koroth	*The Israel Journal of the History of Medicine and Science*
Kinnrot	*Bulletin of the Council of the Regional Jordan Valley*
Latomus	*Revue D'Études Latines*
Laverna	*Beiträge zur Wirtschafts und Sozialgeschichte der alten Welt*
Leshonenu	*A Quarterly for the Improvement of the Hebrew Language*
Levant	*Journal of the British School of Archaeology in Jerusalem*
LCL	*Loeb Classical Library*
LIMC	*Lexicon Iconographicum Mythologiae Classicae*
LMC	*Les Missions Catholiques*
Mada	*A Scientific Journal for Everyone, The Weizmann Science Press of Israel*
Med. Arch.	*Mediterranean Archaeology*
Med. Hist.	*Medical History*
Med. Jud.	*Medica Judaica*
MGWJ	*Monatschrift für Geschichte und Wissenschaft des Judentums*
MHR	*Mediterranean Historical Review*
MHS	*Medical History, Supplement*
Mituv Teveria	*Papers for the Study of Tiberiasd*
ML	*Meida LaRofe*
Mnemosyne	*Bibliotheca classica Batava*
MoA	*Monumenti Antichi*
MOTAR	*Periodical of the Faculty of Arts, Tel-Aviv University*
Nature	*International Weekly Journal of Science*
NEAEHL	*The New Encyclopedia of Archaeological Excavations in the Holy Land*
NEJM	*The New England Journal of Medicine*
NSA	*Notizie degli Scavi di Antichità*
Num. Cir.	*Numismatic Circular*
OGIS	*Orientis Graeci Inscriptiones Selectae*
OJA	*Oxford Journal of Archaeology*
OLZ	*Orientalistische Litteraturzeitung*

OMNIBVS	*OMNIBVS Magazine*
OOr	*Occident & Orient*
PAG	*Pure Applied Geophysics*
Palästina	*Zeitschrift für den Aufbau Palästinas*
Palästinajahrbuch	*Palästinajahrbuch des deutschen Evangelischen Instituts für Altertumswissenschaft des Heiligen Landes zu Jerusalem*
PBSR	*Papers of the British School at Rome*
PEFQSt	*Palestine Exploration Fund Quarterly Statement*
PEQ	*Palestine Exploration Quarterly*
PG	*Patrologiae cursus completus, Series Graeca*
Phoenix	*A Journal of the Classical Association of Canada*
PL	*Patrologia cursus completes, Series Latina*
PRSM	*Proceedings of the Royal Society of Medicine*
PTRSL	*Philosophy Transactions of the Royal Society of London*
Puteoli	*Puteoli, Studi di storia antica*
Qadmoniot	*Quarterly for the Antiquities of Eretz-Israel and Bible Lands*
QDAP	*Quarterly of the Department of Antiquities in Palestine*
Qedem	*Monographs of the Institute of Archaeology, The Hebrew University of Jerusalem*
RB	*Revue Biblique*
RÉA	*Revue des Études Anciennes*
RÉG	*Revue des Études Greques*
RÉJ	*Revue des Études Juives*
RHMH	*Revue d'histoire de la médecine hebraïque*
RhRe	*Rheumathology and Rehabilitation*
RÖJ	*Römisches Österreich, Jahresschrift der österreichischen Gesellschaft für Archäologie*
RP	*Roman Papers*
RPAR	*Rendiconti della Pontifica Academia Romana di Archeologia*
RQ	*Revue de Qumeran*
S	*Syriac*
SCI	*Scripta Classica Israelica, Journal of the Israel Society for the Promotion of Classical Studies*
Sefunim	*Periodical of the Nautical Museum, Haifa*
Semitica	*Cahiers publiés par l'Institut d'études sémitiques de l'Université de Paris*
SH	*Scripta Hierosolymitana*
SHAJ	*Studies in the History and Archaeology of Jordan*
SHH	*Shenaton HaMishpat HaIvri*
Shma'atin	*Journal of Teachers' Union for Holiness Professions*

Sidra	*A Journal for the Study of Rabbinic Literature*
SIFC	*Studi Italiani di Filologia Classica*
SIG	*Sylloge Inscriptionum Graecarum*
Sinai	*Periodical for Torah and Judaic Studies*
SJ	*Saalburg Jahrbücher*
Speculum	*A Journal of Mediaeval Studies*
Syria	*Syria revue d'art oriental et d'archélogie*
Talanta	*Proceedings of the Dutch Archaeological and Historical Society*
Tarbiz	*A Quarterly for Jewish Studies*
Teuda	*Collection of Studies of the School of Judaic Studies, Tel-Aviv University*
Teva Va'aretz	*Nature and The Land, Tel Avivl*
TS Taylor	*Schechter Collection, Cambridge University*
TZ	*Theologische Zeitschrift*
UF	*Ugarit-Forschungen Internationales Jahrbuch für die Altertumskunde Syrien-Palästinas*
Westminster Coll.	*Manuscripts Collection at Westminster College, Cambridge*
WJM	*The Western Journal of Medicine*
ZAW	*Zeitschrift für die alttestamentliche Wissenschaft*
ZBKKH	*Zeitschrift für Balneologie Klimatologie und Kurort-Hygiene*
ZDMG	*Zeitschrift der Deutschen Morgenländischen Gesellschaft*
ZDPV	*Zeitschrift des Deutschen Palästina-Vereins*
Zion	*A Quarterly for Research in Jewish History*
ZPE	*Zeitschrift für Papyrologie und Epigraphik*

LIST OF ILLUSTRATIONS

List of Maps

List of Tables

List of Figures

ACKNOWLEDGEMENTS

It is a pleasant duty to record various debts of gratitude incurred during the writing of the current project throughout the years. I owe a profound debt of gratitude to Prof. Moshe D. Herr of the Department Jewish History at The Hebrew University in Jerusalem, my devoted PhD supervisor, for a staunch support and a fount of inspiration throughout my studies. His intellectual virtuosity, philological expertise, and extraordinary skill in textual analysis of Rabbinic and Classical sources are models to which my own scholarship aspires. It gives a particular pleasure to thank my friend and colleague Prof. Arthur Segal of Haifa University, Department of Archaeology. I have benefited enormously not only as my talented and cordial MA supervisor, but during our mutual work in writing few articles. His fascinating courses, methodological insights, conversations, and encouragement over the years laid the foundation for the current project of thermo-mineral springs in the eastern Mediterranean. I also wish to thank Prof. Ya'akov Meshorer of the Department of Archaeology at the Hebrew University of Jerusalem for his equally invaluable knowledge and inspiration but, sadly, I can no longer express my thanks to him in person. Late Prof. Meshorer first sparked my interest in describing the fascination of ancient coins, taught me the real value of coins, and the attractive way of how to teach numismatics, as I do also nowadays. To them I owe most of my knowledge at its very best. I am extremely grateful to Prof. Martin Goodman of the Oriental Institute and Wolfson College at Oxford University for his friendship, generosity, keen interest, and stimulation during the period of its composition. I am particularly indebted to Prof. Steven King of the Department of History at Oxford Brookes University for unstinting support, confidence and sincere will and efforts in admitting me as a member of staff to Oxford Brookes University and so changed my life for ever.

I have been fortune to have taught at several positions—The Hebrew University of Jerusalem, University of Haifa, The Technion (Israel institute of Technology), Safed Regional College and The Western Galilee College, branches of Bar-Ilan University, and Emek Yizre'el Academic College—richly endowed with colleagues and students whose pointed questions and fresh insights made it fun to work out the argument of the book.

The generosity of editors, scholars and colleagues has also been fundamental for their careful attention to detail and considerable help. I would like to thank all the following: Prof. Henry Near, Prof. Ze'ev Safrai, Dr. Janet DeLaine, Prof. John Humphry, Prof. Yishar Hirschfeld, Prof. Vivian Nutton, Prof. Ronny Reich, Prof. Sebastian Brock, Prof. Felix Jaffé, Prof. Martin Hening, Dr. Dov Levitte, Dr. Arie Kindler, Prof. Roger Hanoune, Prof. Ziony Zevit, Eli Schiler, Dr. Gabi Barkai, Dr. Moshe Hartal, Dr. Shafiq Abouzayd, and Hershel Shanks; and to the physicians Prof. Eran Dolev, Prof. Shaul M. Shasha, Dr. Walter Loebl, Dr. Israel Machty, and Dr. Tamar Armon-Merhav for their suggestions, stimulating discussions, and timely advice. Needless to say, I bear sole responsibility for any remaining errors.

This book came into being after numerous visits to sites and museums in Israel, England, France, Greece, Italy, and Germany during the last fifteen years. It would be impossible to name every site director and museum curator that has shown me their material and bibliography, but above all I would like to thank particularly Dr. Ralph Jackson, curator of Romano-British collections at the British Museum, Mr. Stephen Clews, curator of Bath Spa, England, and Ronny Lothan, former manager of Hammat-Gader Thermo-Mineral Baths Ltd. for their kindness and hospitality.

Several of the ideas and selected portions of this interdisciplinary study have been presented at conferences, seminars and colloquia at the Hebrew University of Jerusalem, Tel-Aviv University, University of Haifa; University College London, Department of Jewish History and The Wellcome Trust Centre for the History of Medicine at UCL; Oxford—Wolfson College, The Oxford Centre for Hebrew and Jewish Studies, and Oxford Brookes University, The Centre of Health, Medicine and Society: Past and Present; University of Manchester, Centre for Jewish Studies; Athens, Cos Island, Greece; and the University of Padua, Italy. I am indebted to the organisers and participants for invitations, their valuable comments, criticisms, and enthusiastic interest.

Financial assistance for continental visits and scholarships were very kindly made available by the Memorial Foundation for Jewish Culture in U.S.A.; Dean of the Graduate Studies Authority at Haifa University; Moris M. Fulber fund; The Centre for the Study of Eretz-Israel and its Yishuv, Yad Izhak Ben Zvi; Hammat-Gader Thermo-Mineral Baths Ltd.; Dean of the Faculty of Humanities and The Institute of Jewish Studies at the Hebrew University of Jerusalem; Safed Regional College; Western Galilee College; Project 2000 and The Jewish Agency; The

Wellcome Trust Centre for the History of Medicine at University College London; and last but not least, Oxford Brookes University.

I also thank the editors at Brill Academic Publishers, Prof. John J. Collins, Prof. Florentino García Martínez, Wilma de Weert, Machiel Kleemans, Michiel Klein-Swormink, and Mattie Kuiper for their confidence and useful work. Their suggestions have made this book more compelling. I also express my appreciation and gratitude for the following publishers who have kindly given permission for their pictures to be reproduced: The British Museum Publications, The Israel Exploration Society, Prof. Yizhar Hirschfeld, The Israel Museum, Prof. J.H. Humphrey, Prof. Martin Henig, Prof. Michele Piccirillo, Librairie Orientaliste—Paul Geuthner, Princeton University Press, Studium Biblicum Franciscanum, and The Open University of Israel.

Many individuals have assisted my work. I am especially indebted to Sonia Gefen, Dr. Tsvia Balsan, Inbal Dvorjetski, Diana Dvorjetski, Malka Eron-Egozi, Kitty and Freddy Liebrich, Miri Fashchik, Mira Waner, Ruti and Noam Or, Dr. Carol Beadle, Dr. Elizabeth Hurren, Dr. Lili Arad, and Miriam Brock-Cohen for all their loving support. Foremost are my husband and friend, Dubi Dvorjetski, who has provided inestimable support in every way, love and devotion all over the years, and our two sons, Meiri and Ariel, who have spent their entire lives with my fruitful prolonged researches. Their remarkable forbearance and novel questions have helped keep my perspective fresh. I have always admired their skillful knowledge in interdisciplinary issues and their control in the computer's hardware functions.

My profound love and respect are for my parents-in-law, Prof. Meir (Mark) and Hasia Dvorjetski. They have encouraged my early steps in the academia wholeheartedly. I wish only that my Professorship awarded by Oxford Brookes University and this book could have appeared before their untimely death.

Kiryat-Bialik, Israel   Estēe Dvorjetski
14th October 2006

PREFACE

This book deals with *Leisure, Pleasure and Healing* in the eastern Mediterranean basin since the Biblical era throughout the Hellenistic, Roman, Byzantine, and Early Muslim periods. It is a monograph of the therapeutic sites in the Levant, which are models for social interaction, especially mutual cultural influences between pagans, Christians and Jews. This study looks closely at the question of whether the spas served as sacred cult places or popular sites of healing, immorality and debauchery.

The main objectives of the book are as follows: • Tracing the process of development of medicinal sites with a distinctly Hellenistic character in a Semitic environment; • Clarifying the leisure-time activities in the therapeutic baths based on Classical and Rabbinic sources, travel-books of pilgrims, Arabic documents, Syriac texts, the *Geniza* fragments, cartographic evidences, and archaeological remains; • Lightening the daily life, healing cults, medical recommendations and treatments at the curative spas; • Investigating Jewish and Christian ethics towards mixed bathing and bathing as a medical measure; • Examining the social history of medicine at the therapeutic thermal baths; • and demonstrating the healing properties of the spas in light of modern medicine.

The book is based upon my PhD dissertation, entitled *Medicinal Hot Springs in Eretz-Israel during the Second Temple ,The Mishna and The Talmud* (1992) and upon my M.A. thesis, entitled *Hammat-Gader during the Hellenistic, Roman and Byzantine Periods: An Historical-Archaeological Analysis* (1988) written both in Hebrew. The current monograph integrates more than dozens of articles and chapters in books published by me since 1991, which deal with medicinal hot springs as a cross-section of socio-economic, cultural and religious history as well as all relevant papers and works published since then. The outcome of this prolonged and interdisciplinary study is presented in this book.

My book was written mainly during sabbatical tenures in England as a Visiting Prof. in the Centre for Health, Medicine and Society: Past and Present at the Department of History at Oxford Brookes University, as a Honorary Research Fellow at the Wellcome Trust Centre for the History of Medicine at University College London (2004–2005), twice as a Visiting Scholar at the Oxford Centre for Hebrew and Jewish Studies

Oxford (2001–2002; 2004–2005), and North Oxford Overseas Centre. These institutions and places provided excellent facilities, congenial hospitality and extensive support during my project. Oxford has been to me and to my husband a haven of academic tranquillity.

While writing my interdisciplinary study, I was assisted by the accessibility to the material and data found in various libraries in England: the unique Wellcome Library for the History and Understanding of Medicine in London, the Oriental Institute library, the Sackler Library and the library of the Oxford Centre for Hebrew and Jewish Studies in Oxford. This accessibility was invaluable for integrating the Classical sources, Talmudic literature, recent archaeological reports, epigraphic findings and contemporary researches, particularly in the Hashemite Kingdom of Jordan.

Although the topics of bathing and medicine in the Roman world have received considerable attention (see bibliography), thermo-mineral baths have remained inadequately studied. Recent research acknowledges the importance of spas, but generally excludes any detailed discussion of the institution. To this day, there has been no study, which surveys the history and archaeology of all spas in the East lightening the issues of daily life, healing cults, medical recommendations and treatments. There has been no systematic collocation of all literary sources and archaeological findings of all spas. No integration of the geological, historical, archaeological, cultural, social and medicinal aspects of the curative sites from the Biblical era until the early Muslim periods has thus far been published as a interdisciplinary monograph of the curative places in the Levant. My book is the first to use and integrate a wide range of evidences, including ancient literary sources, inscriptions, numismatics and archaeological material. This approach provides new insights into *Spa Culture and Medicine in Ancient Eastern Mediterranean*.

In an attempt to do justice to a question of this complexity, each chapter consciously takes a different perspective and approach. Chapter 1 presents the idea behind the book's name; Researches on thermo-mineral springs and baths in Israel and Jordan written by geologists, hydrologists, geochemists, geographers, historians, archaeologists and physicians are reviewed; The source material, goals and methodological issues of the book are described; Etymological and historical investigations of the terms *hot spring, spa, bath, thermae, balnea, miqweh, hammat, hammei, hammtha, hammam, Ba'arah, Emmaus*, and *Kallirrhoe* in Hebrew, Aramaic, Syriac, Greek, Latin and Arabic are discussed extensively; Another issue, which has thus far been neglected by previous scholars, is the traces in the Bible for the existence of hot mineral springs; and finally, all sorts of leisure-time activities and places of entertainment in the eastern Mediterranean in antiquity are demonstrated. In chapter 2 the distribution and identification of the hot springs in the following regions are presented: The Tiberias basin and the Yarmuk Canyon, the western and eastern margins of the Jordan Valley, the Dead Sea basin, the Syro-African Rift, Sinai and more; The formation of thermo-mineral waters, the source of their waters, various models for their creation, and the geothermal energy utilisation in the Jordan Valley since antiquity are also enlightened; The chapter deals too with their use in light of modern medicine for a better comprehension of the spas' qualities, functions and benefits in antiquity. Chapter 3 is a survey of the Medicinal hot springs and healing spas in the Graeco-Roman world, which contributes to a better understanding of the essence of them in the eastern Mediterranean. Thus, five topics are handled: The Original use of hot springs since the days of Hippocrates; Healing qualities and spa therapy; Ritual worship at the sites; The Military presence; and the Roman leisure culture in public baths and spas. Some inquiries face the questions if the term *valetudinarium* is suitable also for health resorts built by the Romans. Were the spas leisure cultural centres or sites to debauch? What functional elements normally existed in ordinary baths, but not in therapeutic baths based on hot mineral waters? Chapter 4 examine an historical-archaeological analysis and healing cults of Hammei-Tiberias, Hammat-Gader, Hammat-Pella, Hammei-Ba'arah, Kallirrhoe, Hammei-Livias, and Emmaus-Nicopolis. In addition, several Talmudic proofs to identify the Waters of Asia and their significance are adduced. In this chapter we present the social, religious, cultural atmosphere and economic life, which prevailed in the spas. The main issues in chapter 5 are as follows: the nature of the therapeutic baths in view of Classical sources; Knowledge and recommendations accord-ing to Rabbinic literature and Cairo *Geniza* fragments; The healing properties in the light of archaeological findings are also displayed. Several common denominators of all literary documents will be shown for classifying the usage of each spa for various ailments. The medical health problems of some personages, like Rabbi Judah the Patriarch and others, who were aware of the reputation of the spas that were regarded highly for their ability to restore health, will be noted. In chapter 6 the daily Life at the spas according to the Rabbinic Literature will be illustrated. Several issues are presented like the *halakhic* rulings of Rabbis towards medicinal springs; *Halakhic* problems in daily life; The

affinity between the Talmudic corpus and Classical sources regarding
the features of these bathing places; and the relationship between Jews
and gentiles at the curative baths; Several imminent problems are
raised. Were they social institutions of bathing, of ritual, of therapy
and of entertainment, including licentious immorality? Did their use
by the Jews create a conflict between the popular need, especially for
healing, and the religious restrictions, which were discussed and decreed
by the Sages? Chapter 7 depicts the intents and actions of the Emperors
Vespasian, Hadrian and Caracalla at the spas as reflected in the Rabbinic
and Classical sources. Their activities at the curative baths enable us
to conclude that it was not merely for military reasons in stationing
at Hammei-Tiberias, Hammat-Gader, and Emmaus-Nicopolis. Their
medical history, which has thus far been neglected by scholars in affinity
with thermo-mineral baths, is illuminated. Chapter 8 is devoted to the
numismatic expression of the spas. Numismatic finds with the ritual
characteristics of the curative sites likewise uncover a veritable treasure
about the therapeutic baths. The ritual worship characteristics of the
spas are expressed in most interesting types of coins from Tiberias,
Gadara and Pella, which represent symbolically the hot springs. Other
issues deal with a reassessment of the nautical symbols of the Tenth
Legion *Fretensis* and their link to Gadara of the Decapolis; The original
name of Hammat-Gader; and lastly, a combination of linguistic,
historical and topographical analysis of Kefar Agon in the domain
of Gadara city offers tangible competitions of leisure and amusement
culture in the vicinity of the Sea of Galilee in particular and in the East
in general. In chapter 9 pilgrimages to the spas in the surroundings of
Sea of Galilee and along the Jordan Valley during the Later Roman
and Byzantine periods are introduced. We will discuss some prominent
inquiries, like for example, if these places were considered as sacred
cult places for healing or popular sites of leisure and recreation; The
Christian sources, which add the most important layer in understanding
the properties of the spas; The Christian ethics toward baths and mixed
bathing, and bathing as a medical measure are reviewed; last but not
least, the contribution of Christian epigraphic finds of nearly 30 Greek
dedicatory inscriptions from Hammat-Gader excavations. Chapter 10
reflects the concept that the many frequent references to the curative
powers of thermo-mineral waters in the texts and the elaborately built
establishments suggest that spas were regarded highly for their ability
to restore health. The integration of sacred springs, healing baths and

cultic installations offered a special combination of religious, medicinal and social conveniences to the many pagans, Christians, Jews and Moslems, who visited the sites during ancient times.

Note: Secondary sources in the footnotes are referred to only by author's name and date, with full citation appearing in the bibliography.

CHAPTER ONE

INTRODUCTION

This is a study of therapeutic sites in the eastern Mediterranean basin based on hot springs. Such springs, which provide relief for many complaints, were well known during the periods of the Hellenistic, Roman, Byzantine and early Muslim periods. The object of the enquiry is to trace the process of development of medicinal sites with a distinctly Hellenistic character in a Semitic environment and is aimed at clarifying many aspects of healing spas.

The three areas containing the best known thermal springs in the eastern Mediterranean basin are situated on the Syro-African Rift, along the Jordan River. Rabbi Yohanan bar Nafha, the greatest of the second generation of Palestinian *Amoraim*, who lived in the third century CE, said of them that of all 'the fountains of the great deep' (*Genesis* 7, 11), three remained of the fountains of the great deep that burst apart at the time of the Flood (*ibid.*): 'The eddy of Gader, Hammei-Tiberias, and the great spring of Biram' (*Babylonian Talmud, Sanhedrin* 108a) (see Map 1).[1]

The conceptual basis of the use of therapeutic springs is to be found in the doctrine of Hippocrates, the great physician of ancient Greece, traditionally known in the history of medicine as 'the father of medicine'. In the area of their conquests the Romans built splendid bathhouses on the sites of hot springs, and virtually all the European spas were built on their remains. The Roman period was one of prosperity for the spas, and many people flocked to them to find succor for their illnesses.[2]

While we have no certain knowledge of the use of thermal springs in Palestine during the period of the First Temple, there is much information about the use of therapeutic baths in the Second Temple

---

[1] On the spreading of the hot springs see the discussion in chapter 2 about the *Geological, Hydrological and Medicinal Aspects of Hot Springs in the Eastern Mediterranean—Past and Present.*

[2] See the extensive discussion in chapter 3 on *the Medicinal Hot Springs and Healing Spas in the Graeco-Roman World.*

period. The culture of bathing was introduced into the Levant at the
beginning of the Roman period. It was developed there in successive
generations, and impressive remains dating from the later Roman and
Byzantine periods still survive.[3]

Sources from the Second Temple period show that the healing
qualities of thermal baths were already known at that time: the First
Book of Enoch says: 'In those days, these waters served kings and rulers and dignitaries and the inhabitants of the land to heal the body
and to heal the spirit'. (67, 8).[4] There is much evidence that various
personages used these sites for medicinal purposes: among others,
Herod the Great in Kallirrhoe (Josephus, *Antiquitates Judaicae* 17.171);
Yohanan of Gischala (*Vita* 17.85–86); Rabbi Simeon ben Yohai and his
son Elazar in Hammei-Tiberias (*Ecclesiastes Rabbah* 10, 8); and Rabbi
Judah Nes'iah and Rabbi Ami in Hammat-Gader (*Jerusalem Talmud,
Avoda Zarah* 2, 2 [40d]).[5]

To this day, only four articles on therapeutic springs in the Levant
have been published. The most recent, by Weber, was written in 1997,
on thermal springs in Roman-Byzantine Jordan.[6] It was preceded by
articles by Hirschberg (1920), Krauss (1907–1908; 1909–1910), and
Dechent (1884).[7] Dechent wrote about therapeutic baths and bathing
customs on the basis of descriptions by ancient non-Jewish historians
alone, and did not use any Jewish sources. He discussed the contribution
to cultural history of the evidence he collected on a rather superficial
level, and did not deal in any depth with its relevance to the cultural
and medical history of the people of Israel and the Land of Israel.
Krauss surveyed natural therapeutic springs, describing the architectural structure of the bathhouses, and the functionaries who worked
there—all this on the basis of descriptions in the Talmudic literature.
He was primarily interested in concrete details, and scarcely mentions

---

[3] See for instance Gichon (1978): 37–53 and the enclosed bibliography there; Tsafrir
(1984): 105–113; See also the review in chapter 4 on *Historical-Archaeological Analysis and
Healing Cults of the Therapeutic Sites in the in the Eastern Mediterranean Basin.*

[4] *Enoch,* I, 67, 8; See also the introduction in chapter 5 on *The Healing Properties of
the Spas in the Eastern Mediterranean in Ancient Times.*

[5] On these persons and others see the depictions in chapter 6 on *The Daily Life at the
Thermo-Mineral Baths according to the Rabbinic Literature* and in chapter 9 on the *Contribution
of Archaeology to the Christians' Deeds at the Spas in the Levant.*

[6] Weber (1997): 331–338.

[7] Hirschberg (1920): 215–346; Krauss (1907–1908): 105–107; idem, (1909–1910):
32–50; Dechent (1884): 173–210.

other aspects of the subject at all. Hirschberg considers the influence of therapeutic sites on the cultural and moral character of the Jews at this period. In his view, life there was distinguished by an abundance of materialism, conviviality, profligacy, licentiousness and immorality. They did much damage to family life and racial integrity among the Jews: so much so that the severe and rigid limitations of religion were unable to resist them at the time. He does not explain why one spa was of more benefit to the invalid than another; what were the differences between the various spas in the Near East; and whether there were centres for the treatment of different complaints. This article, too, contains no comprehensive examination of this question in terms of social history.

All these three scholars are united in the view that the establishment of therapeutic centres in Palestine was not the result of Hellenistic and Roman influence, even though they believe that it had an important effect on cultural life in Palestine. These articles, some of which are now long out-dated, do not discuss the relationship between evidence from ancient historical sources and the archaeological discoveries from Hammat-Tiberias, Hammat-Gader, Hammat-Pella, Kallirrhoe and Emmaus, and the chronological conclusions to be drawn from them. This is because the excavations were conducted after the publication of these articles. Equally, these articles do not attempt to coordinate and combine historical, cultural, archaeological and medicinal aspects of the subject: in short, though they adduce interesting information, until now there has been no systematic collocation of all the literary evidence and certain literary and historical sources have not yet been investigated at all.

Thermo-mineral sites have been mentioned in a number of monographs about the historical geography of Palestine and Jordan, and in topographical, historical and Talmudic encyclopedias, such as Neubauer (1868), Schlatter (1893), Smith (1920), Horowitz (1923), Klein (1925), Abel (1933–1938), Press (1948), Neʾeman (1972), Avi-Yonah (1984) and Schürer (1991);[8] geological, geochemical and geothermal researches

---

[8] Neubauer (1868), in the suitable entries; Schlatter (1893), in the suitable entries; Smith (1920), in the suitable entries; Horowitz (1923), in the suitable entries; Klein (1925), in the suitable entries; Abel 1933–1938, in the suitable entries; Press (1948), in the suitable entries; Neʾeman (1972), in the suitable entries; Smith (1966); Avi-Yonah (1984), in the suitable entries; Schürer (1991), in the suitable entries.

on hot springs have been published since the twentieth century, and
amongst the outstanding were Noetling (1886), Picard (1932), Avnimelech (1935), Eckstein (1976), Levitte and Olshina (1978), Mazor
(1980), Abu-Ajamieh, Bender and Eicher (1989), Greizzer and Levitte
(2000), and Horowitz (2001).[9] The spas are mentioned in published
archaeological reports, as well as archaeological encyclopedias: Dothan
(1983); Dothan and Johnson (2000) on Hammei-Tiberias;[10] Schumacher
(1888), Sukenik (1935), and Hirschfeld (1997) on Hammat-Gader.[11]
The present writer's researches relate to sources from both Classical
and Rabbinical literature, and discuss historical, *halakhic* and archaeological aspects of the site of Hammat-Gader.[12] A survey on 'Thermal
springs, medical supply and healing cults in Roman-Byzantine Jordan'
was done by Weber (1997),[13] while a preliminary treatise on the spas in
the eastern Mediterranean basin—in Israel and Jordan—was done by
the present author in 1992 and up to these days she has written over
twenty five papers and chapters in books on this issue.[14] Monographs on
Pella were written by Smith, McNicoll and Hennessy (1982), McNicoll
et al. (1992), Weber (1993), Walmsley, Sheedy and Carson (2001);[15]
on Emmaus-Nicopolis—Vincent and Abel (1932), Gichon (1979), and
Hirschfeld (1989a).[16] Kallirrhoe's excavations were reported by Donner
(1963), Strobel (1966), and Clamer (1996).[17] All those essays are additional to *The New Encyclopedia of Archaeological Excavations in the Holy Land*
(1993),[18] *The Oxford Encyclopedia of Near Eastern Archaeology* (1997), and
the *Archaeological Encyclopedia of the Holy Land* (2001).[19]

---

[9] Noetling (1886); Picard (1932): 221–225; Avnimelech (1935); Eckstein (1976);
Levitte and Olshina (1978); idem, (1985); Mazor (1980); Abu-Ajamieh, Bender and
Eicher (1989); Greizzer and Levitte (1999); Horowitz (2001); See also the survey in
chapter 2 on the *Geological, Hydrological and Medicinal Aspects of Hot Springs in the Eastern
Mediterranean—Past and Present.*
[10] Dothan (1983); Dothan and Johnson (2000).
[11] Schumacher (1886a); idem (1888a); idem, (1888b); idem, (1890); Sukenik (1935a);
idem (1935b); Hirschfeld (1997); See also the papers written by the latter in the
Bibliography.
[12] Dvorjetski (1988).
[13] Weber (1997): 331–338.
[14] Dvorjetski (1992a); See my various bibliographical items in the *Bibliography.*
[15] Smith, McNicoll and Hennessy (1982); McNicoll et al. (1992); Weber (1993);
Walmsley, Sheedy and Carson (2001).
[16] Vincent and Abel (1932); Gichon (1979); Hirschfeld (1978); idem, (1989a).
[17] Donner (1963); Strobel (1966); Clamer (1997a); idem, (1997b).
[18] Stern (1993).
[19] Meyers (1997); Negev and Gibson (2001).

There have also appeared vast researches on the origins and characters of baths in the Roman Empire like Marquardt (1886), Carcopino (1941), Cowell (1961), Balsdon (1969), Thomson (1978); Manderscheid (1981), Heinz (1983), Merten (1983), Brödner (1983), Pasquinucci (1987), Dunbabin (1989), Jackson (1990a), Yegül (1992), Nielsen (1993a), DeLaine (1993), Toner (1995), Weber (1996), Albu, Banks and Nash (1997); Allen (1998), Fagan (1999), Dalby (2000), Ball (2001), and McGinn (2004).[20] Only few research works have been done so far concerning bath and bathing in the Byzantine Empire and early Muslim period, like Zellinger (1928), Magoulias (1971), Hunger (1980), Berger (1982), Ward (1992), and Constable (2003).[21]

General reports on baths in Palestine, mainly from the archaeological point of view were done by Gichon (1978), Simon (1978), Tsafrir (1984), Small (1987) Kuhnen (1990), Nielsen (1993), and Belayche (2001).[22] Hydrotherapic methods in general and Balneotherapic treatments in particular were being used to treat physical illnesses and eventually they became popular vacation venues for socializing and entertainment. The distinguished researches in this field are as follows: Shew (1845), Trall (1869), Baruch (1897), Kellogg (1918), Ginouvès (1962), Weiss and Kemble (1967), Holden (1970), Aaland (1978), Wright (1980), Kiel (1982), Croutier (1992), Buchmann (1994), de Bonneville (1998), Porter (1997), Campion (1998), Gizowska (1998), Chaitow (1999), and Nolte (2001).[23]

Other scholars have selected sources from the Talmudic literature referring specially to the thermo-mineral baths of Tiberias, Kasher (1934), Udilevitz (1950), Shiponi (1963) and Meiri (1973), and considered *halakhic* aspects of the subject. Yet others have made incomplete

[20] Marquardt (1886); Carcopino (1941); Cowell (1961); Balsdon (1969); Thomson (1978); Manderscheid (1981); Heinz (1983); Merten (1983); Brödner (1983); Pasquinucci (1987); Dunbabin (1989); Jackson (1990a); Nielsen (1990); Yegül (1992); DeLaine (1993); Toner (1995); Weber (1996); Albu, Banks and Nash (1997); Allen (1998); Fagan (1999a); Dalby (2000); Ball (2001); McGinn (2004).
[21] Zellinger (1928); Magoulias (1971); Hunger (1980); Berger (1982); Ward (1992); Constable (2003).
[22] Gichon (1978); Simon (1978a–b); Tsafrir (1984); Small (1987); Kuhnen (1990); Nielsen (1990).
[23] Shew (1845); Trall (1869); Baruch (1897); Kellogg (1918); Ginouvès (1962); Weiss and Kemble (1967); Holden (1970); Aaland (1978); Wright (1980); Kiel (1982); Croutier (1992); Buchman (1994); Bonneville (1998); Porter (1997); Campion (1998); Gizowska (1998); Chaitow (1999); Nolte (2001).

collocations of places in the Rabbinical literature where therapeutic
sites are mentioned.[24] There has also appeared some research on the
attitude of the Sages to the culture of bathing, and to the customs
and *halakhic* decisions concerning idol-worship on the sites, such as
Hirschberg (1920), Urbach (1959), Lieberman (1963), Simon (1978a–b),
Hanoune (1983), Eliav (1993), Hayes (1997), and Jacobs (1997).[25] The
present writer's researches relate to sources from both classical and
Rabbinical literature, and discuss historical, *halakhic* and archaeological
aspects of the curative sites in Palestine and Jordan.[26]

In addition, numismatists have referred to the thermo-mineral springs
in the course of their work on the coins of Palestine and the Decapolis
in the Roman period by de Saulcy (1874), Hill (1914), Seyrig (1959),
Kindler (1961), Spijkerman (1978), Meshorer (1985), and Lichtenberger
(2003).[27]

The physician Dr. Buchmann laid the foundations of the study of
the medical aspects of the baths of Israel. His book, *Tiberias and Its Hot
Springs* (1957), which was translated into four languages, still provides
background material for this subject.[28] He investigated the special characteristics of Hammei-Tiberias, and compared them with those of other
therapeutic springs throughout the world. It should be added that he
was the first to lay down medical rules for those who use therapeutic
springs in Israel. Many articles on this subject have been written, most
prominent among them those of Dr. Kurland, formerly the medical
director of the Tiberias thermal baths (1971a–b).[29] The conclusions
of scientific medical research about the baths of Hammat-Gader and
Tiberias and their therapeutic potential, when combined with textual
analysis of sources from the periods of the Second Temple, Mishnah
and Talmud, may well cast light on events that took place in them in
ancient times.[30]

---

[24] Kaser (1934); Klein (1939), in suitable entries; Udilevitz (1950); Shiponi (1963);
Meiri (1973): 29–35.

[25] Hirschberg (1920): 215–346; Urbach (1959); Lieberman (1963); Simon (1978a);
idem, (1978b); Hanoune (1983): 255–262; Eliav (1993); Hayes (1997); Jacobs (1998a).

[26] Dvorjetski (1988); idem, (1992). See also my publications in the *Bibliography*.

[27] de Saulcy (1874); Hill (1914); Seyrig (1959); Kindler (1961); Spijkerman (1978);
Meshorer (1985); Lichtenberger 2003.

[28] Buchmann (1957); See also his vast publications in the *Bibliography*.

[29] Kurland (1971a); idem, (1971b); See also his publications in the *Bibliography*.

[30] For the full bibliography items for each researcher see the details in the *Bibliography*.

1.1 Source Material

The sources which constitute the basis of this study of the history of therapeutic baths in the eastern Mediterranean, and their place in the daily life of the citizens in the periods of the Second Temple, the Mishnah and the Talmud [= Hellenistic, Roman, Byzantine and Early Muslim periods], are quite varied. The literary sources can be divided into six categories:

A. Classical literature—written in Greek and Latin—by geographers, historians, physicians, Pagans, and Christians, from the second half of the first century BCE up to the eleventh century CE, such as Strabo, Vitruvius, Tertullian, Josephus, Pliny the Elder, Cassius Dio, Galen, Celsus, Ptolemy, Martial, Solinus, Socrates Scholasticus, Soranus, Ammianus Marcellinus, Hierocles, Origenes, Eusebius, Eunapius, Epiphanius, Theodore of Sykeon, Hieronymus [= Jerome], Sozomenus, Theophanes, Saint Willibald, Syncellus, Cedrenus, and others.

B. The literature of the Sages known as the Rabbinic literature, including the *Mishnah*, the *Tosefta*, *Halakhic* and *Aggadaic Midrashim*, the *Jerusalem and Babylonian Talmuds*, and the *Yalkutim* written between the end of the second century CE to the 13th century. This literature is almost totally bereft of chronological and historiographical indicators. On the other hand, for social and economic history, daily life and cultural, spiritual and literary history the literature of the Sages is a treasure trove of sources. The ramified *halakhic* literature reflects all areas of life and gives a full picture of the society and economy of the Jewish people, dealing equally with all the levels and strata of society. Furthermore, the Sages, masters of the *halakhah*, were diligent in transmitting things as they were and in quoting their sources. It is even possible in many instances, therefore, to understand the social or economic reality of which over generation is being reflected by the text. From this point of view, the Rabbinic *aggadah* is entirely different. Here, the historian who tries to separate the historical tradition from the *aggadaic* additions encounters very difficult and complicated problems. There is no tried and true system which can—in the absence of parallel external sources—reveals the actual historical kernel in each *aggadah* and homily with certainty. Therefore, each and every *aggadaic* source requires careful investigation—an investigation which, methodologically, must begin with philological and literary examination of the source, and only thereafter can it be examined from historical perspective; Two Jewish scholars of the twelfth-thirteenth centuries known as Rabbi Moshe

Ben Maimon, Maimonides [= HaRambam] and Rabbi Moshe ben Nachman [= HaRamban], add an important layer by their explanations to the literature of the Sages.

C. *Itineraria*, travel-books of Christian pilgrims to the Holy Land during the Byzantine period, such as the descriptions written by Egeria, Petrus of Iberia, Theodosius, Antoninus Placentinus, Gregory of Tours, Arculfus, Bede Venerabilis, and more.

D. Cartographic evidence from the Byzantine period such as the Peutinger map dates from the fourth century CE, and the Madaba map, of the second half of the sixth century CE.

E. Classical Arabic literature which was written by geographers and historians, who lived between the ninth and thirteenth centuries CE, like Ibn al-Kalbī, al-Yaʾqubi, al-Istahrī, al-Muqaddasi, Nâsir-i-Khusrau, al-Idrīsī, al-Yāqūt, ad-Dimašqī, and others. These authors can assist us to understand the history of the sites.

F. The Cairo *Geniza*, archive of ancient Jewish manuscripts found in the synagogue of Fostat-Cairo, Egypt. The materials are an extremely important resource for the study of Biblical writings and translations, ancient Jewish liturgies and texts. Relevant fragments for this project are dated to the eleventh century.

G. Syriac texts, written by the twelfth century historian Michael the Syrian.

The Archaeological evidences from the excavated thermo-mineral sites—Hammat- Tiberias, Hammat-Gader, Emmaus-Nicopolis, Hammat-Pella, and Kallirrhoe—can be divided into three categories: Excavations' reports; Numismatic evidences of the existence of therapeutic hot springs offered by the coins of their cities: Tiberias, Gadara and Pella; and epigraphical sources, including dedicational inscriptions in Greek, Latin, Aramaic and Syriac dated to the fifth-seventh century CE. Archaeological findings from Hammat-Gader, Tiberias, Pella, Kallirrhoe and Emmaus, will be described in the course of the study, which is also based on scientific medical research in the sphere of balneotherapy.

The research method is interdisciplinary: the combination and coordination of variegated sources and types of research, such as Classical and Rabbinic literature, archaeological reports, epigraphical, and numismatic evidence. Conclusions drawn from these sources will be combined in this work, using both fundamental analysis of ancient sources and contemporary research literature.

1.2   Aims and Methodological Issues

The methodological issues of this study are as follows:

1. The meaning of the term 'therapeutic baths'. The significance of this expression will be examined, using classical Greek and Latin, Syriac and Talmudic dictionaries. Does the term *Hamma* mean only 'heat'? Or does it come from the Semitic root *h-m-i*, whose meaning in Arabic is 'to cover' or 'to protect'? Is the Hebrew term *homa* (wall) derived from this? Moreover, an etymological investigation of the terms *baths, thermae, balnea, spas, hammat, hammei, Emmaus, Kallirrhoe,* and their meanings will be discussed.

2. Various models for the creation of the thermo-mineral waters given by geologists, hydrologists and geochemists in the Jordan Rift Valley. Are there traces in the Bible and in the New Testament for the existence of thermo-mineral springs and geothermal energy utilization in the Jordan Valley?

3. The characterization of the thermo-mineral waters in the Graeco-Roman world. Do we know of specific physicians who developed the ideas of Hippocrates and used thermal balneology systematically? Why do scholars agree that therapeutic baths originated from an ancient Roman tradition, even though there were widespread thermal baths in classical Greece? Were the spas leisure cultural centres for the Romans? Did the Romans themselves denigrate their baths? What functional elements normally existed in ordinary baths, but not in therapeutic baths based on hot mineral waters? Places throughout the Roman Empire that gained great fame because of their healing qualities and their effectiveness in curing various health ailments. Is the term *valetudinarium* [= military hospital] suitable for the health resorts built by the Romans, or were the spas only leisure cultural centres? What are the nearest parallels to the thermal baths of the Levant in the Graeco-Roman world? How can one identify accurately those who established thermo-mineral baths in the Levant?

4. The distribution of therapeutic baths in eastern Mediterranean basin in the periods of the Second Temple, the Mishnah and the Talmud. We shall describe the distribution of hot springs in the Levant and the baths connected with them, examine the references to them in Classical and Talmudic literature, and attempt to give a unified account of them. In the course of the discussion of historical aspects of the subject, we shall consider whether the

historical descriptions accord with the archaeological findings and chronological conclusions derived from the excavations in the baths of Tiberias, Hammat-Gader, Kallirrhoe, Pella, and Emmaus.

5. The therapeutic qualities of the baths of Levant, as attested by the ancient sources. Were the Classical writers acquainted with the healing of the thermo-mineral waters in the Levant? What can be learnt from our information with regard to various personages and their medical problems about the therapeutic qualities of the hot springs? Can we assume, on the basis of various *halakhic* rulings, that the Rabbis were aware of the therapeutic qualities of the baths? Are there common denominators between the Classical sources and the Rabbinic literature about spas being centres of entertainment and social meetings? Have the hot springs been classified by their effectiveness against specific illnesses?

6. Therapeutic baths in Rabbinic literature. Which *halakhic* rulings appertaining to hot springs in connection with acts forbidden on the Sabbath were modified over time to suit the necessities of daily life in the spas? How can it be shown that the Sages disapproved of the therapeutic spas? What was the attitude of the Jews of this period to baths in general, and therapeutic baths in particular? We shall describe both the *halakhic* discussions of bathing in public baths, and the way in which the Sages' viewpoint coped with everyday life in the baths, including therapeutic baths. Which social circles, from among the Jews of Palestine and elsewhere, were accustomed to come to the therapeutic sites in the Roman-Byzantine period?

7. The contribution of modern medicine to the study of therapeutic baths in the Levant. Do we know today most of the components that determine the medicinal characteristics of the therapeutic springs? By analyzing texts in Rabbinic literature, can we trace diseases which required long-term treatment in the therapeutic baths? Moreover, can we learn from the chemical composition of the water in each of the spas which purpose the therapeutic springs served in ancient times? We shall also describe the different approaches and methods of treatment of physicians at the time of the Mishnah and the Talmud.

8. Intents and actions of Roman and Byzantine Emperors at the thermo-mineral baths in the eastern Mediterranean basin.

9. Christian ethics towards the habit of mixed bathing, and bathing as a medical measure during the Byzantine period. What was the perspective of Church Fathers and pilgrims towards the therapeutic baths? Were they sacred places or popular sites of healing?

10. The contribution of archaeology to the study of the spas in the eastern Mediterranean basin. The coordination between the historical descriptions and the archaeological finds and the chronological conclusions drawn from the excavations at the healing sites. How the ritual worship characteristics of the spas are expressed in types of coins of the mother cities Tiberias, Gadara and Pella? Does the evidence of the coins accord that of the literary sources? Aims and deeds of Christians at the thermo-mineral bath of Hammat-Gader according to 24 dedicated Greek inscriptions. Why the inscriptions from private persons on the occasion of their visit at the therapeutic sites are so reliable, so authentic? The magic amulet from Emmaus and the afflictions of a patient. What are the archaeological evidences for local cult at the thermo-mineral springs in the Levant? The contribution of the Madaba map to the study of the thermo-mineral baths. Restoration and reconstruction works at Hammat-Gader during the reign of the Byzantine Emperors. Reopening and renovation of Hammat-Gader according to the dedicatory inscription of Caliph Muʾāwiya, founder of the Umayyad dynasty. What kind of principal findings do we expect to discover during next excavations at the spas in the eastern Mediterranean?

1.3   SEMITIC ORIGIN AND BIBLICAL SURVEY

Varied names are given to places in the Levant that have hot springs. Most of them have the component of the word *Hammei*. Can the expressions *Baluʾah de Gader* [= the eddy of Gader], *Hammtha de* [= of] *Gader, waters of Gader, waters of Hammthan, Hammei-Tiberias, waters of Tiberias, Peḥal* [= *Hammat-Pella*], and *the great spring of Biram* help us to interpret the terms *Hammim* and *Hammei* as components of the phrase *hammei-marpeh* and elucidate its meaning? Which adjective is used of all the sites of hot springs? Can we be certain of the meaning of the noun *Hammat*? Is there explicit mention in the Bible of hot springs? In the course of this study we shall try to find out whether the origin of the name *Hammat*, Ἐμμαθᾶ in Greek, was purely linguistic, or whether this term also signifies municipal dependence, as part of the *chora* (χώρα: territory) of certain city-states (πολεῖς).

The meaning of *hammim* or *hammin* (with the *mem* accented), from the root *h-m-m*, is 'hot water', or hot springs; *hammei-hammim* means 'very hot', 'boiling': 'I thought that you would be scalded with warm water; I see you are not scalded even with boiling hot water' (*Babylonian Talmud,*

Berakhot 16b).[31] Hence, *hammat* is a place with hot springs.[32] In Palestine and Syria there were several towns named Hamath. In most cases the reference is to Hamath (*mem* unaccented)—a big city on the River Orontes in central Syria, the capital of the kingdom of Aram Zobah, where King David defeated Hadadezer the King of Zobah (*I Chronicles* 18, 3). This city was known as Hamath Rabbah (*Amos* 6, 2), after the name of the kingdom, in order to distinguish it from Hamath Zobah, where King Solomon built store cities (II *Chronicles* 8, 3).[33] Its name is preserved by the Arabs as *Ḥama*. The name is apparently derived from the Semitic root *h-m-y* (in Arabic: to cover, to defend); thus, in Hebrew it means 'wall'.[34] 'The Hamathi' is included in the genealogy list descended from Canaan (*Genesis* 10, 18).[35] Riblah was in the land of Hamath (*Jeremiah* 39, 5). In his description of the provinces Ezekiel mentions Hamath, Damascus, Hauran and Gilead—names known to us from the time of the Assyrian conquest (47, 17–18).[36]

Hammat or Hammath (*mem* accented) appears in the Bible as a fortified city in the ancestral territory of Naphtali (*Joshua* 19, 35). In this list, the fortified towns in eastern Galilee are apparently listed from south to north: 'And Hammath, Rakkat, and Kinnereth'.[37] Most scholars believe, therefore, that this Hammath is south of Tiberias—Hammtha—and that this is the site of the thermal baths called Hammei-Tiberias in Rabbinic sources (Arabic: el-Ḥammam).[38] Hammath is also mentioned in the plural, with the *mem* emphasized—Hammoth-Dor—as a city of refuge in the territory of Naphtali which was given to 'the Gershonites

---

[31] Even-Shoshan (1969): I: 401–402.
[32] Gesenius (1899): 213, 287; Steinberg (1960): 252; See below the various dictionaries.
[33] Albright (1965): III: 193–200; Today is el-Hama, 180 kilometres north-eastern to Damascus on the banks of the Orontes River; Steinberg 1960: 252; The Sages interpreted *Amos* 6, 2: 'Pass over to Calneh, and see; and thence go to Hamath Rabbah [= the great]; then go down to Gath of the Philistines. Are they better than these kingdoms?'—'go to Hamath Rabbah this is Hamath of Antioch'; Ne'eman (1971): I: 409; Press (1948): II: 263–264.
[34] Albright (1965): III: 193; See also Negev and Gibson (2001): 214.
[35] Mandelkern (1971): 1405–1406; See Talmon's (1958: 111–113) unique idea.
[36] Aharoni (1987): 308–309, 330; See also Patai (1936): 223; Taylor (2003): 53.
[37] Avi-Yonah (1965): III: 192–193; idem, (1984): 140; Shiponi (1962): 42; Slousch (1921): 5–39; Albright (1925): 10; Abel (1933): I: 445; II: 342; Saarisalo (1927): 128, note 1.
[38] Avi-Yonah (1965): III: 192; idem, (1976): 64; Horowitz (1923): 288–290; Zevin (1980): 44–52.

according to their families' (*Joshua* 21, 32). This was apparently the Hammath which is identified as the Hammath of Tiberias, and is also mentioned in *Joshua* 19, 35 as one of the towns of Naphtali.[39] Levinstam adds that this is the same as the Septuagint's version B of *Joshua* 21, 32 [= Vatican MS.]: την Νεμμαθ (a corruption of την Εμμαθ); therefore, it has been suggested that Hammath rather than Hammath-Dor should be read. But Septuagint's version A [= Alexandrian MS.] reads Εμμθδωρ, and it seems that Hammat is simply an abbreviation of Hammoth-Dor.[40] The name Hammat suggests a hot spring, and the word Dor is interpreted as meaning *dira*, an inhabited place.[41] However, Thomas related it to the Arabic words דּוּאָר, דַּוָּאר, דֻוָּאר [= *dawwar, duwar*, and *duw-war*], which signify the circuits round the *Kaaba* [= the holy black stone in Mecca].[42] He conjectured that the name was connected with the circuits that were made round a holy well. Others identify this city with Hammon, a Levite city in the territory of Naphtali (*I Chronicles* 6, 61), while others again believe that it is the Hammath of *Joshua* 19, 35; and hence the Septuagint version B [= Vatican MS, ed., Lucianus], Χαμωθ: Hammath.[43]

Bar-Droma maintains that it is impossible to know the meaning of the name Hammath for certain, and emphasizes the possibility that it means a city surrounded by a wall, a fortified city (from the root *h-m-h*, meaning to defend, to guard), or a brown city of brown soil (from the root *h-m*, meaning brown); or, possibly, towns were called Hammat because of the *hemmet*, the wild figs which grew around them in profusion, in Palestine and Syria. Bar-Droma maintains, therefore, that it is not necessary to fix their location close to hot springs, or to connect the name with hot baths: this would be neither a means of identification nor an innovation, since there was a bathhouse in every town.[44] This hypothesis is quite extreme: it seems that the texts themselves indicate the position of one Hammath, and even of two. Moreover, not only are the philologists unanimous in their view of the meaning of the various

---

[39] Klein (1934): 83; Abel (1938): II: 341–343; Levinstam (1965d): III: 200; Taylor (2003): 128.

[40] Levinstam (1965d): III: 200.

[41] Levinstam (1965d): III: 200.

[42] Thomas (1933): 205–206; idem, (1934): 147–148; See also Oesterley (1923): 95, 106.

[43] Levinstam (1965c): III: 166; Aharoni (1987): 96, 253.

[44] Bar-Droma (1958): 188–201.

versions of *hammath*, as we shall see below; we may also be able to identify the earliest historical evidence of the existence of these springs in
the Bible. In order to confirm this hypothesis, we shall consider where
the geological conditions for the existence of hot springs are present
in Palestine, the reasons for this, and their characteristics.

Philologists, commentators, and researchers of the historical geography of Palestine throughout the ages, distinguish between Hamath in
Syria and Hammath [= Hammat], a hot spring situated in the tribal
territory of Naphtali. Lexicographers classify the word *hammat* (*mem*
emphasized) together with the nouns *hamma* and *Hammtha* [= *Hammta*],
which signify heat and warmth, and are to be found linked to the names
of several places in which there are springs, such as Hammei-Tiberias,
Hammat-Gader, Hammtha de Peḥal, Hammtan, and more. Gesenius
asserted that *hammat* were 'warm baths', and that the word was derived
from the root *h-m-m*. Thus, we find *ham, hom, hamma, hamman*, and even
individual names such as Hamuel, Hammon and Hammt; the latter is
mentioned as being in the tribal territory of Naphtali (*Joshua* 19, 35),
near Tiberias, which he identifies with Hammoth-Dor in the tribal
territory of Naphtali (*ibid.*, 21, 32).[45]

According to Brockelmann's *Lexicon Syriacum*,[46] and Payne-Smith's
Compendious Syriac Dictionary,[47] the adjective 'warm' (*hamim*) in Hebrew is
in Syriac *hamimtho*, and *hamma*, whose root is *ham*, and thence *hamimtho*,
which means 'warm water' or 'hot spring'. Various commentators also
take this view in their dictionaries, such as Levy,[48] Kohut,[49] Krauss,[50]
Dalman,[51] and Jastrow.[52] Biblical dictionaries, too—Brown, Driver, and
Briggs,[53] Köhler and Baumgartner,[54] Hastings,[55] and Buttrick[56]—interpret the word *hammat* as an adjective for a place in which there are hot
springs, such as Hammath in the tribal territory of Naphtali.

---

[45] Gesenius (1899): 213, 287; See also Zorell (1984): 252.
[46] Brockelmann (1928): 238–239; See also Sokoloff (1990): 204.
[47] Payne-Smith (1902): 145–148.
[48] Levy (1924): II: 68–71.
[49] Kohut (1926): III: 422.
[50] Krauss (1899): II: 58.
[51] Dalman (1922): 153.
[52] Jastrow (1950): I: 480–481.
[53] Brown, Driver and Briggs (1906): 329.
[54] Köhler and Baumgartner (1967): I: 318; Lewy (1943–1944: 436–443) conjectures
that *Hammat* [= חַמַּת] derives from the name *Hamath* [= חֲמָת].
[55] Hastings (1958): II: 290.
[56] Buttrick (1962): II: 516–517.

Modern lexicographers such as Gur and Ben-Yehuda translate *hammim* or *hammin* as 'hot water': 'hot into cold' (*Jerusalem Talmud, Shabbat* 3, 2 [6c]); hot foods, such as those put in the oven on Sabbath eve for consumption on the Sabbath: 'one may keep upon it a dish sufficiently cooked or hot water which is sufficiently heated' (*Babylonian Talmud, ibid.*, 37b); hot springs—those whose waters are hot, *yeimim*. In this connection Gur mentions *Hammei-Tiberias*, the hot springs on the shore of Lake Kinneret, near Tiberias: 'Like a stone in olive-waste, tar, in Hammei-Tiberias' (*ibid., Hullin* 8a).[57] Ben-Yehuda is even more precise: '*hammim, hammin*—natural hot waters which flow from the earth and serve for healing'.[58]

The name of the settlement Hammthan appears in the Rabbinic sources in two forms: Hammthan and Ammto-Ammthan (*Jerusalem Talmud, Shevi'it* 9, 2 [34d]; *ibid., Mo'ed Qatan* 3, 1 [82a]; *Midrash Psalms* 92, 11). *Het* and *ayin* are interchanged in the names of a number of settlements in Palestine: Ofraim-Hofraim (*Mishnah, Menahot* 8, 1; *Tosefta, ibid.*, 9, 2; *Babylonian Talmud, ibid.*, 83b; etc.), and in another group of names which are preserved in the Arabic: Zanoah-Zanoa; Husafiya-Ussafiya; Kefar Hanania-Kefar Anan; Kefar Acre [= Akko]-Kefar Hiko-Hukuk; and others.[59]

To sum up, it may be observed that the earliest historical evidence of the existence of hot springs in the region based on a linguistic approach is to be found in the Book of *Joshua* (19, 35), in the account of the settlement of the tribe of Naphtali, whose borders were 'the fortified cities of Ziddim, Zer, and Hammat, Rakkat, and Kinnereth'. These cities were in the tribal territory of Naphtali, and the name Hammat [= Hammath] apparently denotes the settlement which lies close to the hot springs of Tiberias—Hammei-Tiberias. We shall see below that this identification of Hammat with Tiberias was accepted in the days of the *Amoraim*: Rabbi Yohanan believed that Tiberias was situated on the site of the Biblical Hammat, and that it received its name from the hot springs of Tiberias (*Babylonian Talmud, Megillah* 6a).[60]

---

[57] Gur (Garzovski) (1957): 287.
[58] Ben-Yehuda (1948): III: 1606.
[59] Klein (1924): 42; Damati (1986): 41.
[60] Buchmann (1967): 195–202; Klein (1925): 77; See the discussion in chapter 6 on *Daily Life at the Thermo-Mineral Baths according to Rabbinic Literature*.

There is no real mention in the Bible of therapeutic springs in
Palestine, or even of hot springs.[61] It appears that, in addition to the
phonetic distinction between H'mmath (pointed with *hataf-patah*) and
Hammat (with *patah*), we must reconsider certain Biblical sources in
order to understand why scholars have assumed that the Bible does
mention therapeutic springs.

  A. The earliest allusion to the existence of hot springs is apparently
in *Genesis* 36, 24, where it is said of Anah, the son of Zibeon, one of
the sons of Seir the Horite, that 'he found the *yemim* in the wilderness, as he fed the asses of Zibeon his father'.[62] Ancient and modern
commentators alike have asked what these *yemim* were. The Septuagint
simply transliterates the word: ιαμ(ε)ν; and the translations of Aqilas
and Sumcus read ημιν. They did not translate the word, but copied it
as it was, except for the final letter—n instead of m; apparently they
read it as *heimam*, as if the letter *hey* were part of the root. The Sages'
midrash, quoted in the *Jerusalem Talmud, Berakhot* 8, 6 [12b], and in *Genesis
Rabbah* 82, 15, is close to this reading: they interpreted the *yemim* by the
Greek word ἡμίονος: a mule. The translation attributed to Yonathan
gives *kudaneita*: mules—that is, a mare crossed with an ass. Onqelos
translates *gibaraiya* (heroes). This, too, is based on an interpretation of
the word according to the same reading, as meaning 'terror' (*eimim*). In
the words of the Rabbis, 'Why were the mules called *heimim*? Because
people were in terror (*eimim*) of them' (*Babylonian Talmud, Hullin* 7b). In
the Samaritan Pentateuch, too, *eimim* is apparently the Moabite term
for ghosts (*Rephaim*) (*Deuteronomy* 2, 11). According to Tur-Sinai, the
translations of the Syriac *Peshiteta* (*maya* = water) and of Hieronymus
(aquae calidae = hot water) are also undoubtedly based on a Jewish
interpretation of the word *HaYamim*.[63] Hieronymus translates *Genesis* 36,
24, thus: 'Iste est Ana, qui invenit aquas calidas in deserto' [= This is
Ana, who found the hot springs in the desert].[64] His commentary on
this sentence is:[65]

> Multa et varia apud Hebraeos de hoc capitulo disputantur: apud Graecos
> quippe et nostros super hoc silentium est. Alii putant AIAMIM (הימם)

---

[61] Leibowitz and Kurland (1972): 48; Hirschberg (1920): 217.
[62] Dechent (1884): 173; Krauss (1907): 105; Hirschberg (1920): 217.
[63] Skinner (1963): 432–433; Tur-Sinai (1965): III: 702–703; idem, (1956): 3.
[64] Hieronymus, *Liber Hebraicarum in Genesim* 1043.
[65] Idem, *ibid.*, 1044; The translation is following Tur-Sinai (1956): 3; Meyer (1906:
341) accepts the explanation of hot water; See also Zipor (2005): 447.

maria appellate Iisdem enim literis scribuntur m a r i a, quibus et nunc hic sermo descriptus est. Et volunt illum, dum pascit asinos patris sui in deserto, aquarum congregations reperisse, quae juxta idioma linguae Hebraicae m a r i a nuncupentur; quod scilicet stagnum repererit,cujus rei invention in eremo difficilis est [= The Jews have expressed many varied opinions about this chapter. It is true that the Greek sources and ours are silent on this matter. Others believe that they were called *iamim*, *HaIamim* (יָמִים הַיָּמִים), which is written with the same letters as appear in the text before us. They mean that he [= Anah], who grazed his father's asses in the desert, found pools of water, which are also called seas (maria, יַמִּים) in the Hebrew language. Naturally, he found stagnant water, which was warm because of the heat of the desert, and this is hard to find in the desert].

In his view, therefore, it is not hot springs which were meant, but water which was warmed up by the desert heat. Tur-Sinai adds that this interpretation is based on mispronunciation of the word *heimam* (or *hayamim*), as if it were spelt with a *het* instead of a *hey*; this is a common feature of Rabbinic homilies.[66] None the less, modern commentators are inclined to accept Hieronymus' view, and even find support for it in the Arabic language. *Wama* in Arabic means 'became very hot'. The Arabic *waw* is cognate with the Hebrew *yud*; so the word *yamim* may well mean 'hot water springs'.[67] Hirschberg, Kasher and Steinberg maintain that the meaning of the word *yamim* is based on its meaning in Phoenician: hot springs.[68]

Some Medieval commentators believed that the *yamim* were the people of the Eimim, the heroes (*Genesis* 14, 5 and elsewhere), or, following the Rabbis, mules; this was the view of Rav Saʾadia Gaon, Rabbi Abraham Ibn Ezra and others. Most recent translations accept this interpretation. Ibn Ezra refers to commentators who thought that they were plants. As has been remarked above, some modern commentators amend *eimim* to *hamayim*, or consider that the reference is to animals.[69]

Tur-Sinai assumes that all the interpretations arise from a homiletic interpretation of the text, which also affected the vocalization of the

---

[66] Tur-Sinai (1956): 3.
[67] See for example Braslavsky (1956): III: 332.
[68] Hirschberg (1920): 217; Kasher (1934): 10; Steinberg (1960): 323; Patai (1936): 224; Levy (1856): I: 65; Segert (1976): 290; Luria's idea (1985: 262–268) that it was not a hot spring but a geyser in the Syrian desert on the way from Damascus to Palmyra cannot be accepted for the contradictions with the Biblical details.
[69] Tur-Sinai (1965): III: 702–703.

traditional text of the Bible (*HaYemim*); and it was this which led the commentators astray. However, an examination of the structure of the verse referring to the genealogy of the descendants of Seir the Horite (*Genesis* 36, 20 et seq.) reveals the possibility of another reading of the word *heimam*, which would appear to be closer to the straightforward sense of the Bible. In the verses before the one we are discussing, there are listed among the children of Seir the Horite 'Lotan and Shoval and Zibeon and Anah... and the children of Lotan were Hori and Hemam (Αἱμάν in the Septuagint), and the sister of Lotan was Timna' (*Genesis* 36, 20–22). It is also possible that the word *hayemim* in verse 24 should be read *Heimam*, referring to the incident when Anah found Hemam, his brother's son, wandering in the desert while he, Anah, was grazing the asses of his father Zibeon.[70] As has been remarked, other scholars consider that the reference is to the discovery of hot springs, according to the translation of the Vulgate: *yamim* = hot springs. This accords with the spirit of the account, which extols the discovery of the springs. It is, however, hard to say to which springs the text refers. Some tend to accept Kallirrhoe; but Dechent and Krauss maintain that this was not in the territory of Seir.[71]

Be that as it may, despite the hesitations of the scholars quoted above, who pioneered the research of hot springs and medicinal baths in Palestine, we must consider whether there are in fact hot springs in the border regions of Palestine. Aharoni emphasizes that many names of places and regions have been preserved by their inhabitants almost unchanged over thousands of years, up to our own time.[72] There are apparently two reasons for this: firstly, because during different historical periods most of the peoples of Palestine spoke Semitic tongues, which were related to each other; and, secondly, because, despite the changes in the composition of the population of Palestine, most settlement was continuous, and new inhabitants took over existing names from their predecessors. In other words, the great majority of definite identifications of particular places has been made with the aid of the preservation of the ancient name, usually in Arabic: sometimes the name of the site itself, and sometimes of a ruin or a geographical object close to the spot.

---

[70] Idem, *ibid.*

[71] Dechent (1884): 173; Krauss (1907): 105.

[72] Aharoni (1987): 88; Kliot and Cohen (1984): 316–317, and see the bibliography there.

Thus, it is also sometimes possible to gain topographical information from place-names, and particularly from place-names connected with sources of water, such as *abel, ain, afek, be'er, gevim, hammat*, etc.[73]

Hammam, pl. *hammamat*, is the Arabic word for a bathhouse. *Hamima* is a small bathhouse, and *hammah*—similar to the Hebrew word *hammat*—a hot water spring. Arabic names of hot springs in Palestine and Trans-Jordan are as follows (see Map 2): [74]

Hamma—The Arabic name for the small hot springs on the east coast of Lake Kinneret, 2–3 kilometres north of Ein Gev. They are also known as *al-Ḥamma a-Ẕa'ira*, the small hot spring. One of them is known as Ein Gophra, because of the sulphurous odors which it emits. They emerge at the foot of the Golan Heights, about 200 metres below the level of the Mediterranean.

Hammam al-Malieh—The Arabic name for the hot springs in the mountains of east Samaria, about 15 kilometres south of Beth Shean. The name means hot salt springs, because of the quality of the water. The springs flow in a valley called in Arabic Wadi al-Malieh.

Hammam Ez-Zarqa—The Arabic name for springs in Trans-Jordan. They flow in the *Nahal Zarqa*, which descends from the Mountains of Moab to the Dead Sea, about 4 kilometres from its eastern coast. The spring bears the name of the valley, which means 'blue', and refers to the colour of the water. It is said that a Jew from Jericho 'pitched tents by the hot springs of Ez-Zarqa; and this was of great help to our brethren who wished to visit these places, and also to those who went there to be healed'.[75]

Hammam Musa—A hot spring in the Sinai desert, on the coast of the Gulf of Suez, and close to the town of at-Tur. The spring is situated on the border of the orchards of the monastery of Santa Katherina. On the evidence of a traveler who passed through Sinai in 1722, the Arabs were accustomed to bathe in its waters, and claimed that they found relief from pain through Moses, whom they believed to have bathed there.[76] A Sage from Jerusalem, who sailed to Yemen in the year 1864 and went ashore at at-Tur during the journey, visited the hot spring: 'At a distance of two miles from there, we rode on donkeys, together

---

[73] Aharoni (1987): 90, 97–104.
[74] Vilnaey (1976): III: 2392, 2397.
[75] Vilnaey (1976): III: 2397; Luntz (1904): 196.
[76] Shaw (1738): 350.

with some other travelers, to bathe in the waters of the spring, which
flows out of the mountain like Hammei-Tiberias, and which is called
Hammam Sidna Musa [= Baths of our Lord Moses].[77]

Hammam Phara'on—The Arabic name of a hot spring in Sinai, on
the coast of the Gulf of Suez, close to the road from the Suez Canal
to Abu Zneima and Abu Rodeis. It is named after Pharaoh, *Phara'on* in
Arabic. The traveler Shaw, who passed by the spot in 1722, says: 'Its
waters are so hot that one can boil an egg in them in a minute'.[78]

The author of *Mishpat HaUrim* emphasizes that there were hot springs
in the Idumaean desert south of Moab, which emerged close to the
Dead Sea, flowed into the Wadi al-Achsa, and heated its waters. This
is probably true. The springs in the Dead Sea region are concentrated
in four main blocs:[79] in the *Nahal* Tseret HaShahar pass, also known as
Zarqa Spring (reference point 207.4–113.1), about 4 kilometres east of
the Dead Sea; a group of hot springs, close to the shore of the Dead
Sea (reference point 203.3–111.4); on the western shore, about half a
kilometre north of the tip of the border marked by the cease-fire line
of 1949 (reference point 187.4–100.4); and a cluster of springs near
Hajar ad-D'hor (reference point 186.9–094.4), 3 kilometres south of
David Spring in Ein Gedi.

It should be pointed out that Eisenstein accepts this hypothesis of
Steinberg's.[80] In addition, the Greek name of the hot springs on the
eastern shore of the Dead Sea, Καλλιρρόη, is preserved in the literary sources of the Second Temple, Mishnaic and Talmudic periods.
It seems that the allusion in the important tale about the discovery of
HaYemim inserted into the genealogical table of the children of Seir is
to these springs.[81] Be that as it may, this remark helps us to distinguish
between Anah the son of Zibeon and Anah the son of Seir, who is
mentioned in the following verse (*Genesis* 36, 25). So Weinfeld maintains;
and he adds that were it not for this remark, it would be possible to
conclude, mistakenly, that Dishon and Aholibamah were the sons of
Anah the son of Zibeon, whereas in fact they were the sons of Anah

---

[77] Sapir (1970): 38.
[78] Shaw (1738): 380; See also Mazor (1968c): 297–299; Vilnaey (1976): III: 2395.
[79] Steinberg (1960): 323; Braver (1954): 161–172; Ilan (1972): 44–48; See also the
bibliographical collection on the Dead Sea and its surroundings on various issues: Nir
(1968): 4–18.
[80] Eisenstein (1952): V: 267.
[81] Kasher (1934): 10.

the brother of Zibeon.[82] The Arabic name for the springs of Kallirrhoe is Hammam Ez-Zara; they flow at the foot of the mountains of Moab in the Kingdom of Jordan between the outfall of the Jordan River on the north and *Nahal* Arnon on the south.[83] Klein remarks that north of the spring of Kallirrhoe, today known as Hammam Ez-Zara, east of the Dead Sea, are the hot springs of Hammam Ez-Zarqa, mentioned by Josephus under the name Βαάρας (*Antiquitates Judaicae* 7.186–189), and in the Talmudic literature as Ba'arah [= *bo'er*, burning], viz. 'a place of burning, hot water'; in the course of time the name was corrupted to Mei Ba'arah—Mei Me'arah.[84] It may be assumed that it was this complex that was meant by *HaYemim* of *Genesis* 36, 24.[85] (see Figs. 31–32).

B. The healing of Na'aman, the general of the army of the King of Aram, from leprosy in the waters of the Jordan is described as a supernatural miracle achieved by the prophet Elisha (*II Kings* 3, 6–14). This is one of the stories about the miraculous deeds of Elisha, in the period when the kingdom of Israel was totally subordinate to Aram.[86]

Ever since the people of Israel crossed the Jordan River on dry land this river has been the source of many legends, which apparently derive from the sanctity of the site.[87] Elijah crossed the Jordan by dividing the waters with his mantle, and when he had ascended to heaven his spirit descended on Elisha, who performed the same miracle (*II Kings* 8, 13–14); Elisha brought to the surface an iron axe which had fallen into the Jordan (*ibid.*, 6, 1–7); and, as has been said, Na'aman the Aramaean was cured of his leprosy by bathing seven times in the Jordan, at the behest of the prophet (*ibid.*, 5, 14). Traces of the sanctity of the Jordan River in the Second Temple period may be found in the stories about John the Baptist in the gospels. Thus, for instance, '[They] were baptized of him in Jordan, confessing their sins' (*Matthew* 3, 5–6) or 'They were all baptized of him in the river Jordan, confessing their sins' (*Mark* 1, 5), and more. Further, from the words of Na'aman

---

[82] Weinfeld (1982): I: 125.
[83] Vilnaey (1979): III: 6645–6646.
[84] Klein (1924): 21–22.
[85] Dvorjetski (1992): 5–10.
[86] Levinstam (1965): I: 357; Ahituv (1968a): III: 893; Simon (1978a): 10; Bennahum (1985): 88; Rosner (2000): 43.
[87] Broshi (1965): III: 786; Posner, Paul and Stern (1987): II: 125.

'Are not Aba'na and Pharpar, rivers of Damascus, better than all the
waters of Israel?' (*II Kings* 5, 12) it would appear that the therapeutic
springs of Palestine were not yet known beyond its borders.[88] Shiponi
maintains that the powers of hot springs to heal various diseases were
already known to the early prophets, and that the legend of Na'aman
and the prophet Elisha is proof of this.[89]

Be that as it may, it is important to investigate the geological and
geochemical conditions of the emergence, and perhaps also of the dis-
appearance, of hot springs, since in the period of the Mishnah and the
Talmud therapeutic sites based on hot springs were known in Palestine
and outside it. Why does the Talmudic literature not mention the exact
geographic location of the story of the healing of Na'aman? All the
discussions of the Sages about this incident centre on Na'aman's leprosy
and the reasons for it, and the greatness of the Lord. For instance:
'"And he was a mighty man in valour, a leper" (*ibid.*, 5, 1). Why did
he become leprous? Because a little maid was brought captive from
the Land of Israel'. (*Yalkut Shim'oni*, to *II Kings* 5; *ibid.*, *Zecharia* 14); 'If
anyone says to you that the Lord does not heal leprosy, Na'aman will
come and bear witness that he was healed by bathing in the Jordan'
(*Numbers Rabbah* 14, 4; *Deuteronomy Rabbah* 2, 19).[90] (see Map 1).

C. Despite the uncertainty in relation to the meaning of the word
HaYemim, and our lack of knowledge of the exact part of the Jordan
River where Na'aman was healed, Hirschberg believes that the existence
of therapeutic springs in Palestine can be proved by the allusions to
mineral components of the soil and water of Palestine in Biblical literature. He adds that they may have been used for therapeutic purposes.
The minerals are: *borit* (soap) (*Jeremiah* 2, 22; *Proverbs* 25, 20); *heimar*
(asphalt) (*Genesis* 11, 3; *ibid.*, 14, 10); *melah* (salt) (*ibid.*, 19, 26; *Psalms* 60,
2; *Zephania* 2, 9). He also believes that it is possible to deduce from the
expression 'the springs of salvation' (*Isaiah* 12, 4) that 'at that time there
were springs which afforded help and salvation to human beings'.[91] On
the one hand, Hirschberg adds, it is possible that the sense in which
they afford salvation to mankind may be expressed in their watering the
soil, which makes every tree and every fruit blossom, as does the water

---

[88] Hirschberg (1920): 217.
[89] Shiponi (1962): 1.
[90] Kimhi (1973): II: 643–644; Hyman (1979): 106–107.
[91] Hirschberg (1920): 217.

which comes out of the Temple, in Ezekiel's description (47, 1–12); on the other hand, he adds, it may be that when Ezekiel spoke of every living thing and the fishes, 'he (Ezekiel) did not yet know that water is capable of giving man life, and healing every disease'.

It should be pointed out that many of Hirschberg's theories have no rational basis. In the first place, *borit* is a substance used for cleaning and washing clothes, derived from the ashes of soap plants. The primary meaning of the word *borit* is, apparently, cleanliness, from the root *b-r-r*. The reference in *II Kings* 3, 2 is to laundering soap; *Jeremiah* 2, 22 mentions *borit* together with nitre; and in an obscure passage in *Proverbs* (25, 20), 'vinegar on nitre' is usually taken to mean that the chemical action of vinegar nullifies that of nitre, or that nitre ferments and melts when vinegar is poured on it. In the Talmudic literature, too, *borit* is the name of a plant whose ashes are used to clean and launder (*Tosefta, Shvi'it* 5, 7). It seems that this substance has no connection with the existence of therapeutic springs of Palestine. The same applies to Hirschberg's Biblical references to salt. He refers to the names of a number of places connected with salt: Valley of Salt in the south (*Psalms* 60, 2), to which should be added Tel of Salt and the City of Salt (*Joshua* 15, 62; *II Samuel* 8, 13; *II Kings* 14, 7; *Ezra* 2, 59). All of these places have names which indicate their character and the fact that they are close to a place connected with salt. Hirschberg also adduces *Zephaniah* (2, 9), which shows that, in contradistinction to the blessing which men see in salt, the Bible also sees it as indicating a curse, since Sodom and Gomorrah, symbols of complete destruction, were turned to salt (*Deuteronomy* 29, 22), and the same will happen to the enemies of Israel (*Zephaniah* 2, 9). But in all this there is no hint of the medicinal uses of salt. Moreover, all the stories of the cities of the plain—the tale of Sodom and Gomorrah, which tells that the Lord overthrew these cities and rained brimstone and fire upon them, and 'the smoke of the country went up as the fire of a furnace' (*Genesis* 19, 28), and the story of Lot's wife, who turned into pillar of salt—are influenced by the nature of the Dead Sea region, and its unique phenomena. It seems probable that the pillars of salt in this region were the sources of the etiological legend of Lot's wife.[92] Moreover, Hirschberg's views

---

[92] Goshen-Gottstein (1965a): II: 347; Stern (1968): V: 989–990; Bainart (1963): IV: 1053–1056; Ahituv (1968b): V: 998–1000.

on *hemar* are partially correct. The references to *hemar* in the Bible—in the story of the tower of Babel (*ibid.*, 11, 3), and the description of the battle of Chedorlaomer in the vale of Siddim (*ibid.*, 14, 10)—are not proof positive of the existence of therapeutic baths in Palestine; but they may cast light on the source and uses of asphalt in the Second Temple period. In the Septuagint this material is called ἄσφαλτος, and in the Vulgate Bitumen.[93]

The asphalt of the Dead Sea is pure bitumen, lumps of which float close to the shore in the southern part of the sea, particularly in the vicinity of the outfall of the Arnon and on the Ein Gedi shore. This bitumen is solid, shiny, black and brittle, and it bears signs of flow. It appears that it is forced up from deep layers of the earth, and emerges along the translation near the shore. In the area surrounding the southern part of the Dead Sea liquid asphaltic bitumen is to be found. In the places where bitumen emerges on land it merges into the dust, or flows, or collects in puddles. Sulphur, which accompanies the bitumen as it surfaces, is formed from gypsum by a process of reduction, which is induced by the bitumen. Light oil or gas which comes out of the soil can easily burst into flame. If it does so, an undying flame, fed by the bitumen which emerges continuously from the soil, is produced. These phenomena have been known in many parts of the East since ancient times, as is shown by the poetic description in *Isaiah* 34, 9–10, which contains a geological explanation: 'And the streams thereof shall be turned into pitch, and the dust thereof into brimstone [= Sulphur], and the land thereof shall become burning pitch; it shall not be quenched night or day'. The words of the Bible about the wells of asphalt near Sodom show that the bitumen in the vicinity of the Dead Sea was known in the Biblical period. Classical writers have frequently written about the asphalt from the Dead Sea and its uses. Thus, for instance, the Greek geographer Strabo, the Greek historian Diodorus Siculus, the Roman historian Tacitus, and Josephus Flavius, who says that it can be mixed with many medicines.[94]

In short, the Bible contains no explicit reference to hot springs. Only the name Hammat (*Joshua* 19, 35), which was connected with the hot springs of Tiberias—Hammei-Tiberias—hints at their existence. It

---

[93] Abramski and Parness (1965): III: 187.
[94] See e.g. Josephus, *Bellum Judaicum* 4.485. Abramski and Parness (1965): III: 188; Blake (1930): 26, 32; Forbes (1936); Almog and Eshel (1956): 36–38; Klein (1968): 893–894; Ilan (1972): 33–35.

may be that a reference to the Trans-Jordanian hot springs is hidden in the passage: 'and this was Anah [= of the children of Seir] who found the *yemim* in the wilderness, as he fed the asses of Zibeon, his father' (*Genesis* 36, 24); Hieronymus translates this, in Latin, as: 'This was Anah, who found the hot springs in the desert'. Moreover, the word *yemim* is found in the sense of 'hot springs' in Phoenician, a language cognate to Hebrew.

In our view, the Bible alludes to the existence of hot springs between the border with Sidon and the east of the Dead Sea—the area of Moab and Edom—by the use of expressions which attest to the characteristics of therapeutic springs, as detailed below:

A. *Misrephoth Mayim*. This place, on the border of Sidon, is mentioned in the description of the borders of the 'land which remains': the region which was not settled by the tribes of Israel, and to which part of the Canaanite army fled after the battle of Mei Merom (*Joshua* 11, 8). Some scholars see in this name evidence of a hot [= burnt] spring, whereas others think, following Noth, that it should be read not *Misrephoth Mayim*, but *Misrephoth Miyam* [= from the sea = from the west], since the other directions of the flight were towards Sidon Rabbah, and to the Valley of Mitzpeh in the east. Accordingly, some scholars seek Misrephoth (Mayim) in the northern part of the Valley of Acre, and identify it with Hirbet al-Mesherpeh, south of Rosh Hanikra, also known as Tel a-Tabaik. This identification is possible, considering that the springs there are rather warm.[95] If *Misrephoth Mayim* is identical with Hirbet Mesherpeh the border of the 'land which remains' was in the northern part of the Valley of Acre.[96]

B. It seems that in Isaiah's prophecies of the destruction of the Assyrian army and Edom there are allusions to the hot springs east of the Dead Sea. The texts read as follows:

> For *Tophet* is ordained of old; yea, for the king it is prepared; he hath made it deep and large; the pile thereof is fire and much wood; the breath of the Lord, like a stream of brimstone, doth kindle it.
>
> (*Isaiah* 30, 33)

---

[95] Noth (1958): 43; See also Patai (1936): 224; Aharoni (1968): V: 641; Press (1952): III: 606; Yeivin (1956: 37–38) notes that at Tel a-Tabaik remains from the Middle Bronze age were found; According to Maizler-Mazar (1954: 24) the citizens in this city adored the local god by the title Asraf (Saraf), and the local ruler was named Afru-Asraf, which indicates his service in worship. This name means a servant of the god Asraf; For the hot water there, see Garstang (1931): 190; cf. Luria (1990): 187–188.

[96] Aharoni (1987): 203–204.

And the streams thereof shall be turned into pitch, and the dust thereof
into brimstone, and the land thereof shall become burning pitch. It shall
not be quenched night nor day; the smoke thereof shall go up for ever;
from generation to generation it shall lie waste; none shall pass through
it for ever and ever.

(ibid., 34, 9–10)

Most civilized nations have always known of sulphur. In the Bible it
is alluded to as inflammatory and destructive material, together with
fire (*Genesis* 19, 24) and salt (*ibid.*, 19, 26; *Deuteronomy* 29, 22). Hence
the descriptions of raining fire and brimstone (Sulphur) (*Genesis* 19, 26;
Ezekiel 38, 22; *Psalms* 11, 6), of turning streams of water to streams of
fiery Sulphur (*Isaiah* 34, 9, and, similarly, *ibid.*, 30, 33), and of the sowing
of Sulphur on field and meadow as a means of destroying crops (*Job*
18, 15). These descriptions arose from the custom of using sulphur as
a means of spreading fire, and that this is common to sulphur and to
pitch, of which Isaiah also speaks (*Isaiah* 34, 9).[97] Sulphur is found in
Palestine south of Gaza (near Be'eri), as a deposit of sulphurous fumes
which arise from the depths of the earth and penetrate the sandstone.
It is also found dispersed in small quantities in the marlstone of the
Jordan Valley and the Dead Sea. There, knots of Sulphur the size
of nuts are formed from the gypsum in the marlstone strata. The
sulphur in the hot springs on the border of the Jordan Valley south
of the Dead Sea has some therapeutic value. Sulphur, a non-metallic
chemical element, is easily separated out, and sulphur dioxide, which
has an unpleasant smell, is created when it is burnt. Sulphur deposits
accumulate in an extremely volcanic process of crystallization. The
Sulphur deposits exuded from hot sulphurous springs are associated
with asphalt, tar, pitch, earth-wax, petroleum and the like. It may well
be that the 'streams of sulphur' are springs and streams of hot water
which discharge sulphur into the environment, and spread the strong
odour of the Hydrogen Sulphide which accompanies it. 'Kindled them':
for their temperature reaches 60°C and more.[98] Strabo is not unjustified
in calling them 'boiling streams which stink afar'.[99] In Braslavsky's view,
it is quite possible that the prophet Isaiah was influenced by the name

---

[97] Ben Shamai (1960): XI: 149; Goshen-Gottestein (1965b): II: 545; See also Frass
(1879): 113; Blanckenhorn (1896): 44.
[98] Parness (1965): II: 545–546.
[99] Strabo, *Geographica* 16.2.44.

'Ba'arah' [= burnt], which was common in the First Temple period, since the springs of Ba'arah, which are first mentioned by Josephus, are the hottest in the whole of the Dead Sea region, and are indeed boiling hot.[100] It may be mentioned that three kilometres before the outfall of the stream of Zarqa-Ma'in, on the further side of the Dead Sea, in a direct line east-wards from the springs of Awir and Thorba, there emerge hot springs with therapeutic qualities, known as Hammam Zarqa-Ma'in. These springs are identified with the bath of Ba'arah, which is mentioned by Josephus (*Bellum Judaicum* 7.186–189) as well as in the Rabbinic literature, and appears in the Madaba map.[101] We may surmise that when the prophet wrote 'the breath of the Lord, like a stream of brimstone, doth kindle (*ba'arah*) it', (*Isaiah* 30, 33), he was referring to sulphurous springs of this type, which are to be found on the shores of the Dead Sea.

It should be emphasized that the therapeutic effects of Sulphur baths—that is to say, immersion in springs or baths of sulphides—on arthritic pains, rheumatism and the like were well known in antiquity. Many therapeutic sites in Western Europe will be discussed later in this study.[102]

1.4 TERMINOLOGY

The issue of bath, bathing and spa-bathing terminology is a particularly knotty one especially in the Levant concerning very many sources written in Hebrew, Aramaic, and Syriac further to the intricate evidences written in Greek and Latin. Technical terms in any society often have fluid applications, and they frequently change by region and/or over generations, particularly when such a subject handle since Biblical days through the twelfth century CE.[103]

The practice of Hydrotherapy, which involved various activities and methods of applying water at baths of any kind, early on became part

---

[100] Braslavsky (1956): III: 333.

[101] See the discussion in chapter 4 on *Historical-Archaeological Analysis of Hammei-Ba'arah*.

[102] See the discussion in chapter 3 on *The Medicinal Hot Springs and Healing Spas in the Graeco-Roman World*.

[103] For the important rôle that the bathhouse played in the life of the Romans, see the discussion in this chapter on *Leisure-Time Activities and Places of Entertainment*.

of Roman medicine, and can be distinguished from the use of mineral
spring water applied for therapeutic purposes. There is no question
that hydrotherapy, which took place in ordinary baths, formed a larger
portion of medical treatment than any curative thermo-mineral springs.
The differences between spa-bathing and ordinary hydrotherapy are
most visible in the earlier stages of development. Spa-bathing, at its very
core, relied on the use of spring water. It was not, as in regular bath
therapies reportedly given by Asclepiades, the result of using hot or
cold baths. The benefits achieved at a spa relied on the actual perceived
properties of the water—more so than on the activity of bathing.[104]

By definition, a *spa* is a place or resort that is built around a mineral
spring. Nowadays, it is a commercial establishment offering health
and beauty treatment through such means as steam baths, exercise
equipment, and massage. Spa bathing, at its very core, relied on the
use of spring water.[105] There are several possible origins for the word
Spa. It is supposed to be from the Latin words 'Espa' [= fountain] and
'Sparsa' from spargere [= to bubble up]. The initials *S P A* from the
Latin expression *Salus per Aquis* mean several ideas. Latin for enter by
means of water and Latin for health or relaxation through water. It
was found in graffiti in Roman baths. The interpretation of the Latin
expression *SPA* [= health by or through waters] was used by the Romans
to point out that thermal balneotherapy can help people maintain their
bodies in good shape, prevent diseases, and sometimes restore function
to parts of the body. It eventually became the word *spa*, used today to
signify a thermal spring, resort, or similar facility. Respectively to the
International SPA Association [= ISPA], the glossary of spa water terms
of modern times are as follows:[106]

1. *Hydrotherapy*: Generic term for water therapies using jets, underwater
   massage and mineral baths (e.g. Balneotherapy, Iodine-Grine therapy,

---

[104] A number of studies have been carried out on the interaction between bathing and health. See, for instance, most recently, Allen (1998): 40–41; Fagan (1999a):
128–155; Yegül (1992): 352–355; Garzya (1994): 109–119; D'Amato (1989): 10–16;
Jackson (1988); Di Capua (1940).
[105] Pearsall (1998): 1782; Allen (1998): 14–15; Nolte (2001): 26; Wood (2004): 30.
[106] Martin (1998): 63; See also http://spas.about.com/gi/dynamic/offsite.htm?
site=http://experienceispa.com/

Kneipp treatments, Swiss Shower, Thalassotherapy and others. It also can mean a whirlpool bath, hot Roman pool, hot tub, Jacuzzi, cold plunge and mineral bath. These treatments use physical water properties, such as temperature and pressure, for therapeutic purposes, to stimulate blood circulation, dispel toxins and treat certain diseases.

2. *Crenotherapy*: All types of treatment carried out with mineral water, mud and vapor.

3. *Thalassotherapy*: An ancient Greek therapy (θάλασσα = sea), these treatments use the therapeutic benefits of the sea, and sea water products for their vitamins, minerals and trace elements, which can heal and reinvigorate skin and hair.

4. *Balneotherapy*: A generic term for mineral water treatments, balneotherapy is the traditional practice of treatments by waters, using hot springs, mineral, or sea waters to restore and revitalize the body. Since antiquity, Balneotherapy has been used to improve circulation, fortify the immune system, as an analgesic (pain reliever) and as an anti-stress treatment. In other words, it is the treatment of disease by bathing, usually in the mineral containing waters of hot springs.

The expression *hot spring* may be interpreted in several ways, in accordance with the various topics of interest to those who deal with this subject. Ordinary people think that a hot spring is a spring whose temperature is greater than that of their own body. This approach is close to that of the balneologists. According to them, any mineral spring above a certain temperature which can be comfortably bathed in is a hot spring. Thus, a person's subjective feeling determines what a hot spring is. This is not scientifically exact. Geologists and hydrologists define a hot spring as a spring with a permanent temperature higher than the average annual temperature of the area in which it is situated. According to this definition, springs in Arctic and mountainous areas, whose temperature is, in effect, no greater than that of cold springs in temperate and tropical regions, are considered hot springs. From the biological point of view, the most important factor relating to the fauna in the springs is the prevailing temperature inside the spring. For hot springs, as distinct from other watercourses, whose temperature varies daily or seasonally, the permanent level of temperature is particularly important. The heat of the springs is the result of a number of causes: The depth from which the water rises and the penetration of magma close to the surface.[107] Hot springs are divided into four groups, according to their temperature:[108]

1. Lukewarm (Cliarothermal), 18°C–28°C.
2. Warm (Euthermal), 29°C–44°C.
3. Hot (Akrothermal), 45°C–65°C.
4. Boiling (Hyperthermal), 66°C and over.

The analysis of mineral waters provided a rationale for their use in medicine which supported the enthusiastic recommendations of physicians. Even where there seemed to be no obvious connection between the chemical constituents of the water and the medicinal virtues claimed for it, the very existence of a chemical analysis gave the water added appeal as a curative agent and many physicians were able to turn this to good advantage in attracting patients to the spas in Britain, France, Germany, and throughout Europe. Thus while mineral water analysis certainly proved to be most difficult, the efforts of physicians and chemists to perfect it in the eighteenth and nineteenth centuries yielded benefits of various kinds for the improvement of inorganic chemical analysis in general and for some medical practitioners.[109]

Natural mineral springs were used empirically throughout the centuries, perhaps for thousands of years, before being used under medical indication and direction. Empirical treatment similarly preceded scientific use of many internal medicines and this common practice should by no means be deprecated. Thermal baths using natural springs of hot water are mentioned repeatedly in the ancient sources stated before, particularly those at Tiberias, Gadara, Pella, and Kallirrhoe.[110]

The terms *Hammat, Hammtha,* or *Hammthan,* are linked to several sites in the Levant: Hammat near Tiberias, Hammat near Gader, Hammat in Judaea, Hammtha de Peḥal, and Hammthan. Their Greek names Ἐμμαθά, or Ἐμμαοῦς, or Ἀμμαοῦς, or Ἀμμαθοῦς are derived from the Hebrew, Syriac and Aramaic languages. They are written exactly as the phonetical spelling in the Greek language.[111] Already in Josephus

[107] See, for example, Kahan (1963): 1–2; Mazor (1968a): 65–80; idem, (1980): 300; Garg and Kassoy (1981): 57–59.
[108] Vouk (1950): 36–42.
[109] Coley (1990): 56–66; idem, (1982): 123–144.
[110] See for instance, Buchmann (1928a): 28–34; idem, (1928b): 364–371; Kottek (1994): 61.
[111] Rapoport (1857): 196–201; Gesenius (1899): 213; Krauss (1899): II: 58; Brown,

one can learn about the phonetic connection between Hammat and Ammathous or Hammthan, and the literal meaning of the word. In the *Bellum Judaicum* (4.11) he says:[112]

> Vespasian now broke up the camp which he had pitched in front of Tiberias at Ἀμμαθοῦς. This name may be interpreted as 'warm baths', being derived from a spring of warm water within the city possessing curative properties, and proceeded to Gamala.

The meaning of the name θέρμαι or θερμά in Greek, as also of *'aquae calidae'* or *'thermae'* in Latin, is 'hot springs' or 'hot baths'.[113] Hieronymus helps to illustrate the connection between these terms: 'Gadara city over the Jordan, opposite Scythopolis and Tiberias..., in the hill, at the foot of which hot springs burst forth and over which bathhouses were built'.[114]

The different names of the therapeutic sites in the Levant hint at the question of the creation and source of the waters of these springs. Even the name of *Ba'arah*, for instance, is related to the verb bet-'ayin-resh [= burn], and there are traces of a subterranean fire there.[115] The name *Kallirrhoe* in Greek means a fine stream and was of an applied to hot springs and healing installations in the ancient Mediterranean world—the most famous of which was the Kallirrhoe spring near the Acropolis in Athens.[116]

All the sites reviewed in this study are described by Greek and Roman writers in almost set terms since they are the dominant, inseparable component of each of the mother cities. Thus, for instance: τὰ τῶν θερμῶν ὑδάτων λουτρὰ [= the hot water baths]; τὰ τῶν θερμῶν ὑδάτων θερμὰ λουτρὰ [= the hot baths of the hot waters]; or also: τὰ τερμὰ ὑδάτα [= the hot baths]; or: θερμῶν ὑδάτων πηγαί [= the hot water springs].[117] Later on, it seems, sites of cold therapeutic springs were also

---

Driver and Briggs (1906): 329; Krauss (1910): I: 214–216; Klein (1924): 42–43; Kohut (1926): III: 441; Schocett (1936): 166; Eisenstein (1952): II: 78; Weiss and Kemble (1962): 11; Köhler and Baumgartner (1967): I: 318; Eisenstein (1952): II: 78; Negev and Gibson (2001): 214.

[112] See also *Antiquitates Judaicae* 18.36; Kottek (1994): 136.

[113] Liddel and Scott (1985): 363; Lewis and Short (1951): 1867; Glare (1976): II: 1937.

[114] Hieronymus, *Onomastikon* 75.

[115] Dechent (1884): 202.

[116] Dechent (1884): 198; Pauly and Wissowa (1919): 1669; Smith (1922): 149, 244–248; Donner (1963): 60.

[117] Dvorjetski (1992a): 53, 64–65, 73, 105–106, 108, and especially 115; idem, (1999): 122.

called *Emmaus*, and one cannot therefore deduce from this common
name the existence there of specifically hot springs. The testimony of
Ammianus Marcellinus of the fourth century CE, makes this very clear.
He pointed out that in Mesopotamia, the very place where the springs
are found is called in Syriac both cool waters and Emmaus.[118]

The Latin words normally used to indicate a thermo-mineral spring
are *fons* and *aquae*. The word *aquae* can refer not only to the springs
at a spa, but to the actual spa itself, so that it is sometimes obscure
which is meant.[119] There is less confusion in the Greek texts because
the writers tended to refer to a spa by name and to identify specific of
springs available at a spa.[120] Despite the lack of clarity in terminology,
some patterns regarding the vocabulary of springs at spas are evident.
Locations could be designed as *aquae*. Thus, when indicating spa location, the texts refer, for instance, to Aquae Albulae, Aquae Auguriae,
Aquae Cutiliae, Aquae Aponi, Aquae Sinuessanae, Aquae Mattiacae,
and Aquae Tauri. If particular springs ere referred to, it was likely that
the term *fons* would be used. But sometimes after a location became
known specifically as either fons or aquae, it retained that designation.[121]
In a few cases, however, the terms are inter changed, but for the most
part the designations remained constant.[122]

Our intention in this study is not to deal with all kinds of washing
and cleansing, but only with the thermo-mineral public baths, namely
spas. The main function of a bath complex of this kind was to provide
access to the spring waters for therapeutic purposes. The natural springs
usually supplied hot water, but it was also possible for cold spring water
to feed the pools of the baths. A bathhouse which received its water
supply from a nearby spring may be considered a spa if one or more
of the following occur:[123]

---

[118] *Res Gestae* 18.6.16.

[119] See, for example, Aquae Sinuessanae: Livy, *Historia Romana* 22.13.13; Pliny,
Naturalis Historia 31.4; Tacitus, *Annales* 12.66; Aquae Albulae: Pliny, *Naturalis Historia*
31.6; Aquae Aponi: Pliny, *Naturalis Historia* 2.106.227; Aquae Cumanae: Livy, *Historia
Romana* 41.16.3; See also Allen (1998): 17–18; On other terms and verbs for using
thermo-mineral waters, see idem, (1998): 103–106.

[120] See, for example, Galen, *De method medendi* X.536; Strabo, *Geographica* 5.2.3; Cassius
Dio, *Historia Romana* 66.17.1; For the Roman classification of thermo-mineral springs,
see chapter 3 on *Medicinal Hot Springs and Healing Spas in the Graeco-Roman World*.

[121] Allen (1998): 18.

[122] Cutiliae was known sometimes as *fons* (Celsus, *De Medicina* 4.12.7) but more
regularly as *aquae* (Pliny, *Naturalis Historia* 31.6; Caelius Aurelianus, *De Acutis Morbis*
3.1.10, 3.2.45, 5.4.77).

[123] Allen (1998): 15.

1. The spring is warm and mineral, although in a few cases the spring could be cold.
2. There is sufficient archaeological evidence to suggest a healing function.
3. An ancient source identifies the site as a healing establishment.

Spas were a variation on regular bathing establishment which entailed a different architecture appropriate to their specific health function. Nevertheless, we do have to recollect some entries relating to Roman and Muslim baths from methodological and didactical point of view.

The term *Thermae* is applied to bath buildings, usually used to denote richly decorated establishments, especially large Imperial baths. Unlike the smaller bathing establishments, the *balneae*, which were often privately owned, *thermae* were owned and operated by the city or the state and were open for all. *Thermae* of the 'imperial type' are exceptional in their formal and grandiose plans, characterized by bilateral symmetry about a main axis created by four standard rooms or units: *apodyterium* [= dressing room], *tepidarium* [= warm bath], *caldarium* [= hot bath], and *frigidarium* [= cold bath].[124]

Balnea and *balneae* (pl.) are terms denoting bath buildings. It is used to refer to small city baths, as distinct from the great public baths, and of the type found at Pompeii. An abundance of written evidence makes it clear that the Romans used these terms interchangeably with each other and with *balneum* to denote bath buildings, both public and private, and segregated and mixed. The term *balneum* is applied liberally in the written sources both to bath buildings, private and public, to the act of bathing itself, and to bathing tubs. In its purest form it seems to denote a private bath and the act of bathing, but it is often found in reference to public bathing establishments. The *balneator* means 'bath-man', or 'bath-master', and is broadly defined. His role and duties are most unclear and appear to have varied from place to place. In some instances, the *balneator* seems to be the manager of a facility, in others he is a minister performing a host of tasks: collecting

---

[124] More detailed discussions on terms can be found in Fagan (1999a), s.v. 'Terminology'; Nielsen (1990): I: 3–4, 153–166; Yegül (1992): 487–489; Croutier (1992) provides a non-academic approach to the subject); Allen (1998): 1–19 (spas in Italy); Wood (2004): 32; For the early provincial baths, see Nielsen (1999): 35–43; See the glossary on Ancient Baths Resource Site in the internet: http://www3.la.psu.edu/cams/Baths/gloss.html#frig organized by G.G. Fagan.

money at the door, pouring water over customers, anointing, keeping the cloakroom, and even stoking the furnaces and procuring. What all of these notices take for granted, however, is that the *balneator* is very much on-the-spot, a visible representative of the management, if not the actual management.

Public baths and public hostelries were other institutions pointing to the influence of Hellenism in the Levant. For a warm bath, the general term *Merhatz* is used; for a bathhouse *beth merhaz*, less often *bé bâne* (*Babylonian Talmud, Shabbat* 41a) or *bé bane* (*ibid., Berakhot* 60a), both contractions of the Greek βαλανεία. The title of the 'bath-master', βαλανεύς, also indicates its Greek origin. Quite rare is *balne* (*Jerusalem Talmud, Ma'aser Sheni* 4, 2 [54d]). In the *Jerusalem Talmud* the word *sachi* is used mostly for bathing, from which are said to be derived the terms *mis'chuta* (*Babylonian Talmud, Qiddushin* 33a) or *bé mesutha* (*ibid., Baba Metzia* 6b; *ibid., Shabbat* 140a; *ibid., Berakhot* 22a; *ibid., Hullin* 45b) for a bathhouse. Otherwise, one attempted to connect *bé mesutha* with *assi*, to heal. The terms *tebila* (immersion) or *miqweh* (collection basin) are used exclusively for a ritual bath. There were no separate establishments for cold baths; bathing in cold water is not considered a bath, *rechitza* (*Jerusalem Talmud, Berakhot* 2, 7 [5b]. Where the Rabbinic literature differentiates between community baths and those of private enterprise, the former is called *demosia* (public), whereas the latter retains its ancient name *merhaz* or *merhatzaah* (*Babylonian Talmud, Shabbat* 33b), and is rarely called *privata* (*Jerusalem Talmud, Shevi'it* 8, 11 [38b]. The thermo-mineral springs of Tiberias are also called *demosin* [= *demosia*] (public) (*ibid., Sanhedrin* 7,13 [25d]; *ibid., Avoda Zarah* 4, 4 [43d]; *ibid., Berakhot* 2, 8 [5c]; *ibid., Peah* 8, 9 [21b]), and Emmaus-Nicopolis is mentioned as *demosith*, which served as a place of recreation (*Avot de Rabbi Nathan*, Version A, 14, Schechter ed., p. 59).[125] It is very important to point out that the usage of the term *demosin* or *demosith* in the Rabbinic literature has been blurred throughout the ages for baths in general and therapeutic baths in particular.

Miqweh is a Jewish ritual bath, and means in Hebrew 'collected water'. The *miqweh* is used for ritual cleansing after menstruation or contact with the dead. Proselytes to Judaism are immersed in it as part

---

[125] Preuss (1993): 533; 535, 541; See also Krauss (1910): 224–225; Schürer (1991): II: 55; Kottek (1985): 149; Eliav (1995): 22–32; Schocett (1936: 166–167) believes that *demosin* is a general term for any public institution for pleasure.

of the conversion ceremony and vessels are dipped in it. A *miqweh* must contain enough water to fill a square cubit up to the height of three cubits. The water must come directly from a spring or be rainwater—it cannot have been previously drawn into a receptacle. The *miqweh*, or community bath, arose perhaps because the virtues of cleanliness were bound together with spiritual considerations, forming both a practical and an ethical code of conduct for Jewish people. The literary and the archaeological evidence make it clear that the synagogue and the *miqweh* emerged as buildings constructed for the service of the Jewish community in the Second Temple period.[126]

As the Arabs picked up foreign bathing habits, they were quick to tailor them to their own ways. The *hammam*, which means in Arabic 'spreader of warmth', gained religious significance and became an annex to the mosque, used to comply with the Islamic laws of hygiene and purification. Physical and intellectual development was deemphasized, and only the massage remained. Once the delight of the warm water sunk in, the cold water bath or shower after sweating no longer appealed to the Arabs. The *hammam* developed into a quiet retreat—an atmosphere of half-light, quiescence and seclusion. Architecturally, vaulted ceilings shrank as the buildings became smaller and modest. While the Romans built enormous central baths, the Arabs preferred several small baths throughout their cities, comparable to the Roman *balnea*. They still followed a progression through a series of hot rooms as in the *thermae*, but with different emphasis. In the *hammam* the Roman *tepidarium* dwindled to a mere passageway leading from dressing room to *harara* (hot room) where, unlike the Roman caldarium, special massages were administered. A small steam room adjoining the *harara* replaced the *laconicum* [= the hot, dry-steam sweat chamber in Roman baths]. While the Roman bather finished with a stay in the library or study, the *hammam* bather ends where he or she began, lounging on couches in the rest hall while servants bring drinks and cool the bather with fans. The hypocaust heating systems remained, but in some regions Arabs followed the Roman example of utilizing heat from their many hot springs. These *hammams*, called *kaplica* or *ilica*, have no sweat platform

[126] Reich (1988): 102–107; idem, (1995): 289–297; Sanders (1994): 222–229; Regev (2000a): 184–185; idem, (2000b): 234–236; Berlin (2005): 450–452; For the resemblance between the terraced pool in the bathhouse and the *Miqweh* in Palestine, see Grossberg (1991): 171–184.

in the center of the hottest room. Instead, a pool of natural hot water
heats the *hammam*. Because the water bubbled and flowed, the Arabs
could take a dip in those pools without bathing in their own filth. In
Sum, the Muslim world adopted the Romano-Byzantine taste for steam
baths and the tradition still exists in the form of the Turkish bath.[127]

1.5   Leisure-Time Activities and Places of Entertainment

Leisure is a system of symbols which acts to establish a feeling of
freedom and pleasure by formulating a sense of choice and desire. It is
perceived as being a style of behaviour, which may occur in any activity outside of obligations, rather than a definite category.[128] In other
words, leisure is activity—apart from the obligations of work, family,
and society—to which the turns at will, for either relaxation, diversion,
or broadening his knowledge and his spontaneous social participation,
the free exercise of his creative capacity.[129] Leisure cannot be tied down
to a precise period of time. Its moods and perceptions can be created,
and experienced, at any point. Free time not only appears as a social
construction, but it can also perform a wide variety of functions at both
societal and individual levels. This also means, according to Toner, that
leisure cannot be confined solely to the 'non-serious', for to engage in
something seriously is merely to adopt a certain mood of participation,
and that can be directed towards any activity.[130] The amount of time
available for recreation for most people in antiquity was not unduly
small and could be spent in a number of ways. Many of leisure-time
activities took place within the private house or residence. Places of
entertainment were of a very varied character, which gave architects
every opportunity to demonstrate heir artistic skills. The buildings
associated with public entertainment and leisure were distinguished by
their function and the activities that they housed, as much as by the
building technology employed to construct them. Some structures had

---

[127] Louis (1971): 139–146; Yegül (1992): 339–351; Croutier (1992): 91–93; Newmyer
(1988): 81; Fagan (1999a): 3–4; Ball (2000): 303–304; Lee (2004): 44; See also Aaland
(1997): http://www.cyberbohemia.com/Pages/Islahammam.htm
[128] Toner (1995): 17, 143; See also Goodale and Godbey (1988): 4–9.
[129] Dumazedier (1967): 16–17; See also Haywood et al. (1995); For the Jewish society
that was not exceptional in leisure-time activities, see Crabtree (1983).
[130] Toner (1995): 18–21; For the contribution of the *Jerusalem Talmud* to leisure time
activities in Roman Palestine, see Schwartz (1998a): 313–325.

a very long history and were adapted over time as cultural and social changes occurred. Buildings for public entertainment remain some of the most spectacular monuments to survive from the Roman Empire. There was also wide variation in the provision and form of these facilities across the Empire. The great age of public entertainment was not the great age of social improvement, nor was it only the age in which Rome's neighbors began to acquire greater force. It was also the period of Roman history where alternative ideological systems began to spread and gain adherents—the most important of these being the Christian Church and Judaism. Human institutions are, by their very nature, unstable and persistently evoke diverse responses to them. As the Roman world changed, so did its entertainments, until both ceased to exist.[131] (See Map 3).

The importance of entertainment and leisure in the Roman world can be judged by the plethora of theatres, amphitheatres, bath buildings, and the like that survive across the Empire. While the activities of the theatre, amphitheatre and circus were not every day activities, those of the baths were. The juxtaposition of temple and theatre was common in the Graeco-Roman world, and usually indicates the presence of a deity popular enough to attract large crowds on festival days. The amphitheatres were used not only for entertainments, but also for training exercises, drills and parades. The types of displays performed in amphitheatres had varied enormously, ranging from gladiatorial combats to cock-fighting or bear-baiting. Sometimes, also, animals may have been tamed to perform *circuses* acts, and it should not be forgotten that public executions were often carried out in the arena. Scenes from theatrical and amphitheatrical performances were used to decorate pottery and glass vessels, wall paintings and face-masks or mosaics depicting different types of combats and gladiatorial battles. The Roman *circus* was the large entertainment building used first and foremost for chariot races, most commonly with four-horse (*quadrigae*) or two-horse (*bigae*) chariots. By the time of the Empire the *circus* had taken the form of a hairpin shape, but early on it had a far less formalized layout. Estimates of seating capacity vary from 150,000 to 350,000.[132]

---

[131] Dodge (1999): 205–206; Potter (1999b): 256, 325.
[132] Plommer (1983): 132–140; Barton (1995): 98–166; Wacher (1998): 284–291; Dodge (1999): 236–241; 255; Weeber (1999): 4–39; Köhne and Ewigleben (2000); The most

Less bloodthirsty were the horse and foot races in *stadia*, which were more highly favoured sports than the slaughter of men and animals in the eastern part of the Empire. *Stadia* were to be found in cities where games were celebrated, and they were eventually used for other sorts of athletic contests as well. The *stadium* was a well-established Greek type. In plan it often resembled the *circus*, though on a much smaller scale. Only the very largest cities during the Roman period would have possessed both a *circus* and a *stadium*. In general, with some major exceptions, those in the west would posses only a *circus*, whereas those in Greece and Asia would possess only a *stadium*. It was always possible for a *circus* to double as a *stadium* if necessary. The only cities which possessed a Greek style *stadium* were Samaria-Sebaste and possibly the Phoenician site Marathus-Amrit. The best example is the *stadium* built by Herod in the northern section of Samaria-Sebaste and renovated during the third century CE. This *stadium* was apparently connected with the local cult of Kore.[133]

It appears that—unlike in the Latin West—no clear distinction was made in the East between the use of an amphitheatre, *stadium* and hippodrome. Furthermore, hippodromes had a much greater variety of use than in the West as places for civic functions, caravanserais, and as factories. The first hippodromes were built by Herod the Great in Jerusalem, Caesarea, and Jericho.[134] *Circuses*, or hippodromes, as they were called in the East, were known to have existed in Antioch, Laodicea, and Beirut. Remains of other hippodromes also exist at Bosra, Gadara, Tyre, Gerasa, Caesarea, Shechem-Neapolis, and possibly

---

thorough treatment of the subject on the *circus* and chariot racing is Humphrey (1986); For the performers, performances and participants in the arena or *circus*, see Cameron (1976); Golvin (1988): 149–152; Wiedermann (1992): 120–124; Roueché (1993): 49–80; For the gladiatorial displays, see Humphrey (1988): 1159–1163; Wiedermann (1992): 1–54; For amphitheatres in the west provinces, see Golvin (1988): 117–118, 225–236 and supporting including bibliography; Grenier (1958): III: 880–975; For amphitheatres in the eastern provinces, see Dodge (1999): 233–234; Drinkwater (1983: 179–181) suggests that these sanctuaries, which also have baths and other Roman urban-style facilities, provide a place for the rural population to enjoy such amenities.

[133] Grant (1995): 57; Dodge (1999): 241–242; Weeber (1999): 40–69 (*circus*) 70–87 (*stadium*); There are instances in Asia Minor of theatre-stadium complexes. See Vann (1989): 59–65 for a general discussion of this arrangement; For Palestine see Tsafrir (1984): 121; Schwartz (1998): 169; Ball 2000: 305.

[134] *Antiquitates Judaicae* 15.268 (Jerusalem); *ibid.*, 16.137; *ibid.*, 17.175–178; Although Josephus terms the structures amphitheatres, they should be regarded as hippodromes; See also Netzer (1980): 104–106; Weiss (1998): 99.

Shahba-Philipopolis. Most of the hippodromes in the region date from the second and third centuries CE and were built beyond the city limits. The Tyre hippodrome was one of the largest in the Roman world, and the Gerasa hippodrome, although one of the smallest, is one of the best preserved. Both Gerasa and Bosra might also have functioned as caravanserais, or at least as 'corrals' outside the cities where animals would be quartered. It is noteworthy that the hippodrome at Constantinople came to form the ceremonial heart of the city, functioning as a stage-setting for imperial pageantry and as the city assembly area, in addition to its conventional function as staging chariot races.[135]

One of the earliest entertainments to be found in the Roman world is drama, and it was the popularity of drama, and of its near relations like mime and pantomime, which led to the evolution of the Roman theatre-building. Under the Empire, plays such as tragedies were written more and more for recitation at gatherings of the intellectual elite not for performance, while in the live theatre the old mimes and their more sophisticated cousins, pantomimes, held ever-increasing sway. Theatres of more Greek design were still built in the eastern provinces in the Roman period. All over the Roman world, every sizeable town had at least one theatre, and these were frequently enlarged, modernized or adapted to the changing fashions in theatrical entertainment, and were kept in good repair until the end of the Roman world.[136]

It is reasonable to assume, not only because of their different populations, that the theatres did not fulfill the exact same function in the eastern part of the Roman Empire nor that they addressed their audiences in the same language, or even transmitted a single uniform message. In the second and third centuries CE, classical plays were still being presented, but during the course of the third and fourth centuries CE tragedy and comedy gave way to more popular forms of entertainment. Mimes and pantomimes became very popular throughout the Empire. Oriental audience, which was satisfied with mime presentations, may never even have watched a classical tragedy or comedy. Mime was notable for its licentiousness, its crude and daring humour. The

---

[135] Ball (2000): 305–306; Schwartz (1998): 170; Goodman (1983): 82.

[136] Bieber (1961) is the only standard work on the subject of Greek and Roman theatre. It is still useful but now rather out-of-date; See also Brothers (1989): 97–112; Sear (1990): 376–383; Mitens (1993): 91–106; Weeber (1999): 88–124; Akurgal (2002); On the affinity of theatres and temples see Hanson (1959).

actors and actresses did not wear masks. Mime actors even allowed
themselves to voice criticism of the Emperors and the members of the
ruling class, by hinting at what was happening in the imperial family.
There were also some agonistic performances, acrobats, jugglers, and
clowns.[137] The most surprising feature of the Roman theatres of the
East is that there is not a single Greek theatre in the East. All conform
to the Roman style: semicircular, rather than horseshoe in plan, with a
scenae frons or stage backdrop, rather than open.[138] Theatres were built
in Hellenistic-Roman cities, in Jewish cities, in Nabataean cities, and
even in the countryside removed from cities. Josephus mentioned three
earliest theatres, which erected at the initiative of Herod the Great
and were funded by him: Caesarea, Jerusalem and Jericho.[139] The
theatres can be divided into two primary categories: urban theatres,
such as: Philipopolis, Sepphoris, Qanawat, Gadara, Abila, Dor, Legio,
Bosra, Beth Shean-Nysa-Scythopolis, Pella, Caesarea, Gerasa, Samaria-
Sebaste, Shechem-Neapolis, Aphek-Antipatris, Amman-Philadelphia,
and recently Tiberias; and the urban ritual theatres: Hammat-Gader,
Elusa in the Negev, Petra, Sahr in the Trachon, Birketein near Gerasa,
Shuni near Caesarea and others, dated to the late second century or
third century CE and particularly during the reign of the Severans.
Every large city had at least one theatre, and some, like Gadara, Gerasa,
Amman-Philadelphia, and Petra had two or three.[140] The most dramati-
cally different of the eastern theatres is the one at Petra which uniquely
in the Roman world, is entirely rock-cut in the local style. The theatre
at Batrun in Lebanon is also partly rock-cut.[141] (See Map 3).

The *odium* (Greek ᾠδεῖον) was essentially a small scale theatre building that was entirely roofed. The incidence of *odea* is far less than
that of theatres, and they tend to be more common in the east. More
serious cultural performances, such as concerts, lectures, and poetry

---

[137] Bieber (1961): 238, 238; Beare (1963): 238; Jory (1986): 145–146; Beacham (1991): 150; Segal (1995a): 3–15; Weiss (1998): 83.
[138] Grainger (1990): 85; Sear (1998); Ball (2000): 305; The only exception is Byblos which appears to incorporate some Greek features: Jidejian (1968): 115.
[139] *Bellum Judaicum* 1.415 (Caesarea), *Antiquitates Judaicae* 15.268 (Jerusalem), *ibid.*, 17. 161 (Jericho); The theatre in Jerusalem has never been found although two 'tickets' were discovered in the Upper City of Jerusalem; Segal (1995a): 4–7; Butcher (2003): 258.
[140] Goodman (1983): 81–82; Segal (1995a): 16–34; Weiss (1998): 79–85; Butcher (2003): 256–257; For the theatre at Tiberias, which was located at the foot of Mt. Berenike, see Hirschfeld (1991a): 32–35.
[141] Boulanger (1966): 178; Ball (2000): 305.

readings with musical dimensions, were the domain of the *odea*, though these buildings could also serve public or civic functions.[142] One of the best preserved and excavated buildings of this type was found in Aphek-Antipatris, lies near the source of the Yarkon River and built by Herod. The *odeion* was never completely finished. The *scaenae frons* which was to face the *cardo* was hardly built at all. The same was true for the orchestra and other parts of the building. The earthquake of 363 CE probably destroyed the building before it was completed. The lack of a real theatre in this city and the existence of only an *odeion*, and an incomplete one at that, does not say much for the cultural level of Antipatris.[143] An interesting combination of theatre and ᾠδεῖον is found at Gerasa, where an *odeion* is located to the east of the northern theatre. Such a combination of the two institutions is unique in the eastern Mediterranean. It could hold 800 spectators at the most.[144] However, a somewhat similar phenomenon has been uncovered at Beth Shean-Nysa-Scythopolis, in which an *odeion* has been discovered near the north-east corner of a large bathhouse.[145] Qanawat in Syria only had an *odeion* and no theatre.[146]

Seating arrangements for theatre or amphitheatre performances reflected the social organization of the city. Each segment of society had its own assigned area. *Decurions, magistrates* and senators sat in the *orchestra* [= the front], most conspicuous part, of the theatre. The charter of Carthage imposed fines of 5,000 *sesterces* on those who sat in areas to which they were not entitled.[147] The seating arrangement in Roman theatres was based on rank. Prominent people sat in the *orchestra*, and the others, according to their rank in the *cavea*. This also applied to the theatres of Roman East. While the masses gained access to the *cavea* through the various *vomitoria*, the *parodoi*, on the side of the building, led distinguished guests directly to their seats in the *orchestra*. Among the inscriptions unearthed at the theatre of Shechem-Neapolis, as at

---

[142] Dodge (1999): 223; On the distinction between theatre and *odeion*, see Segal (1995a): 85.

[143] Kochavi (1989): 103–109; Segal (1995a): 81–82; See also Bieber (1961): 220–222.

[144] Browning (1994): 175; Segal (1995a): 74.

[145] Mazor (1987–1988): 18–19; idem, (1988): 9–10; Bar-Nathan and Mazor (1992): 40; Segal (1995a): 60–61.

[146] Ball (2000): 304.

[147] Allison (2003): 211.

the north theatre of Gerasa, the names are found of the patriarchal
families or tribes of these cities, the φυλαί.[148]

Some theatres were adapted even further so that they could be
flooded and provide a venue for aquatic displays. At a later date a high
wall was placed around the orchestra and an aqueduct was provided
to flood the arena. In addition to theatres, other buildings could also
be adapted for arena games such as *stadium* surrounded by a wall, or
basins of amphitheatres, or sea battles, or 'water ballets'—often involved
nudity and themes of love and sex.[149] At Birketein theatre at Gerasa in
Jordan a large double pool outside the city was used for aquatic displays
of a particular nature. A small theatre formed part of the complex.
The pool in fact supplied water to the main *nymphaeum* [= monumental
fountain] in the city and was the location of the celebration of the
notorious festivals of *Maiouma*. A sixth century inscription found at a
small theatre dated to the late second or early third century CE, refers
to the festival of [M]αειουμᾶς. It apparently provided for shows of the
same name, which were of ill-repute because of their licentiousness.[150]
The *Maiouma* was probably of Phoenician origin, and by the late Empire
it seems to have gained a reputation for promiscuous goings-on. The
Byzantine chronicler of the sixth century CE John Malalas described it
as 'theatrical festival by night', and he thought its name meant that the
festival was celebrated in May.[151] The derivation is more likely to be from
the Semitic word *mai*, meaning 'water'. In the light of archaeological
remains and literature evidence it is assumable that several sites in the
Levant such as Maioumas-Shuni, Maioumas-Gaza, Maioumas-Ascalon,

---

[148] Weiss (1998): 82–83; For Shechem-Neapolis see Magen (1984): 275; ibid. (2005):
119–124; Segal (1995): 80; For the north theatre at Gerasa, see Clark, Bowsher and
Stewart (1986): 205–270, especially p. 229; Segal (1995a): 72–74; Butcher (2003):
257.

[149] For this practice see Traversari (1960); Kraeling (1962): 91–92; Golvin and Reddé
(1990); Welch (1991): 277–279; Dodge (1999): 234–236; Butcher (2003): 257; For the
naumachiae in general, see Golvin (1988): 50–51, 59–61; On themes, subjects, and range
of the aquatic displays see Coleman (1993); There are numerous mosaics, reliefs and
inscriptions testifying to the use of other buildings for arena displays. See Hornum
(1993): 52–54; Cozzo (1971): 60–71; Connolly and Dodge (1998): 199–208.

[150] Ball (2000): 188; Segal (1995a): 44; Browning (1994): 211–215; Schürer (1991):
II: 48, 155; Lankester-Harding (1990): 99; Khouri (1986): 134–136; MacMullen (1981):
21; McCown (1938): 159–167; For the [M]αειουμᾶς inscription, see Welles (1938):
470–471, no. 279.

[151] Malalas, *Chronographia*, 18.232; Roueché (1993): 188–189; See also Sawyer (1996):
62–65; Perles (1872): 251–254; Belayche (2001): 249–255.

Ein Harun near Sebaste, Beida northern to Petra, Hammat-Gader, and more, celebrated the Maioumas festivals.[152]

Festivals were established as state holidays, *feriae*, days spent in devotion to the gods. Some of them were annual festivals, other marked special occasions, particularly a military victory. Throughout the duration of the festival all other activities ceased, while the priests carried out the requisite. The triumphs allowed numerous secular elements to creep into the traditional Roman festivals. The triumph ended with public games, which were set in motion by a procession (*pompa*) from the Capitol to the place where the games were to be held. Gradually these games differed from the war celebration, the triumph, and became purely popular entertainment. The games were called *ludi*, and this became the common term for free time and entertainment as well. At first they lasted one day only, but this increased in the course of time to several days, and under the late republic seventeen days, in the year were devoted to public games. There were three types of performance: games in the *circus*—*ludi circenses*, games with animals—*venations*, and theatrical performances—*ludi scaenici*.[153]

This type of entertainment, which provided 'blood' for the masses, was incongruous with the mores of the East in general and thus not many amphitheatres have been discovered so far. Furthermore, these buildings in the East were not always used for their original or started purpose even when they did exist. Amphitheatres are known at Antioch, Beirut, Caesarea, Beth Shean-Nysa-Scythopolis, Jerusalem-Aelia Capitolina, Jericho, Beth Guvrin-Eleutheropolis, Dura Europos, and possibly Qanawat and Bosra.[154] The one at Antioch, ordered by Caesar, was one of the earliest in the Roman world.[155] The unusually large occurrence of amphitheatres in Judaea was probably the result of a deliberate Romanization of the area following the two great Jewish Revolts.[156] (See Map 3).

---

[152] See my forthcoming study [c] on the Maioumas festivals and their affinity to Maioumases and theatres in the eastern Mediterranean basin; see also Dvorjetski (2001a): 99–118 on Maioumas Ascalon.

[153] See, for instance, Olivová (1984): 163–171; Fowler (1969): 40–65; Bunson (1994): 156; Potter (1999a): 159–164; Weeber (1999): 125–144; Coulston and Dodge (2003): 160–161.

[154] Goodman (1983): 83; Kloner (1988): 15–24; Kloner and Hübsch (1996): 85–106; Gatier (1990): 204; Porat (1995): 15–27; Ball (2000): 305.

[155] Downey (1961): 156–157; Although it may have been a hippodrome, like Caesarea.

[156] Ball (2000): 305.

We today, from a moral point of view, find it difficult to appreciate, by way of contrast, the finer aspects of Roman civilization, given the appalling love of its people for the slaughter of gladiators and wild animals. There is no avoiding the fact that public slaughter, for the Romans, was an essential institution. This slaughter did provide lessons regarding pain and death, and regarding the fragility of life. It was a horrifying demonstration of the fates which could befall those who did not manage to please their masters. It was institutional terror such as was never seen before. We can only sum up by concluding that this was the disease of Rome, the infection of the Empire. But did it relieve, or intensify, social tensions? It remains doubtful whether it effectively relieved them.[157]

In contrast to the theatres, amphitheatres and *circuses*, which were places of occasional entertainment, the baths were an integral part of Roman urban life. It was one of the commonest ways of relaxation. Baths were one of the most characteristic and widely distributed types of Roman buildings, had their origins in the Greek world where public baths were common from at least the fourth century BCE. Bathing occupied a central position in the social life of the day. By the second century CE, any community of any substances, civil and military, had at least one set of public baths, while private baths are common in country villas and in wealthier town houses. Larger towns often had one or more substantial buildings (*thermae*), which were show-pieces for the community as well as a number of smaller, privately owned *balnea* to serve everyday needs. Most bathhouses in the Roman world were equipped with an open space, the *palaestra*, or, a covered hall, in which a variety of ball-games could be played or very strenuous exercise indulged in, such as running, wrestling and boxing. After this exercise a bath would be taken in the normal manner, or, a dip in an open air swimming-bath.[158]

Bathing became a symbol of being Roman, and thus the structures themselves became a symbol of Rome. Bath-buildings were habitually combined with structures and spaces devoted to other leisure activities: libraries, lecture-halls, lounges, sports grounds, gardens and paths for walks, all put together in a clever homogeneity and symmetry of design.

---

[157] Weeber (1994): 145–155; Kiefer (1994): 161–163; Grant (1995): 55; Purcell (1997): 144–145; See also Wells (1992): 248, 254; Wilkinson (1981): 163.
[158] Wacher (1998): 279; DeLaine (2004): 113–115; See also Newby (2002): 20–21.

Quite early in the first century CE, baths formed an essential and inevitable part of public buildings. And a century later they proliferated in a wide variety of forms. The Romans deserve the credit for combining the spiritual, social and therapeutic values of bathing and exalting it to an art. Baths were the focus of communal life, offering a place for relaxation, social gathering and worship. Emperors seeking popularity built *thermae* for their people and soon philanthropists followed, building their own elaborate baths as a sort of public relations gesture. Thus the bathhouse evolved from simple, wood-enclosed, single-function unit, small and austere, into a complex, luxurious, spacious, multi-functional establishment. The intricate architectural layout of the *thermae* gave birth to an elaborate bathing ritual.[159]

Men, and increasingly women, spent a great deal of their time every day bathing and swimming in these thermal centres, and engaging in the various kinds of social life that were available there. In order to satisfy the Romans' predilection for such activities, and their keen attention to the water supply which was so essential to this sort of activity, many of the baths at Rome and other centres were artificial, fed by water which was brought from elsewhere. But in other places, outside Rome itself, baths were created out of existing spas and springs. Often they had started as sacred springs where people worshipped, and like similar sanctuaries in other provinces provided a remarkable, versatile blend of religious, curative and social welfare. This was notable in Roman Gaul and in Britain, too. The thermal establishment at Bath Spa (*Aquae Sulis*), the most imposing known in Western Europe, formed just such a complex, with many rooms containing spacious plunge-baths full of water that came direct from the springs and helped to counteract rheumatic and lymphatic illnesses. So it provided agreeable bathing in addition to its healing capacity. A sacred spring was developed into a famous and magnificent thermal establishment, of which the principal feature can still be seen today. The whole plan was ambitious and contained a high degree of luxury. To the Romans the spring was not

---

[159] For a very useful discussion of bath studies see DeLaine (1988): 11–32; Nielsen (1990); Yegül (1992); DeLaine (1993): 348–358; idem, (1997); Weeber (1999): 125–144; Fagan (1999a); Dodge (1999): 243–251; For the different methods of heating walls see Brodribb (1987): 67–70; Yegül (1992): 192–196; For the baths in the provinces see Nielsen (1990): 84–118; Yegül (1992): 193–196, 201–206, 250–313; Dodge (1999): 251–255; See also Grant (1995): 50–51.

merely a source of hot water but a sacred place where mortals could communicate with the deities of the underworld. An important function of the sacred spring was to bring retribution to one's enemy. The Bath curses are extraordinary documents, giving us a glimpse into the hopes, expectations and piety of a society during the Roman occupation. Beyond all doubts the baths at *Aquae Sulis* followed a widespread, Rome-centred taste for thermal establishments, and yet placed this within the framework of a local worship and spring.[160]

Located in the forum and near *gymnasia* [= *palaestra*] baths were popular places, where men could watch others train, listen to music, discuss politics, gossip or listen to philosophers. The curative powers of mineral waters were undisputed, as worship and healing intermingled, until the fifth century CE. The popularity of warm bathing gradually faded away and, as elsewhere in Europe, seemed to disappear with the advent of Christianity. In Eastern Christianity throughout the Byzantine period, however, warm bathing was common among the aristocracy—although not so common among the rest of the population—despite hostility to it by monks and religious hermits, who considered care of the body the door to indulgence and sin.[161]

The Roman baths, above all in their public, imperially funded form, were pleasure palaces dedicated to the principle of enjoyment. Most importantly, they celebrated beauty, luxury, love, and sexual charm. This means that food, drink, and sex were all for sale. Even smaller, privately owned operations might offer a taste of these attractions.[162] Commercial sex was only one of several sensual pleasures that were associated with the bath.[163] Prostitutes might visit the baths strictly as bathers, a fact that helps raise the crux of the problem of respectability. The sources transmit some very mixed signals on the subject of women and men bathing together. It is unsurprising that *balnea, vina, venus* served as a Roman slogan for the good life.[164]

---

[160] For the different rooms of a Roman bath building and their technical terms and facilities, see Nielsen (1990): I: 153–166; For the ritual bathing see Yegül (1992): 30–47; See also Grant (1995): 51–53, 59; Croutier (1992): 81–86, 116–123.

[161] Gatier (1999): 227; Dritsas (2002): 195; For bathing during the Byzantine period, see Berger (1982) and the discussion in chapter 9 on *Pilgrimage to the Spas in the Eastern Mediterranean during the Later Roman and Byzantine Periods.*

[162] McGinn (2004): 23–26; Kardos (2001): 411; Dalby (2000): 237 240; Fagan (1999a): 32–36; Dunbabin (1989): 19–20, 23–24, 28, 32.

[163] Zajac (1999): 99–105.

[164] Sources and discussion in Merten (1983): 79–100; Ward (1992): 139–142; Fagan (1999a): 26–29; McGinn (2004): 24–25; For evidence and discussion on this slogan, see Kajanto (1969): 357–367; On bathing and society, see DeLaine (1999): 7–16.

The massive bathing establishments are often the most conspicuous monuments still standing in many Roman sites, both East and
West. In the East they range from very modest, local bathhouses such
as those at Serjilla, Babisqa or Barad in northern Syria, to elaborate
multi-functional complexes that can compare to those in North Africa
and Rome. Gerasa has two such baths, as does Bosra. Other large bath
complexes survive at Shahba-Philipopolis, Gadara, Hammat-Gader,
Beth Shean-Scythopolis, Palmyra, and Apamaea. At least five were
known to have existed at Antioch.[165] In addition to obvious functional
purposes related to bathing and hygiene, it served as a place of gathering, facilitating social and business intercourse. The large bathhouse
near the southwestern corner of the Temple Mount in Jerusalem and
dating to the period of Aelia Capitolina and afterwards have been for
the use of Roman legionaries as well as other sites.[166] There were types
of Roman style bathhouses in the region, such as bathhouses or units
of bathhouses in private houses, Hasmonean and Herodian bathhouses
in palaces of the Second Temple period, public hot bathhouses, and
thermo-mineral baths. Alongside the introduction of the hot bathhouse
in Palestine in the second half of the second century BCE, another
water installation was introduced: namely the *miqweh*, ritual immersion
pool.[167] A fairly coherent mosaic 'bath life' can be reconstructed from
the Rabbinic sources as well as the Classical literature.[168]

Music or visiting the library must also have played its part in leisure
hours. Bone pipes, mouthpieces from bronze trumpets or horn-like
instruments, stringed instruments, and more turn up from time to
time. It is probable that apart from the army, most musical activities
would have been restricted to religious ceremonies or theatrical perfor-

---

[165] Charpentier (1994): 113–142; Butcher (2003): 259 (Serjilla); Butler (1903) (Bosra
and Shaba); Kraeling (1938) (Gerasa); Browning (1994); Downey (1963) (Antioch);
Browning (1979): 139–142 (Palmyra); Balty (1981): 53–55 (Apamaea); Nielsen, Andersen
and Holm-Nielsen (1993); Holm-Nielsen, Nielsen and Andersen (1986): 219–232
(Gadara); Hirschfeld (1997) (Hammat-Gader); Foerster and Tsafrir (1993) (Beth Shean);
Mazor (1999) (Beth Shean); See also Ball (2000): 303; Dodge (1990); Ward-Perkins
(1981): 325, 345; Goodman (1983): 83–84; For the baths in mixed gentile-Jewish cities
and the pagan cult atmosphere, see the descriptions in chapter 6 on *The Daily Life at
the Thermo-Mineral Baths according to Rabbinic Literature.*
[166] Gichon (1978): 37–53; Tsafrir (1984): 105–111; For Jerusalem see, for instance,
Mazar (1999): 52–67; Stiebel (1999): 68–103; Mazar (2000): 87–102; ibid. (2006):
53–58, 82–83.
[167] Reich (1988): 102–107; Netzer (1999): 45–55.
[168] For the Classical literature see, for instance, Yegül (1992): 30–47; Fagan (1999a):
7–39; Eliav (2000): 416–454; idem, (2002): 411–433.

mances.[169] Libraries were fully developed in imperial Rome, although no trace of them is now extant in the city. Public libraries for book-scrolls were built not only at Rome itself from the beginning of the Imperial epoch, but at other points throughout the Empire. The extensive remains of the second century CE Library of Celsus, in Ephesus in Ionia, the Roman imperial province of western Asia Minor—give a good idea of what the libraries in the principal cities of the Roman world were like. People admired the well-planned unity and balance of this sort of elaborate façade, which aimed at a three-dimensional, undulating effect, and created an illusion of protecting and receding at one and the same time.[170]

Various games of skill or chance were also played extensively among, seemingly, all classes of society including children. In play, the outcome was always in doubt. Often play was highly competitive and utterly absorbing. There is also no doubt that play must be defined as a free and voluntary activity, a source of joy and amusement. It is simultaneously liberty and invention, fantasy and discipline. As an obligation or simply an order, it would lose one of its basic characteristics: the fact that the player devotes himself spontaneously to the game, of his free will and for his pleasure, each time completely free to choose retreat, silence, meditation, idle solitude, or creative activity. In effect, play is essentially a separate occupation, carefully isolated from rest of life, and generally is engaged in with precise limits of time and place. The point of the game is for each player to have his superiority in a given area recognized. That is why the practice of *agon* presupposes sustained attention, appropriate training, assiduous application, and the desire to win.[171] It is difficult to visualize the game played but several possibilities can be imagined. Board games of various types existed, and gambling pieces of glass, pottery, stone, bone and lead occur widely and usually in quite large numbers, although such objects could also have been used as aids in arithmetical calculations.[172] Different games were held periodically at the public buildings in the Roman East. In the second and third centuries CE cities organized these events in honour of

---

[169] Wacher (1998): 282.

[170] Brown (1961): 30–31; Robertson (1971): 29–33; Andreae (1978): 56 60, 805; Grant (1995): 48–50; Ramage and Ramage (2005): 105, Fig. 727.

[171] See, for instance, Huizinga (1955); Caillois (1961); Pieper (1963); Goodale and Godbey (1988); For leisure-time activities in Jewish children society, see Schwartz (2003): 132–141.

[172] Wacher (1998): 281.

the Emperors and local entities. The cities provided the facilities and awarded prizes to the winners even for some athletes who participated in the contests and came from abroad.[173]

Another, more polite way of enjoyment among the wealthier classes in Rome was the fashionable dinner party, given at the ninth hour, in the afternoon. It was customary in the better circles for readings or recitations to take place during dinner, or for dancers, jugglers or acrobats to perform afterwards. It was also customary after a dinner party to spend the evening drinking. Since, however dinner was the only real repast of the day, and was restricted to no more than three courses, the popular idea of orgiastic gluttony, often attributed to the Roman world. For the less well-to-do, who could not afford, or did not belong to the social class that gave dinner parties, there was almost certainly an abundance of restaurants, taverns, and brothels. The women of the taverns were musicians, dancers, waitresses and prostitutes. The bars and taverns in and around the great baths were the nearest thing that Rome had to restaurants. In some you could choose either to sit or to recline; and in some you could spend serious money.[174]

Business establishments serving as fronts for prostitution is a fairly universal phenomenon, and it is not therefore surprising to find this reflected in the Rabbinic literature. The Aramaic translation of the Hebrew prostitute is a mistress of the πονδοχεῖον, the tavern. We can find many references to markets, brothels, and taverns, which were notorious as places of prostitution. They are well attested to in literary sources.[175] Thus, for example, a marketplace with stalls or shops selling a variety of products. Some of these shops front for brothels (*Sifre on Numbers* 131, Horowitz ed., pp. 170–171). In *Babylonian Talmud, Shabbat* 33b we find Rabbi Simeon ben Yohai (mid-second century CE) accusing the Romans of building market-places only to be able to establish houses of prostitution. And in *Babylonian Talmud* (*Pesahim* 113b) we read of Rabbi Hiyya and Rabbi Oshaya, two early third century CE authorities, working as cobblers in the market of prostitutes, probably

---

[173] Holum et al. (1988): 116–117; Weiss (1998): 86–89; On games in the Roman East, see Jones (1940): 227–235; Pleket (1975): 49–89; White (1985): 30–40. See also the *agones* in chapter 8.5.

[174] Martial *Epigrammata* 5.70; See also Wacher (1998): 280–281; Dalby (2000): 220; For the role of the banquet in Roman life, see Dunbabin (2003).

[175] Krauss (1929): I: 135; Safrai (1984): 146; Sperber (1998): 15–17; For the taverns as the main places of prostitution, see MacMullen (1967): 338; idem, (1974): 86–87, 182; Balsdon (1969): 152–154; Hermansen (1982): 197–198; Gager (1992): 153; Dalby (2000): 217.

Tiberias, and making shoes for the prostitutes without actually looking at them.[176]

It is possible that certain types of buildings or structures that have been discovered and identified in the eastern Mediterranean could have also served as taverns, brothels or the like. This may have been the case, for instance, in the Byzantine period bathhouse in Beth Shean-Scythopolis, in Ascalon or in the Roman period bathhouse to the west of the Temple Mount in Aelia Capitolina and used by Roman soldiers.[177] The portico at Beth Shean where the girls strolled in the hope of attracting passers-by from the impressive street of Palladius as well as the neighbouring Byzantine Baths were part of a fascinating network: soliciting at the Baths, in the portico and in the exedra courtyard, followed by sex in the cabins, which are reminiscent of the cells of the Pompeii; and at the back of the building, an entrance-and-exit system for supposedly 'respectable clients'.[178] Archaeologists have raised the possibility that a fourth century CE bath at Ascalon might have functioned as a brothel. The bathhouse was built over several earlier villas, including a villa with erotic lamps. Their hypothesis, whether the upper structure was a small public bath or a large private one, is supported both by a fragmentary Greek inscription found on a plastered panel of a bathtub that read εἰσέλτηε ἀπολαύσον καὶ [...] ([= Enter, enjoy, and [...]), which is identical to an inscription found in a Byzantine bordello in Ephesus and by a gruesome discovery.[179] Nearly 100 infants' skeletons were crammed in a sewer under the bathhouse, with a gutter running along its well plastered bottom. The good condition of the bones indicated that the infants had been tossed into the drain immediately after birth. This manner of disposal of the infants shows a rather callous attitude, suggesting that these might represent abortions or infanticide, rather than death from natural causes. Thus, the prostitutes of Ascalon used the Baths not only for hooking clients

---

[176] Sperber (1998): 16.

[177] Schwartz (1998b): 183; Dauphin (1996): 52, 62.

[178] Dauphin (1996): 53–54; See also Mazor (1987–1988): 18–19; Bar-Nathan and Mazor (1993): 43–44.

[179] Stager (1991): 45–46; Dauphin (1996): 62; idem, (1998): 189–190; This inscription may have been simply a warm welcome and not a hint of illicit pleasures to be found: Stager (1991): 46; McGinn (2004): 209; For Ephesus see Jobst (1976–1977): 63–64; The inscription from Ephesus is ambitiously reconstructed by Fagan (1999a): 335–336, who risks making a functionalist confusion of bath with brothel.

but also for surreptitiously disposing of unwanted births in the din of the crowded bathing halls.[180]

The evidence for prostitution differs from place to place. To admit a bath as a brothel, we would almost have to identify all baths in the Roman world as brothels. Sometimes we are not even certain whether the bathhouse was public or private. To make a point that is explored at great length by McGinn—baths were, apart from the issue of prostitution, highly sexualized places, and they might easily acquire a reputation as centres of prostitution, especially if both sexes were present. It is plausible that the Church Fathers and the Rabbis were aware of this and not only the fear of temptation was their main reason for equating baths with lust.[181]

The activities at the medicinal hot baths in the vicinities of the mother cities in the Levant were somewhat different from those at regular city bathhouses. It seems that the fourth century CE Church Father Epiphanius's evidence, for instance, is one of the illustrative, vivid, and remarkable depictions of the atmosphere at most of the spas. He mentions that men and women bathed together not only at festivals at Hammat-Gader. Even among the Jews, this misconduct threatened to become ingrained. This is an image of daily life of leisure and pleasures at the thermo-mineral sites, which integrate also therapeutic activities. They developed from popular recreational venues to multipurpose entertainment centres.[182] At this point, it may be of interest to illuminate that the spa institution has been a unique subject worthy of study. It has served a different purpose, and has a different architectural form. These baths were dependent on the presence of hot and/or mineral springs, which means that they were independent of the towns and arose where nature allowed them to. Moreover, the treatments found in spas were aimed at specific needs and focused on the thermo-mineral springs. They primarily served medical purposes, although they were also social resorts, like present-day spas.[183]

---

[180] Stager (1991): 45–46; Smith and Kahila (1991): 47; Dauphin (1996): 62–63; McGinn (2004): 209, 221.

[181] McGinn (2004): 210; See also Dauphin (1996): 63.

[182] Epiphanius, *Panarion, Adversus Haereses* 30.7; See Dechent (1884): 192; Abel (1938): II: 458–459; Sukenik (1935a): 21; idem, (1935b): 111; Hirschfeld and Solar (1981): 202; Rubin (1982): 110–111; Hirschfeld (1987): 105; Dvorjetski (1988): 93–94; idem, (1992a): 106–107; Preuss (1993): 539; Dvorjetski (1994a): 17–18; ibid. (2004): 16–27.

[183] Nielsen (1990): I: 5.

GEOLOGICAL, HYDROLOGICAL AND MEDICINAL
ASPECTS OF HOT SPRINGS IN THE EASTERN
MEDITERRANEAN—PAST AND PRESENT

Hot springs have been a subject of interest since ancient times because
of the therapeutic qualities attributed to them. From the geological point
of view, the phenomenon of hot ground-water is of great interest. All
over the world, hot springs are concentrated in geological rifts. In the
eastern Mediterranean basin, the Jordan Valley is part of a rift valley
which extends from the Lake District in the southern part of East Africa
in the south to Turkey, in the north. In this area, the rift was formed by
tectonic movements during the Tertiary and Quaternary ages. During
the Diluvial period the Jordan Valley filled with water, which turned
into a great lake stretching from the Sea of Galilee [= Lake Kinneret]
as far as the Arava Valley. The water level was high, and, for instance,
in the area of the Sea of Galilee it was 170 metres higher than today's
water level. When the amount of rainfall lessened, the waters receded,
and two lakes were left—the Dead Sea and Lake Kinneret, joined by
the Jordan River. Taken as a whole, the Jordan Valley represents the
deepest depression on Earth, reaching −210 metres (below sea level)
at Lake Kinneret and −400 metres at the Dead Sea. Hence, all the
hot springs in this region considered in this chapter are well below sea
level. The last stage of the rift development occurred in the past 4–5
million years, during which the change in the poles of plate motion
led to the development of oblique stresses and to the formation of the
Dead Sea transformation trough-morphology.[1]

Israel and Jordan are rich in springs containing minerals, but the
conditions for the creation of springs rich in minerals with special
properties, such as heat—which gives the mineral springs their healing properties—are to be found particularly in the geological rift of
the Jordan Valley. Between the point where the Jordan flows out of

---

[1] Kahan (1963): 1–2; Mazor (1968a): 65–80; idem, (1980a): 300; Bartov, Arad and
Arad (1992).

the Huleh Valley and the southernmost tip of the Dead Sea there are
many hot and cold sulphurous springs and other mineral springs.[2] The
waters of these springs, which are distinguished by the strength of their
Sulphurous gases, are principally effective against various rheumatic
complaints. They can also help those who suffer from ailments of the
circulation of the blood or the respiratory system, from skin diseases
and other complaints. The waters of the particularly saline springs
are effective in treating women's complaints. It should be emphasized
that today a thermal centre is the most up-to-date stage in the use of
therapeutic springs.[3]

The Kinnerot Valley is part of the Jordan-Arava rift Valley, which
runs the whole length of Israel, and is itself only a section of one of
the youngest and most prominent lines in the tectonic structure of the
earth—the Syro-African Rift, which runs from the southern border of
Turkey in the north to the Zambezi River in Africa to the south. The
mountainous escarpments west and east of the Kinnerot Valley consist
mainly of basaltic rocks and Neogenic limestone. Like other parts of
the Jordan Valley, the Kinnerot Valley is distinguished by three features
of tectonic origin:

A. Hot springs rich in minerals, both in the Valley and in its vicinity.
B. Seismic sensitivity: frequent earthquakes.
C. Basaltic areas in the Valley or close to it.

The temperature of the waters of the thermal springs in Hammei-
Tiberias is 65°C and in Hammat-Gader is 39°–42°C. There are also
springs in the seabed of the Kinneret, especially near the north-east
shore. The hot springs contain minerals, particularly Sulphur, and also
radioactive material, which proves that they originate in the depths of
the earth and that there is tectonic activity at their point of origin.[4] It
appears that the radioactivity of the therapeutic springs increases their
therapeutic value.[5]

The whole of the Jordan Valley is known to be a place of great
seismic activity, and earthquakes take place quite often in the region;
their main centre is in the towns of Tiberias and Jericho. Various

---

[2] Atlas (1970): 166.
[3] Kurland (1982): 20.
[4] Ben-Arieh (1973): 17–28; Mazor (1980a): 93–112.
[5] Kurland (1971b): 44.

historical sources speak of fourteen earthquakes, many of them severe and lethal: for instance, in 363, 749, 1033, 1759, 1837, and 1927 CE.[6] As has been remarked, the third tectonic feature is the fact that there are broad areas of basalt in and around the region. The volcanism began during the Middle to Upper Miocene in the west and continued in the Pliocene on both the eastern and western shoulders of the rift. Volcanism, however, took place in younger times in the northeast, away from the rift. The geological features on the two flanks of the Dead Sea transform display an interesting asymmetry, which cannot be explained entirely by the significant north-south displacement. In the Dead Sea area, for instance, the eastern flank is raised 1–2 kilometres.[7] In the Zarqa Ma'in region, eight post-Eocene to recent Olivine basalt plugs and several flows of similar rocks are to be found, while across the Dead Sea, volcanic formations are unknown.[8]

The volcanic areas are not confined to the narrow strip of the Valley, but are particularly extensive on both its sides: in the Golan, east of the Jordan, and in the hilly areas in the east of Lower Galilee, as well as in Korazim, the basaltic area to the north of the region. The many hot springs in the Jordan Valley are also volcanic phenomena. Many more than those that exist today disappeared long ago, in prehistoric times. Their residue, lime or gypsum sinter, still covers broad areas and bears witness to their past existence. Hot water is better able than cold water to dissolve solid substances. When it cools down, it spreads over the surface and discharges some of the solid matter in solution. This matter settles round the springs. It is known as sinter sediment, and its presence proves the existence of hot springs which no longer exist. In the sinter of the lower Jordan Valley there are thin layers and nut-sized lumps of Sulphur.[9]

---

[6] Ben-Arieh (1973): 17–18; On the earthquakes in the region, see Amiran-Kallner (1950–1951): 225–228; Brock (1977): 267–286; Karcz and Kafri (1978): 237–253; Russell (1985): 37–59; Tsafrir and Foerster (1989): 362–357; Karcz and Elad (1992): 67–83; Amiran, Arieh and Turcotte (1994): 261–305; Amiran (1996): 53–61.

[7] Jaffé, Dvorjetski, Levitte, Massarwieh and Swarieh (1999): 37–38; Girdler (1990): 1–13; Freund, Garfunkel, Zak, Goldberg, Weissbrod, and Derin (1970): 107–130; Greitzer and Levitte (2000): 209–212; See also a general survey in van Rose and Mercer (1999): 34–43.

[8] Abu-Ajamieh (1980); Hakki and Teimeh (1981); Galanis, Saas, Munroe and Abu-Ajamieh (1986); Swarieh (1990); Swarieh and Massarweh (1995); Swarieh (2000): 469–474.

[9] Braver (1928): 10; Shalem (1956): 159–170.

These springs are 'Juvenile', in geological terms: that is to say, they were created from the magma which is found in the depths of the earth, and thence rise to ground level for the first time. But mineral springs may also be 'Vadose': their water, like any ordinary water, originates in precipitation, such as rain, which entered the soil a long time ago, sank down, remained in the depths of the earth for long periods, and gradually rose to the surface.[10]

The source of the heat of the springs which emerge in the Jordan Valley is connected with the depth from which they rise. There is no proof of the existence of a special source of heat, such as a mass of basalt sunk into the earth and still hot. The source of the salts is still controversial. Some scientists believe that Hammei-Tiberias, Enot-Tsukim and others originated in sea-water which filled the Jordan Valley (by way of the Yizre'el Valley) at some geological period, and descended to its lowest point; today it rises to ground level, and merges with the local groundwater on its way. Others believe that this is water from the mountains which has penetrated deep into the earth, dissolving various salts on its way.[11]

The controversy between geologists on the nature of the springs is still unresolved, and perhaps both schools are correct. In the course of this study we shall demonstrate how enlightening was the approach of the Sages of the *Mishnah* and the *Talmud* to the question of the source and attributes of the thermal springs. They asked whether they were derived from *ur* (light) or from *hama* (heat), until it was decided that they were derived from heat, since 'they passed over the entrance to Gehenna' (*Babylonian Talmud, Shabbat* 39a). It is clear that the Sages relate this to volcanic processes, as does modern science.[12]

2.1   DISTRIBUTION AND IDENTIFICATION

We shall now give a concise description of the thermal springs of the Levant, based primarily on the works of a number of the remarkable geological and hydrological scholars, dating from beginning of the 20th

---

[10] Buchmann (1956): 16–17; idem, (1968): 195; Shiponi (1963): 1–2; Kasher (1934): 8–10.

[11] Mazor (1980a): 306; idem, (1966): 72.

[12] See chapter 6.1 on *The Halakhic Stance of the Sages towards Curative Springs and Baths.*

century up to date, such as Blanckenhorn,[13] Friedman,[14] Lachman,[15] Brzezinski,[16] Yaron,[17] Ekerstein,[18] Mazor,[19] Abu-Ajamieh,[20] Bender,[21] Levitte,[22] Salameh,[23] Swarieh and Massarweh,[24] and Horowitz.[25] The springs will be described in order from north to south, according to the following geographical classification: The Tiberias basin and the Yarmuk Canyon; The western margins of the Jordan Valley; The Dead Sea basin; The eastern margins of the Jordan Valley; Hot springs within the Syro-African Rift in Sinai; and Thermal springs in other places in Palestine. (See Tab. 1 and Map 2).

2.1.1   *The Tiberias Basin and the Yarmuk Canyon*

The mountainous area on the west descends to the Tiberias basin in a series of tiered faults built of layers of limestone, from the Cenomanian to the Eocene period, covered with the residues of Neogene watercourses and deposits of basalt ranging from the Neogene period to the Pliocene. The eastern part of the Golan Heights is built of a similar sequence of rocks, with a foundation of Eocene rocks covered with Pleistocene basalt in the upper half of the region. There are many thermo-mineral springs spread out along the coast of Lake Kinneret and on the sea-bottom. The most prominent are Hammei-Tiberias (the Tiberias Springs), Ein Folia, Ein Nun, Ein Kinar, Ein Ravid, and the springs of Tabgha (Heptapegon), which are situated along the western system of faults of the Jordan Valley. They flow out of isolated tectonic

---

[13] Blanckenhorn (1912).
[14] Friedmann (1913).
[15] Lachman (1933): 221–235.
[16] Brzezinski (1934).
[17] Yaron (1952): 121–128.
[18] Eckstein (1975); idem, (1979a); idem, (1979b).
[19] Mazor (1980a); Mazor, Levitte, Truesdell, Healy and Wissenbaum (1980b): 1–19.
[20] Abu-Ajamieh (1980); Abu-Ajamieh, Bender and Eicher (1989).
[21] Bender (1974); idem, (1975).
[22] Levitte (1966); Levitte and Olshina (1978); Levitte and Olshina (1985); Levitte and Greitzer (1997).
[23] Salameh and Udluft (1985); Rimawi and Salameh (1988); Salameh (1990); Salameh and Bannayan (1993).
[24] Swarieh (1990); Swarieh and Massarweh (1995); Massarweh and Swarieh (1995); Swarieh and Massarweh (1997); Swarieh (2000): 469–474.
[25] Horowitz (2001).

masses, raised and inclined, surrounded or covered by Neogene residues and volcanic streams.[26] The principal hot springs are as follow: (See Map 2).

HAMMEI-TIBERIAS—These are situated on the shore of Lake Kinneret, about two kilometres south of Tiberias, at the foot of the Mount of Herod, some 200 metres below sea level. The waters are very hot. They are radioactive, and contain considerable quantities of salts, ions and gases in solution. There are nineteen well-heads. The temperature of the water is 59°C in the wellhead by the main fountain, and about 62°C in the fountain which emerges close to the ancient Roman bathhouse.[27] The fountains emerge through a system of fractures in the Cenomanian-Turonian limestone and dolomite strata spread over a 20 metres strip some 30 metres from the Sea of Kinneret. The source of the water in Hammei-Tiberias is, in general, rainwater. Only a small proportion of the waters in hot springs throughout the world have proved to be magmatic, i.e., derived from vapour within the magma. Since neither arsenic nor boron has been found in the hot springs of Tiberias, and since the quantity of the flow varies over time, it is clear that the source of the water is rain rather than magma. This water seeps through cavities and cracks in the rocks, and reaches a great depth. At this depth it heats up, according to the geothermal gradient; on its way it dissolve various salts, and, also, apparently, passes through saline strata derived from the residue of the Sea of Thetis. The pressure brings the water to the surface, where it appears in the form of springs. According to the data derived from analysis of the water which has been found in various drillings in the vicinity, it is supposed that the mineral waters are also diluted with a small quantity of sweet water. As for the chemical composition of the waters of the springs of Tiberias, analysis shows that they contain the cations: Potassium, Magnesium, Sodium, Calcium, Iron, Lithium and Strontium, and the anions: Chlorine, Sulphate, Bromine, Bicarbonate, Silicon dioxide and Hydrogen Sulphide. In addition to the saline elements the waters also contain free Sulphur. Because of the high proportion of minerals in the water, it is hypertonic, i.e., it contains more salts than blood serum. Its electrical conductivity is high, as a result of the great quantity of electro-

---

[26] Eckstein (1975): 7–8.
[27] Scherrer (1936): 5–8; Buchmann (1928a): 28–31; idem, (1956): 43–46; idem, (1971): 90; Melamed (1971): 13–17; Pines (1979): 181.

lytes dissolved in it. The highest concentration of salts in the water is of Sodium Chloride and Calcium Chloride; it also contains liquefied gases, primarily Radon. It has a high specific gravity—about 3.3%—because of the concentrated salts. The special characteristic of the springs of Tiberias is the mixture of a great many calcareous materials with a high proportion of Sodium Chloride, a rare combination in mineral springs. In view of their chemical composition, Hammei-Tiberias may be defined as hot, saline, calcareous and sulphurous—or, in other words, hyperthermic, hypertonic and radioactive.[28] In practice, they have been used in the course of generations for the cure of rheumatic conditions, women's complaints, chronic skin diseases, nervous disorders, disorders of the respiratory system and infertility. Today, they serve as a centre for the treatment of rheumatic complaints.[29]

HAMMAT-GADER—Hammat-Gader is located in a small Valley on the banks of the Yarmuk, between the Golan Heights and the Mountains of Gilead. In this Valley, about 600 dunam in area, there are five springs with different degrees of heat. The most southerly is 'Ain el-Maqle, also known as Hammat-Selim. During the Roman period therapeutic baths were built round this spring, which reaches a temperature of 52°C. The waters of Hammat-Selim are the richest in therapeutic properties. 200 metres to the east is situated 'Ain er-Rih, the temperature of whose waters is 34°C. In the north-west of the Valley there are two more springs, next to each other: 'Ain eğ-Ğarab, whose waters reach 42°C; they are clear and transparent, but emit a strong odour of Hydrogen Sulphide. The second, 'Ain Būlus (25°C), whose waters are cool and potable. The fifth spring, 'Ain es-Sāhne, is located in the north-eastern corner of the Valley. Its waters are lukewarm (28°C), and today are used to replenish the nearby crocodile pools.[30] The source of the springs of el-Hamme is connected with volcanic activity: they are situated in the east of a rift in the deep picturesque canyon of the Yarmuk River. The steep cliffs of the canyon are made

[28] Eggel (1839); Golani (1962); Kahan (1963): 9–12; Mazor and Mero (1969): 276–288; Melamed (1971): 15; Buchmann (1971b): 84–94; Kurland (1971a): 649–655; idem, (1976): 21–31; Meiri (1973): 32; Rosenthal (2001): 263–264.
[29] Buchmann (1928a): 32–33; idem, (1933): 303–304; idem, (1971a): 29–43; Kurland (1977): 27; idem, (1980): 44–60; Segev (1989): 149–153; Margalit (1976): 141–143.
[30] Mazor (1969): 272; Mazor and Molcho (1970): 260–263; Karson (1970): 122–123; Levitte, Olshina and Wachs (1978); Mazor, Kaufman and Carmi (1981): 289–304; Hirschfeld (1989) c: 141.

up of streams of young basalt, resting on a course of Eocene limestone. These springs, therefore, constitute the final stage of this activity.
Traces of lava can still be distinguished in the Hauran and in various
parts of the Golan. The springs of Hammat-Gader differ from those
of Hammei-Tiberias in that they have a higher proportion of Sulphur,
and a lower proportion of salts—a little more than one percent—and
a lower temperature. The waters are radioactive, as are those of most
of the mineral springs in the Jordan and Kinnerot Valleys. The source
of the radioactivity is in two isotopes, Radium and Radon, which
are created by the decomposition of the Uranium in the rocks. The
Radium is solid, and it is similar to Calcium, and, like the other salts,
its distribution changes with the changes in temperature. Radon is a
gas, and its distribution is the opposite of that of Radium: it is richer in
cold water than in hot. Thus, there exists here a mechanism for mixing
two types of water—hot water, containing salts, Hydrogen Sulphide
and Radium, and cold water containing little chlorine, but relatively
rich in Radon. The waters from these two sources combine close to
the surface, at the last moment.[31] These thermo-sulphurous radioactive
springs are used to cure rheumatic complaints, ailments of the joints and
muscles, various skin diseases, and obstructions of the digestive system.
The mineral composition and therapeutic qualities of the springs of
Hammat-Gader are different from those of Hammei-Tiberias; hence
their special importance, since they are capable of healing ailments
which the hot springs of Tiberias cannot.[32]

THE SPRINGS OF NUQEB AND GOPHRA—Two small springs
on the shore of Lake Kinneret, north of Ein Gev. At the spot where
they flow into the Kinneret they create white fans, as a result of the
Sulphur they contain. Their waters have a strong odour of Hydrogen
Sulphide. Their chemical make up is similar to that of Hammat-Gader,
but it is more concentrated, though still less so than Hammei-Tiberias.
They have a high proportion of Radon, as do most of the springs in
this region.[33]

---

[31] Noetling (1886): 59–88; Picard (1932): 221–225; Sukenik (1935a): 101–108;
Schulman (1968): 179–181; Mazor and Molcho (1970): 261–263; Eckstein (1975): 8;
Levitte, Olshina and Wachs (1978); Starinski, Katz and Levitte (1979): 233–244; Nir
(1985).
[32] Buchmann (1933): 305; idem, (1971): 90–92.
[33] Mazor (1980a): 304, Fig. 381; On the chemical composition of Nuqeb and Gophra
springs, see Mazor and Molcho (1970): 263.

2.1.2   *The Western Margins of the Jordan Valley*

Many scholars have investigated the geology and hydrology of this region. Most of the thermal springs in this part of the rift are connected with secondary fault systems, which spread out in the shape of an arc to the north-west of the main structures of the rift. The water is relatively sweet. It is also colder, since it is diluted with the cold contents of shallow aquifers. The most prominent of these springs is Hammam al-Malieh (Hammei-Malha) about 15 kilometres south of Beth Shean, which is fed by deep Jurassic aquifers. At the end of the Jurassic era and the beginning of the Lower Cretaceous there occurred a number of volcanic eruptions, which created alternating layers of basalt and tuff. Some of the volcanic eruptions were subaqueous; therefore, in these marine layers there are fossils of fish and shells, whereas in the terrestrial strata there are remains of plants, frogs, and terrestrial insects. The basalt is dark and hard, as distinct from the tuff, which is particularly friable. In the layers of tuff there are to be found many 'volcanic explosions', formed by the penetration of water into the cracks in the surface of the fault in which volcanic activity took place. As a result, a great quantity of gas was created, and this caused an explosion and threw the basalt to a distance. The temperature of the waters of Hammei-Malha reaches 39°C, and they smell of Hydrogen Sulphide. The water is not very saline, but is rich in Sodium and Carbonate.[34]

The thermo-mineral springs in this group are: 'Ain Um-Tiunh, 'Ain Jamal, 'Ain el-Ḥamma, Ein Ash-Shak, Ein Haim and 'Ain Amal, and their chemical composition are similar to that of Hammam al-Malieh. A survey of Wadi Malieh shows that several booths containing hot water pools were built over the springs of Hammam al-Malieh; however, as a result of severe floods and years of neglect they are today blocked up with silt. It is with good reason that Hammam al-Malieh is called 'the deserted Hammam'.[35] (See Map 2).

---

[34] Picard (1932): 221–225; Schulman (1959): 63–90; Burdon (1959); Flexer (1961): 64–72; Bender (1968); Eckstein (1975): 7; Mazor (1980a): 197.

[35] Ozerman (1980); idem, (1982): 72–74; Mimran (1984).

2.1.3   *The Dead Sea Basin*

The Dead Sea is part of the Syro-African Rift. In the Israeli section, the direction of the rift is north to south, and it is bounded on both sides by fault cliffs. The fragmented terraces which create the western fault cliffs are built primarily of strata of limestone and dolomite, alternating with strata of clay and marlstone, most of them dating from the Cenomanian and Turonian periods. Above them there are strata of limestone alternating with layers of flint and Phosphorate from the Senonian period. The remains of Bitumenic shales from the Maastrichtian-Paleocene period are to be found on the faulted masses of rock. To the north, along the Jordan, the western fault cliffs of the rift are made of crystalline limestone of the Eocene era. Round the sea there lies exposed the sediment of the rift, covering the low tectonic masses in disconformity.[36]

Along the southern part of the Dead Sea there are several springs, whose therapeutic properties are well known. Their waters contain a high proportion of salts, and their temperature is high, as is the relative degree of radioactivity. Scientists propose various explanations for these phenomena. Most of them presume the existence of extremely saline water trapped underground, resulting from the penetration of the waters of the Dead Sea or a prehistoric sea, or of a mass of salt like the Mount of Sodom. It appears that pure groundwater flowing under pressure in the lower aquifers rises along the faults, bringing with it to the surface some of the salt waters imprisoned there. On their way to the surface, some of the water passes through strata of Senonian rocks, which contain Phosphate and Bitumenic shales. It absorbs radioactive components associated with the phosphates and sulphurous elements found in the Bitumenic shales, and thereby acquires a certain degree of radioactivity, as well as Hydrogen Sulphide gas (H_2S).[37]

The Dead Sea is a sea of salts. Its water contains a high proportion of Calcium, Magnesium, Potassium, Bromine and Sulphur. The

---

[36] Neev (1965); Neev and Emry (1967); Eckstein (1975): 5; Schulman and Bartov (1978): 37–94; Bartov (1983): 30–35; Nir (1989): 323; Garfunkel (1997): 36–56; Shapira (1997): 82–88; Niemi and Ben-Avraham (1997): 73–81; Ben-Avraham (1997): 22–35; Bowman (1997): 217–225.

[37] Kolton (1973): 61–67; Yechieli and Gat (1997): 252–264; Mazor (1997): 265–276.

composition of the waters of the springs in this area is not uniform: they generally contain the same minerals as in the Dead Sea, but in different proportions (a higher proportion of Sulphur), as well as Iodine, Strontium Fluoride, and radioactive materials. The site has been known for generations as a therapeutic region for rheumatic diseases, skin complaints, and disorders of the respiratory system. It has been proved that there is estrous hormone in the water, the seabed, and the salts of the Dead Sea.[38] Dr. Buchmann, a medical doctor, defines the Dead Sea as 'a reservoir for the residues of all the mineral springs', and adds that it is used to deal with organic and functional nervous complaints, premature old age and general weakness.[39]

The thermo-mineral springs in this group are as follows: Ain Jazal, Ain Tanur, Ein Feshkha, Einot Kane and Samar, Ein Turba, Hammei-Shalem, Hammei-Yesha, Ein Nu'it, Hammei-Zohar, Hammei-Mazor, Ein-Gedi, 'Ain Mumila, Ein Tamar and Ein HaKikar. The best known and most important are:[40] (See Map 2).

EIN FESHKHA (EINOT TSUKIM)—A complex of springs, spread over about 3 kilometres in the northern part of the western shore of the Dead Sea, between the cliffs of the rift and the sea. The water in most of the springs is of moderate salinity, but in some of them it is merged with a considerable amount of Dead Sea water. The Feshkha springs were the subject of much attention in the 1940s, as a result of their high degree of radioactivity. As remarked above, this is produced by two isotopes, of Radon gas and Radium, which are generated by the decomposition of natural uranium.[41] In his article, 'The Radioactivity of Springs in the Jericho Region', Blake maintains that the radioactivity of one of the springs of Ein Feshkha is dangerous to animals or humans if drunk regularly.[42] Mazor strongly denies this theory, and claims that the Feshkha springs contain only a thousandth part of

---

[38] Blake (1930); Elazari-Volcani (1936); idem, (1940); Almog and Eshel (1956); Nir (1968); Machtey (1977): 28; Tweig (1979): 28–29; Kurland (1982): 23; Nishri and Stiller (1997): (199–204; For the estrous hormone in the water, see Tzondak (1938): 428–432.

[39] Buchmann (1933): 306; idem, (1971): 90; See also Thomson (1978): 62, 66, 69, 171–172.

[40] Eckstein (1975): 5.

[41] Mazor (1980a): 305, Figs. 382–383; idem, (1969): 272; idem, (1968b): 387; Mazor and Molcho (1972): 37–47; Ilan (1972): 125–128; For the archaeological excavations at Ein Feshkha, see Hirschfeld (2004): 37–74.

[42] Blake (1967): 86–97.

the degree of radioactivity liable to be harmful.[43] From the point of view of their chemical composition, the Feshkha springs fall into two groups. The first, which includes most of these springs, is very similar to those of Hammei-Tiberias; their source is apparently in seawater which was trapped in the substratum in ancient times, and now rises to the surface and mingles with the groundwater which collects as a result of the rains. The second group is composed of several small springs at the south of the area. They are distinguished by their high concentration of salts, and their composition is similar to that of the Dead Sea. Their source is the waters of the Dead Sea, which filter through to the shore and mingle with the waters of the first group as they rise from the depths. The temperature of Ein Feshkha varies between 26°C and 31°C. At this spot no distinctive remains of ancient baths have been found, but it may be that the pools in the north-eastern section of the complex of buildings in this area served for therapeutic bathing.[44] De Vaux, who conducted excavations here in 1956 and 1958, concluded that the pools were used for processing the skins which the men of the Judean Desert sect used for writing their scrolls.[45] Other scholars reject this possibility. Zeuner made various scientific tests of materials taken from the pools, and found no traces of the processing of leather. He believed that they were too big for this purpose, and were used for the artificial breeding of fish. Other scholars have surmised that they were used for soaking flax, since it is known that the men of the sect wore clothes made of flax.[46]

EINOT KANE AND SAMAR—An area of springs about 2 kilometres in length, south of Einot Tsukim. Some are sweet water springs. The source of most of the waters is in the Judean Hills, and they are drinkable; but when they reach the Dead Sea Valley there is a small admixture of water from the Dead Sea.[47]

HAMMEI-YESHA—A group of springs on the western shore of the Dead Sea, south of Ein Gedi. The temperature of the water, measured on the spot, reaches 40.5°C. There is a very strong odour of Sulphur

---

[43] Mazor (1968b): 387; idem, and Molcho (1972): 37–47; Mazor (1997): 265–276.
[44] Ilan (1972): 125–132.
[45] de Vaux (1956): 575; idem, (1959): 225–255.
[46] Zeuner (1960): 33–36; See also Poole and Reed (1961): 114–123.
[47] Mazor, Nadler and Harpaz (1973): 255–262; Mazor (1980a): 306, Fig. 384; Dothan (1986): 51.

in the vicinity. The water is rich in salts. Some of the springs have a greenish-yellow colour, because of the Sulphur and algae they contain. There are facilities for bathing and treatment at this location.[48]

EIN NU'IT—This mineral spring, which belongs to the group of springs of Ein Bokek, possesses a unique structure, which it distinguishes it from most of the springs of the Dead Sea basin. It is separated from the Dead Sea and the Rift by masses of faulted rocks, covered with thick opaque Maastrichtian-Paleocene bituminous shales. The water of Ein Nu'it is brackish to slightly saline and it stands out by its relatively low pH [= level of acidity], high Iron content, and high Sulfate concentration. It is distinguished by its brown colour, and its temperature is 39°C. Signs of tectonic and volcanic activity associated with the Rift system are plentiful in the region. There is archaeological evidence indicating the water of Ein Nu'it was diverted by an aqueduct to the nearby fortified settlement of Bokek which was erected as early as the Hellenistic period. At a later stage, because of above human body temperature of the spring water, excessive salinity, sulphurous odor and Iron content, Rosenthal claimed that the Romans developed Ein Nu'it as a spa, which was used by the garrison of Bokek. It became a military outpost, later to become a part of the *limes* [= strategic military fortifications protecting the eastern borders of the Roman Empire].[49] Despite the fact that no report has ever been published on this spa, balneologists suggested that Ein Nu'it waters could be therapeutically exploited both by bathing to treat various skin ailments and by ingestion to treat chronic constipation. In the past Bedouins from all over the Negev, Sinai, and Tran-Jordan made the strenuous journey through the desert and the exhaustive climb of the escarpment to enjoy the curative properties of the spring. They used to tell of the therapeutic qualities of the waters, which they drank when ill.[50]

HAMMEI-ZOHAR—A group of springs, including three underground springs, in the southern part of the west coast of the Dead Sea, between the outflow of *Nahal* Zohar on the south and that of *Nahal* Bokek on the north, about 20 kilometres south of Masada. Its waters are rich in minerals and salts, sulphurous and radioactive. Their

---

[48] Kahan (1963): 7; Eckstein (1975): 1; Margalit (1976): 144; Mazor (1980a): 306.

[49] Rosental (2001): 258–262; Illani (1985): 197–206; Mazor (1981a): 4; Eckstein (1975): 6; Kolton (1973): 67; Ilan (1972): 188; Eckstein and Rosental (1965): 3; Doron (1965).

[50] Atlas: (1970): 166; Margalit (1976): 145; Rosental (2001): 262.

composition is very similar to that of the Dead Sea, but less concentrated. Their natural temperature is 28°C–37°C. There are facilities for bathing and treatment at this location. The waters of Hammei-Zohar have a marked therapeutic effect on rheumatic complaints and various skin diseases.[51]

HAMMEI-MAZOR—A hot spring and bath on the shore of the Dead Sea, close to Kibbutz Ein Gedi. The spring waters are mineral, rich in Sulphur, and their odour can be sensed in the vicinity. He who bathes in them is healed and soothed, and thence the modern name (*mazor*, Hebrew = healing). In the past, the Bedouins bathed here, and rested their backs on a nearby rock for relief; this rock was, therefore, known as Hajar Abu ad-D'hor—the stone which is the father of backs. The water contains more salts than that of Hammei-Zohar, the temperature is higher and it is more radioactive.[52]

EIN GEDI—Geological observations of Ein-Gedi 3 borehole over the years 1962–1983 have pointed out distinct trends of decrease in overall salinity and changes in water composition. Analysis of the data indicates that the heat source of the Ein Gedi 3 water are presumably brines that rise from a depth of 1200–1300 metres, with initial temperatures of 47.7°C–49.3°C. These brines rise along border faults of the Dead Sea Graben, from whence they mix with surface waters of the Dead Sea. The actual mixing takes place at an interface within the gravel mar aquifer of the Lisan Formation on the shore where the borehole and the spa are situated. In proportion to the change in the mixing ratio, ions such as Magnesium and Potassium decrease in comparison to Dead Sea waters, and Sulfate, Bicarbonate and Sodium increase. The thermo-mineral reserve of Ein Gedi 3 is unrestricted for balneological purposes.[53]

---

[51] Eckstein (1972): 9–11; Margalit (1976):144–145; Mazor (1980a): 306; idem, (1981b); Yakobovitz (1981): I: 195; See also Kahan (1963): 7; Atlas (1970): 166; Buchmann (1971): 91.

[52] Almog and Eshel (1956): 168; Atlas (1970): 166; Kolton (1973): 67; Vilnaey (1977): 2407; Dothan (1986): 30, 51.

[53] Raz (1989); idem, (1993): 97–114, 189–192.

2.1.4 *The Eastern Margins of the Jordan Valley*

This group includes Hammam ad-Dable, the el-Mahruk spring, the el-Ḥammam spring, ʿAin Sweimeh, Hammam Zarqa Maʾin, and the Kallirrhoe springs.[54] (See Map 2).

HAMMAM AD-DABLE—South of the el-Ḥamma springs, also known as Hammam el-Paḥel, Hirbet Fâḥil, and Hammat-Pella. Water temperature: 37°C. The water smells of Sulphur. It is mentioned in the historical sources as a location of hot springs. The local inhabitants frequently use its waters.[55]

THE EL-MAHRUK SPRING—On the southern tip of the Yabok Valley, debouches into a pool. Water temperature reaches 34.5°C, and the water smells of Sulphur. It contains a considerable amount of Iron, which colours the plants and rocks with a brown residue.[56]

THE EL-ḤAMMAM SPRING—East of Jericho. Its waters are saline, and reach a temperature of 36°C. An analysis of the spring shows a marked presence of organic matter—more than 2%—including algae and bacteria.[57]

ʾAIN SWEIMEH—In the north-east corner of the Dead Sea. The water, whose temperature reaches 27°C, is rich in Calcium, drinkable but rather saline.[58]

HAMMAM ZARQA MAʾIN—A group of springs on the east coast of the Dead Sea. They flow from between the basalt strata, creating beautiful waterfalls. Each spring has a different temperature. In the historical sources they are also named Biram, Baaras, Baris, Bare, Baar(o)u, Baʾar, and Baʾarah, because of their 'burning' waters . The temperature of the hottest spring is 57°C. The local inhabitants use it to treat rheumatic complaints and nervous disorders. In Wadi Zarqa Maʾin, above these thermal springs, are to be found ochre and umber, which are used in manufacturing paints.[59]

---

[54] Kahan (1963): 4–6; Dermage and Tournage (1990); Salarneh, Rimawi and Hamed (1991).

[55] Kahan (1963): 4–5; Lachman (1933): 181.

[56] Kahan (1963): 5; Lachman (1933): 181.

[57] Kahan (1963): 5.

[58] Kahan (1963): 5.

[59] See especially note 24 above; Rimawi and Salameh (1988): 147–163; See also Lachman (1933): 181; Braslavski (1951): III: 222–223; Kahan (1963): 5–6; See the discussion in chapter 4.5 on *The Historical-Archaeological Analysis of Hammei-Baʾarah.*

THE KALLIRRHOE SPRINGS—A group of springs, south of
the Zarqa springs, also known as Tseret HaShahar and Ain Wafiah. It
contains several springs, some cold and some hot. The hot springs Ez-
Zara reach a temperature of 62.8°C. Braver maintains that the waters
of Tseret HaShahar are drinkable, and can alleviate constipation.[60]

2.1.5 *Hot Springs within the Syro-African Rift in Sinai*

There are also hot and saline springs in the Suez Valley. The most
prominent is Hammam Fhara'on [= Pharaoh's Bath]. The temperature of its water reaches 72°C, and its composition is very similar to
that of Hammei-Tiberias, though less concentrated. It emerges from
the sand, close to the Gulf of Suez. On a cliff a few metres above the
spring is a cave in which the temperature reaches 52°C, whose heat is
derived from the waters of the fountain flowing below it. The water
of the principal spring is clear, but in some of the minor springs with
lower temperatures black, green and white algae grow. Jebel Hammam
Fhara'on (the hill close to the well) is built of limestone, but its slopes
are coloured in light hues of brown, purple and red, originating in iron
solutions which have risen to fill the fissures. The source of the mineral
waters is sea-water, and not the salts dissolved in the rocks. According
to the Bedouin of the tribe which lives in the date plantations of *Nahal*
A'randel, north of the spring, in the recent and more distant past many
sufferers have visited this spring. The therapeutic characteristics of
the bath were so famous that pilgrims on their way to Mecca would
go out of their way for a day or two in order to bathe in the spring
and bask in the heat of the cave. It appears that bathing in Hammam
Fhara'on cures all ills: aching bones in the winter, itching skin and sores
and other undefined pains. Along the Gulf of Suez there are several
more hot wells and springs. The most famous is Hammam Sidna Musa
[= the Baths of our Lord Moses], north of the town of at-Tur. The
waters of this spring, which is relatively sweet, reach a temperature of
32°C, and have a sulphurous odour. It lies on the border of the date
farms of the monks of Santa Katherina monastery. Of recent years artesian wells have been discovered along the Gulf of Suez. Their waters

---

[60] Braver (1928): 10–11; Kahan (1963): 6; See above, note 58; See also the discussion
in chapter 4.4 on *The Historical-Archaeological Analysis of Kallirrhoe.*

contain little salt, but have a sulphurous odour; their temperature is more than 30°C.[61]

2.1.6   *Thermal Springs in Other Places in Palestine*

Volcanic phenomena between the Judean hills and the coastal plain indicate the occurrence of earthquakes in this region, too. There is evidence of this in the sediments of the thermal springs which have been discovered south of the village of Beth Jiz. Hall's book on the geology of Palestine (1886) and Conder's on Palestine (1891) mention the existence of basaltic rocks between Jerusalem and Jaffa, but later geological maps make no mention of the existence of volcanic formations in the region of Beth Jiz and Gezer.[62] Near Beth Jiz there is silicon rock coloured like baked brick. It originated from limestone which changed its original form under the influence of the intense heat of gases and hot water containing various minerals. This red rock is covered with a sort of hard silicon crust, which is sediment caused by the heat, or sinter. The geologist Avnimelech raises a historical question connected with the thermo-mineral springs. He claims that there are heat-caused sediments close to Emmaus, the ancient spa which is also mentioned in the Talmudic literature as Hammat or Hammtha.[63] Since Emmaus lies at the entrance to the Vale of Ayalon, it may be that there is a link between this volcanic phenomenon and the words of the book of *Joshua* (10, 11), 'And it came to pass as they fled before Israel, and were in the going down to Beit Horon, that the Lord cast down great stones from heaven upon them unto Azekah... Sun, stand thou still upon Giv'on; and thou, moon, in the Valley of Ayalon' (*ibid.*, 10, 12).

There is a region of therapeutic baths in the south of Israel, about 200 metres from the road between Ascalon and Kiryat-Gat: Hammei-Yoav, which was first operated in 1989. The water is pumped from an artesian well, 1,500 metres deep, into the pools. Its temperature reaches 42°C, and it is recommended for skin diseases and rheumatic complaints.[64]

---

[61] Mazor (1970): 297–299; Mazor, Nadler and Molcho (1973): 289–309; Mazor (1980a): 703, Figs. 385–386; Yakobovitz (1981): I: 197; LaMoreaux (2001): 24–26.
[62] Hull (1889).
[63] Avnimelech (1935): 60–63.
[64] According to internal reports of Hammei-Yoav.

It may be said, in short, that wherever marked thermal anomalies
have been recorded they are connected with fault systems. Most of
the springs flow from the meeting point between secondary faults and
the main lines of the fissure connected with the Jordan Valley—Dead
Sea—Red Sea system. The depth of the underground flow of groundwater of meteoric origin before it appears on the surface as a hot spring
is connected with the source of the heat, and that is still a matter for
speculation.[65]

Geologists, hydrologists and geochemists have been attempting to
solve the problem of how these springs were created, and what the
source of their waters is. They have suggested a variety of mecha-
nisms, including: a magmatic source—vapours and gases rising from
the boiling lava inside the earth; a primeval salt lake, whose waters
have been imprisoned and preserved in deep subterranean reservoirs,
and are now rising in the form of a hot salt solution: the residue of
oceanic waters, which percolated to the fault valleys during the period
when the sea reached the Jordan Valley through the Yizre'el Valley
or the Valleys of Be'er Sheba and Dimonah; rainwater, dissolving
strata or granules of salt dispersed among the rocks which constitute
the Jordan Valley.[66] The most likely explanation seems to be that the
thermal springs are by products of extinct volcanic activity.[67] It is not
surprising that the number of hot springs varies as between historical
periods, since earthquakes and soil erosion have wrought changes in
the number of springs. Some springs have been blocked up; in several
places—but not all—new ones have appeared in their place.[68] It may
be pointed out that in all the discussions and disputations of the Sages
of Tiberias in the Talmudic period there is no mention of the number
of hot springs in the region, and we do not know how many fountains
there were at the time. In subsequent periods, however, the descriptions
of chroniclers and travellers who visited the spot give several numbers.
Some exaggerated the number of springs, while others found only one.
For example, in his description of the great earthquake in Palestine in
749 CE, Michael the Syrian speaks of one spring in Tiberias, whereas
al-Muqaddasi, writing in 985, speaks of eight hot springs there. The

[65] Eckstein (1975): 8–12.
[66] Mazor (1969): 272.
[67] Avnimelech (1935): 62–63.
[68] Hirschberg (1920: 225) thinks that it regards to all places by the name *Emmaus*.

Persian traveller Nâsir-i-Khusrau, writing in 1047, says that there is one spring, with very hot water, in Tiberias, whereas the Muslim traveller al-Idrīsī, who visited Tiberias in 1154, speaks of 'springs' in the bath-houses of the town; it seems that these were brought into Tiberias by means of conduits. When the Arab traveller Ali Mahirat came to the town in 1173, he wrote that in the front of the palatial bathhouse the water flowed forth from twelve (sic) fountains. In 1522 Rabbi Moshe Bassula wrote that he saw two springs, each of which flowed out of the wall of a different bathhouse. In 1769 Rabbi Moshe Yerushalmi mentioned one spring which came out of the ground. The traveller Abraham Israel Rozanis, who visited the place in 1867, said that there were three springs there. In 1883 Rabbi Yehiel Brill said that there were five springs in the Tiberias spa.[69]

Some homiletic remarks of the Sages show that it was generally believed that there were hidden subterranean caverns connected with the Jordan River and Tiberias. Thus, for instance:

> "What aileth thee, O thou sea, that thou fleest? thou Jordan, that thou turnest backward?... At the presence of the God of Jacob, etc" (*Psalms* 114, 5, 7). Rabbi Levi said: 'There is a place where the Jordan falls with a roar into Hammei-Tiberias.; in his great trepidation Jacob entered there and Esau shut him in, but the Holy One, blesses be He, dug an opening for him at a different point, so that he got through. Thus it is written, "When thou passest through the waters, I will be with thee, and through the rivers, they shall not overflow thee" (*Isaiah* 43, 2)'.
>
> (*Genesis Rabbah* 76, 4–5)

or the version of the *Midrash Tanhuma, Wayyetse*, 3 (Buber ed., p.146), which is as follows and demonstrate the idea:

> So Esau was waiting on the way, but Jacob did not pass on the way. When Esau perceived that Jacob had fled and crosses the Jordan, what did he do? He pursued him and found him in a cave, a place like the bath that is in Tiberias.[70] Jacob had said: 'There is no bread and no food at hand. I shall go in and get warm in the bath.' Esau the Wicked came and had the bath surrounded the bath, so that he would die in it... Immediately the Holy One said to Jacob: 'What are you afraid of? See, I am with you.' Jacob said to him: 'Sovereign of the World, inasmuch as I trust you

---

[69] Meiri (1973): 29–30.
[70] On the similarity between 'cave', *Mea'rah*, and Ba'arah, see the discussion in chapter 1.4 on *Terminology* and in chapter 4.5 on *The Historical-Archaeological Analysis of Ba'arah*.

and you are making me a promise, I will have trust and set out (*Genesis* 28, 10). And Jacob set out from Be'er Sheba <through a subterranean cavern which brought him to Be'er Sheba>.

It may be assumed that in ancient times there were therapeutic sites with hot springs whose sources dried up or were blocked over the years. It is natural for changes in the flow and quality of the waters to take place in the course of generations. Geological research has also proved that springs have been blocked up as a result of earthquakes.[71] Be that as it may, nobody doubts that Hammei-Tiberias, Hammat-Gader and the Dead Sea were, and still are, balneological units with therapeutic qualities.[72] It seems that the unambiguous contemporary evidence of Hammam el-Malieh, 'the deserted Hammam' shows that there have existed in Palestine more baths than exist today; but it is very doubtful whether there was a tradition of the use of thermo-mineral sources for treatment before the Roman conquest.

2.2 Geothermal Energy Utilisation in the Jordan Valley

Numerous small and a few major hot springs are the main manifestations of geothermal energy in the Jordan Valley. Since only four major thermo-mineral springs are known to have been utilized intensively in antiquity, this review will be restricted to their description: Hammei-Tiberias on the western flank and Hammat-Gader, Ez-Zara (Kallirrhoe) and Zarqa Ma'in (Ba'arah) on the eastern flank. (See Tab. 1 and Map 2).

Much information about these springs has been provided by the regional studies in the Lake Kinneret and the Dead Sea areas. The economic importance of these conspicuous fresh and saltwater springs spurred vigorous hydrological, hydrogeological, and hydrogeochemical investigations, as well as studies in related fields, such as isotope geology and heat flow.[73]

The existence of well developed rift fracture-zones accounts for an easy ascent of the thermal waters from deep layers and for their outflow at the surface. The variability that has been documented in temperature

---

[71] Shalem (1953): 419; Gilad (1985): 1–27.
[72] See chapter 5 on *The Healing Properties of the Spas in the Eastern Mediterranean in Ancient Times.*
[73] Jaffé, Dvorjetski, Levitte, Massarwieh and Swarieh (1999): 37–38.

and chemical concentrations among the various spring systems, and also among the individual springs in a given spring cluster, leads one to think that different confined aquifers with thermal water exist at depth and that a variable dilution of this water occurs with colder water of meteoric origin circulating in shallow aquifers.

Preliminary studies on the low enthalpy geothermal potential of the thermo-mineral springs in question, and of the confined aquifers existing in their surroundings, have been carried out and submitted with specific recommendations for further work, mainly on the eastern flank of the Jordan Valley.[74]

Obviously, no quantitative data are available on the utilisation in antiquity of thermo-mineral springs in the Jordan Rift Valley as will be shown obviously in the following chapters. There is, however, sufficient information to surmise that conditions and applications have not changed significantly over last 2,000 years. Quite to the contrary: the spas just described were far more important in antiquity than in the last few centuries and at present.

It can be reasonably assumed, though, that a major change may take place in the next century. Then the geothermal potential of the springs' area and of the whole surrounding region is expected to be harnessed, not only for classical balneological purposes but for new and challenging low enthalpy applications.[75]

2.3   EXAMINATION OF THEIR USE IN THE LIGHT OF MODERN MEDICINE

The therapeutic springs in Israel and Jordan have a special place among the natural resources.[76] Their use is still empirical, and their mode of operation somewhat obscure. In the eyes of contemporary medicine, the fact that the therapeutic springs in Europe and Israel are ancient does

---

[74] Eckstein (1979a): 150–159; idem, (1979b): Gat, Mazor and Tsur (1979): 334–352; Galanis, Saas, Munroe and Abu-Ajamieh (1986); Gavrieli and Bein (1995): 174–176; Bein (1976); Mazor, Levitte, Truesdell, Healy and Wissenbaum (1980): 1–19; Serruya (1978); Vengosh, Starinksy, Kolodny and Chivas (1994): 165–169.

[75] Abu-Ajamieh (1980); Abu-Ajamieh, Bender and Eicher (1989); Allen (1988); Galanis, Saas, Munroe and Abu-Ajamieh (1986); Myslil (1988); Tournaye (1990); idem, (1992).

[76] Kurland (1971): 44–45.

not afford them any privileges. In the nineteenth century, when medicine
was being developed on the basis of the exact natural sciences, many
doctors scoffed at the idea that bathing in or drinking their waters could
have a therapeutic effect. This led to the development of the science of
balneology, whose object is to investigate the special nature and effects
of therapeutic springs. It removed the mists of mysticism from mineral
waters, and investigated them as pharmacological phenomena.[77] In this
connection, some interesting questions may be mentioned:

1. Are all the constituents of the hot baths which determine their
   therapeutic qualities known?
2. What are the different theories relating to treatment in therapeutic
   baths?
3. How does medical science relate to treatment in therapeutic
   baths?
4. How are therapeutic springs classified?
5. How can minerals influence the body while bathing?
6. What are therapeutic centres combined with hot springs?
7. Do the main therapeutic sites in the eastern Mediterranean compete
   with each other, or supplement each other?

Today, most of the components which determine the therapeutic
effects of the baths are known. Apart from the chemical elements, heat
and radioactivity are important, as are specific gravity, the degree of
hardness, osmotic pressure, and degrees of acidity and colloidality. In
modern times many theories about methods of treatment in therapeutic
springs have been developed, among them hydrotherapy, balneotherapy,
and more.[78]

Therapeutic baths are classified according to their most characteristic uses, i.e., their effectiveness against particular complaints including
fatigue, headaches, rheumatic complaints, disorders of the respiratory
system, diseases of the digestive and urinary systems, dermatological
and venereal diseases, women's complaints, nervous disorders, and nose,
ear and throat complaints.[79] (See Tab. 2).

---

[77] See, for example, Nováček (1966): 5–16; Albu, Banks and Nash (1997): 26–33.
[78] Leibowitz and Kurland (1972): 47; Pines (1979): 181; Buchmann (1956): 49; idem,
(1957): 35–36.
[79] See, for example, Leibowitz and Kurland (1972): 47; Buchmann (1948): 130–131;
Weiss and Kemble (1962): 11–12; Thomson (1978): 189–199.

It is known that three factors have a positive influence in mineral springs: water pressure, chemical composition and temperature.[80] The pressure of the water on the intestines, the skin, and the veins of the hands and feet causes the blood to flow from the blood vessels in these limbs to the right atrium. Pressure on the chest limits its expansion and reduces the area of ventilation of the lungs; The influence of the chemical composition of the water depends on its constituents (Carbon dioxide, Sulphur, salts, etc.), which will not be discussed in detail here; The heat of the water is also important. Hot and warm water, acting through the skin, expand the blood vessels, and cold water contracts them. This results in part from direct contact, and in part from the secretion of Histamine, Acetylcholine and Adenosine.[81]

It appears that bathing in mineral waters influences the heart and the circulation of the blood. Observation of groups of patients who have come to Hammei-Tiberias for the treatment of rheumatoid arthritis, liver complaints, diseases of the peripheral nerves and light arteriosclerosis leads to the conclusion that from the point of view of the blood vessels and the heart treatment in the Tiberias baths should not be undertaken in cases of high blood pressure, advanced arteriosclerosis, weak blood circulation, choking feelings while resting, and irregularities of the heart beat.[82]

The mineral contents of the water also affect the circulation. This may be proved objectively by the fact that patients are able to withstand greater heat in the Hammei-Tiberias than in ordinary water. Accurate measurements have shown that a process of exchange of anions and cations takes place. The question is not whether the ions pass through the skin, but whether they enter the skin cells. The process differs in accordance with the concentration and reaction of the solution which comes into contact with the skin. In dilute solutions, for instance, only cations pass through in both directions, whereas in concentrated solutions both cations and anions pass through. The thermal, physical-chemical and mechanical elements in combination undoubtedly affect the functioning of the body.[83]

---

[80] Boren-Borenstein (1971): 57–59; Buchmann (1971): 84–87.
[81] Atlas (1971): 78; Weiss and Kemble (1962): 16–20; See also Baudisch (1939): 440–448.
[82] Boren-Borenstein (1971): 57–59.
[83] Buchmann (1971): 84–89.

The first person to take note of the great therapeutic value of the
Hammei-Tiberias was Frumkin. In 1885, after a visit to the site, he
wrote in the Hebrew journal *HaHavatzelet*:[84]

> In the town of Tiberias there is a precious treasure. The hot springs
> contain a high proportion of Sulphur, salt and Iron, and cure nervous
> weaknesses, etc. If there were to be found there a competent doctor to
> observe the complaints of the invalids who come to bathe, and to give
> them orders as to what they should do… Tiberias would be one of the
> best known medical centres throughout the world, and thousands would
> be saved from death and destruction.

A development of great significance for the special characteristics
of Hammei-Tiberias took place in 1912, with the publication of the
research of Friedmann, the first to test the mineral components of the
springs in a well equipped laboratory.[85] Their medical importance was
increased in 1956 with the publication of Buchmann's comparative
analysis of the waters of Tiberias, Wiesbaden and Aachen in Germany
and Piestany in Czechoslovakia.[86] In 1969, Melamed made a fundamental analysis of the hot water using up to date methods, including tests of
its radioactivity and its gaseous components. These tests proved that the
waters of the Tiberias are hyperthermal (hotter than body temperature),
acidic (as a result of the carbon dioxide they contain), hypertonic (containing more salts than the blood) and radioactive.[87] The considerable
body of research on thermal sites in Europe where there are springs
with a high degree of radioactivity, such as Badgustin, Lison, a centre
of natural medicine with high Radon content, and Aix-les-Bains, where
there is radioactivity similar to that in hot springs of Tiberias and well
known to all those who suffer from arthritis, proves that the natural
radioactivity of therapeutic springs increases their medical efficacy.[88] We
may sum up by saying that Hammei-Tiberias are hot and radioactive,
and contain a high proportion of salts and ions. They contain gases in
solution and trace elements. Comparison between recent analyses and
earlier research proves that the proportions of salts, ions and liquefied
gases changes from time to time, within certain limits, but that these

[84] *HaHavazlet* folio 36, *Adar* 1846.
[85] Friedmann (1913a); idem, (1913b): 429–436.
[86] Buchmann (1928a): 28–30; idem, (1956): 46.
[87] Melamed (1971): 13–17; Kurland (1971): 44–45; Meiri (1973): 31.
[88] Kurland (1971): 44–45.

changes do not affect the chemical reaction of the water. It is at present still impossible to single out any particular element which affords mineral waters their therapeutic properties.[89]

In modern times the baths of Hammei-Tiberias have become comprehensive medical centres. Apart from baths, pools and showers, they provide additional forms of treatments such as subaqueous massage, subaqueous exercise, inhalation, physiotherapy, electrotherapy and mechanotherapy. Fangotherapy, the use of mud for rheumatic diseases, women's diseases and contusions, has a special place.[90] In addition to research on the hot springs of Tiberias, *Peloma*, the unique natural mud which is used to dress infirm parts of the body, has been the subject of analyses and fundamental research. It is inorganic sediment which appears in volcanic areas or in the form of geological strata in prehistoric river-beds. Its unique quality is that it is permeated with minerals, and conducts heat slowly, and therefore becomes a sort of accumulator of heat, at a temperature of up to 55°C. It cools down extremely slowly. It is applied as a hot poultice directly to the skin of the painful limb, or on an unhealthy joint or a deformed muscle. When *Peloma* is applied to the affected limb, heat and various chemicals are slowly absorbed from it into the bodily tissues through the skin, and this relieves the pain and heals the limb. The *Peloma* stimulates the blood vessels of the affected limb, whose blood circulation is increased, and this expedites the cure.[91] Comparative research by Buchmann and the Hebrew University of Jerusalem on *Peloma* in Czechoslovakia, Italy and Russia proves that the heat conductivity of the Tiberian *Peloma* is slow, and it can be applied to the body, even at a high temperature, for 20–30 minutes.[92] *Peloma* is soaked in water from the therapeutic springs so that it absorbs the ions and assumes the characteristics of the mineral waters.[93]

Buchmann, who conducted a great deal of research on the special characteristics of the hot springs of Tiberias, and played a central role in formulating the medical instructions for those who use thermal baths,

---

[89] Meiri (1973): 31; Buchmann (1971): 29–43; Kurland (1977): 27; Segev (1989): 151.
[90] Leibowitz and Kurland (1972): 47; idem, (1982): 21–22; Buchmann (1971): 67–70; idem, (1962): 100–101.
[91] Buchmann (1955): 287–291; idem, (1971): 48–49; Pines (1979): 181.
[92] Buchmann (1956): 50–56; Meiri (1973): 31–32.
[93] Segev (1989): 150.

claims that the waters may be defined, according to their chemical composition, as 'saline, calciferous, sulphurous, and unlike virtually all the hot springs in the world'.[94]

It is universally agreed today that balneological centres specialize in particular areas of healing. The thermal centre of Hammei-Tiberias, in its current state of the art condition, is designed primarily for treatment of rheumatic complaints, defects in the motorial system, posttraumatic disturbances, skin diseases, gynecological and prostate gland treatments. It is particularly effective of Hammei-Tiberias thermo-mineral baths in dealing with the following complaints: Rheumatic complaints: Arthritis; Rheumatoid arthritis; advanced chronic Polyarthritis; Ankylotic spondylitis; Articulated rheumatism; aftereffects of infectious arthritis, whose causes are many and are often difficult to diagnose, such as Tuberculosis, Syphilis, and Gonorrhoea; Arthrosis, degeneration of the cartilage and the bones which appears after the age of 40, slowly and unperceived; Gonitis, water on the joints, arthritis of the knuckles of the hands; rheumatic injury to the tendons, the muscular tissue and the nerves; inflammation of the connective tissue round the joints of the thigh and the knees; and myalgic pains, including Lumbago and stiff neck; Traumatism: fractures; Periostitis; lameness of the hip, whether through natal dislocation or inflammation of the bone; Diseases of the joints; Podagra; After effects of Poliomyelitis; Peripheral inflammation of the nerves; After effects of Phlebitis; Women's complaints: Dysmenorrhea; Parametritis; Salpingitis; Infecunditas; Inflammation of the Prostate gland; Skin diseases: Eczema; Acne; Psoriasis; Urticaria; Chronic complaints of the respiratory tract: Nasopharyngitis; Laryngitis; Sinusitis; Bronchitis and Emphysema; Allergic conditions of the nose: nasal allergy, attacks of sneezing, itching of the nose, badly running nose.[95] (See Tab. 2).

It should be added that, in addition to whichever of the means of treatment described above is most suited to the specific case, treatment is always combined with hydrotherapy or *Peloma*. It is, of course, adapted to the patient's general state of health, his/her age, the progress of

---

[94] Buchmann (1971): 18–28; idem, (1956): 45.

[95] Buchmann (1928b): 368–369; idem, (1933): 303–304; idem, (1956): 57–64; Atlas (1970): 79; Buchmann (1971): 22–28; Poldi (1971): 60–66; Meiri (1973): 32; Margalit (1976): 137–146; Kurland (1980): 44–46; idem, (1982): 20–21; Machtey (1986): 12–13, 115–116; Segev (1989): 152.

the disease and the stage it has reached, and the degree of his/her endurance. During treatment the patient is under continuous medical observation: individual reactions are noted, and suitable changes made in the therapeutic programme.[96]

Patients who suffer from disorders of the heart, the kidneys, the liver or the endocrine glands, such as thyroid or kidney excess, should not be sent for thermal treatment; nor should those with a tendency to bleed or who suffer from stomach ulcers. Those who suffer from cancer, diabetes, disorders of the blood vessels or the myocardium, or tuberculosis should also not undergo thermal treatment. It is also considered undesirable for those who suffer from inflammatory skin conditions, particularly when these cause secretions, or in chronic cases with a tendency to recurrent inflammation, such as eye infections, abscesses, and fungal inflammation of the skin. A pregnant woman may receive treatment in the baths for the first six months of her pregnancy, provided that she does not have a tendency to haemorrhage or miscarry. Thermal treatment during menstruation is forbidden. The duration of the treatment is 21 days, in chronic cases; in sporadic and first time treatment, 8–12 days. In Europe, plans of treatment usually call for one treatment per year for the first two years, and four weeks every two years thereafter. Chronic and allergic cases in which medicaments are ineffective or may not be used can best be dealt with by treatment once every year.[97]

The constituents of the waters of the springs of Hammat-Gader and Hammei-Tiberias, which are close to each other, are very similar, but their attributes are quantitatively different. The waters of Hammat-Gader are poor in minerals and contain more Hydrogen Sulphide, and their natural temperature is lower. They are effective against almost the same illnesses. Some doctors prefer one spring or another in accordance with different diseases, the gravity of the illness, and, primarily, the state of the patient.[98]

There are a number of springs in Israel with therapeutic qualities from which drinkable mineral water is obtained. It is used for the treatment of disorders of the digestive and urinary tracts. The waters of

[96] Kurland (1977): 27.
[97] Kurland (1977): 27; idem, (1980): 44–46; Buchmann (1956): 4–65; Margalit (1976): 137–139; Segev (1989): 153.
[98] Buchmann (1971): 92; Selomi-Friedmann (1936): 175–177, Pl. VI; Margalit (1975).

the Tiberias baths are rich in Calcium, which is important in treatment
by drinking. It may be that this water also has a salutary influence
on the gall bladder, and its laxative effect is well known. The water
of Hammat-Gader is also drinkable, and is effective against chronic
constipation.[99]

The Dead Sea and its shore also possess healing qualities. There
are two reasons for the growing interest in this region as a therapeutic
site: the ancient tradition regarding the effectiveness of mineral waters
against various illnesses; and personal experience, passed on by word of
mouth. The coast of the Dead Sea serves as a therapeutic region for
several types of patient: those who have rheumatic diseases, skin diseases
(Psoriasis) and disorders of the respiratory tract. Psoriasis, which is not
contagious but cannot be permanently cured, brings many tourists to
Israel.[100] Buchmann emphasized that bathing in the Dead Sea allevi-
ates organic and functional nervous disorders, paralysis, weakness of
the nervous system, destructive metabolism, and states of premature
aging and general weakness.[101]

The Dead Sea is unique in that it contains many elements used in
thalassotherapy, climatotherapy, and balneotherapy. The air is fresh,
dry, and free from smoke and industrial waste, and there are few
variations in temperature at different times of day; certainly there are
no sudden changes. The atmospheric pressure is higher than that of
the Mediterranean coastal plain, since the region is 400 metres below
sea level. The deep atmospheric layer, rich in Oxygen, filters out the
sun's rays and reduces the danger of sunburn even when the sun is
at its highest. Because of the great depth of the Dead Sea, the solar
radiation which reaches the ground and the bodies of the bathers
contains few Ultra Violet rays. The distance from the main centres of
population fosters tranquility, detachment from day to day problems,
and completes rest.[102]

There seem to be three reasons for the effectiveness of the Dead Sea
in treating various rheumatic disorders—particularly Arthritis—and

---

[99] Leibowitz and Kurland (1972): 47; Buchmann (1942): 140; idem, (1971): 21;
Shelomi-Friedman (1936: 171–174, Pls. III, IV, V; Kasher (1934): 10–13; Atlas (1951):
157–159; Tweig (1979): 28; Preuss (1993): 531–532.
[100] Machtey (1979): 8–11; idem, (1977): 28; Margalit (1976): 143–144; Tweig (1979):
28; Yaron (2001): 27–28.
[101] Buchmann (1933): 306.
[102] Machtey (1986): 12–13, 115–116.

Psoriasis: they are thermal, chemical and mechanical. The hot water of the sea and the springs round it is able to expand the blood vessels and speed up the circulation. Some believe that this may reduce blood pressure, but as yet there is no proof of this. The hot water may bring about relaxation of tense muscles, which is much practised in physiotherapy. We have very little knowledge of the effect of chemical factors on different illnesses. Various materials penetrate beneath the skin only to a minor degree. The concentration of radioactive materials in the water is apparently too small to be active, and it is therefore not dangerous. None the less, it is not impossible that the high concentrations of Bromine in the Dead Sea (and in the air, as a result of evaporation) have a soothing influence the nervous system; this, too, however, has not been scientifically proved. From the point of view of rheumatic complaints, the most important influence is that of mechanical factors. It should be recalled that a body in water loses as much weight as that of the water it repels. If that is so in normal water, it is even truer of mineral water, and primarily of the Dead Sea, where the concentration of minerals is as high as 30%. The relative gravity of a body in the Dead Sea is so small that it floats on the surface of the water and is almost unsinkable. Under these conditions it is easier to move limbs and execute physiotherapeutic treatment, while the heat of the seawater helps to relax the body and reduce pain.[103]

The calculations of Tzundak are very important. He proved that there is oestrous hormone in the Dead Sea and in the mud of the seabed. As early as 1929 he discovered that this hormone enters the body through the skin, and in his experiments in 1935 he proved that this process has therapeutic value. Therefore he posited that bathing in the Dead Sea, the use of mud from its seabed, and the use of *Salsana*, are effective in curing hormonal complaints. For the sake of comparison he also tested the waters of the Jordan River, Hammei-Tiberias and Lake Kinneret, but found no hormones in them.[104]

The waters of the therapeutic springs on the coast of the Dead Sea—particularly Ein Bokek, Hammei-Zohar and Ein Gedi—have particularly strong sulphurous gases, which are especially helpful to those with arthritic complaints. They are also helpful to those who suffer from

---

[103] Machtey (1986): 28–29; Tweig (1979): 28.
[104] Tzundak (1938): 428–432; See also Almog and Eshel (1956): 35, 42–43.

heart complaints, disorders of blood circulation and the respiratory tract, and skin diseases, particularly Psoriasis. Because of their high salinity, these springs are also effective against women's complaints.[105]

It is important to point out that the use of therapeutic baths is a medical procedure, and should be undertaken only at the detailed instructions of a doctor and under his supervision. Because of the complex medical problems involved in this treatment, a new medical specialization with its own experts has come into being: hydrotherapy. There is no doubt that over the generations the combination of observation and tradition has led to the accumulation of much empirical evidence which has proved the value of the springs as effective means of dealing with many diseases, and particularly those of the limbs, the joints, the respiratory system, and infertility.[106]

More than two thousand years ago Enoch of the pseudepigrapha declared that these springs give 'healing to the flesh and healing to the spirit'.[107] His words are echoed in the norms of contemporary medicine, according to which the aim of all medicine is to heal both the body and the mind. Modern medical practice in some countries continues to advocate the use of balneotherapy and thermo-mineral springs.[108]

[105] Atlas (1971): 166; Margalit (1976): 144–145.
[106] Leibowitz and Kurland (1972): 47; Meiri (1973): 9.
[107] See the reference and contribution of Enoch in chapter 5 on *The Healing Properties of the Spas in the Eastern Mediterranean in Ancient Times*.
[108] See, for example, Porter (1990); Agishi and Ohtsuka (1995); Campion (1996); Nováček (1966); de Zanche (1988); Lichet (1963).

CHAPTER THREE

MEDICINAL HOT SPRINGS AND HEALING SPAS
IN THE GRAECO-ROMAN WORLD

si primum omnibus templis saluberrimae regiones aquarum que fontes
in hic locis idonei eligentur, in quibus fana constituantur, deinde maxime
Aesculapio, Saluti, et eorum deorum quorum plurimi mediccnns aegri
curari videntur [= In the case of all sacred precincts we select very healthy
neighborhoods with the suitable springs of water in the places where the
fanes are to be built, particularly in the case of those to Aesculapius and
to Salus, gods by whose healing powers great numbers of the sick are
apparently cured].

Thus did the first century BCE Roman architect Marcus Vitruvius Pollio
explain the basis for the correct selection of a site for a new sacred
precinct. He recommends choosing a healthy spot with a spring for
all gods but especially for those connected to healing when planning
a new temple.[1]

Most sacred buildings at the sites of medicinal hot springs, known
from antiquity, cannot be identified nowadays. Some of the springs were
blocked and others dried up. Where they have remained in use, the
ancient structures have usually been subsequently modified or replaced
by later buildings.[2]

The following is intended merely as some general observations on
the original use of hot springs for medicinal purposes; the healing
qualities of such springs; ritual worship of the therapeutic sites; the
military presence at these sites; and the archaeological finds in the
Graeco-Roman world. This chapter will focus on a historical cross
section of the socio-economic, cultural and religious aspects of these
places. Bath Spa in Gloucestershire, Britain, will function as a model
for those fascinating aspects. (See Figs. 1, 2 and 3).

---

[1] Vitruvius, *De Architectura* 1.2.2; See also Allen (1998): 49.
[2] Jackson (1990a); Dvorjetski (1992a); idem, (1992b).

3.1   The Original Use of Hot Springs for
Medicinal Purposes

As early as the era of Hippocrates (ca. 460–370 BCE), who is traditionally regarded as 'the father of medicine', bathing was considered
not simply as a measure of hygiene. Its properties of cleaning and
refreshing were augmented by more general effects, particularly its
healing and curing qualities. Bathing was considered one of the means
by which a person could both maintain and restore health. The use
of hot springs for medicinal purposes originates in the teaching of
Hippocrates. In his day, the method became practical and of benefit
to the sick.[3] Hippocrates' ideas were developed mainly by Galen, the
Greek physician, anatomist and writer on medicine and philosophy
(129–ca. 199 CE), who does not elaborate at length on the benefits
of spring water and bathing, but his medical advice includes the use
of thermo-mineral waters.[4] Others were Celsus, the encyclopaedist,
whose writings on medicine are extant (ca. 25 BC–50 CE); Soranus of
Ephesus, the most famous physician of the Methodist sect, who studied
in Alexandria before going to Rome to practice during the reigns of
Trajan and Hadrian (90–150 CE); Oribasius, the Greek physician and
medical writer from Pergamon of the fourth century CE; and Caelius
Aurelianus, who lived in the fifth century CE and preserved Soranus'
treatise.[5]

Medicinal hot springs were recommended for the treatment of specific
complaints, such as disturbances of paralysis, muscle disorders, and
diseases of the joints, most notably gout; urinary diseases, including
bladder stone; digestive disorders and internal ailments, including colic,
liver abscess and 'wasting' diseases; skin diseases, including psoriasis
and ulceration; eye diseases, head pains, and insanity; female disorders,
including infertility; fevers, pneumonia, respiratory problems and chest

---

[3] Hippocrates, *Regimen in Acute Diseases* 65–68; Leibowitz (1960): 341–348; Cohen and
Drabkin (1966): 507–508; Fytikas, Leonidopoulou and Cataldi (1999): 86, 89.
[4] Hippocrates, *Places in Man* 43; Galen, *In Hippocrates De Natura Hominis* 15–21;
See also Ginouvès (1962): 21–225; Leibowitz (1969): 911–915; Villard (1994): 41–60;
Jouanna (1994): 25–40; Buchman (1994): 8; Ruoti, Morris and Cole (1997): 3; Allen
(1998): 36–37; Nolte (2001): 7.
[5] Fontanille (1985): 15–24; Yegül (1992): 15–24, 352–355; Heinz (1996): 2411–2432;
Jackson (1999): 107; Allen (1998): 102–103; Nolte (2001): 6–7.

pains; convalescence, including recovery from wounds and surgery.[6] Such illnesses as these, though not psychological in causation, would certainly have been alleviated by faith, warmth and relaxation.[7]

Asclepiades, the first century BCE Greek physician, who introduced medical methods to Rome, stubbornly extolled the use of the baths for the sick as well as for the healthy. He widely used cold water for external and internal therapy;[8] as a result, Pliny the Elder named him *frigida danda praeferens*, the giver of cold water.[9] While many despised his teaching, many others esteemed his methods, and hydrotherapy became popular during the first century BCE. Less extreme were the treatments recommended by Celsus, who wrote his treatise *De Medicina* some decades after the cure of Augustus by Antoninus Musa, one of Asclepiades' pupils.[10] Celsus's book gained wide recognition as a valuable source of Hellenistic medical knowledge. He specialized in the doctrines of Asclepiades and regarded the use of baths as an integral part of treatment for fatigue, chills, high fever, and especially for diseases of the skin or sinews, Podagra [= Gout], wounds, digestive disturbances, weakness, eye disease and post-operative convalescence.[11] It should be noted that despite the successful treatment of Augustus by Musa, Celsus recommended hot baths rather than cold ones for sufferers from liver abscesses and warned against all cold things.[12] The Greek physician Soranus of Ephesus, in his work Γυναικεῖα βιβλία, regarded baths as particularly valuable for the relaxation of physical and mental tensions. He believed that while such relaxation was very beneficial during the later stages of pregnancy, it was detrimental early on, when the seed or embryo could be expelled from a relaxed uterus. Bathing in natu-

---

[6] See, for example, Hippocrates, *Aphorisms* 5.25; idem, *Regimen in Acute Diseases* 66; Celsus, *De Medicina* 1.1–4.7; 2.14.17–18; 3.6.12.15.20.22.27; 4.2.12.15.31; 5.26–28.30; 6.6; 7.26; Soranus, *Gynaecia* 1.46.54–56; 3.10–16.28.32.38.44; 4.38; Caelius Aurelianus, *De Acutis Morbis* 5.4.77; See Temkin (1991): 48, 55–56, 135–142, 152, 159–160, 167–168, 205; Jackson (1990a): 1–2; idem, (1999): 108–109; Dvorjetski (1994a); idem, (1997): 463.
[7] Cruse (2004): 112.
[8] Rawson (1982): 358–370; idem, (1985): 170–184; Vallance (1990); Jackson (1990a): 3; Vallance (1993): 693–727; Jackson (1999): 108.
[9] Pliny, *Naturalis Historia* 26.
[10] Suetonius, *De Vita Caesarum, Augustus* 80.1; See Allen (1998): 31, 122; Nolte (2001): 9.
[11] Celsus, *De Medicina* 1.1–3; 2.17; 3.12.20.22; 4.15.31; 5.26–28; 6.6; 7.26; See also Allen (1998): 31.
[12] Celsus, *De Medicina* 2.14.17–18; 3.2.7.

ral waters relieves the *status strictus*—narrow state of women suffering
from menstrual or uterine disturbances.[13] Galen is somewhat cautious
in prescribing spa visits and thermo-mineral water use. He is aware
of the potential harm caused by springs as well as their benefits, and
therefore tends to advise bating and water in general rather than any
specific location and type of spring.[14]

In the absence of any considered account from antiquity of the
functioning of a spa,[15] Soranus' description of the special arrangements to be made for patients suffering from leg paralyses is nonetheless
illuminating:[16]

> Have the patient use mineral waters, especially warm springs... and
> prescribe swimming in the sea or in these springs. At first an inflated
> bladder should be attached to the paralysed parts to reduce the effort
> required in swimming. Also direct a stream of water... upon the para-
> lysed parts, for the impact of the water is very effective in altering the
> condition of the body.

Like Soranus, Celsus stipulated the form of treatment for paralysis
and other disorders of the stomach with some precision:[17]

> But the commonest and worst complaint of the stomach is paralysis, when
> it does not retain food, and the nutrition of the body is wont to cease,
> and so it is consumed by wasting. In this sort of disease the bath is most
> harmful; reading aloud and exercise of the upper limbs are needed, and
> also anointing and rubbing; it is good for the patient to have cold water
> poured over him, and to swim in cold water, also to submit his stomach
> to jets of it, especially at the back of the stomach from the shoulder-
> blades downwards, to bathe in cold medicinal springs, such as those at
> Cutiliae and Simbruinum.

Pliny the Elder and Vitruvius recognized various types of hot and
medicinal springs.[18] Their classifications do not differ from those of
the modern era. They list sulfurous springs, whose waters 'refresh the

---

[13] Soranus, *Gynaecia* 1.46.54–56; 3.10–16.28.32.38.44; Temkin (1991): 48, 55–56,
135–142, 152, 159– 160, 167–168; Jackson (1990a): 4; See also Edelstein (2003):
851.

[14] Allen (1998): 43–44.

[15] Jackson (1999): 114.

[16] Caelius Aurelianus, *De Acutis Morbis* 2.44–48.

[17] Celsus, *De Medicina* 4.12.

[18] Pliny, *Naturalis Historia* 31.3–8.33.45; 32.32–33; Vitruvius, *De Architectura* 8.4–5;
See also Healy (1986): 111–146; Rowland (1999): 97; Allen (1998): 21–22, 24, 34–35,
113.

weakness of muscles and tendons' by heat; aluminous springs, immersion in which served to treat palsies, because the water opens the skin pores; bituminous springs which provided water for the irrigation and healing of 'internal deficiencies'; alkaline springs; and acid springs, whose water, when imbibed, dissolves bladder stones. Pliny the Elder even collected references that contained instructions for the healing of wounds, dislocations, fractures, gout, foot conditions, fever, sciatica, headaches, psoriasis, diseases of the eyes and the ears, insanity, and infertility of women.

As in more recent times, the drinking of mineral water for health purposes was a major activity and integral part of spa therapy. The water functioned as either a purge or an emollient for many internal ailments. Vitruvius, Pliny, Seneca, and others, were dealing with a specific malady or range of diseases. Seneca the younger, for instance, recommends drinking thermo-mineral water to relieve internal pain and to alleviate problems of the lungs and bowels.[19]

Spa water was sometimes consumed in legendary quantities, on the assumption that if a little did you good a lot must do you a lot of good. Pliny the Elder castigated not just those who bathed overlong in hot Sulphur springs, but also those who through ignorance or bravado drank excessive quantities of medicinal waters:[20]

> Many people make a matter of boasting the great number of hours they can endure the heat of these Sulphur waters—a very injurious practice... Those make a like mistake who boast of the great quantity they can drink. I have seen some already swollen with drinking to such an extent that their rings were covered by skin, since they could not void the vast amount of water they had swallowed.

Excepting such occasional excesses, the therapeutic use of water at spas was probably often beneficial and equally important, seldom detrimental to health. As such, hydrotherapy and balneology as well can reasonably be regarded as two of the milder and more positive aspects of whole medicine in the ancient world.

---

[19] Vitruvius, *De Architectura* 8.3; Rowland (1999: 99–103; Pliny, *Naturalis Historia* 31.3–8. 32–33; Seneca, *Quaestiones Naturales* 3.1.2; See Thomson (1978): 8–9; Garbrecht and Manderscheid (1994): I: 85; Allen (1998): 109–111; Manderscheid (2000): 531.

[20] Pliny, *Naturalis Historia* 31; 32; For a similarly excessive zeal in the use of cold baths, see also *ibid.*, 29.5; Jackson (1990a): 12; idem, (1999): 116; On the presence of physicians at the spas, see chapter 3.4 dealing with *The Military Presence at the Medicinal Sites and the Archaeological Finds.*

3.2   Healing Qualities and Spa Therapy

In the lands which they conquered, the Romans systematically developed
hot springs in general and thermo-mineral springs in particular. They
were attracted by the curative properties of thermal springs and often
settled in their vicinity, and erected magnificent bathhouses as they
encountered them in newly conquered provinces. Most of the therapeutic sites in Europe were, in fact, built upon their remains. Certain
sites became famous for their healing properties, as at Aix-en-Provence
(Aquae Sextiae), Vichy (Aquis Calidis), of Aix-Les-Bains in Savoy
(Aquae Gratianae), Baden (Aquae Helveticae), Baden-Baden (Aquae
Aureliae), Wiesbaden (Aquae Mattiacae), Aachen (Aquae Granni),
Bath (Aquae Sulis), and many others. Although not all were directly
associated with healing cults, the majority were already presided over
by a native deity or spirit, for the phenomenon, especially, of hot water
bubbling up from the depths of the earth must always have inspired
a sense of wonder and a belief in the limitless powers of the divine
spirits.[21]

By the Roman Imperial era, baths in general were available not
just to a wealthy elite but to many people at most social levels. In the
absence of a proper understanding of the causes and communicabil-
ity of diseases, the sick appear not to have been segregated from the
healthy in the communal bathing facilities at baths and spas. Jackson
assumes that certainly there is little evidence to suggest that they were.
Even the well known regulations attributed to Hadrian in the *Historia
Augusta*, 'No-one except the sick is allowed to bathe in public before
the eighth hour' [= before about 1.00 pm], which might be explained
as a piece of positive discrimination in favour of the sick. It seems that
after that time all, healthy and sick alike could bathe.[22]

Certain sources were especially renowned for their healing properties and were singled out for mention. Thus, for example, the intensely

---

[21] Smith (1922): See the sites' names in the index; Jackson (1988): 162; King (1990):
37, 68, 92, 142; Albu, Banks and Nash (1997): 4–7; Authier and Duvernois (1997),
s.v. 'Aix-en-Provence'; Wohnlich (2001): 164–165; Kellaway (2001): 242–256, with an
intensive bibliography; Wood (2004): 31; Manderscheid (2004): see the sites' names in
the index; For the chronological development of ancient scientific though on geothermal
heat (6th century BC–4th century CE), see Cataldi and Chiellini (1999): 165–178.

[22] Jackson (1999): 107, 109; On Hadrian's regulations see *Historia Augusta, Hadrian*
22.7–8.

cold waters of Aquae Cultiliae, near Rome. They were praised by Pliny the Elder and by Celsus for their effectiveness in healing paralysis and other disorders of the stomach disorders;[23] and the sulfurous springs of Aquae Albulae, between Rome and Tivoli, described by Vitruvius, the geographer Strabo, and the Roman poet Martial, recommended by Pliny the Elder for the healing of wounds.[24] Suetonius mentions that Emperor Augustus frequently attended the hot springs of Albulae 'every time that his nerves required relief' and when he was troubled with rheumatism, 'contented himself with sitting on a wooden bath-seat... and plunging his hands and feet in the water one after the other'.[25] Although the waters at Albulae were usually classified as cold, Caelius Aurelianus describes them as hot springs which can provide treatment for arthritis or for paralysis.[26]

The largest island of the Grecian archipelago, near the town of Aedepsus, modern Lipsos, was known as 'The Baths of Heracles'. The Greek biographer Plutarch mentions its therapy by the dictator L. Cornelius Sulla:[27]

> During Sulla's stay about Athens, his feet were attacked by a heavy benumbing pain, which Strabo calls the first inarticulate sounds of the gout. Taking, therefore, a voyage to Aedepsus, he made use of the hot waters there, allowing himself at the same time to forget all anxieties, and passing away his time with actors.

These springs, strongly sulphurous with outflow temperature of 78°C, rise a short distance inland at several points, and at last pour steaming over the rocks, which they have yellowed with their deposit, into the Euboic Sea. They are still frequented by the Greeks for the cure of gout, rheumatism and digestive disorders.[28] For bladder troubles, the waters of Aquae Auguriae were recommended by Caelius Aurelianus.[29]

---

[23] Pliny, *Naturalis Historia* 31A; Celsus, *De Medicina* 4.12; See also Tacitus, *Annals* 11. 13; See Allen (1998): 14, 31; On sacred springs to be cold waters, see Croon (1967): 225–246.

[24] Vitruvius, *De Architectura* 8.3.2; See Rowland (1999): 99; Allen (1998): 21–22, 26; Strabo, *Geographica* 5.3.2; Martial, *Epigrammata* 1.12; Pliny, *Naturalis Historia* 31.6.

[25] *Suetonius, De Vita Caesarum, Augustus* 82.2; See also Allen (1998): 26, 32, 104.

[26] Caelius Aurelianus, *De Acutis Morbis* 5.2.40; See also 2.1.48.

[27] Plutarch, *Vitae Demetrius et Antonius Pyrrhus et Caius Marius* 34.2; Ginouvès (1962): 362; Croon (1967): 244.

[28] Frazer (1951): 211–212; Fiedler (1840): 487–492; Neumann and Partsch (1885): 342–344; Croon (1967): 230, 246; Krug (1993): 183–184; Fytikas, Leonidopoulou and Cataldi (1999): 86–87, 90.

[29] Caelius Aurelianus, *De Acutis Morbis* 5.4.77.

We can infer that the natural hot mineral springs at Bath Spa in
Gloucestershire, Britain, had been venerated from very early times. Such
sites have universally been held in awe and respect. After the Roman
conquest, the place was rapidly magnificent classical buildings.[30] Of all
Roman-British towns, the most bath-conscious was Bath (Aquae Sulis)
where people arrived—as they do today—to take waters. In spite of
this well known fact there are no historical evidences from the Roman
period to demonstrate the specific site. During the third century CE,
Solinus, the Roman author of *Collectanea Rerum Memorabilium*, a descrip-
tive book about places, recorded the luxurious furnishings of the springs
at Britain and also commented: 'there are many great rivers and hot
springs richly adorned for the use of men. The patron godhead over
these springs is Minerva, in whose temple perpetual fires never whiten
into ashes'. Minerva was conflated with a local healer, Sulis, who presided over the great sanctuary.[31] At Bath Spa the waters are said to
benefit those suffering from rheumatism, gout, dyspepsia, skin diseases,
anaemia, and diseases of the nervous system.[32] (See Fig. 1).

Allason-Jones has recommended that doctors were present at the
sanctuary at Bath and the practice empirical medicine went hand in
hand with spiritual healing. Stamps for eye-physician, Janianus, may
have held a regular clinic there. The many women who patronized
Sulis' shrine perhaps found especial help for child-bearing disorders.
The model bronze and ivory breasts offered to the goddess may have
been associated with lactation.[33] Henig has suggested that the ivory ones
may have been worn as an amulet by a woman until she had success-
fully weaned her infant when, in thanksgiving for the vital supply of
milk, she gave the models to Sulis.[34]

One of the more famous ancient healing places was Baiae, on the
coast of Campania, at the northern end of the bay of Naples. Plutarch
relates that Marius, who fought against Jugorta, the king of Numidia,
was advised to go to the hot springs of Baiae for treatment of his failing health: 'he had been weakened by age and rheumatism'.[35] Baiae

---

[30] Potter and Johns (2002): 174; Kellaway (1991).
[31] Solinus, *Collectanea Rerum Memorabilium* 22.10; According to him the shrine was
called *fons Minervae*; See also Smith (1944): 15; Grant (1995): 50–53; Henig (1995): 43;
Adkins and Adkins (2000): 211–212; Wacher (2002): II: 791.
[32] Jackson (1999): 109, note 20; Smith (1944): 11–12, 14–15.
[33] Allason-Jones (1989): 156–157; Green (1995): 95.
[34] Henig (1988): 5–6.
[35] Plutarch, *Vitae Demetrius et Antonius Pyrrhus et Caius Marius* 34.2; See Smith (1922):

became the most fashionable Roman place of healing. Celsus advised sweating in hot vapour baths, especially the sulfur baths at Baiae, and Strabo described the site and its hot springs, which were appropriate both for the tastes of the discerning, and for the curing of diseases.[36] The wealthy upper classes and the crippled frequented the place in multitudes to utilize the waters and to take part in the social activities. Baiae became famous not only for its springs but also for its debauchery. Martial was one of many who described its temptations, which lured the virtuous.[37] Josephus describes the varied facilities of Baiae when recounting the visit of Caius Caligula:[38]

> There are in that place royal palaces, with sumptuous apartments, every emperor still endeavoring to outdo his predecessor's magnificence; the place also affords warm baths, that spring out of the ground of their own accord, which are of advantage for the recovery of the health of those that make use of them, and, besides, they minister to men's luxury also.

The activities taking place in the baths at Baiae are described by the younger Seneca, whose rooms were adjacent to a bathing establishment:[39]

> So picture to yourself the assortment of sounds, which are strong enough to make me hate my very powers of hearing! When your strenuous gentleman, for example, is exercising himself by flourishing leaden weights, when he is working hard, or else pretends to be working hard, I can hear him grunt; and whenever he releases his imprisoned breath, I can hear him panting in wheezy and high-pitched tones. Or perhaps I notice some lazy fellow, content with a cheap rub down according as the hand is laid on flat or hollow. Then, perhaps, a professional comes along, shouting out the score; that is the finishing touch. Add to this the arresting of an occasional roisterer or pickpocket, the racket of the man who always likes to hear his own voice in the bathroom, or the enthusiast who plunges into the swimming-tank with unconscionable noise and splashing. Besides all those whose voices, if nothing else, are good, imagine the

---

621–622; D'Arms (1970): 23–28; Comfort (1976): 137–138; For a preliminary investigation of the spas in Campania, see Houston (1992): 356–379; Yegül (1996): 137–161; cf. Allen (1998): 10–11.

[36] Celsus, *De Medicina* 2.17.1; Strabo, *Geographica* 5.4–5.

[37] Martial, *Epigrammata* 1.42; See also Maiuri (1989); McKay (1989): 155–172; Amalfitano, Camodeca and Medri (1990): 183–234; For the upper class Romans' visits at Baiae and the surrounding area, see Allen (1998): 126–131.

[38] Josephus, *Antiquitates Judaicae* 18.249; Neuburger (1919): 71.

[39] Seneca, *Epistulae Morales* 56.1–2; See also Shelton (1988): 314.

hair-pluckier with his penetrating, shrill voice—for purposes of advertise-
ment—continually giving it vent and never holding his tongue except when
he is plucking the armpits and making his victim yell instead. Then the
cake-seller with his varied cries, the sausage-man, the confectioner, and
all the vendors of food hawking their wares, each with his own distinctive intonation.

However, the experience not exactly enjoyed by Seneca may not
have been typical of all bathing establishments. According to Pliny
the Younger, other healing places were more modest than Baiae.[40] The
fourth century CE Greek biographer Eunapius notes that the thermal
baths of Hammat-Gader were:[41]

> Second only to those at Baiae, with which no other baths can be compared
> throughout the Roman world.

The Classical writers were acquainted with the curative springs of
Hammei-Tiberias, Hammat-Gader, Hammat-Pella, Hammei-Ba'arah,
Kallirrhoe, Emmaus-Nicopolis and Hammei-Livias. All of them will
be demonstrated later on.[42]

3.3   Ritual Worship

Many medicinal hot springs through the Graeco-Roman world were
dedicated to Heracles, to the Nymphs and to gods with healing capabilities, such as Apollo, Aesculapius, Hygieia, Zeus, Jupiter, Vulcan,
Artemis, Mars, Athena, Minerva, Venus, Mercury, Dionysus, Silvanus
and the Three Graces.[43] All of those are evidenced by sculptures of
the gods, votive offerings, and literary sources, including texts and
inscriptions, which provide further information about the existence of

---

[40] Pliny the Younger, *Epistulae* 8.8.
[41] Eunapius, *Vitae Sophistarum* 459; Dechent (1884): 190–191; Sukenik (1935a): 21;
Lieberman (1946): 354; Hirschfeld and Solar (1981): 202; Hirschfeld (1987): 104;
Geiger (1986): 375–376; Dvorjetski (1988): 92; Yegül (1992): 121; Dvorjetski (1994a):
16–17; Hirschfeld (1997): 5; Dvorjetski (1997a): 465; idem, (2001–2002): 492; idem,
(2004): 19.
[42] See the intensive discussion in chapter 4 on *The Historical-Archaeological Analysis and
Healing Cults of the Therapeutic Sites in the Eastern Mediterranean Basin.*
[43] Smith (1922): 393; Frazer (1951): 209–213; Weiss and Kemble (1962): 11; Croon
(1967): 230, 244; Jackson (1990a): 5–9; Dvorjetski (1994a): 16–19; idem, (1997a):
465–468; Albu, Banks and Nash (1997): 4–5; Fytikas, Leonidopoulou and Cataldi
(1999): 84–85, 91–94; Cataldi and Burgassi (1999): 152.

religion in spas. Notwithstanding these do not provide a clear picture of the religiosity of a spa.

The choice of Heracles, the mythological hero, as patron of hot springs, and subsequently of medicinal hot baths, was based on a combination of the elements water and fire, fertility and destruction, which are apparently contradictory but are linked to his life and death. According to the second century CE Greek author Lucianus of Samosata, Heracles refused to make way for Aesculapius. They quarreled over this and Zeus decided in favor of Aesculapius, who was the senior of the two: 'It is only logical, Heracles, that Aesculapius should be placed above you, because he died before you.'[44]

The hot springs of Thermopylae were among those that were dedicated to Heracles. Strabo explains that the name means hot gates,[45]

> Because there, near the place, there are hot springs which are dedicated [= by the local inhabitants] to Heracles.

Herodotus described the site in the fifth century BCE, emphasizing that an altar to Heracles stood there.[46] His contemporary Aristophanes, in his treatise, Νεφέλαι, 'The Clouds', alludes to the tradition of the period by asking rhetorically: 'Have you ever seen baths of Heracles that were cold?'[47] The anonymous author of the notable tenth century Greek lexicon *Suidae* deduces from the expression Ἡράκλια λουτρά that these baths were given to Heracles as a gift by Hephaestus.[48] In accordance with this expression, it can be assumed that the Greeks usually termed natural hot springs *Heracleia*.[49] Two other sites of medicinal hot springs were consecrated to Heracles. One is in Hierapolis (Pamukkale) southeast of Sardis. It gained wide publicity due to the reputed healing properties of its springs, which are still in use.[50] The other is the spa

---

[44] Lucianus of Samosata, *Dialogi Deorum* 15.13.238; On Heracles' capabilities as the god of hot springs, see Frazer (1951): 209–213; Boardman (1988): 787; Moitreux (1992): 67–76.

[45] Strabo, *Geographica* 9.4.13.

[46] Herodotus, *Historiae* 7.176.

[47] Aristophanes, *The Clouds* 1050–1052; See also Croon (1967): 244.

[48] *Suidae Lexicon* 581.

[49] Diodorus Siculus, *Bibliotheca Historica* 4.23.1; Leutsch and Schneidewin (1958): 174; Frazer (1951): 211.

[50] Strabo, *Geographica* 13.4.14; Vitruvius, *De Architectura* 7.3.10; Chandler (1776): 228–235; Davis (1874): 97–112; Kekeç (1989): 15–46; Dvorjetski (1992a): 38; Özgüler and Kasap (1999): 58–62.

of Aedepsus, on the west coast of Euboea Island, in a volcanic region which is subject to frequent earthquakes.[51]

The link between hot springs and the worship of Heracles was not confined to Greece alone. The Greek influence spread to Dacia—present-day Romania—Italy, and Sicily.[52] An interesting legend has been preserved by the first century BCE Greek historian Diodorus Siculus about the association of the deeds of the Nymphs with Athena and Heracles, with regard to the springs of Himera in Sicily:[53]

> In the region of Himera, where the Nymphs, in order to find favor with Athena, caused the hot water springs to erupt and flow forth vigorously when Heracles visited the island. And the inhabitants dedicated a town and a tract of land, which is called until now Athena.

The Greek poet Pindaros (520–442 BCE) calls Himera 'the hot baths of the Nymphs'.[54] The city's coins bear the figure of Heracles, as a youth or bearded, as well an image of a Nymph sacrificing at an altar. Behind her is a satyr standing in a basin below a fountain which pours from a lion's head spout. These baths which are partially preserved are known by the modern name Thermi Imerese.[55]

The beliefs of the healing powers of the local spring traveled with the Greek colonists to, for example, the Provence region. The Greeks had become established at Glanon, near Saint Remy-de-Provence, by the end of the third century BCE. There was already a Celto-Ligurian settlement here with a shrine dedicated to the curative waters and now a beautiful Hellenistic city was built, which reached its peak in the second century BCE. The city centre was dominated by a monumental temple built close to the miraculous fountain, which was dedicated to the Nymphs and to Apollo the Healer.[56]

---

[51] Strabo, *Geographica* 1.3.16.20; Thucydides, *Historiae* 3.87.89; Neumann and Partsch (1885): 321–323; Smith (1922): 392–393; Ginouvès (1962): 362, notes 11–13; Croon (1967): 244.

[52] For Dacia, see for example Dessau (1902): *ILS*, II/1: no. 3891; For Italy see Wilmanns (1873): 227: no. 735c; Nissen (1885): 798; Frazer (1951): 213, and for Sicily, see Baedeker (1880): 356–357.

[53] Diodorus Siculus, *Bibliotheca Historica* 4.23.1; 5.3.4; See also Fytikas, Leonidopoulou and Cataldi (1999): 84.

[54] Pindaros, *Odes* 1.19.

[55] Ziegler (1929); Frazer (1951): 213; Krug (1993): 181–182; Penn (1994): 29, 139; Belvedere and Alliata (1988–2002): III.

[56] Lévêque (1987).

The relationship between the Etruscans and active geothermal manifestations included religious aspects, such as divination based on the shapes of the steam plumes from fumaroles, a unique belief in the afterlife, and the formation of cults for subterranean divinities. The worship of Velchans, the equivalent of the Greek God Hephaestus, keeper of fire and volcanoes, seems a practice initially borrowed from the Hellenic world. However, the Etruscans elaborated on it and brought the cult first to Etruria proper and afterwards to Southwestern Italy, site of trading outposts, such as Capua and Cumae at the Campania region.[57]

The Celts of the third to the first century BCE worshipped curative springs and the goddesses associated with them. They used the waters of the thermal spring, for example, at Teplice, the German Teplitz, in northern Bohemia, and elsewhere for bathing therapy.[58]

In several cases, votive offerings have been discovered in Italy, which demonstrate a pre-Roman cult use at sites with thermo-mineral spring. Three were found near Montegroto Terme (Aquae Aponi). Several bronze figurines, including a group of small horses, nearly 4000 clay vases together with a few bronze and gold vessels were found in the area where the spring waters are known to be collected—attest to religious activity. The small bronze feet and arm also provide evidence of making anatomical votive offerings at a healing spring which latter became a spa.[59] At Aquae Sinuessanae, some of the ex-votos of around 5000 statuettes are believed to be pre-Roman.[60] At Vicarello, a collection of votive offerings, including many vases and coins, was found in the basin around the spring. Most of the objects belong to the Roman period and some indicate that the cult began earlier. Republican coins were recovered from the spring, silver goblets, and a large number of metallic vases made of gold, silver and bronze. Many of them are inscribed with dedications to Apollo, Numphs, Silvanus, and Aesculapius.[61] A series of votive reliefs found on the island of Aenaria (Ischia), date from

---

[57] Cataldi and Chiellini (1999): 170–171.

[58] Drimba (1987); Albu, Banks and Nash (1997): 5; Chyský, Skalník and Adamec (1967).

[59] Lazzaro (1981): 31–44, 105–106; Migliolaro (1956): 35; Zanovello and Basso (2004).

[60] Arthur (1991): 111.

[61] Heurgon (1952): 39–50; Colini (1968): 35–56; Künzl and Künzl (1992): 273–296; Allen (1998): 178, 182–183; Fytikas, Leonidopoulou and Cataldi (1999): 91–92.

the first century BCE through to the fourth century CE, are similar in style and probably are products of a local workshop. The inscriptions specially refer to the Nymphs and Apollo.[62]

The literary sources from the Roman period reveal little about the nature of cult activity or religious belief at spas. The texts are as follows: A letter from Seneca to Lucilius reveals the religious belief which could exist with respect to springs. He says that springs of hot water are worshipped as devine.[63] He apparently sees no contradiction between the belief in the divinity of springs and his interest in natural science and rational medicine. Seneca efforts to explain the cause of thermo-mineral springs as part of natural science arise from his Stoic philosophy.[64] Martial mentions several times the Nymphs in their healing capacity. They are identified as having a role in the healing of a visitor named Philostratus at the baths of Aquae Sinuessanae. The thermo-mineral waters at Baiae are associated by him to Venus and Mars. Venus was typically found in contexts of bathing and health while Mars also had a role as healer, but is not normally found at baths.[65] Claudian attributes the heat of the springs at Aquae Aponi to Vulcan.[66] Allen points out that the lake of references to divinities at spas is somewhat curious. It would appear that in the descriptions of activity in spas, there was a much greater interest in the rational procedures which occurred. The few allusions to gods at the therapeutic sites are found almost only in the poets, who regularly make mythological references without clear cult implications.[67]

Sculptural material recovered from several spas in Italy:[68] Agnano, Teanum Sidicinum, Aquae Vescinae, Aquae Tauri, Vicarello, Baiae, and

---

[62] Forti (1951): 161–191.

[63] Seneca, *Epistulae Morales* 41.3.

[64] Seneca, *Quaestiones Naturales* 3.1–16; See also Griffin (1992): 40–42; French (1994): 166–178; Allen (1998): 197.

[65] Martial, *Epigrammata* 6.47; 9.58; 11.82; For Venus and Mars at Baiae, see *ibid.*, 11.80; See also Jayne (1962): 432–433.

[66] Claudian, *Carmina Minora* 26.17–18.

[67] Allen (1998): 199.

[68] The survey from Italy is based mainly on Allen (1998): 176–192; For Aesculapius, see Kerényi (1960); Hart (2000); Fulvio (1887): 409; For Apollo, see Künzl and Künzl (1992): 274; For the Nymphs, see Fulvio (1887): 409–410; Bastianelli (1933): 398–421; For a discussion of the popularity of statues of Venus in baths, see Dunbabin (1989): 24–25; and for Venus at spas see Jayne (1962): 306; Robertson (1975): II: 390–391, 548–549; Ridgway (1990): I: 355–356; Allen (1998): 186; For Dionysus see Burkett (1985): 158; Jayne (1962): 318; Macchioro (1912): 284; For a discussion of Hermes as a healing god, see Jayne (1962): 331–332; On the spread of Egyptian cults at those spas, see Allen (1998): 188–190.

Aquae Aponi. Aesculapius is the most prominent as the best known of the healing gods. Several fragments from Aquae Vescinae preserve his arm, foot, and staff with an entwined serpent and other statues from Vicarello and Aquae Aponi; A statue of Apollo was found in a *nymphaeum* associated with the baths at Vicarello and from the Baths of Mercury at Baiae; The Nymphs' association with healing springs and Aesculapius made then appropriate for display at spas. Female figures identified as Nymphs are known from Agnano, Aquae Vescinae, and Aquae Tauri; Venus is regularly found in baths and also appears in healing spas as she is associated with ideas of beauty, luxury and health. At Agnano, the goddess is portrayed preparing for a bath and resembles to the Cnidian Aphrodite and to the Capitoline Venus. Another statue of Venus which is related to that of Capitoline Venus comes from the baths at Teanum Sidicinum. A third statue of the goddess was found at Agnano, and she has been identified as representing a Venus Armata. A small figure of Eros was beside her feet. In the Baths of Sosandra at Baiae there was a statue known as Aphrodite Sosandra; Each of two small figures from Teanum Sidicinum may be identified as Eros; Dionysus is also an appropriate figure to have in a spa. As the god of wine and intoxication he is the god who is capable of freeing the mind from cares and troubles. But he also had specific associations with healing. A statue of infant Dionysus and Hermes is known from Agnano as well as two statues of satyrs with Dionysus or with the Nymphs. At Aquae Tauri the bearded head of Hermes was found. As god of the *palaestra* and *gymnasium*, Hermes represents youth and vigour. Allen is absolutely convinced by clarifying that his image was viewed as an inspiration to those using the spa. He adds also that Hermes role as a leader of souls to the Underworld also had obvious implications for those seeking health, and in this function Hermes can be seen to have some association with healing as a guardian of life.[69]

A number of gods who do not necessarily have a primary role as healers are also indicated in dedicated inscriptions from the spas in Italy. Thus, at Aquae Caeretanae, one inscription refers to Jupiter and another refers to Jupiter and Hercules.[70] In contrast with this, the most common reference to divinities in inscriptions is to Nymphs. Dedication

---

[69] Allen (1998): 187.
[70] *AE* (1989): no. 305.

on an alter and inscriptions on votive reliefs are known from Aquae
Tauri, Aquae Sinuessanae, Puteoli, Vicarello, Aenaria, and Aquae
Apollinares.[71] Apollo could also be invoked together with the Nymphs
as in Aenaria and Vicarello.[72] In the latter site, an attempt was made
to include as many gods as could be propitiated in a single dedication.
Thus, Apollo, Silvanus, the Nymphs, and in one case, Aesculapius were
named together in the inscription.[73] At Aquae Vescinae, an inscription
dedicated to Hygieia, was found in the outlet of a thermo-mineral
spring.[74]

    Throughout the Roman Empire, a deity of local or general repute
was combined with the parallel Graeco-Roman deity in accordance
with its power and influence. The healing gods of both Gaul and
Germany were frequently identified with Apollo the Healer, as at the
shrines of Essarois near Dijon, where an inscription records Apollo
Vindonnus.[75] At Aachen, Apollo was affiliated with the local god,
native deity, Grannus as the central deity of a group of medicinal hot
springs.[76] Apollo Grannus was an especially popular healing deity of
springs in the Rhine, Moselle region. Sometimes he had a divine partner, the goddess Sirona, who fulfilled the same role as Hygieia. Thus
on a statue from the shrine of Apollo and Sirona at Hochscheid near
Bernkastel, Sirona is depicted in the guise of Hygieia feeding a snake
which is entwined around her forearm. An altar found in Aachen possibly depicts the image of Apollo Grannus sitting on a throne holding
a lyre and a plectrum and carrying a quiver of arrows on his right
shoulder. Its inscription indicates that the altar was dedicated 'to fulfill
a vow' by Latinius Macer from Verona, who served as *praefectus castrorum*
[= senior officer] of the Legion IX *Hispania*, who may have been restored
to health or healing for recuperation at the spa.[77] Another high-ranking
visitor to this site could have been Caracalla. Apollo Grannus was a
famous healing deity, and the sick Emperor visited sites dedicated to

---

[71] Mengarelli (1923): 343; *CIL* 10.4734; *CIL* 10.1592; *CIL* 11.3290.
[72] *CIL* 10.6786; *CIL* 10.6787; 10.6788; *CIL* 3287—There is a direct reference to
health in an offering *pro salute* (Vicarello).
[73] *CIL* 11.3289; *CIL* 11.3294.
[74] Fulvio (1888): 460; Giglioli (1911): 39–87; Sobel (1990).
[75] Hatt (1985): 205–238; Dehn (1941): 104–111, Pl. 14; Krug (1993): 176–177.
[76] Jackson (1990a): 8; idem, (1988): 163; Cüppers (1982); Hugot (1963): 188–197.
[77] Dehn (1941): 104–111, Pl. 14; Nesselhauf and Petrikovits (1967): 268–279; Jackson
(1988): 163; Goethert (2001): 28; Wood (2004): 33–34.

him during his 'temple tour' between 211 and 217 CE, according to the evidence of Cassius Dio.[78] (See Fig. 4).

There is a connection of a votive inscription found at al-Harra in southern Syria to the local cult of Hammei-Ba'arah, known as Baaras springs, situated in Wadi Zarqa Ma'in in the eastern shore of the Dead Sea. The altar was dedicated by a certain Diomedes Charetos, a Roman official of the Bataneae in the rank of a governor (*eparches*) and military commander (*strategos*). For the sake of his recovery he donated the votive offering to Zeus Beelbaaros, the local god of the curative place of Hammei-Ba'arah. Unfortunately, no imagery representations survived to explain the features of this deity.[79]

Before the penetration of Roman influence, the Dacians practiced balneal therapy and internal cures with mineral waters.[80] In Roman Dacia, thermal waters were used for therapy at places well known, such as Ad Mediam (Băile Herculane) and Germisara (Georgiu). Of these, the most important was undoubtedly Ad Mediam, where the springs were tapped and pipes, pools and buildings for balneal treatment were constructed. The curative qualities of the waters were acknowledges in dedications to the healing divinities Hercules, Aesculapius and Hygieia, 'dis et numinibus aquarum', to the warm springs 'fontibus calidis' and to the spirit of the place Genio Loci.[81] Germisara, with the renowned 'Thermae Dodonae', was equipped for curative baths by a detachment of the Legion XIII *Gemina* from Apulum.[82]

One of Baiae's impressive edifices is the Temple of Mercury, a vaulted circular building with high windows that served for illumination and ventilation. The water entered the structure of a *nymphaeum*. Statues decorated the niches. Nearby are two other bathing complexes: the baths of Sosandra on three levels, and the baths of Venus. The Temple of Venus is a huge vaulted building, reminiscent of the unique vaulted

---

[78] Cassius Dio, *Historia Romana* 78.15.3–7; Engelmann (1980): no. 802; Jackson (1990ª): 8; Drug (1993): 175; See also the discussion in chapter 7 on *The Roman Emperors at the Spas in the Eastern Mediterranean.*

[79] Sourdel (1952): 45–46; Hübner (1995): 252–255; Weber (1997): 332–333; On Hammei-Ba'arah and the identification of the local god Zeus Beelbaaros, see the discussion on *The Historical-Archaeological Analysis of Hammei-Ba'arah* in chapter 4.5.

[80] Drimba (1984).

[81] Macrea (1969); Ardet (1996): 3; Sauer (1996): 68; Cohut and Árpási (1999): 244–245.

[82] Szabó (1978); Albu, Banks and Nash (1997): 5; Cohut and Árpási (1999): 243–244.

structure in Pergamon dedicated to Aesculapius which is associated with therapeutic bathing or some similar form of hydrotherapy.[83]

Four deep-bowled pans were found at Baden. Two of them were dedicated to Mercury by T. Cammianius Bacchus 'gladly and willingly in fulfillment of a vow', perhaps after a successful treatment;[84] and one from Augst in Switzerland inscribed with a dedication to the Gallic healing pair Apollo and Sirona.[85]

One of the principal Roman imperial medicinal hot baths in Britain was at Bath Spa, also known as Aquae Sulis. The predominant local deity was Sulis Minerva—a combination of the Celtic Sul or Sulis and Minerva, the Roman goddess of wisdom, invention, the martial arts and crafts, who also had a healing aspect as Minerva Medica. She may have been invoked at Bath as a spirit of the craft of medicine, in other words, associated with both healing and craft-skills. First and foremost Sulis was the native goddess of the curative hot springs beside the River Avon at Bath. The numerous inscriptions on stone and lead or pewter attest to her equation with Minerva. As happened with Mars in Celtic Europe, the war-element in Minerva's cult may have been transmuted to guardianship against disease. The cult of Sulis flourished because of her reputation as a goddess of healing and because the springs produced curative hot water, which could ease gout and rheumatism.[86]

Two of the impressive finds from Bath are a life-size gilded bronze head of Minerva from a life-size statue, probably the cult figure itself, and a sculptured cornice which features two winged figures near a Gorgon's head—a classical motif which is presented in Celtic style. This blend of two entirely different iconographic traditions reflected very well the identity of Minerva and Sulis. Furthermore, the Gorgon sculpture has several characteristics which are reminiscent of the deities of sun and water. Above the monumental opening between the temple *temenos* and the holy spring, the relief on the cornice shows the head of

---

[83] Behr (1968): 27–28; Ziegenaus (1981): 76–100; Yegül (1992): 106–108; idem, (1996): 93–110; Allen (1998): 82–101; Jacobson and Wilson-Jones (1999): 57–71; Branda, Luciani, Costantini and Piccioli (2001): 609–614.

[84] Wiedemer (1967): 91–92; Jackson (1990a): 12.

[85] Staehelin (1948): 538–541.

[86] Green (1995): 93–94; Grant (1995): 50–53; See also Smith (1922): 501; Smith (1944): 17–18; Neville Havins (1976): 13; Sauer (1996): 63–68; Adkins and Adkins (2000): 212.

the sun god, Sol, being held by two water Nymphs above a rock from which the spring water gushes.[87] (See Fig. 2).

The spring in Bath Spa was always the dominant component of the bathing complex and the focus for personal contact with the goddess, where vows, prayers, requests and thanksgiving took place. Grateful suppliants and others could reach the spring from the temple to bathe, to contemplate the sacred waters, and to cast gifts into the spring-water, including money and more personal objects such as brooches, pins, shoes, spindle-whorls, and their votive offerings in gratitude for the healing bestowed by Sulis-Minerva. The ailments from which the people suffered can be surmised from the artifacts that have been found at Aquae Sulis, such as a fragment of a bronze breast and a carved ivory cameo featuring breasts and the vows of those treated. More than 20 Roman vessels with flat handles, made of pewter, copper or bronze, were found in the vicinity of the spring. Six of them bear dedicatory inscriptions to the local gods Sulis or Minerva. This type of pan was used in cultic ceremonies such as libations and the serving of wine, but could certainly have been utilized at Bath for drinking water as a remedy. Jugs or deep jars have been found at other medicinal sites and temples, such as four from Baden, two of which are dedicated to Mercury 'joyfully and willingly in fulfillment of a vow'.[88]

We know of some employees of the Temple of Sulis Minerva. One of them was the temple augur Lucius Marcius Memor, whose inscribed statue base in its original position was uncovered on the precinct floor. As a *haruspex* [= gut-gazer] he would have been a member of an elite class of augurs who officiated in the principal temples of the Empire, foretelling the future through their closely guarded knowledge of omens. There is some direct evidence for ritual activities associated with the veneration of Sulis: a priest of the cult, Gaius Calpurnius Receptus, served at the temple until his death at Bath Spa aged 75. His wife, Calpurnia, who had once been his slave, set up his tombstone, a simple affair carved piously in the form of an altar. Two other dignitaries connected with the temple were Claudius Ligur and Gaius Protacius. They were responsible for the restoration and repairing of a monument or

---

[87] Richmond and Toynbee (1955): 97–105; Cunliffe and Davenport (1985): 114–115; Yegül (1992): 117–119; Cunliffe (1984): 40, Fig. 40.
[88] Cunliffe (1995): 16–60; Davenport (1999): 84–89; See also Green (1995): 96; Jackson (1990a): 11–12; For Baden see Wiedemer (1967): 91–92.

building belonging to the temple. Cunliffe records that both of them were probably public-minded citizens willing to show their devotion to the gods, and incidentally to their fellows, by making a donation in aid of good works.[89]

People would have flocked to Bath from other parts of the Roman Empire and from all over the Celtic world in search of divine aid. Some erected alters or tombstones to the gods for their safe journey or their recovery or for some other service. Thus, Peregrinus son of Secundus, a Treveran from Gallia Belgica, brought with him his local cult and offered an altar to his two favourite deities, Loucetius Mars, god of war, and his consort Nemetona, goddess of the sacred grove. She was Gaulish and British goddess whose name appears in many ancient inscriptions and was venerated by the Celto-Germanic people called the Nemetes, whose name shares her root name. Loucetius was the epithet of Mars. A *lapidaries* [= stonemason] from Chartres from northwestern France, Priscus son of Toutius, dedicated the inscription to Sulis, while the offering of Sulis, which may also have come from the main temple, was dedicated to a collection of local deities, the Suleviae. Altar to the Suleviae was also erected by the sculptor Sulinus son of Brucetius. Suleviae is the Latin name given to a Triad of Deae Matres [= the three mother goddesses] known in many parts of the Roman Celtic world. Iconographic and epigraphical evidence suggests that the goddesses were linked to cults of healing, regeneration, fertility, and maternity.[90] Dedications to gods other than Sulis Minerva, suggesting as Cunliffe has stressed, a separate shrine, a place where travelers could thank their own patron gods without risk of disrespect to the presiding deity.[91]

Inscriptions and curses that were written on metal tablets are perhaps the most revealing artifacts from the hot spring at Bath Spa. The evidence for the healing beneficence of Sulis at Bath is counterbalanced by a more sinister aspect of her character, namely her role as an avenger of wrongs. 130 *defixiones* or curse-tablets, small sheets of pewter or lead inscribed with messages to the goddess, telling her the nature of the wrong done, the name (if known) of the evil-doer,

[89] Cunliffe (1995): 102.
[90] Mackillop (2004): 303, 344–345, 393; Adkins and Adkins (2000): 143–144, 212; Wacher (2002): II: 731, 790.
[91] Cunliffe (1995): 106.

and graphic details of the desired retribution. Most of the complaints involved theft of personal property, particularly cloths. Presumably these were items shed by bathing pilgrims and left unattended: cloaks, a cap, bathing-costumes, a bath towel, a bracelet, and even a pair of gloves are recorded. Unlike the stone dedications to Sulis, not a single Roman citizen is mentioned on the curse inscriptions. Many names were of Celtic derivation. The message, appealed 'to the goddess Sulis' or 'to Sulis Minerva', often ask for revenge to affect the victim's blood, eyes, fertility, sleep or bodily functions. Another course requests vengeance from Sulis through the victim's blood and health and those of his family, so that they should be able neither to eat, to drink, to urinate nor to defecate. The language used by the cursers was often savage and emotional. Thus, for instance, 'May he who carried off Vilbia from me become liquid as the water. May she who so obscenely devoured her become dumb'; 'be cursed in their blood, eyes, and every limb, and have all intestines eaten away'. Another translates to 'I curse Tretia Maria and her life and mind and memory and liver and lungs mixed up together, and her words, thoughts and memory; thus may she be unable to speak what things are concealed, nor be able'.[92]

The goddesses were often requested to damage the physical or mental wellbeing of the perpetrator by lack of sleep, cessation of bodily functions, or death. The wretchedness could stop however, if the belongings were returned to the owner or sacrificed to the gods as requested. For example, one tablet translates to 'Solinus to the goddess Sulis Minerva. I give to your divinity and majesty my bathing tunic and cloak. Do not allow sleep or health to him who has done me wrong, whether man or woman, whether slave or free, unless he reveals himself and brings those goods to your temple'.[93]

These texts provide a fascinating insight into provincial life in all its pettiness, what it was that made people irate and how they relied heavily on the presiding deity to help them every turn. For a miscreant, even if undetected, to suspect that he had been named and cursed must have been a fearsome uncertainty to live with.[94] Historians believe

---

[92] Green (1995): 97–98; See also Cunliffe (1995): 53–54; Gager (1992): 21; Tomlin (1988): no. 41; Adams (1992): 1–26.
[93] Fagan (1999a): 37; See also Cunliffe (1995): 34.
[94] Cunliffe (1995): 54.

that many of these curses were written backwards in order to yield extra-potent magic.[95]

Another of Bath's major religious might be learnt by several archaeological remains. In the year 1885, a carved block was found in a cistern of one of the thermal springs from a depth of 6 metres, depicting scenes from the Aesculapius legend. The block of stone carved was carved with three scenes: a naked woman standing by a reclining male; a quadruped walking beneath a tree; and a snake curled round a tree. This is a very appropriate fitting for a curative spring as Aesculapius was a deity associated with healing.[96]

Apart from a dozen altars and other inscribed stones dedicated to the patron goddess Sulis Minerva, there are other known altars to other pagan deities. The sacrificial altar was the focus for public worship where priests conducted ceremonies and animal sacrifices. An altar to the *Genio Loci* or Local Spirit also one shared with Sulis Minerva, and an altar rededicated to the *Numen Augusti*, the Living Spirit of the Emperor; An altar or statue base to goddess of the hunt, Diana, which reads: 'To the goddess Diana the most holy, Vettius Benignus, freedman, fulfilled his vow'; Altars to Jupiter holding a trident in one hand while at his feet stands an eagle and to naked Hercules Bibax holding a large drinking vessel in one hand, the other resting on a knobbed club. Over his soldiers he wears a cape made of lion's skin, the paws of which are knotted over his chest; and alters for Apollo playing his lyre; and god Bacchus, who holds a *thyrsus* and pours a drink to a panther squatting at his feet; Stone relief of the god Mercury and relief carving of the Roman god Mercury and his Celtic consort Rosnerta. Beneath them are three hooded deities the *genii cucullati* and an animal; Another one is a goddess that cannot be identified, but the cornucopia which she holds and the libation flowing from the upturned vessel suggest that she is connected with fertility.[97]

In short, then, temples were erected at these spas. Each site had a spring that served as the dominant part of the bathhouse complex and was dedicated to a God of Healing. Within the boundaries of the

---

[95] See http://faculty.vassar.edu/jolott/clas217/projects/bath_project/Tablets.htm; Allason-Jones (1999): 136.

[96] Cunliffe (1984): 157–158.

[97] Cunliffe (1995): 37–39, nos. 22–25; See other explanations in Cunliffe (1984): 51–53, nos. 24–26; See also in this chapter on the section of *The Military Presence and Archaeological Finds*.

Roman Empire local deities were integrated with their parallel deities in the Graeco-Roman world. One of the significant factors contributing to the Roman use of spas was a deeply embedded religious conviction about divinities associated with healing and springs. The main purpose for seeking a spa was to use the appropriate waters necessary for a cure—not to worship a god. Yet it cannot be overlooked that certain aspects of activity at the healing spas did have a religious content and that healing for the Romans belonged to the realm of the divine.[98] (See, for instance, Fig. 3). The curative springs in the eastern Mediterranean especially those located along the Syro-African Rift in the Jordan Valley are integrated to the typical elements of those places by their ritual worship to the gods with healing powers as well as by their unique names. Roman coins of the mother cities Tiberias, Gadara and Pella with their depictions, as well as engraved gems, enable us to reveal the worship of Athena, Heracles, Hygieia, Aesculapius, the Three Graces and other deities in their suburbs, the thermo-mineral baths. These spas will be enlightened extensively in the following chapters.[99]

3.4   THE MILITARY PRESENCE

It is very rare for our literary sources to go into much detail about the location of the units of the Roman army at any fixed period. Even when they do so, these authors tended to be mainly concerned with the locations of the legions and are particularly vague about the garrisons provided by the *auxillia*. A large number of military sites have been located and a reasonable number partially excavated, although it should be noted that some regions, notably Britain and Germany, have received far more attention, and are therefore much better known, than others. The movements of legions, given their sheer size, status and frequent appearance in the epigraphic record, and comparatively straightforward to trace, although even so there is often doubt about the circumstances in which a few of these units disappeared. The Roman army—and especially in Europe—was spread around the frontier provinces. Deepest within the province were often the great fortresses of the legions usually lying on the most important route of communication,

---

[98] Allen (1998): 176.
[99] See chapter 8 on *The Numismatic Expression of the Medicinal Hot Springs.*

whilst auxiliary forts and small outposts were mainly dotted around the periphery. In the eastern provinces a significant number of military garrisons were based in or near cities. The continued good health and fitness of its soldiers was essential for maintaining the army's effectiveness. Roman bases and temporary camps were supposed to be sited as healthy a location as possible. Bathhouses were provided to keep the soldiers clean, and drains and latrines to ensure reasonable standards of hygiene.[100] The allocation of considerable military resources to the construction of facilities at medicinal sites was motivated not by public concern, but by the army's self-interest. The military sick or wounded were sent to these places, which also served as rest and recreation centres for healthy soldiers.[101]

The presence of soldiers spurred the economic growth and prosperity of the medicinal sites.[102] There were not a few clashes developed between the soldiers and the local population. A fascinating document, dating from 238 CE illustrates the sufferings of the inhabitants of the village of Scaptopara in Thrace (Bulgaria) at the hands of the Roman soldiers, 'because of the hot springs' in the vicinity of their village. In a letter of complaint and supplication to the Emperor Gordianus III, the inhabitants complained that soldiers from two nearby forts made deliberate detours to take advantage of their excellent hot springs. What is more, they demanded food and hospitality and refused to pay for them, despite an order of the governor:[103]

> We are land-owners and inhabitants of a village close to two army camps, to which many come because of the hot springs... A great and famous fair is held every year two miles from the village. Those who come to the fair force us to give them lodging and other services without payment; and the military do likewise. Many of the governors of the region and many of your inspectors come here because of the hot springs. We shall

[100] Goldsworthy (2003): 99, 142–143; For the medical provision for the military in general, see Boon (1983): 1–12: Jackson (1993): 84; idem, (1996): 2228–2251; Cruse (2004): 204–207.

[101] Collingwood and Wright (1965): nos. 139, 143–144, 146, 147, 152, 156–160; Scarborough (1969): 109–121; Davies (1970): 84–104, especially p. 100; Webster (1979): 248–254; Jackson (1988): 136.

[102] See for example, Milne (1907): 144–145; Mylius (1936); Staehelin (1948): 487; Wiedemer (1967); Davies (1970); Unz (1971); Künzl (1986); Jackson (1988): 112–147; idem, (1990b): 5–27; Cunliffe (1995); Sauer (1999): 53–54.

[103] *CIL* III, no. 12336; Rostovtzeff (1957): 478–479; Alon (1971): 186–187; Dvorjetski (1992a): 165: idem, (1997): 468.

accept them, but we are unable to accept the others. We have several times told the governor of Thrace that we cannot stay in our village, and that we are forced to abandon it because of this exploitation... and that we, too, like many before us, are about to leave the village, the foundation of our homeland. Therefore we ask you to direct that we be not harassed by demands for lodging, since the bishop has given orders that only the emissaries of the governor and the inspectors should be given accommodation. If not—we shall flee our ancestral homes, and the royal treasury will suffer a great loss.

Friction between soldiers and civilians is clearly nothing new. At another spa, Hammat-Gader, Roman military interference in the therapeutic baths, is shown clearly in the *Jerusalem Talmud, Eruvin* 6, 4 [23c]. There is an interesting distinction between the arbitrary and 'legal' actions of the officials.[104]

If the provincials sometimes had cause for complaint against the army, then they also had reason to be thankful. Many advantages accrued to those who lived in the neighbourhood of military garrisons, not least the opportunity to profit, by trade and services, from the presence of large numbers of well-paid soldiers. Beyond this the army participated in many 'community projects', especially the construction of roads, civic buildings, aqueducts, sewers and more. Many commanders no doubt made a conscious effort to establish and maintain good relations with the local population. They would certainly have worked together with the local aristocracy and town councils, while through common-law marriage of the other ranks; we may assume, according to Jackson, that there was normally a rapid integration of static garrisons.[105]

A military presence was the key to the development of Aachen, as in many other places of healing in the Roman Empire. An altar found in Aachen possibly depicts the image of Apollo Grannus sitting on a throne holding a lyre and a plectrum and carrying a quiver of arrows on his right shoulder. Its inscription indicates that the altar was dedicated 'to fulfill a vow' by Latinius Macer from Verona, who served as *praefectus castrorum* of the Legion IX *Hispania* which had come to this place of healing for recuperation.[106] (Fig. 4).

---

[104] Lieberman (1946): 354; Urbach (1976): 125–126; Dvorjetski (1997): 468; idem, (2001–2002): 499.
[105] Jackson (1988): 136–137; See also Nutton (2003): 49–51.
[106] Nesselhauf and Petrikovits (1967): 268–279.

At the end of the first century CE, units of the Legion VI *Ferrata* and Legion XXX *Ulpia Victrix* stationed across the River Rhine at Novaesium, the modern Neuss, near Düsseldorf, and at Vetera, present day Xanten on the lower Rhine, built two bath complexes above the sulfurous hot springs, which were called Buchelthermae and Münster thermae. A *temenos* with two Roman Celtic temples, located within the site of the therapeutic Grannus springs, emphasizes the importance that was attributed to divine influence. Xanten might be an example for the presence of diagnostically medical artifacts that provide a glimpse of the healing aspect of baths. Surgical instruments, including two scalpels and a pair of bone chisels, permitted at Xanten the tentative identification of a suite of rooms as a surgery or *taberna medica*.[107] The most complete plan, with a systematic layout modified, is that of the *valetudinarium* [= hospital] in the double legionary fortress at Vetera, built in stone in the time of Emperor Nero. The hospital is described as possessing colonnaded rows of rooms, a reception ward and an operating theatre. Next to this was a room where there had been hearths which could also have served a number of purposes in connection with the functioning of a hospital. A corridor ran from one side of the long hall to the other where there may have been kitchens, cooking ranges and pantries. On the west side were hot and cold baths, latrines and rooms that could have served as treatment areas. A small set of surgical instruments found in a room at the Roman baths. The provision of these facilities meant that the hospital could be almost independent of the main garrison, making life easier for patients and also minimizing the spread of disease.[108]

Military involvement is evident at Aquae Helveticae, the Swiss healing site of Baden, whose god was Mercury. It served the Roman legionnaires stationed in Vindonissa, modern Windisch in Switzerland. A building discovered there yielded numerous medical instruments, as well as tiles bearing the seal of the legion. This building has been identi-

---

[107] Gask and Todd (1953): 123–124; Hugot (1963); Cüppers (1982); Jackson (1990a): 8; idem, (1999): 109–110; For other archaeological evidence suggesting medical treatment at baths, see Künzl (1986): 491–509; idem, (1989–1990): 147–152; idem, (1996): 2433–2639.

[108] An excellent examination of Roman military hospitals, with the ground plans of several, is provided in Majno (1991): 381–390; See also Scarborough (1969): 66–75; Jackson (1988): 129–137; Newmyer (1996b): 78, 82–85; For the legionary fortress at Vetera, see Oelmann, Bader and Hagen (1932): 273–278; Jackson (1988): 48; Cruse (2004): 99.

fied as a military hospital and clinic.[109] Some of the instruments might have been for cosmetic use, while others included bronze catheters for males, most appropriate medical instrument to have been found at a spa: urinary complaints must have been commonly treated and relieved by spa therapy, then and now. Furthermore, the catheters also serve as a reminder that spas attracted physicians as well as patients, just as physicians were drawn to the crowds of potential customers at town baths. As yet no lithotomic instruments have been found in a baths context, but it is likely that lithotomists will have been drawn to baths and spas. These finds indicate that physicians were present at the healing sites.[110] The excavations at Baden revealed a bath complex built on the slope from which the hot springs emerge. A system of conduits conveyed the hot spring water to a series of basins and pools. One of the pools was provided with stepped sides permitting perhaps as many as 100 bathers to sit immersed in the 45°C water. The arrangement is similar to that at the spa of Badenweiler, in the Black Forest.[111]

Four doctors are known from inscriptions at the spas in Italy dated between the first and the third century CE. Three are from a collection of votive reliefs from Aenaria (Ischia). The first one is named Menippos, enslaved doctor, who traveled far to reach the place. He must have been a successful doctor who was able to offer a dedication. Two others were Aurelius Monnus and Numerius Fabus and their status is *alumnus*, indicating a student of medical knowledge, as in the following inscription. Another doctor is named Charinus in a funerary inscription found in the vicinity of Aquae Caeretanae.[112] Allen emphasizes that in none of these examples there is a clear suggestion of the role that a doctor might have had at a spa. He adds that it is worth nothing, however, that the presence of doctors at spas confirms the idea that spas were considered to be beneficial in essentially rational medicine. The dedications to the appropriate gods, the Nymphs and Apollo, which

---

[109] Hartmann (1973): 45–51; Wiedemer (1967): 83–93; Staehelin (1948): 487; Unz (1971): 41–45.

[110] Milne (1907): 144–145; Künzl (1986): 491–509; Jackson (1990a): 9; idem, (1999): 112; On Roman lithotomy instruments, see Künzl (1983): 487–493; Jackson (1994): 167–209, especially p. 190, Fig. 2.

[111] Mylius (1936); Jackson (1990b): 5–27; Yegül (1992): 119–121; Krug (1993): 173–175.

[112] *IG* 14.892; *CIL* 10.6792; *AÉ* (1989): no. 307.

were offered also, demonstrate that the role of the doctor and the role of the god could live together.[113]

The occurrence of collyrium-stamps [= oculists' stamps] at Bath Spa, the Wroxeter baths, the Lydney healing temple complex north-east of Chepstow, and the Trier Barbarathermen may signify the activities at these places of doctors who treated eye diseases. Eye diseases were a common and troublesome affliction, and literally hundreds of ointments were used to treat them.[114]

It seems that the work of military physicians would not be restricted to the soldiers alone. Either on a formal or, more probably, an informal basis, people from surrounding farms, small towns or villages may often have come to the fort, fortress or spa for treatment by the medical staff. There were a range of medical staff supporting the legions. The most important was the doctor (*medicus*), at least some of whom seem to have ranked with centuries (*medicus ordinaries*). A good number of these men appear to have been from the Hellenistic provinces, and some at least were highly skilled. Beneath the *medici* were a range of personnel, including the *optio valetudinarii*, who seems to have overseen the administration of the hospital. Celsus' manual *De Medicina* provides detailed descriptions of treating various wounds, methods which were only a little less advanced than any employed until recent centuries.[115] They must frequently have continued to practice, and also in a civilian setting. In this way the army spread knowledge of Graeco-Roman medicine in general and hydrotherapy and balneotherapy in particular throughout each new province of the Empire. As in other matters, this was not a one way process. At the same time as knowledge, experience and techniques were disseminated, new information and traditions of the local population were collected, which were constantly adding to the existing medical corpus.

Equally popular were the neighboring health facilities of Cumae and Puteoli [= Pozzuoli], as were the baths of Naples which, according to Strabo, are 'not inferior to those of Baiae'.[116] For a long time, the coast from Naples to Misenum served as the preferred visiting place

---

[113] Allen (1998): 152–154; On the use of the term *almnus*, see Nielsen (1987): 141–158.

[114] Frere and Tomlin (1992): nos. 2246.9–2246.10; Künzel (1986): 495–498, Fig. 4, H2; Jackson (1999): 110.

[115] Goldsworthy (2003): 101.

[116] Strabo, *Geographica* 5.4.7.

for Roman Emperors and for the wealthy, not only on account of its natural beauty and favorable climate, but mainly because of its medical facilities. Imposing buildings are located to this day on the volcanic slopes of Baiae, including the hot baths' *stoas* and colonnades.[117]

Archaeological evidence for drinking at thermo-mineral baths is provided by some of the finds associated with spas. The striking archaeological discovery at Tunisia in North Africa of glass bottles bearing engraved schematic scenes enables us to envision the magnificent architectural highlights of Baiae and neighboring Puteoli. Among the featured buildings are a sun terrace (*solar[ium]*) and a temple portico, in which stands a statue of the rayed sun god Sol. These bottles were probably manufactured locally in the third-fourth centuries CE for sale to visitors who wished to drink the site's healing water.[118] These objects, like the many small cups from Bath,[119] and the numerous drinking vessels from Aquae Helveticae,[120] could have been used for consuming thermo-mineral waters at a spa. They may have also been souvenirs of visits and, as such, would have been particularly appropriate for a treatment which centred on drinking the water.[121] (See Fig. 5).

Fascinating artifacts found at other medicinal sites illustrate the nature of hot springs in the Classical world. A silver and gilt *patera* handle from the Capheaton hoard in Northumberland, dating from the second-third century CE, shows Minerva presiding, with her foot on an upturned pot from which the sacred spring is gushing, symbolizing her power over the healing waters, possibly Bath Spa. Below, a figure takes a draught of the healing water from a fountain in front of a classical temple.[122] (See Fig. 6). Silver and gilt bowl from Otanẽs, near Castro Urdiales in northern Spain is ornamented in low relief with scenes of the Spanish spa of Salus Umeritana, as recorded by the encircling inscription 'Salus Umeritana.' Salus was equated by the Romans with Hygieia, the Greek goddess of health. The medicinal site

---

[117] De Franciscis (1967): 212–214; D'Arms (1970): 119–120; Borriello and d'Ambrosio (1979): 59–73; Ling (1979): 33–60; Yegül (1988): 282; idem, (1992): 93–110; Krug (1993): 182–183; Medri, Soricelli and Benini (1999): 207–2(19.

[118] Painter (1975): 54–67; Ostrow (1979): 77–140; Jackson (1990a): 7; For the bottling of mineral spring waters, see also Thomson (1978): 10.

[119] Henig (1988): 5–36.

[120] *LA* (1893): no. 59; *ibid.*, (1966): no. 610; *ibid.*, (1980): no. 621.

[121] Allen (1998): 116.

[122] Walters (1921): 48–51; Henig (1995): 43, Fig. 8; idem, (1999): 154, Fig. 7; Cruse (2004): 112.

of Umeri in the Pyrenees became famous on account of its waters, which were bottled for dispatch to those who were unable to visit the place. The scene within the bowl depicts Salus reclining on top of the medicinal spring, her left hand symbolically directing the water that is flowing from a jug into a container. There is also an old man clad in a toga sitting in a chair and next to him stands a young servant who has brought him water from the spring. Another old man in a toga is seen sacrificing on the altar in gratitude for his cure. Finally, pair of mules is waiting patiently while a couple of barrels on their cart are being filled with the spring's water by a youth, perhaps a temple servant, carrying an amphora.[123] (See Fig. 7).

At Bath Spa the curative waters of Sulis Minerva were enjoyed not just by civilians but by the military too, as the many altars and tombstones of serving soldiers testify. There were the retired soldiers living in and around the town, soldiers on leave visiting the spring, and a constant stream of tourists from Britain and abroad. Some of the soldiers, like the cavalryman Lucius Vitellius Tancinus, a Spaniard from Caurium serving with the *ala Vettonum*, who died at the age of 46 after twenty-six years of service, may possibly have been stationed at the supposed fort at Bath. The same may also be true of Marcus Valerius Latinus and Antigonus, both soldiers of the Legion XX. Neither of the last two tombstones bears the words *Valeria Victrix* after the title of the legion, a fact which suggests that the tombs were erected at an early date in the first century, before the legion had won the honours, at which time the two soldiers may well have been on active service. Whatever may have been the position of these three, other soldiers recorded from the town were visitors or retired veterans choosing the enervating atmosphere of Bath in which to spend their declining years. Some of the soldiers died at an unnaturally early age, people such as Julius Vitalis, an armourer of the Legion XX *Valeria Victrix* recruited in Gallia Belgica, who died after only nine years' service, aged 29; and Gaius Murrius Modestus, of the Legion II *Adiutrix*, from Forum Julii, in southern France, who died aged 25. They must have been ailing from disease or wounds when they visited Bath, never to return to their legions. Vitalis belonged to a craft guild. When he died his members of the craft guild to which he belonged paid for his cremation and tombstone, carefully record-

---

[123] *CIL*, II: no. 2917; Rostovtzeff (1957): Pl. XXV, 2; Jackson (1990a): 12–13; Baratte (1992): 43–54; Krug (1993): 180–181.

ing on it, 'with funeral at the cost of the Guild of Armourers'. Even a young soldier could be assured of a decent burial if he belonged to a guild.[124]

Other soldiers settled in Bath Spa after demobilization. Altar to the goddess Sulis was erected for Marcus Aufidius Maximus, a retired centurion of the Legion VI *Victrix*, by 'his freedman.' By this time he was probably a probably a prosperous local figure living in comfortable retirement. Another soldier, unnamed, probably settled in the north suburbs of the town, where he lost his bronze diploma issued to all soldiers on their retirement. He had served in a cavalry regiment, the *ala I Gallorum Proculeiana*, early in the second century CE and like all time-expired veterans was granted the right of citizenship after twenty-five years' service. As a man in his mid-forties, he and possibly his family chose Bath as a congenial town in which to begin his new life, perhaps as a farmer, a craftsman or a merchant. Cunliffe assumes that there must have been many more like him living and working in the surrounding countryside. Another altar was dedicated by 'the centurion in charge of this region', Gaius Severius Emeritus, recording his act of piety in cleansing afresh the spot which was 'wrecked by insolent hands'. He may have been a military administrator, perhaps responsible for a nearby imperial estate. The Roman settlement at Combe Down, near Bath, has produced an inscription recording a *principia* which is thought to refer to the headquarters of local procuratorial administration, and a lead seal found on the same site, stamped *P(rovinciae) Br(itanniae) S(uperioris)* shows that official parcels were passing through. It may be, according to Cunliffe, that Emeritus ran the establishment for a while.[125]

Finds from several military baths as well as ordinary spas show that they were used by women as well as soldiers, although it is possible that there were set times for different groups. The Roman army also appears to have taken a keen interest in the development of baths at spas sites, such as Bath Spa (Aquae Sulis) in Britain. This complex was constructed relatively soon after the conquest of the area and it is likely that the legionary garrisons at other places in Western Europe and in the eastern Mediterranean basin were closely involved in its construction. The healing power of hot springs was highly valued by the Romans,

---

[124] Smith (1944): 17; Collingwood and Wright (1965): 139, 143–144, 146–147, 152, 156–160; Cunliffe (1995): 102–103.
[125] Cunliffe (1984): 187.

and almost certainly employed for aiding the recovery of the sick and
wounded. One altar from Bath recording the reconstruction of a *locus
religiosus* [= religious place] was set up by Gaius Severius Emeritus, the
centurion charged with the administration of a region.[126]

There is an overwhelming male representation in the inscriptions
recovered from the spas in Italy. Out of 65 individual examples, only
8 dedications were made by women.[127] This is not surprising in a social
world largely dominated by men.[128] But there is a definite presence of
women which cannot go unnoticed according to the Greek and Latin
authors. Thus, for instance, Seneca expresses strong opinions about
the moral laxity of the resort at Baiae although he believes that there
might be some benefits to be gained from the natural setting of the
resort.[129] Martial offers valuable insight into the use of spas by the upper
classes during the early Empire. He presents an image of the luxurious
and, at times, infamous activities for which the resort was renowned.
The formerly chaste Laevina often came for the *Baianis Aquis* and, as
a result, succumbed to the temptations of the place. Furthermore, he
encourages an unfaithful wife, Paula, to go alone to the baths of Aquae
Sinuessanae for curing hysteria.[130] Some of Martial's friends are hoping
for relaxation and pleasure, 'a difficult pursuit without abundant financial resources', due to Allen's remark.[131] This, together with evidence
of epigraphical inscriptions from Hammat-Gader and especially the
frequent recommendations of Soranus to use mineral spring water to
relieve gynecological disorders—reveal that women were among the
regular visitors to spas.[132]

The epigraphical documents from the thermo-mineral baths at
Hammat-Gader reflect also the involvement of the military presence.
Except for the small group of building inscriptions, most texts written
by private persons open with the words Ἐν τῷ ἁγίῳ or (ἰερῷ) τόπῳ
μνησθῇ [= in this holy place may someone be remembered]. According
to this term, the baths were viewed as a healing place endowed with

---

[126] Goldsworthy (2003): 107.
[127] Allen (1998): 155.
[128] See some of the fundamental studies on women in antiquity: Balsdon (1974);
Pomeroy (1976); Fant and Lefkowitz (1992); Allason-Jones (2000); Fraschetti (2001).
[129] Seneca, *Epistulae Morales* 51.4; See also Wood (2004): 33–34.
[130] Martial, *Epigrammata* 1.62, 11.7; See also Howell (1980): 253–257.
[131] Allen (1998): 129; See Martial, *Epigrammata* 3.20; 6.43.
[132] Soranus, *Gynaecia* 1.56; 3.16; 3.28; 3.32; 3.38; 3.44.

a God-given power of restoring health.[133] (See, for instance, Figs. 16, 17, 18, and 20).

An inscription, which was placed in a prominent spot near the entrance, reads: 'In this holy place may Theosebius the *singularis* be remembered'. Under the Principate the *singulares* were among the selected soldiers second to the military *officia* of prefects, proconsuls and legates from unites under their command in order to take care of the judicial and sometimes the financial affairs of their jurisdiction. In the Byzantine period the *singulares*—although still formally enrolled as soldiers and drawing rations as such—were in fact clerks in the sub-clerical branch of the civil service both in the military and the civil administration. Cases are known of retired members of the sub clerical grades who owned land and were wealthy enough to enroll a son in the *curia* of their town.[134] The same style occurs in another inscription in Area A, Hall of Inscriptions, indicates that 'In this holy place may Leontius the notary be remembered, (the son) of Droserius, *tribunus* of Damascus'. *Tribunus* was a military rank, denoting the commander of a regiment or any commanding officer. As the civil service was also organized as a *militia*, members of the corps of notaries could rise to the tribunate. Customarily service in the *militia* was passed on from father to son, and since Leontius was a notary, his father was probably a senior member of the same service.[135] There is an appeal to Christ in an inscription, surmounted by a palm leaf and a similar decoration closes the last line, which runs as follows: 'Christ, help Siricius the Gazean *magistrianos*'. (See Fig. 16). The imperial couriers, *agentes in rebus*, were known by the term μαγιστριανοί, as they were closely attached to the *magister officiorum*. They formed a *militia palatina* and were organized as a cavalry regiment, starting as troopers (*equites*) and passing through the noncommissioned grades up to *ducenarius*. Soon they became important as confidential agents of the imperial government, especially the senior members of the corps, who were sent out to the provinces as inspectors of the post (*curiosi*). As such, they earned the reputation of government spies and were much hated by the provincials. Among the task of the *agentes in rebus* was also the control of maritime traffic.[136]

---

[133] Di Segni (1997): 185, 253.

[134] Jones (1964): 563–566, 590–596; Di Segni (1997): 192, no. 3; On another *singularis* named Domninus, see idem, (1997): 212, no. 27.

[135] Jones (1964): 573–574, 640; Di Segni (1999): 207, no. 22.

[136] Jones (1964): 103–104, 128–129, 547–549, 578–581; Di Segni (1997): 210–211, no. 26; On another *agens in rebus* named Philologius, see idem, (1997): 214, no. 32.

In the centre of the pavement in The Hall of Inscriptions, there is an appeal to God and a title of 'Zenon the patrician': 'God, he who created all things, help Zenon the patrician and his servant Alexander...' The ancient title of *patricius* was revived by Constantine. One of the two distinguished Isaurian generals by the name of Zeno who held the consulate during the fifth and sixth centuries CE, and is very suitable in this case is Flavius Zeno. He was *magister militum per Orientem* between 447–451 CE, and achieved the patriciate on leaving his post in early 451 CE. Zeno retired under a shadow and held no other office under the new Emperor, Marcianus. Members of the aristocracy, who had become *persona non grata* at the Byzantine court, were often bundled off to Palestine. Thus in all likelihood Zeno came as a private citizen after his retirement, and his visit must be dated between 451 CE and his death in 457 CE.[137]

In conclusion, although it is possible at many of these sites to make a good argument for the identification of a hospital, there is virtually no unequivocal evidence in any of them to prove the case. However, the presence of surgical instruments as evidence for the recognition of hospital buildings carries some weight. Unfortunately, we ought to wait for the forthcoming excavations at the curative sites in the eastern Mediterranean for verifying our assumption and point of view.

3.5   Public Baths and Spas: The Roman Leisure Culture

In the Graeco-Roman world the properties of various kinds of water were held in great esteem. Hot springs and mineral contents were particularly appreciated. The main remedial sites attracted very large numbers of visitors. Medicinal spring water, like medicinal mud, was applied to painful areas of the body. Regular bathing and drinking of the water were practised routinely—many internal diseases were treated by drinking the water. In addition, people in antiquity regarded water in general, and that of medicinal baths in particular, as a source of enjoyment.[138]

The practice of taking hot baths, which seems to us a typical Roman custom and necessitated the construction of the most grandiose build-

---

[137] Di Segni (1997): 218, no. 34.
[138] Jackson (1990a): 13; See also Pliny, *Naturalis Historia* 31.32.

ings in Rome, was another of the customs introduced into Italy from Greece towards the end of the third century BCE, the century which was the decisive age for penetration of Greek civilization into Italy. The Greeks developed bathing centres near natural springs and rivers. They encouraged bathing for physical health, recreation, and for relaxation and mental well-being. Water was prized as a health-giving gift from the gods. Bathing played an important role in the lives of ancient Greeks, and the Greek bath became an addendum to the gymnasium. The baths were used to prepare and stimulate the athletes before the games. Often the baths were quick and cold and sometimes followed by a warm bath after the athletic events. The Romans were greatly influenced by the Greeks, extending their belief of water's healing uses into their own culture. The Romans deserve the credit for combining the spiritual, social, and therapeutic values of bathing and exalting it to an art. In the warm Roman climate, *thermae* were a welcome part of the day; going to the baths became a social pleasure. Baths were the focus of communal life, offering a place for relaxation, social gathering, and worship.[139]

Bathing was a recreational activity enjoyed by people of all ages, sexes, and social classes. The wealthy might have bathing facilities in their own homes, but most people used public establishments which were operated either by the state or by a private, profit-making company. So popular were these baths that throughout the Roman Empire, almost every town and every village had at least one public bath building and by the fourth century CE there were almost 856 public bath buildings in Rome alone. Baths and bathing provided a range of services far beyond simple hygiene. For the Romans bathing was an important ritual, a process which involved passing through a series of bathing areas maintained at different temperatures.[140]

Much has been written of the luxuriousness of the baths, the bathing procedures, and other practices. The purpose of the classical Roman public bath installation was to cleanse the body by perspiration and washing, similar to the 'Turkish bath' or the sauna in later times. Baths

---

[139] Paoli (1958): 221; Licht (1963): 131–133; Aaland (1978): 28–32; Croutier (1992): 79–81; Ruoti, Morris and Cole (1997): 3; Nolte (2001): 5–7; Lee (2004): 39–43; For the transition from Greek to Roman preferences and methods of bathing, see mainly DeLaine (1989): 111–125; Nielsen (1985): 81–112.

[140] Shelton (1988): 311; Nolte (2001): 9; Goldsworthy (2003): 106.

demanded specialized techniques of building and engineering, the existence of an effective method of heating and a reliable and abundant
water supply. The Roman bathing establishments varied considerably
in their layout but in all of them the following essential elements are
found: The building included an entrance hall, which served as a
dressing room (*apodyterium*), from which one could enter a courtyard or
exercise hall (*palaestra*), or directly into one of the sweating chambers
(*sudatoria*). Sometimes a cold pool (*frigidarium*) preceded the sweating
chamber, whose floor was elevated on brick pillars (*suspensurae*) that were
60–90 cm high. Hot air from a furnace (*furnarium*) circulated among the
pillars under the floor, and also in the walls, which incorporated square
vertical pipes with perforations (*tubulatio*). This 'burning from below' is
therefore known as the hypocaust heating method. In the more sumptuous baths the floor and walls were lined with marble. From the sweating
room, the bather proceeded to the tepid room (*tepidarium*) and thence
to the hot room (*caldarium*), which was vaulted and had particularly
thick walls, with washing tubs recessed into them. This was followed
by a massage, and the exit was through the tepid and cold rooms.[141]
Externally the enormous quadrilateral was flanked by porticos full of
shops and crowded with shopkeepers and their customers; inside it
enclosed gardens and promenades, *stadium* and rest rooms, gymnasiums
and rooms for massage, even libraries and museums. The baths in fact
offered the Romans a microcosm of many of the things that make life
attractive. Here the alliance between physical culture and intellectual
curiosity became thoroughly Romanized.[142]

When the plans of such installations are known, it is possible to
reconstruct the bathing procedures and the methods employed by
the architects to facilitate them. In Pompeii, for example, the rooms
are arranged in one line next to the *palaestra*, whereas at Thamugadi
(Timgad) in Libya, they are arranged in a circle and the first *sudartorium*
is connected to the entrance hall and to the cold room. There were
baths with twin installations arranged symmetrically. The twin installations not only offered facilities for more numerous bathers but also
enabled men and women to bathe separately and simultaneously. Apart

---

[141] Paoli (1958): 222–223; Guthrie (1960): 81; Weiss and Kemble (1962): 11; Gichon (1978): 37–38; Aaland (1978): 33–35; Henig (1983): 59–60; Grimal (1983): 68–69; DeLaine (1988); Nielsen (1990); Yegül (1992): 30–47, 92–127; Ring (1996): 717–724; Gizowska (1998): 9; Manderscheid (2000): 484–535; Nolte (2001): 8.
[142] Carcopino (1991): 279–280.

from periods of extreme decadence, women usually bathed in separate locations or at special times. Emperor Hadrian decreed that women should use the baths in the hours of the morning ('until the seventh hour,' in Roman nomenclature), while the men should bathe in the afternoon until darkness. When men and women did bathe together in the public baths, they were naked. The custom of joint bathing by men and women, which was prevalent in the first to third centuries CE, was abolished by Hadrian. The fact that in the following generation Marcus Aurelius again had to forbid the practice, as did Alexander Severus in the third century CE, testifies both to the prevalence of the phenomenon and the scandals which it engendered.[143]

The method of bathing naturally varied according to taste, age and health, but the object was always to alternate hot and cold baths. A cold bath, whether simply washing or swimming and diving in the *piscinae natatoriae*, was only taken when the body was heated and the pores open from the hot bath, a longer or shorter stay in the *laconicum* or a vigorous game in the *sphaeristerium*. Less energetic people took a long sun bath (*apricatio*) before entering the cold water.[144]

The sphere of Roman manners with baths and bathing had connection with sexual life. Ovid, The most elegant and productive of Roman poets, observes:[145]

> What is the use of guarding women?... When, even although the girl's guardian keeps her clothes in safety outside the baths, hidden lovers lurk safe within?

Kiefer believes that this shows that assignations with lovers must frequently have been made in one or other of the baths. He adds that this took place, not in the great baths of later times, but in smaller establishments built or rented by private individuals, who managed them and charged visitors a small sum.[146] According to Martial there must have been special baths for prostitutes, which were visited by no respectable women. They must have been visited by men, wishing not so much to bathe as to have a convenient opportunity of visiting their mistress.[147]

---

[143] Carcopino (1991): 293–304; Cowell (1973): 144–147; Balsdon (1969): 26–32; Dilke (1975); Howell (1980): 157–158, 307–308; Dvorjetski (1992a): 43–45; Croutier (1992): 85–86; Guhl and Koner (1994): 395–406; Williams (1999): 69–70; Nolte (2001): 9.
[144] Paoli (1958): 224.
[145] Ovid, *Ars Amatoria* 3.633–634; See also Hazel (2002): 217–219.
[146] Kiefer (1994): 161.
[147] Martial, *Epigrammata* 11.47.

Every time a Roman went to the baths he further endangered his sex life. Most men went there every day. Unfortunately, hot baths appear to have the effect of reducing fertility by inhibiting sperm production The normal temperature of the testicles is lower than that of the rest of the body (37°C or 98.4°F). The Roman *caldarium* appears to have maintained a temperature of something in the region of 43°C or 110°F.[148]

The difference between conventional baths and therapeutic baths can be seen in the architecture and the technical fixtures involved with heating. The thermal baths did not follow the normal pattern of water management. The conventional functional elements, particularly the *caldarium* and the hypocaust, are not to be found in medicinal hot baths. Therapeutic baths often had, in addition to the *piscinae*, which were operated with thermal water, a conventional bathing section. Manderscheid assumes that since thermal baths were usually located outside cities, accommodations for housing and feeding patients must have been furnished. According to him, since the relative temperatures of the springs vary considerably between circa 26°C and circa 70°C, there must have been some provision for cooling the water down to a temperature which was beneficial or perhaps comfortable to the human body. Indeed, in only a very few cases would the water have 'automatically' cooled off sufficiently on its way from the source to the bathing pools. The archaeological evidence reveals two possibilities; first, an installation of cooling basins into which the water would flow before being introduced into the *piscinae* (Baden-Baden). Secondly, the mixing of hot thermal water with fresh water (Fordongianus), which must have been transported separately over a relatively long distance by means of an aqueduct for this and other purposes.[149]

The primary consumers of fresh water in the healing baths were as follows: the mixing system for cooling off water which was too hot; a fountain for drinking water; the facilities of the conventional bath wing, that is to say, the cold *piscinae*, the boiler installation for the *caldarium* pool, and the latrine; overall cleaning of the complex; the food and lodging accommodations for the patients, in which water was needed for drinking, food preparation, hygienic fixtures, and cleaning purposes.[150]

---

[148] Tannahill (1980): 132–133.
[149] Manderscheid (2000): 511–513; See also Garbrecht and Manderscheid (1994): I: 83–87; Czysz (1994): 115–117; Romanelli (1970): 170.
[150] Manderscheid (2000): 513.

The thermal bath installations at Hammat-Gader near the famous *polis* Gadara of the Decapolis, which were renowned throughout the Roman world, constitute a very distinct complex. With its wide lavish halls and spacious pools, it resembles the large *thermae* of the Roman Empire and in particular the famous installations at Aquae Sulis (Bath Spa).[151] The uncovered hypocaust of the main *tepidarium* and the *caldarium* in Bath, for instance, might demonstrate that alterations have been added to the facilities of the complex according to the demand of the citizens or the municipal council's determination.

Apart from frequenting the forum and the temples, the Romans liked to spend their time at the baths and at public places of entertainment, which formed the basis of the Roman leisure culture. In place of the former sport education in the Greek gymnasium, and immersion in modest baths, the Romans deliberately promoted bathing. They turned it into the dominant, or even the sole, form of body care. The main merits of the baths for the Romans lay in prompt enjoyment and self indulgence, bordering on exaggeration and vanity, to which was added a modicum of social intercourse. All citizens, and not only the wealthy, frequented the baths. The bathers either brought slaves with them to carry their towels, to scrape, and to rub them down, or they hired such services at the baths where there were also masseurs, anointers, depilators and perfumers. The poor, who could afford none of these attentions, rubbed and scraped themselves by hand or against a wall. The places served also for the display of works of art. Famous statues often adorned the edifices, which were themselves richly decorated. In the adjacent buildings and *stoas*, lectures and poetry readings took place; and philosophers held their discussions there in the certain knowledge that a large audience would come to listen.[152]

It should be noted that in the Greek literature and in the writings of the Jewish Sages, the projects undertaken by the Roman Empire, including its baths, have been subjected to numerous and diverse evaluations—both complimentary and critical. The Romans themselves denigrated their baths. They were well aware that beneath the tall *stoas* there

---

[151] Tsafrir (1984): 110; Dvorjetski (1988): 135–136; idem, (1997): 472; For Bath Spa complex, see, for example, Cunliffe (1995); Yegül (1992): 117–119.
[152] Carcopino (1991): 277–286; Cowell (1961): 144–147; Balsdon (1969): 26–32; Tsafrir (1984): 110; Dunbabin (1989): 6–15.

teemed peddlers and pimps, and that many people were frequenting the site in order to gorge, to guzzle and to debauch themselves.[153]

Yegül sums up the variety of bathing choices provided for a visitor at *Aquae Sulis* bath complex, which can be a model for spas during the height of the Roman Empire:[154]

> Entering the complex from the northwest and southwest, he could take a regular hot bath in the *tepidarium* and the *caldarium* and finish his ablutions, as accustomed, in the *frigidarium*, a square room with a round pool of fresh, unheated water. Alternatively, he could spend some time in the circular *laconicum* before taking the cold plunge; or he could omit the artificially heated baths altogether and go for a treatment in the hot and tepid thermal pools of the Great Bath or the Lucas Bath. As yet another option he could combine the two modes of bathing, regular and thermal, in any order he pleased or as his doctor recommended. During the third period, a pair of small, tepid chambers built to the west of the *laconicum* may have served for the individual treatment of patients. Although the entire complex seems to have been supplied copiously with hot mineral water, it is likely that fresh, cold water was also piped into the establishment.

Yegül has identified three stages of development of thermo-mineral sites: a simple pool with very few architectural features fed by a spring; a more elaborate structure with a central pool-hall as its focus; and an integrated building which had both natural and artificially heated elements. He suggests that a site might either progress through each stage or remain at a particular phase of development. In any case, the terminology established for ordinary bathing is often not appropriate for describing spa facilities.[155] A large pool hall, which contained a pool for thermo-mineral water, is a very significant feature of a spa site. The large dimensions of the main pool halls highlight the importance thermo-mineral bathing had for therapeutic measures. The most common form for these pools is either rectangular or apsidal, but round pools offered a variation on the traditional shape. While not all spa establishments have clear evidence for sweating rooms dependent on natural hot springs, it is clear, according to Allen, that their use formed part of the therapy expected to be available at one of these centres.

---

[153] Hahn (1906); Carcopino (1939): 293–304; Fuchs (1964); Friedländer (1964): 318–320; Herr (1970): 95–108; Dunbabin (1989): 6–46.
[154] Yegül (1992): 110–111, 117–119.
[155] Rebuffat (1991): 1–32; Allen (1998): 74–75.

In addition to bathing facilities, which made use of naturally heated spring water, a number of spas also had artificially heated rooms. These rooms are sometimes later additions to the original core of the structure and functioned alongside the already-present thermal baths. There are examples of large artificially heated pools—Vignale Baths at Velia, Suburban Baths at Herculanum, Small Baths in Villa Adriana at Tivoli, Babni di Nerone at Massiciuccoli (near Pisa) in Italy and Bath Spa in Britain—but there are, on the whole, rather rare and tend to be restricted to luxurious establishments. As the focus of the spas was on the resources of the thermo-mineral springs, the main aim of the design was to create access to the waters. This led to an architectural type that can clearly be seen as related to normal bath buildings, but with variations as necessary.[156]

Healing spas formed an important component of health and hygiene in the Roman world. Spas provided a new method for improving health which combined the comforts of the bath with innovative treatments based on rational and logical medicine. The treatments found in spas were aimed at specific needs and focused especially on thermo-mineral springs. At a spa a visitor could partake of the restorative measures available by bathing in or drinking the waters of a spring. A belief in the effectiveness of the water lay at the centre of the use of thermo-mineral springs for healing. Although there was an undercurrent of religious belief at spas, the main healing activity focused on what was considered to be a rational use of the thermo-mineral waters. Information concerning the staffing of a spa is sadly lacking in the literary record. It is likely that the non-medical staffing needs of a spa were similar to those of an ordinary bath. Although there is little in the evidence to confirm it, there must have been doctors or attendants in the establishments who could treat clients at the spas.[157]

In conclusion it is important to point out that the testimony offered by the numerous dedicatory inscriptions, frequent recommendations by medical writers and non-specialists, and the existence of many thermo-mineral establishments throughout the Graeco-Roman world provide an unequivocal demonstration of the important role spas had in antiquity.

---

[156] Allen (1998): 56–67, 74–75–81; Nielsen (1990): II: 7, Cat. no. 39, 52; 9: Cat. no. 55; 10, Cat. no. 61; See also Grenier (1960): 409—for Amelie-les-Bains.
[157] Allen (1998): 1, 45, 205.

CHAPTER FOUR

HISTORICAL-ARCHAEOLOGICAL ANALYSIS AND HEALING CULTS OF THE THERAPEUTIC SITES IN THE EASTERN MEDITERRANEAN BASIN

Following our survey of the locations, the names and the identification of the hot springs in the Levant, we shall now discuss the history and the archaeology of the most important and best-known of them.[1] We shall use references in classical literature by Greek and Roman historians and other writers, and in Rabbinic and Christian literature, and attempt to integrate them to form a unified picture. In our discussion of the historical aspects of the subject, we shall consider whether the historical accounts accord with the archaeological findings and chronological conclusions to be drawn from the excavations in Hammat-Tiberias, Hammat-Gader, Hammat-Pella, Kallirrhoe, and Emmaus-Nicopolis. In addition, we shall adduce historical evidence to identify the Waters of Asia and their importance. Illustrating the archaeological material, epigraphic documents and the little finds from the curative thermo-mineral baths in the eastern Mediterranean basin, we shall present the social, religious and economic life in the spas during the Hellenistic, Roman, Byzantine and Early Muslim periods.[2] (See Map 1).

4.1   Hammei-Tiberias

Hammat was the most southerly of the fortified towns of the tribe of Naphtali on the coast of Lake Kinneret: 'And the fortified cities are Ziddim, Zer, and Hammat, Rakkat and Kinnereth' (*Joshua* 19, 35).[3]

---

[1] For the names, locations and the identification of the thermo-mineral springs in the East, see the discussions on *Terminology* in chapter 1.4 and in chapter 2 on *The Geological, Hydrological and Medicinal Aspects of Hot Springs in the Eastern Mediterranean—Past and Present*.

[2] On the effects of the contacts between Jews and non-Jews in the spas, see also chapter 6 on *Daily Life at the Thermo-Mineral Baths according to Rabbinic Literature*.

[3] This identification is uncertain since no remains from the Hellenistic period were uncovered in the excavations at Hammat: See Dothan (1983): 3; idem, (1993): II: 573; Anyway, the real thing depends on the fact that nearby those springs, which were called

Even before the conquest of Palestine by Joshua the region round Hammath was known as an area of recreation and healing because of its hot springs and the landscape of the Kinnereth. The Anastasi Papyrus I, dating from the days of Ramses II in the thirteenth century BCE, which describes the major routes of Canaan, mentions Hammath after Hazor, as 'a place for excursions'.[4] Other traditions give an early date for the use of Hammei-Tiberias, and emphasize its origins in volcanic processes at the time of the Flood. Among them are: 'All the fountains of the great deep broke up' (*Genesis* 7, 11); 'Rabbi Yohanan said: "Three remained of the fountains of the great deep that burst apart at the time of the Flood (*ibid.*): The eddy of Gader, Hammei-Tiberias, and the great spring of Biram. 'For all flesh had corrupted his way upon the earth'" (*Babylonian Talmud, Sanhedrin* 108a); the *Midrash* even connects Jacob with Hammei-Tiberias: *Genesis Rabbah* 76, 5 (Theodor-Albeck ed., p. 901) says that when Jacob fled from Esau, on his way to the Hauran he went into Hammei-Tiberias; and in *Midrash Tanhuma, Vayehi* 6, we find: 'Rabbi Yohanan said: "Jacob's arms were like two pillars in the *demousin* of Tiberias'"; it is said that Job's house of study was in Tiberias, and it may be assumed that this legend was derived from the tradition that Job was cured there of 'evil scabs' (*Babylonian Talmud, Baba Bathra* 15b, and more).[5]

One of the 24 Priestly Courses named Ma'aziya (*Nehemiah* 10, 8; I *Chronicles* 24, 18) lived in 'Hammat, Ariah and Kafarnia', at the south of the Sea of Galilee, and not in Tiberias itself.[6] It appears that this

---

later Hammei-Tiberias, a site has been existed and already mentioned in *Joshua* (19, 35); See also *ibid.*, 21, 31; It seems that the conditions to recognize and utilize the hot springs were known. Buchmann (1967: 196) is convinced that this was the very ancient therapeutic place in the world; Aharoni (1957: 80) assumes that the Israeli settlement is buried deep under the later layers, because by Hammei-Tiberias remains from the Chalcolithic and Bronze ages were discovered; See also Dvorjetski (1992a): 48, 93; Dothan (1993): 573.

[4] Aharoni (1957): 123, 128; idem, (1963): 160–162; Itshaki (1978): 199; Although Ahituv (1984: 113) is correct when he describes Hammat's location, near the hot springs south of Tiberias, he has made a severe mistake in the punctuation of the word Hammat. By this fact it seems that Ahituv is not aware of the meaning of the term and contradicts himself by adding the word 'Ammathus'; See the discussion on *Terminology* in chapter 1.4.

[5] On the various names and traditions of Hammei-Tiberias, see Kasher (1934); Margalit (1976): 141; Weiss (1986): 175–179; Dvorjetski (1992a): 47–52; See also the discussion in chapter 5 on *The Healing Properties of the Spas in the Eastern Mediterranean in Ancient Times*.

[6] For the Priestly Courses see, for example, Klein (1909); Sukenik (1926): 16–17; Klein (1939): 162–165; Avi-Yonah (1964b): 25–28; Urbach (1973): 304–327; Ilan (1974):

was because of the impurity attributed to the town, or to sections of it, which precluded many people from settling there.[7] According to Rabbi Yohanan, Tiberias is situated on the site of the town of Hammat, and the name *Hammat* is derived from the hot springs (*hammei*) of Tiberias (*Babylonian Talmud, Megilla* 6a).[8] It should be pointed out that only the latter statement is correct, since Hammat continued to exist as a distinctive settlement even after it had been incorporated into Tiberias.[9]

The growth and fame of this therapeutic site was expressed in the sources after the foundation of the town of Tiberias. The proximity of the therapeutic springs was undoubtedly one of the reasons why Herod Antipas established his capital there. He ruled under the tutelage of the Romans, and, though he was a Jew, his outlook on life was Hellenistic-Roman. Like Herod, his father, he saw town building as an important part of his capacity to rule. So as a Roman client-prince, Herod Antipas obsequiously named his newly built city, in honour of the Emperor Tiberius—Tiberias. The kings of the Herodian dynasty appreciated that they must combine Jewish and Hellenistic culture if their dynasty were to survive. To this end they established urban centres with a mixed population of Jews and non-Jews.[10] A great increase in population, some of it voluntary and some compulsory, opened up a new era in the life of the town and its baths, Hammei-Tiberias.[11]

225–226; Naveh (1978): 87–92, 140–143; Kahana (1979): 9–29; Fleischer (1986): 47–60; Levine (1989): 171–172, 174; Eshel (1991): 159–161; Oppenheimer (1991): 53–57; Slouschz (1993): 65–77; Walner (2000): 125–141.

[7] Safrai (1982a): 159, 167; The *Masora's* authors [= traditional text of Bible] called the town of Tiberias by the name of the Priestly Course of Ma'aziya; See Klein (1967): 62–68; Assaf (1958): 142–144; Oppenheimer (1991): 53–57; Gil (1981): 67; See also the discussion below.

[8] On the explanation and origin of the term *Hammei* and *Hammat*, see the *Terminology* in chapter 1.4; The Talmudic sources identify generally Rakkat with Tiberias (*Jerusalem Talmud, Megilla* 1, 1 [70a]; *Babylonian Talmud, ibid.,* 6a; *ibid., Sanhedrin* 12a); But according to Rabbi Yohanan, which is the individual opinion, Rakkat is Sepphoris (*ibid., Megilla* 6a; Rakkat is identified with Tel el-Qaltia known also as Tel el-Kneitra and located about 2 kilometres north-western to Tiberias on the way to Migdal; Throughout the ages, Tiberias inherited the status and role of Rakkat. See Amir (1976): 437; Sohat (1926): 165; idem, (1936): 165; Aharoni (1957): 80–81, 123; Landau (1967): 176–177; Press (1955): IV: 371.

[9] See *Tosefta, Eruvin* 5, 2 (Liberman ed., p. 111); *Jerusalem Talmud, ibid.,* 5, 7 [22d]; Buchmann (1967): 196; Dvorjetski (1992a): 47–52; See also the discussion below.

[10] Dechent (1884): 179; Avi-Yonah (1950a): 162–163; idem, (1967a): 164–165; Hoehner (1972): 91–100; Rosenfeld (1983): 13; Schürer (1991): I: 342–343; II: 17; Horsley (1995): 169–171; For the comparison between the literary sources and the numismatic evidence, see Kindler (1961): 15.

[11] See Josephus, *Antiquitates Judaicae* 18.36–38; See also Kasher (1988b): 3–5.

Soon after the foundation of Tiberias, Pliny the Elder knew of its
therapeutic springs as 'aquae calidae salubrae' [= healthy hot waters].[12]
Pliny's *Historia Naturalis* provides valuable information about Palestine at
the end of the Second Temple period. He never actually visited Palestine, however, but relied on the records of the Roman administration
from the Herodian period, with later additions.[13]

One of the main reasons for the opposition of broad sectors of the
Jewish population to the foundation of Tiberias was based on *halakhic*
arguments. It appears that from its beginnings the establishment of
the town involved a bitter controversy connected with impurity, since
it was situated on the site of graves which, according to the Talmudic
tradition, belonged to the Biblical town of Rakkat or its neighbour
Hammat (*Jerusalem Talmud, Megilla* 1, 1 [70a]; *Babylonian Talmud, ibid.,* 6a;
ibid., Shabbat 33b–34a, and more).[14] According to Josephus, this did not
deter Herod Antipas, who ordered that the graves should be removed
from the building site. He had to give incentives to the lower classes
to encourage them to settle in the town. It is clear that there were also
observant Jews who settled in Tiberias, and as early as the period of
Jabneh there were synagogues in the town, Rabbis were active there,
and even Rabban Gamaliel of Jabneh visited the town in his tours of
the country (*Tosefta, Shabbat* 13, 2–3).[15] Rabbi Eliezer, Rabbi Joshua and
Rabbi Akiva are said to have bathed in Hammei-Tiberias (*Jerusalem
Talmud, Sanhedrin* 14, 19 [25d]), and it may be conjectured that they
came to the town in the course of their journey to Antioch as envoys
of Rabban Gamaliel on behalf of the Rabbis (*ibid., Horayot* 3, 7 [48a]).

In the course of time Tiberias was cleansed of its impurity. The
Talmudic tradition attributes this deed to Rabbi Simeon ben Yohai,
the disciple of Rabbi Akiva, and one of the senior Rabbis of Usha.
He hid from the Roman authorities in one of the caves in the vicinity.
After hiding for some time covered in sand up to his neck, when he
left the cave his body was covered in sores; but when he bathed in

---

[12] Pliny the Elder, *Historia Naturalis* 5.71; See also Stern (1974): I: 469.
[13] Stern (1974): I: 465–466; idem, (1968): 216, 219–224.
[14] Kasher (1988b): 8; Klein (1967: 100–101) impugners Josephus's testimony and
remarks that the forbidden dwelling in an impure place is existed only for priests;
Oppenheimer (1991: 57) comments that this argument is derived from the approach,
which decreases the affinity of the range of purity only to priests, but this access does
not resist the criticism and in any case ought to be rejected.
[15] Oppenheimer (1991): 53–57; Rosenfeld (1983): 20; idem, (1985): 11–13; idem,
(1988): 25; Dudman and Balkhorn (1988): 37–38.

Hammei-Tiberias with his son he was cured of them. Then he decided to cleanse the town of its pollution, and put an end to the disruptive controversy on the matter. Kasher maintains that to a great extent it was the special characteristics of the town, and its world-wide fame as a therapeutic site, that prepared the way for its purification.[16] Oppenheimer maintains that the purification of Tiberias was a reflection of the increase in its population in the wake of the Bar Kochba revolt, and the need to prepare the town for the arrival of refugees from Judaea, among whom were doubtless to be found people for whom its purity was an important factor. Even so, as Oppenheimer points out, the later Talmudic evidence shows that there were Rabbis who were opposed to the purification. Even after Rabbi Simeon ben Yohai declared that the town was pure, priests did not settle there; and, indeed, no name of any order of priests is connected with the town.[17] Evidently the purification of the town took place at the time when Jews left Judaea for Galilee, after the Bar Kochba revolt, as is seen in the evidence for the extension of the town and the increase in the number of its Jewish inhabitants. Thus, for instance:

> In the past the people of Tiberias used to go as far as Hammat, but the people of Hammat did not come to them beyond the place of the dome; but now the people of Tiberias and of Hammat have once again become one town.
> (*Tosefta, Eruvin* 5, 2, Lieberman ed., p. 111; *Jerusalem Talmud, ibid.*, 5, 7 [22d]).

Oppenheimer says that the time when this *halakhic* decision was made is not clear, since the expression 'in the past' makes it more probable that the *halakhic* decision was made in the period of Usha; this decision makes it clear that Tiberias was extended, and they were both surrounded by a single Sabbath boundary. It is, however, unlikely that Hammat was

---

[16] For the several sources for purifying Tiberias, see *Jerusalem Talmud, Shevi'it* 9, 1 [38d]; *Genesis Rabbah* 79 (Theodor-Albek ed., p. 941); *Pesikta de Rav Kahana, Besalah* 17 (Mandelbaum ed., p. 191); *Eccelesiastes Rabbah* 10, 8; See also Hirschberg (1920): 237–240; For the traditions' analysis see Levine (1978): 173–179; Rabban Yohanan was prior to Rabbi Simeon ben Yohai in trying to purifying the site, see *Babylonian Talmud, Shabbat* 33a; Kasher (1934): 10; idem, (1988b): 3–5; Dvorjetski (1992a): 50, 95; For different reasons of Rabbi Simeon ben Yohai's concealment see Herr (1970): 192–193; Buchmann (1967: 196) indicates that we have to add the commercial and economic reasons for purifying Tiberias; Leebner (2004: 182) thinks that eating Gidoran carobs of a low quality caused Rabbi Simeon and his son such a problem in their body; For *The Healing Properties of Hammei-Tiberias*, see chapter 5.

[17] Oppenheimer (1991): 53–57; See also Alon (1967): I: 162–163; Safrai (1958): 206–207.

actually merged with Tiberias, since the *Amoraim* of the fourth century
CE speak of Hammat and Tiberias as separate settlements (*Jerusalem
Talmud, Megilla* 1, 1 [70a]; *Babylonian Talmud, ibid.*, 2b).[18]

It appears that villas were built in the space between the town of
Tiberias and the spa, like those of Baiae, by the bay of Naples.[19] It
may well be that Herod Antipas' memories of the days of his youth
in Rome strengthened his decision to build the spa.[20] In the course of
time the bathhouses of Tiberias created a new culture, the culture of
bathing, for the inhabitants of the town and those who visited it. This
culture also influences their lives at various levels, and was the subject
of profound and lengthy discussions among the Rabbis of Tiberias as
will be seen later on.[21]

Josephus frequently mentions the Tiberias thermo-mineral bath in
several of his works. Among other matters, he describes an incident
in his life connected with this site: John of Gischala planned to kill
Josephus, the governor of Galilee, whom he suspected because of his
moderate attitude to the Romans and the fact that he took insufficient
precautions for the defence of the region. In order to reach Tiberias
unhindered John claimed to be ill and wrote to Josephus asking to be
allowed to bathe in the therapeutic springs. When he arrived there,
he began to incite the crowd and create a riot, in order to get the
governor to come to calm the disturbances; he would then be able to

---

[18] Oppenheimer (1991): 59, note 40; See also Lieberman (1962): III: 387; Safrai
(1982a): 159; Rosenfeld (1988: 29) remarks that since this *Tannaitic* tradition and the
word 'now' is emphasized it means that it was agreed in the close of the period and
opposed to the earlier situation; The results of the archaeological excavations in the
southern gate of Tiberias strengthen also the conclusion that Tiberias was connected
to Hammat only in the Geonitic era; See Foerster (1977): 87–91; Setefanski (1983):
24–28.

[19] Dechent (1884): 180; For the remains related to Herod Antipas era, see Smith
(1920): 290–291; For additional information on the character of the area from more
recent excavations, see Hirschfeld, Foerster and Vitto (1993): 1464–1473; Hirschfeld
(1991c): 15–50; idem, (1994): 122–134; Stacey (1995): 15–37.

[20] Meiri (1973): 29; Furrer (1879): 54; The resistance to the buildings built by Herod
Antipas in Tiberias found expression in the strict criticism by wide circles because
of the royal palace he built for himself. The palace was decorated with animals'
picturesque, which was against the Torah laws; See Stein (1968): 122; Kasher (1988:
9) assumes that the resistance towards him was a consequence of the drawing of an
eagle which ornamented the palace for the reason of flattering to Rome by adopting
her symbols; On these tensions in particular and during the war against Rome in 70
CE, see Rajak (1973): 345–368.

[21] See the discussion in chapter 6 on *Daily Life at the Thermo-Mineral Baths according
to Rabbinic Literature*.

murder him. According to Josephus, he was saved by fleeing to Lake Kinneret. This story shows that it was normal to use the therapeutic springs at this time, and, therefore, that John's request to stay there did not arouse Josephus's suspicions.[22]

A short time after this a Roman military camp, commanded by Vespasian, was erected near Hammei-Tiberias.[23] In Dechent's words, 'The terrors of war erupted in this calm spot'.[24] The story of the surrender of Tiberias is told in details in *Bellum Judaicum* 3.445–461: the people of the town opened its gates before Vespasian, and the townspeople, who were rent by dissension between those who favoured the Romans and their opponents, greeted him with applause. Before Vespasian's arrival he sent ahead of him the commander of the Legion X *Fretensis*, Trajan, and his cavalry.[25] It is not impossible that, in the course of time, soldiers of the Tenth Legion and others helped to create the baths, which were built, as we shall show in our reconstruction, below, in contemporary Roman architectural and technical style. Before Hammat and Tiberias were joined together, there was an empty area between them which was used for burials, as is attested by the inscriptions found on this spot, which confirm our contention that Roman forces were based in Hammat, close to the thermo-mineral springs. Two Latin funerary inscriptions connected with the Roman army were built into the town wall. One is engraved in magnificent monumental script within a *tabula ansata*, whose borders are decorated with four ivy leaves. It reads 'To the gods of the dead. [Here lies] Titus Artenius Augurinus, who lived for 22 years.' Schwabe conjectures that the dead man was one of the soldiers who were encamped on the site.[26] Di Segni, on the other hand, points out that from the wording of the inscription it is clear that the dead man came from one of the imperial provinces, which supplied not only legionaries, but also officials of high and middle rank; it will also be recalled that officials, many of them civilians, were attached

---

[22] Josephus, *Vita* 17.85–86; See also chapter 5, note 27.

[23] Josephus, *Bellum Judaicum* 4.11.

[24] Dechent (1884): 180; Krauss (1907–1908: 108) asserts that because of the Roman camp near the springs of Hammei-Tiberias it caused damage to the site. This fact is quite possible although no written documents and archaeological proofs have been survived.

[25] See Avi-Yonah (1967b): 158–162; See also Rajak (1973): 351–358; Bar-Kochva (1980): 188; Rappaport (1988): 19–20.

[26] Schwabe (1949): 230–231, nos. 18–19; Avi-Yonah (1946: 88) assumes that the date of the inscription is the end of the second century CE or the beginning of the third century CE.

to all the Roman legions.[27] The second inscription, also inside a *tabula ansata*, is incomplete. It reads: 'Pompeius Catullus [?], centurion of the Legion VI *Ferrata* from Orphos'.[28] At the time of Bar Kochba's revolt, the main encampment of the VI Legion was in Kefar Otnei-Legio (Lejjun), but units belonging to it were stationed in various parts of Palestine.[29] In addition, four sarcophagi from the second and third century CE with Greek inscriptions have been discovered. On one of them is a long inscription in the form of a lament in an archaic lyrical style, about Amandos of Tiberias, who served as a junior officer in the Roman army, loved the town and died, apparently, after he had retired and returned to his homeland.[30]

Coins of Tiberias from the time of the Emperor Trajan (99/100 and 108/109 CE), also bear witness to its importance as a famous therapeutic site. On them is engraved the figure of Hygieia, the goddess of health, together with a snake, the symbol of Aesculapius, the god of medicine.[31] Dechent maintains that the many non-Jews living in Tiberias worshipped the daughter of Aesculapius, as was done in many therapeutic sites in Greece and Rome.[32] It seems that the Romans turned the town into a therapeutic centre in the first century CE, and they built magnificent baths, as they did wherever there were hot springs in the lands they conquered.[33] In the time of the Roman Emperor Commodus (188/189 CE) Hygieia again appears, as in the coins from the time of Trajan, sitting on a rock from which flows a spring, and feeding a snake from a bowl.[34] These coins undoubtedly served as a means of advertising the thermo-mineral baths of Hammei-Tiberias,

---

[27] Di Segni (1967): 79.

[28] Avi-Yonah (1946): 91; This inscription is dated to the second half of the second century CE.

[29] Di Segni (1967): 80.

[30] Schwabe (1949): 222–223, 225–226; Di Segni (1967): 89–90; See also Ovadiah (1972): 229–232; For other inscriptions written in Aramaic and Greek and the affinity to Jews and non-Jews, see chapter 5 on *The Healing Properties of the Spas in the Eastern Mediterranean in Ancient Times* and chapter 6 on *Daily Life at the Thermo-Mineral Baths according to Rabbinic Literature.*

[31] For the Tiberias coins and their significance, see chapter 8.1 on *The Numismatic Expression of the Medicinal Hot Springs of Tiberias*; See also de Saulcy (1874): 335; Kindler (1961): 30, 52; idem, (1973): 50, 56; Meshorer (1985): 34; idem, (1988): 98; Dvorjetski (1990): 134–135; idem, (1992a): 187–189; idem, (1994a): 11–15; Meshorer (2000): 50; Wallack-Samuels, Rynearson and Meshorer (2000): 119; Dvorjetski, (2001–2002): 500–501; idem, (2004): 26.

[32] Dechent (1884): 180–181, note 1.

[33] Buchmann (1967): 196.

[34] Meshorer (1985): 34–35; idem, (1988): 100; Dvorjetski (1992a): 97–98.

in order to encourage people to come for treatment, and thus aid the town's economy.[35] (See Fig. 8).

The non-Jewish population and those whom they influenced also made their mark on Tiberias and its suburb, Hammat. They built temples and set up statues. One of the statues, the *Hadorei (Dorei) Tsalma*, stood over one of the springs, and served as an outlet for its waters *Dorei's penis* (*Jerusalem Talmud, Avoda Zarah* 3, 13 [43b]; *ibid., Shabbat* 14, 4 [14d]; *ibid., Berakhot* 2, 1 [4d]; *ibid., Sheqalim* 2, 7 [47a]). This statue apparently stood in front of the *Hadrianium*, a pagan shrine within the area of the thermo-mineral springs where Hadrian was worshipped.[36] Furthermore, Emperor Hadrian intervened in the administration of the towns of Galilee. From the early years of his reign the coins of Tiberias began to bear a sacred character, suggesting a process of Hellenization, and the transfer of the local authorities to the hands of non-Jewish elements.[37] In the coins dating from the town's 110th year [= 119 CE], during Hadrian's reign—one of their most prominent symbols is a temple faced with four pillars, and a statue of Zeus inside it. In that year Hadrian visited Palestine; this shrine, which the Emperor named the *Hadrianium*, was apparently built in his honour, and Zeus-Jupiter was worshipped there, as depicted in the coin.[38] Oppenheimer is of the opinion that the Talmudic tradition in the *Babylonian Talmud, Yevamot* 96b, linked to the name of Rabbi Yosse ben Qisma, who lived at the time, which speaks of a synagogue in Tiberias which became a place of idol-worship, is an allusion to Hadrian's establishment of the temple.[39] This story is connected with the *halakhic* question concerning a certain type of bolt, and whether it is permitted to lock a door with it on the Sabbath. Rabbi Elazar and Rabbi Yosse held to conflicting traditions concerning the way in which Rabban Gamaliel of Jabneh decided this question during his visit to Tiberias. It may well be that the conversion of the synagogue to a place of idol-worship was the result of Hadrian's policy, as indicated in the evidence adduced above.[40]

---

[35] Meshorer (1985): 35; Yankelvitz (1988): 17; See chapter 8 on *The Numismatic Expression of the Medicinal Hot Springs of Tiberias*.

[36] Klein (1967): 99–100; Ginzberg (1941): I: 244–246; On the non-Jewish population, see also Dvorjetski (1992a): 98; and the discussion in chapter 6 on *Daily Life at the Thermo-Mineral Baths according to Rabbinic Literature.*

[37] Jones (1971): 278; Issac and Roll (1979): 63–64; Oppenheimer (1991): 34.

[38] Meshorer (1985): 34, no. 81; Kindler (1975): 62.

[39] Oppenheimer (1991): 34, note 15.

[40] Oppenheimer (1977): 61–62.

The *Hadrianium* temple is again reproduced in the coins of Commodus, and in other types of coin, in which the figure of Sarapis is
prominent. Sarapis became the subject of one of the most popular
pagan cults in the Roman world. Aesculapius, the god of medicine,
was also identified with several Eastern gods, including the Egyptian
god, Sarapis. Sarapis's distinctive medicinal aspect is also indicated by
a considerable number of marble votive feet found in Palestine and
Trans-Jordan.[41]

Epiphanius, the Church Father of the fourth century CE, attests to the
position of the statue in front of the *Hadrianium* in the area of the hot
springs. He writes of Joseph the Comes, who was sent by the Emperor
Constantine to establish churches in Galilee—among other places,
in the unfinished *Hadrianium*; the local inhabitants, however, wanted
to turn it into a *demousin*, a public bath.[42] Some trustworthy evidence
emerges from this story. In the first place, Tiberias is depicted as a
Jewish town, in which the activities of the proselyte Joseph encountered
effective resistance on the part of the citizens. Secondly, the *Hadrianium*
is described as much bigger than the small church whose construction he managed to complete in a small section of the pagan temple.
Thirdly, after the remarkable miracle attributed to Joseph at the time
of the building of the church we would have expected more impressive
results; but Epiphanius' evasive words indicate that Joseph's initiative
was unsuccessful.[43] We may conjecture that the waters of Hammei-
Tiberias helped him to present his actions as miraculous; it is hard to
explain his success in any other way. Epiphanius' words also cast light
on Joseph the Comes' order 'to build many furnaces outside the town'.
It appears that there is here some evidence of rules and customs which
were practised in Palestine, the beginnings of which can be seen in the
Tosefta (*Baba Bathra* 1, 10, Lieberman ed., p. 131): 'Rabbi Nathan says
that furnaces must be kept 50 *amah* from the town'.[44]

---

[41] Meshorer (1988): 100; Kindler (1961): 21; See also the references to Serapis and
Aesculapius in chapter 8 on *The Numismatic Expression*; For votive feet, see for example
Weber (1993): 93–94; Bagatti (1969): 315–316; Avi-Yonah (1952): 118–119; Dussaud
(1921): 29.
[42] Epiphanius, *Panarion, Adversus Haereses* 30.12; Klein (1967): 72–73; Tzafrir (1967):
81–82; Rubin (1982): 110–111.
[43] Rubin (1982): 113; On Jewish Tiberias and the confrontation between Jews and
Christians during the Byzantine period, see Tsafrir (1967): 79–90.
[44] The reality of the municipal laws such as building rules and prohibited constructions is shown in Julianus's essay from the sixth century CE. See Lieberman (1971):
409–417.

Tiberias has a prominent place in Jewish life and thought because, for a longer period than any other place in Judaea and Galilee, it was a great centre of Torah teaching, the meeting-place of the Sanhedrin, and the residence of the Rabbis.[45] Dechent emphasizes that even to its suburban section 'there was imparted some of the splendour which encompassed Tiberias'. Thus it was, for instance, when Rabbi Meir was accustomed to preach in the synagogue of Hammat 'Knishta de Hammtha' every Sabbath eve (*Jerusalem Talmud, Sotah* 1, 4 [16d]).[46] We possess no later literary evidence about synagogues in Hammat. Two synagogues have, however, been discovered there, one north of the baths of Hammei-Tiberias, and one south of them. They were founded in the third century, and, according to Safrai, from the numerous repairs and alterations made to them it can be deduced that they were in use for an extended period.[47] Slouschz identified the northern synagogue with Knishta de Hammtha, and dated it to the early Roman period.[48] Vincent disagrees, basing his arguments on a comparison with early synagogues and on the original dimensions of the building. In his view, the main stage, and the latest, was executed in the fourth and fifth centuries CE.[49] Dothan claims that by comparison with synagogues which have been discovered since, it seems that this building, which still lacks an apse but has an entrance on the north side, facing Jerusalem, dates from the fourth century CE.[50] The northern synagogue, situated to the south of the town wall of Tiberias, was partially excavated again by Oren in the early seventies. It served the Jewish congregation of Hammat continuously from the third century CE until the beginning of the eighth century CE. Some of the most important findings here were: a latticed column with a relief portraying a menorah, a capital decorated with a menorah, and a 'seat of Moses'.[51] Dothan discovered another

---

[45] Safrai (1982a: 164) claims that in the *Jerusalem Talmud, Avoda Zarah* 4, 4 [43d] there is a continuation to Joseph the Comes narrative: Rabbi Yohanan ordered a gentile to break all the statues in the baths, and so was executed. According to Safrai Rabbi Yohanan exploited the flabbiness of the authorities during the anarchy of the third century CE; For Tiberias in the third and fourth centuries CE, see Neubauer (1868): 208–214; Bacher (1899), s.v. 'Tiberias'; Rosenfeld (1988): 29–31; Oppenheimer (1991), s.v. 'Tiberias'; Schürer (1991): II: 181.

[46] Dechent (1884): 181–182; See also Safrai (1982a): 167; Dothan (1993): 574; Yudelevitz (1950): 9; See also the notes below.

[47] Safrai (1982a): 167.

[48] Slouschz (1921): 5–39; idem, (1925): 49–52.

[49] Vincent (1921): 438–442; idem, (1922): 115–122.

[50] Dothan (1983): 66–67; idem, (1993): 574.

[51] Oren (1971a): 277; idem, (1971b): 234–235; idem, (1971c): 435–437; Weiss (1988):

synagogue south of this one, which had been excavated by Slouschz. On this spot there were two synagogues, one on top of the other, each with a different plan. Both of them had undergone a number of internal modifications, and they served the Jewish congregation of Hammat from the middle of the third until the eighth century CE. Here were found inscriptions in Greek and Aramaic, and a lattice-work marble tablet decorated with a seven-branched menorah and doves, and a relief portraying a menorah, a ram's horn and a palm frond.[52]

In addition to these archaeological remains, which attest to the cultural and spiritual life of Hammat, it should be remarked that the *Tannaim* and *Amoraim* sometimes used the expression *Hammei-Tiberias* [= the thermal baths of Tiberias] as a metaphor for hot baths in general: 'Why are there no baths of Tiberias in Jerusalem?' (*Babylonian Talmud, Pesahim* 8b); or, for instance: 'The Passover sacrifice which was cooked in the baths of Tiberias' (*ibid.*, 41a)—that is to say, in hot springs, not necessarily those of Tiberias, as will be shown below.[53]

The people of Tiberias were accustomed to bathe in the hot springs and baths of the neighbouring Hammat, both on weekdays and on Sabbaths (*Tosefta, Eruvin* 7, 5). Bathing on the Sabbath raised a number of *halakhic* questions, but the Rabbis saw that 'they could not withstand it', and permitted it in Hammei-Tiberias (*Babylonian Talmud, Shabbat* 40a; and cf. *Mishnah, ibid.*, 22, 5; *Tosefta, ibid.*, 16, 20; *Babylonian Talmud, ibid.*, 109a). Poor people from Tiberias used to frequent the baths to ask for charity (*Jerusalem Talmud, Pe'ah* 8, 9 [21b]). The people of Hammat itself used the baths not only as a place of entertainment, but as a work-place and source of income, and sometimes even used the hot water for cooking (*ibid., Shabbat* 7, 2 [10b]; *Babylonian Talmud, ibid.*, 40b; *ibid., Pesahim* 41a; cf. *Mishnah, Shabbat* 3, 4; *Babylonian Talmud, ibid.*, 39b). It is of very great importance to take into account the fact that in Rabbinic literature the many Rabbis who came to Hammei-Tiberias baths for medical treatment are not mentioned.[54] Moreover,

35; Dothan (1993): 574; Narkiss and Eshkoli (1935: 175–196) published architectural details and a number of objects found in the synagogue and its vicinity; See also Sukenik (1930): 145–151.

[52] Dothan (1968): 116–123; idem, (1981): 63–69; idem, (1983); Weiss (1988): 35–46; Hirschfeld (1992): 37–41; See also Naveh (1978): 47–50; Roth-Gerson (1987): 65–75; Milson (1987): 303–310; Dothan and Johnson (2000); Milson (2004): 45–56.

[53] See Zevin (1980): 44–52; Kasher (1934); Weiss (1986): 175–179; Dvorjetski (1999a): 117–129; See also the discussion in chapter 6.1 on *The Halakhic Stance of the Sages towards Curative Hot Springs and Baths*.

[54] See Dvorjetski (1992a): 150–153.

the Talmudic literature mentions the internal arrangements of the bathhouses only incidentally. By using the plans of the Roman baths, which have been more completely preserved, it is possible to reconstruct the configuration of the ancient baths of Tiberias to a certain extent. The walls of most of the halls were covered with polished white marble and contained rooms and halls, each of which had a specific function. One hall was a dressing-room (*apodyterium*); others housed the cool water bath (*tepidarium*), the hot-water bath (*caldarium*), and the cold water bath (*frigidarium*).[55]

The halls of the bathhouses were decorated with many statues and 'images', as we learn from Rabbi Yohanan's injunction to Bar Drosai to break up the graven images in the public bathhouse of Tiberias (*Jerusalem Talmud, Avoda Zarah* 4, 4 [43d]); from this passage we also learn that during this period the bathhouses ceased to be 'bathing houses' in the Roman style, and became Jewish establishments under the supervision of the Rabbis. We also learn of the existence of a 'cupola', an alcove in which an idol was erected—apparently a statue of Hygieia, the goddess of health, the patron of the hot springs.[56] From another source we learn that there were tall and impressive columns on the site: 'Jacob's arms were like the two pillars in the *demosin* of Tiberias' (*Tanhuma, Vayehi* 6). Judging from the archaeological remains found on the site, Meiri conjectures that these great columns supported the roof of the bathhouse, and that they also served as colonnades.[57]

The hot water which filled the pools was brought from the springs of Hammat through a 'pipe of hot water' (*Babylonian Talmud, Shabbat* 38b)—that is to say, an artificial channel. In addition to these pools were pools of cold sweet water (*ibid., Shabbat* 6a). In order to cool the water, water was brought in a pipe from the Yavne'el valley, Wadi Fajas, about 18 kilometres south of Tiberias.[58] This, too, was a serious matter, which was discussed on the therapeutic site: was it permissible

---

[55] Buchmann (1967): 197; Meiri (1973): 32; Dvorjetski (1992a): 174–176; For the technical terms, see also Gichon (1978): 37–53.

[56] Schwartz (1988): 106; See also Buchmann (1940): 95; Dvorjetski (1992a): 173–179, 187–189.

[57] Meiri (1973): 32; See also Horowitz (1923): 288.

[58] The stone pipe which branched off the aqueduct taking water to one of the bathhouses of Hammat is described by Saarisalo (1927): 53. He notes that the segments of the pipe were cylindrical on the interior and also the exterior. According to Winogradov (2002): 302, the few remaining segments have an internal diameter of 30 centimetres; See also Yanklevitz (1988): 17, 20; Dvorjetski (1999a): 123–124.

to bring cold water in a pipe through the bathhouses of Tiberias on the Sabbath in order to cool them? 'The people of Tiberias brought a stream of cold water into a channel of hot water'. Ulla said that the *halakhah* supported the people of Tiberias. Rav Nahman answered that 'the Tiberians have already broken it into its channels' (*Mishnah, Shabbat* 3, 4; *Babylonian Talmud, ibid.*, 39b). The men of Tiberias broke up the device, thereby determining that water should not be warmed with waters from the hot springs.

The course of the aqueduct inside the limits of Hammat may be traced. A complete section is visible below and south of the burial cave associated with the name of Rabbi Kahana and west of the Ganei-Hammat hotel. Sections are found inside ancient Tiberias.[59]

Today only a few poor remnants of thermo-mineral baths of Hammei-Tiberias dating from the Roman period have survived. (See Fig. 9). South of Tiberias, in Beit Yerah, the remains of a bathhouse to which a branch of the ancient aqueduct of Tiberias led have been discovered. Near the southern wall of Hammat-Tiberias have been discovered a few remnants of hot baths which apparently belonged to a private villa.[60] In Tiberias impressive remains of a bathhouse of the Roman period have been found. The site was excavated by Rabani in three seasons, but as a result of his sudden death the complete findings have not been published. The bathhouse was built at the end of the first or the beginning of the second century CE. Nine strata can be distinguished, of which the latest is from the fifth century CE. It is about 150 metres east of Mount Berenice. At an early stage two pools of plastered rough stones were dug. The building was destroyed in the second century, under unknown circumstances. This bathhouse reached the peak of its magnificence in the Byzantine period. The caldarium, two hypocausts, two deep pools, a mosaic floor and water-channels dating from this period have been discovered. This bathhouse, too, received water from the ancient town aqueduct.[61] Kallner connected

---

[59] The sections that are found inside ancient Tiberias are as follows: one is found near the south gate and was evidently connected to pools and installations excavated there by Foerster. It was dated to the Late Byzantine and Early Muslim period (1977: 87–91); In the excavations conducted by Hirschfeld a square structure that seems to be a *castellum* of this water system was exposed (1998: 104); Rabani excavated a network of pipes which joined the aqueduct to a large and elaborate bath building in the centre of the city (1953: 265); See also Avissar (1973): 49; Winogradov (2002): 302.

[60] Winogradov (1988): 151–165; idem, (2002): 295–304; Dothan (1983): 6.

[61] Scherer (1936): 5–8; Rabani (1953): 265; Photos of the reports are kept in the archive of the Tiberias Research Centre; See also Dothan (1983): 6, note 61.

the date of the building of the aqueduct with that of the bathhouse, and maintained that 'the building of the bathhouse must be linked with the construction of the Roman camp at the time of the revolt of the '70s'.[62] It should be pointed out that, despite the large number of remains, we do not possess enough data to reconstruct the appearance of the bathhouse.[63]

From the beginning of the Byzantine period, at the end of the fourth century CE, the sources relating to the baths of Hammei-Tiberias become more scant. It seems, however, that throughout all the later periods—Muslim, Crusader, and Ottoman—it was reported that the therapeutic site retained its good name despite the vicissitudes of the times. The sick people who came to the site still looked for succour, even in the half-ruined baths.[64]

The Italian Christian pilgrim Antoninus of Placentia, of the sixth century CE, observed that in his day that there were saline and sweet pools next to each other. He praised the curative properties of the hot saline waters.[65] A contemporary of Antoninus was the Byzantine historian John Malalas, known as John 'Rhetor' or 'Scholasticus'. His knowledge differs from previous traditions although he provides a useful information for everyday life of Hammei-Tiberias:[66]

> Tiberius built by the lake in the land of Judaea a city which he called Tiberias. Having discovered hot springs in the area, he built a public bath for the city which was without furnaces but which served the needs of the city from the hot springs.

Arculfus, a Christian pilgrim who visited Palestine in about 670 CE, makes similar comments, saying that Tiberias promotes health by means of its hot springs.[67] In about 749 CE the Bede Venerabilis, one of the earliest English scholars, wrote in Latin about the holy places of Palestine: 'Ab occidente Tiberiade, aquis calidis salubri' [= And Tiberias,

---

[62] Kallner (1947): 133–140; For the remains of a temporal Roman camp, see the conjecture of Meisler and Stekelis (1945): 81.

[63] Yankelevitz (1988): 18.

[64] Buchmann (1947): 101; idem, (1967): 200; Dvorjetski (1992a): 101.

[65] Antoninus, *Itinerarium* 10; Stewart (1896): 6; See also Wilkinson (1977): 81; Leyerle (1996): 355; For the analysis of the salted springs, see Anonymous (1964): 1–6.

[66] Malalas, *Chronographia* 304; Jeffrey, Jeffrey and Scott (1996): 125.

[67] Arculf, *De Locis Sanctis* 26–27; Macpherson (1896): 40–41; Margalioth (1941): 104; Buchmann (1947): 101; Kindler (1961): 31; Dvorjetski (1992a): 101; Dothan and Johnson (2000): 5.

with its hot salubrious waters, in the west]. Bede collected the material for his work *De Locis Sanctis* from earlier sources, particularly from a book written by the Frenchman Arculfus; but here it is obvious that he is quoting from Pliny the Elder, of the first century CE.[68]

In 749 CE there was a great earthquake in the Levant, which destroyed also Tiberias. It is referred to in an antique poetry, by the poet Rabbi Pinhas ben Rabbi Ya'akov, who stressed the force of the earthquake:[69]

> And the town of Tiberias was wroth and alarmed, suddenly it fell into profound darkness, the people of the upright congregation were shut in and raged...they were oppressed and worn down to the gates of Hell...women and children and preachers of the Bible and Mishnah were drowned. The strong were overcome by smoke. They cried, 'Wake, O Lord, why do you sleep?'

The twelfth century CE historian Michael the Syrian, the head of the Christian congergation of Antioch, also recalls this earthquake in his *Chronicle*. We learn from his account that the earthquake destroyed thirty synagogues as well as the baths. Hotels and inns were close to the curative baths:[70]

> This earthquake destroyed the whole of the town of Tiberias, apart from the house of one man, whose name was Issa. It also destroyed thirty Jewish synagogues, and wonderful natural objects; also bathhouses built by King Solomon the son of David. Marvellous buildings, in which there was a fountain of purifying water, collapsed and was destroyed; over and around it were wonderful buildings, and hostelries on all sides, for those who wished to be cured. There were also artistically worked earthenware vessels, and on each one was written how often it activated the stomach of whoever drank from it; everyone would choose a vessel according to the amount he wanted. All of these things were destroyed.

Michael's account of the earthenware vessels artistically wrought and in exemplary order, attests to the unique value of the waters of the baths of Hammei-Tiberias as medical potions. The waters were drunk from very thin transparent cups, known as *Kasaia Tiberiah* [= Tiberian glasses], manufactured in Elusis, a suburb of Tiberias (*Jerusalem Talmud,*

---

[68] Bede Venerabilis, *De Locis Sanctis* 316; See also Dechent (1884): 184; Dvorjetski (1992a): 101.

[69] Zulay (1937): 154; Margalioth (1941): 97–104; Assaf and Meir (1944): 10; Press (1955): I: 69, IV: 371; Klar (1967): 230; Gil (1992): 89, 178–179.

[70] Michael the Syrian, *Chronicles* 466; See also Assaf and Meir (1944): 10; Buchmann (1956): 24; Meiri (1973): 32; Dvorjetski (1992a): 102; idem, (1994b): 40; idem, (1999a): 119; idem, (2000b): 87; Dothan and Johnson (2000): 5.

Nida 2, 7 [50b]; *Babylonian Talmud, ibid.*, 21b]). This may give us a better understanding of the term *fahortha* [= earthenware pitchers], and its everyday use, in the context of Tiberias and its suburb (*Jerusalem Talmud, Eruvin* 5, 1 [22b]).[71]

During the reign of the Umayyad Caliphs new bathhouses were built, though not, as previously, at the site of the springs, but within the town.[72] The Egyptian Muslim historian and geographer al-Ya'qubi expressed wonderment at the attributes of the springs. In his *Book of the Lands* (891) he writes that the hot waters are brought to the bathhouses in pipes.[73] The Persian Muslim al-Istahrī in his *Book of the Ways of the Regions* (951) describes their location and their characteristics. He stresses that even when the water reaches the town, despite the length of the connecting channel, which cools them down, they are still so hot that the skin of hides thrown into them drops off. It is impossible to use them for bathing without mixing them with cold water.[74] Dechent says that al-Istakhrī's remark about the hides thrown into hot water shows that tanners used the waters of the hot springs for their work, as was done in antiquity in other places where there were hot springs.[75]

In a book completed in 985 CE, al-Muqaddasi, one of the greatest medieval Muslim geographers, gives a description of Palestine, Syria and Lebanon and their inhabitants. He says that Tiberias was the capital of the northern region, and that there are hot springs alongside Tiberias that supply most of the water for the bathhouses in the town. A pipe brings the water to the many bathhouses, and the hot steam heats every building, so that no artificial heating is required. According to him in another building there is cold water, a certain amount of which has to be mixed with the hot water when one wants to bathe. The same applies to the water, which is used for cleansing the mosques. Within the town he found eight bathhouses, whose hot waters were brought through canals from a site south of the town and they had no need of kindling material.[76]

---

[71] Vohalman (1939): 208; Dvorjetski (1992a): 129; cf. Schwartz (1988): 104, 109, note 14; See also the discussions on the glasses of Tiberias and the earthenware vessels in chapter 5.4.3.
[72] Buchmann (1967): 200; Kindler (1961): 32; Meiri (1973): 32–33; See the discussion below and the references to the Umayyad geographers and historians in chapter 5.1.
[73] al-Ya'qubi, *Kitab al-buldan* 115; See also Le Strange (1865): 334.
[74] al-Istakhri, *Suwar al-aklim* 58; See also Le Strange (1865): 334; Gildemeister (1883): 5; Buchmann (1967): 200.
[75] Dechent (1884): 185.
[76] al Muqaddasi, *Ahsan al-taqasim fi ma'rifat al-aqalim* 185; See Le Strange (1865): 335–336; Sukenik (1935a): 21–22; Buchmann (1967): 200–201.

The Persian traveller Nâsir-i-Khusrau visited Tiberias in 1047. He writes in his diary that 'the water of the lake is sweet and of good flavour. The waters from the hot springs near by, and the drainage-water of the houses, all flow into the lake'. Moreover, he saw at the gate of the mosque in the town a spring over which was built a hot bath. The water of this spring was so hot that until it had been mixed with cold water none could bear to have it poured over himself. 'They say this hot bath was built by Solomon, the son of David...and I myself did visit it'.[77]

During this period Jews and many other 'sufferers' from many places continued to come to Tiberias to obtain relief for their illnesses in its baths. There are appalling descriptions of this in the letters sent in 1034 to the Jews of Fostat, in Egypt, by the invalids, who call themselves 'the inhabitants of the shore of Rakkat', the ancient name of Tiberias. Letters found in the Geniza show that most of them suffered from leprosy, and that they lived in a separate camp close to the thermo-mineral springs. One of the letters, sent in order to solicit monetary contributions, describes the state of 'the sufferers from evil scabs, some deaf, some blind, some lame, and some crippled in the state of Tiberias'.[78]

The Spanish Muslim geographer al-Idrīsī wrote in 1154 about the many sufferers who apparently lived in a separate camp near the thermal springs outside the town and on other sick people: 'and sick people from all neighboring countries stream to these springs, especially those who are exhausted, lame, paralyzed, wounded, rheumatoid, and those with boils and eczema. They stay in the waters for three days and become well with Allah's help'.[79]

To this list of healing indications, one should add what Maimonides, known as Rabbi Moshe ben Maimon [= HaRambam], who lived in the twelfth century and was one of the most prominent Jewish Medieval physician. He states in his explanation to *Mishnah* (*Machshirin* 6, 7), that the quality of Hammei-Tiberias is that it is a purgative when

---

[77] Nâsir-i-Khusrau, *Tahlil-i Safarnāmah* 16; See also Le Strange (1865): 336–337; idem, (1893): 16–17; Buchmann (1967): 200.

[78] See the discussion in chapter 5.3 on *The Cairo Geniza Fragments*; See also Mann (1922): II: 193, 196–197; Assaf and Meir (1944): 11; Assaf (1958): 144–145; Buchmann (1967): 201; Gil (1981): 67; Avissar (1973): 381–382; Meiri (1973): 31; Gil (1992): 183–184, 495; Dvorjetski (1992a): 103; idem, (2000b): 85–91; Dothan and Johnson (2000): 7.

[79] al-Idrisi, *Kitāb nuzhat al-mushtāg fi ikhtirāq al-'afaq* 347.

drunk.[80] Rabbi Moshe ben Nachman, the thirteenth century Jewish scholar known as HaRamban, and one of Judaism's primary Torah commentators, notes that the water is bitter, and it is drunk by rheumatics and epileptics.[81]

The healing qualities of this site will be described below.[82] There is much truth in the descriptions of travellers, geographers and pilgrims—only a tiny selection of which has been quoted here, because of chronological limitations—claiming that the baths of Hammei-Tiberias are effective against many varied complaints, and that their efficacy in reducing pain and afflictions is well-known.[83]

4.2 HAMMAT-GADER

One of the most impressive monumental bathing complexes in the eastern Mediterranean Basin was revealed in the course of the excavations in Hammat-Gader. We shall reconstruct the history of these baths in the light of ancient historical sources, and then consider whether the historical accounts tally with the archaeological finds and the chronological conclusions which have been drawn from which these finds. (See Map 4 and Fig. 10).

Already in the Hellenistic period Gadara seems to have been a city where medical therapies were practiced. The Philinna Papyrus of the first century BCE preserves an incantation in metrical Greek prose against every type of inflammation. This charm was ascribed to a 'Syrian Gadarene woman' (Σύρας Γαδαρηνῆς).[84] The curative site at Hammat-Gader has often been described in the literature. The existence of mineral waters within the mother city of Gadara was first

---

[80] Maimonides to *Mishnah Machshirin* 6, 7.
[81] *The Babylonian Talmud* with Rav Elfas, *Shabbat* 18a.
[82] See the intensive discussion in chapter 5 on *The Healing Properties of the Spas in the Eastern Mediterranean in Ancient Times.*
[83] A partial description of Hammei-Tiberias spa in modern times was published by Robinson and Smith (1841): 258–260; For the spa's surveys since the 10th c. CE till the end of the 20th century, see Dechent (1884): 185–187; Buchmann (1947): 102–106; idem, (1956): 32–43; Buchmann (1967): 200–202; Meiri (1973): 29–34; Simon (1978a): 57–62.
[84] Maas (1942): 33–38; Koenen (1962): 167–174; Henrichs (1970): 204–205; Daniel (1988): 306; Graf (1992): 33, note 99; Weber (1992): 266, note 35; Schürer (1991): II: 135; Dickie (1994): 119–120; See especially Weber (1997): 335.

mentioned by the Greek historian and geographer Strabo, of the second half of the first century BCE. According to him, the springs were situated in a marshy region, a place where animals wallowed and drank:[85]

> In Gadara, too, there is a noxious pool; when cattle drink its waters they lose their hair, their horns and their hooves.

This state of affairs apparently continued until the time of Josephus. Although he mentions the town of Gadara, there is no mention of Hammat-Gader and its curative baths in his writings; the only hot baths east of the Jordan of which he knows are Hammei-Ba'arah and Hammei-Kallirrhoe.[86] From his silence we may conclude that the massive operation required to build the infrastructure of the bathing area had not yet been begun. It is virtually certain that the development of the spa was initiated in the second century CE, the golden age of the cities of the Decapolis, of which Gadara was one.[87]

The earliest reference to Hammat-Gader as a settlement inhabited during the bathing season is in the *Midrash Ecclesiastes Babbah* 5, 10:[88]

> He [= the Samaritan] said to him [= Rabbi Meir]: 'Have you ever been to Hammat Gader?' He replied: 'Yes'. He said, 'In the season, or not in the season?' He said, 'And how is food to be found there?' He replied 'Because the masses bring [= food] to buy and sell.'

Here, these words are attributed to Rabbi Meir, of the mid-second century CE. From his time onwards Hammat-Gader is described in the Rabbinical literature as a bustling spot, with inns, shops and living quarters. Many Rabbis visited the spa. Among them were Rabbi Judah the Patriarch, Rabbi Hanina, Rabbi Ze'ira, Rabbi Yonathan, Rabbi

---

[85] Strabo, *Geographica* 16.2.45; See also Stern (1974): I: 298; Today, there is no doubt that what happened to the animals was caused because of the chemical composition of the water. It seems that from the pharmacology analysis, the Sulphur is almost effectless on the skin and on the mucous membrane of the mouth and the stomach. The chemical composition of the liquefactive Alkaline Sulfides scorching the skin and liquefying horn tissues such as hair, nails, etc. They are used nowadays as ointments for removal of warts and treatment for several skin diseases.

[86] Schalit (1968): 22, 30, 70; See also Dechent (1884): 189; Sukenik (1935a): 20; idem, (1935b): 110.

[87] Hirschfeld (1987): 103; Dvorjetski (1988): 90–91; idem, (1992a): 104; Hirschfeld (1997): 4.

[88] This description reminds Epiphanius's report on the annual festive assembly at Hammat-Gader; For details see the discussion below and in chapter 5 on *The Healing Properties of the Spas in the Eastern Mediterranean in Ancient Times*.

Hama bar Hanina, Rabbi Ami [who went there] with Rabbi Judah Nes'iah, and more. These Rabbis also discussed the question of the Sabbath boundary and the *eruv* between Gadara and Hammat, which lies below it. It should be pointed out that in none of these writings is there an explicit reference to the complex of baths on the therapeutic site of Hammat-Gader. Inscriptions from the synagogue of Hammat-Gader also indicate that there were many visitors to the place.[89]

The first writer to mention the bathhouses of Hammat-Gader explicitly is the Church Father Origenes, of the third century CE. On verse 6, 41, of the gospel of St. John, 'The Jews then murmured at him, because he said "I am the bread which came down from heaven" ', he comments: 'Gadara is a city in Judaea close to which there are famous baths'.[90] This proves that the baths were in use at the middle of the third century CE. We may deduce, therefore, that the baths of Hammat-Gader were constructed at the beginning of the third century CE, or even earlier, during the second century, and that they were already famous at that time.[91]

The baths are mentioned again in Eusebius' *Onomastikon*, at the beginning of the fourth century CE. According to him, the baths were situated in Hammatha, or Emmatha, a village within the boundaries of Gadara: 'Gadara (*Matthew* 8, 28), a city east of the Jordan opposite Scythopolis and Tibererias to the east, on the mountain below which are the hot baths'.[92] Elsewhere in this book Eusebius again mentions the proximity of the mother city, Gadara, to its suburb: 'And there is another village near Gadara: Emmatha, where the hot water baths are situated'.[93]

Cyril, a bishop of Jerusalem of the fourth century CE, states that there was a devastating earthquake in Palestine in the year 363 CE. Among the places which were destroyed and turned into blood he includes *Aina de Gader* [= the spring of Gader], the Aramaic-Syriac name of Hammat-Gader.[94] Modern eyewitnesses of such natural catastrophes

---

[89] Naveh (1978): 54–64; Avi-Yonah (1993): II: 566–569.

[90] Origenes, *Commentaria in Evangelium Joannis* 6, 41, p. 150.

[91] Hirschfeld (1987: 103–104) believes that the evidence for constructing the *thermae* at the beginning of the mid third century or even in the second on century CE is the mention of Emperor Antoninus Pius (138–161 CE) in Empress Eudocia's dedicatory inscription.

[92] Eusebius, *Onomastikon* 74.

[93] Idem, *ibid.*, 22; See also Schürer (1991): II: 133; Sukenik (1935a): 20.

[94] Brock (1979): 273, no. 10, 276; For the explanation, see Jastrow (1950): 1072.

confirm our assumption that this apocalyptic metaphor might be explained by the red soil of the area mixed with groundwater during seismic activities.[95]

In the fourth century CE the Greek biographer Eunapius wrote:[96]

> After a certain time they saw Gadara; there are situated the Syrian hot baths, second only in the whole Roman world to those of Baiae [= in the Gulf of Naples], to which no other can be compared.

Eunapius' literary account adds that people flocked in groups to the site to bathe. One such group was that of his revered teacher, the neo-Platonist philosopher Iamblichus, and his disciples, who made the long journey from Athens to the spa of Hammat-Gader. In his words can be sensed the mystic atmosphere in which the site was shrouded. There were many accounts of miracles linked to the fountains of Hammat-Gader, which in his day were also known by the mythological names of Eros and Anteros. While they were bathing the people of the group discussed the two springs. Iamblichus touched the spring water, and to the astonishment of the onlookers a child sprang up from the water and embraced him. This phenomenon was repeated in the other spring. Thereafter, he let the two children return from whence they came. From then on, his companions had no doubt of the philosopher's ability to perform miracles.[97]

Dechent maintains that images of the guardian gods of the spa were engraved on coins of the Roman period. He maintains that the coins from Gadara which bear the image of the goddess Ashtoreth, the Syrian counterpart of the goddess Aphrodite, are proof that Eros was worshipped in the town of Gadara because of his links with Aphrodite.[98] Moreover, Geiger points out that Eunapius' exact description of the location of Gadara, and the names of the two springs, are based on local tradition. In his view, an epigram about Eros written by Meleager, an epigrammatic poet poet who lived in Gadara in the first half of the

[95] Weber (1997): 335.
[96] Eunapius, *Vitae Sophistarum* 459.
[97] Sukenik (1935a): 21; Lieberman (1946): 354; Hirschfeld and Solar (1981): 202; Dvorjetski (1988): 92; idem, (1992a): 105; Yegül (1992): 121; Hirschfeld (1997): 5; Belayche (2001): 269; On Eros and Anteros in the Greek mythology see, for instance, Rose (1989): 123; Mulas (1978); On the close affinity between Eros, the baths and the Three Graces, see Dunbabin (1989): 13–16; Dvorjetski (1999a): 127–128; See also *The Numismatic Expression of the Thermo-Mineral Hot Springs at Gadara* in chapter 8.3.
[98] Dechent (1884): 190–191.

first century BCE, was derived from an ancient tradition which was the source of Eunapius' information.[99] This hypothesis may be confirmed in the light of a hoard of jewels recently discovered in Gadara. The image of Eros is engraved on eighteen jewels dated between the first century BCE and the third century CE.[100] Hirschfeld identifies Eros with the hot spring of 'Ain el-Maqle, which reaches a temperature of 51°C, round which the therapeutic baths were constructed, and Anteros with 'Ain Būlus, whose temperature is 25°C, and is the only spring of Hammat-Gader whose waters are drinkable.[101] (See Map 4).

The Church Father Epiphanius, a contemporary of Eunapius, describes the colourful atmosphere of the Hammat-Gader thermal baths. A festive gathering, an annual fair, πανήγυρις in Greek, used to take place there, and people from all parts of the empire would gather there to bathe. Men and women bathed together, and the curative site was exceedingly crowded:[102]

> Well, they went to Gadara for the hot baths. There is an annual gathering there. Persons who wish to bathe for a certain number of days arrive from every quarter, to rid themselves of their ailments, if you please—though it is a trick of the devil. For where God's wonders have been, the adversary has already spread his deadly nets—men and women bathe together! There happened to be an unusually beautiful free woman in the bath. With his accustomed licentiousness the young man brushed against the Girl's side as he strolled about in the hot-air room. But being Christian, she naturally made the sign of the cross. There was no need for her to break the rules and bathe in mixed company. These things happen to simple laypersons, from the laxity of the teachers who do not forewarn them through their instructions. Still, that God might make his wonders manifest, the younger, I mean the Patriarch, failed in his enterprise. For he sent emissaries to the woman and promised her gifts, but she insulted his messengers and did not yield to the pampered youth's futile efforts. Then, when his helpers learned of the passion the boy had betrayed for the girl, they undertook to equip him with more powerful magic—as Josephus himself described to me minutely. After sunset they took the unfortunate lad to the neighboring cemetery. In my country there are

[99] Geiger (1986): 375–376; Merrill (1944): 268–269.

[100] Henig and Whiting (1987): 19–21, nos. 166–184.

[101] Hirschfeld (1987): 104, note 16; idem, (1989c): 141–143; On the folklore of 'Ain Būlus, which was known by the Christians as the spring of Paul, see Ben-Ami (1984): 18–19.

[102] Epiphanius, Panarion, Adversus Haereses 30.7; Williams (1987): 125; See also Rubin (1982): 108–109; Abel (1938): II: 458–459; Sukenik (1935a): 21; idem, (1935b): 111; Hirschfeld and Solar (1981): 202; Hirschfeld (1987): 105; Dvorjetski (1988): 93–94; idem, (1992a): 106–107; idem, (1994a): 17–18.

places of assembly of this kind, called 'caverns', made by hewing them
out of cliff sides. Taking him there the cheats who were with him recited
certain incantations and spells, and did some things, with him and in the
woman's name, which were full of impiety.[103]

Epiphanius' account is incomplete, and part of it is suspect, but his
description of the baths is accurate in the main.[104] Safrai maintains that
the fair was centred on a regional festival in honour of Heracles, the
patron and guardian of the merchants.[105] We shall see below that an
analysis of a *baraitha* in the *Jerusalem Talmud* (Tractate *Shabbat*) shows that
the pagan fair was primarily in honour of the τρεῖς χάριτες: The Three
Graces, after whom the Hammat-Gader baths were originally named.[106]
The fact that there was an annual fair on the site recalls the saying in
Midrash Ecclesiastes Rabbah 5, 10, in which Hammat-Gader is mentioned
as a place where crowds come to buy and sell. (See Fig. 22).

We know of the prohibition of mixed-sex bathing at the time of
Hadrian, and it was renewed during the reign of Elagabal. The church
enforced this prohibition strictly, and permitted the use of the baths
for therapeutic purposes only.[107]

The Church Father Hieronymus, who lived at the end of the fourth
and the beginning of the fifth century CE, mentions the bathhouses
under the entry 'Gadara' in his *Onomastikon*. His description explicitly
explains the connection between the hot springs and the baths:[108]

> Gadara urbs trans Iordanem contra Scythopolim et Tiberiadem ad ori-
> entalem plagam sita in monte, ad cuius radices aquae calidae erumpunt,
> balneis desuper aedificatis [= Gadara, a city beyond the Jordan opposite
> Scythopolis and Tiberias to the east, is situated on a mountain at whose
> foot hot springs, on which baths have been built, erupt].

---

[103] According to Rubin (1982: 111–112) from the chronological point of view the
Patriarch Judah III, who is known as Rabbi Judah Nes'iah, is more suitable than Hillel;
cf. Schwabe (1949): 236–237; idem, (1968): 187, who is confident that hermaphrodites
bathed there and not men and women together; See also Tsafrir (1968): 81–82; Herr
(1985): 63–64; The caves around the site were documented by the German engineer
Schumacher (1886b: 298–300), who fulfilled an intensive survey in the Golan.

[104] Efron (1988): 317; See especially Rubin (1982): 105–106, 111–112.

[105] Safrai (1984): 158.

[106] See for instance Dvorjetski (1994c): 100–115; idem, (1999a): 127–128; idem,
(2004): 25–26; See also the discussion on the τρεῖς χάριτες in chapter 8.3 on *The
Numismatic Expression of the Medicinal Hot Springs of Gadara*.

[107] Dechent (1882): 193; Jones (1964): 976–977; Yegül (1992): 314–320; Dvorjetski
(1992): 107; See also the survey in chapter 3 on *Medicinal Hot Springs and Healing Spas in
the Graeco-Roman World* and in chapter 9 about *Pilgrimage to the Spas in the Eastern Mediterranean during the Later Roman and Byzantine Periods*.

[108] Hieronymus, *Onomastikon* 74; See also Dechent (1884): 191–192; Sukenik (1935a):
20.

In another place in the *Onomastikon*, in the entry 'Ammatha', Hieronymus gives a literal translation of Eusebius' words, with no comment:[109]

> Est et alia uilla in uicinia Gadar nomine Ammatha ubi calidae aquae erumpunt [= And there is another village, called Ammatha, near Gadara, and there hot waters erupt].

The Christian pilgrim Antoninus from Placentia in northern Italy, who travelled in the Holy Land in about 570 CE, documented his visit in a book describing his pilgrimage. His accounts of the name and location of the baths, the method of treating lepers, the lepers' pool and their quarters, are of great importance.[110] According to Antoninus, invalids who came to the baths stayed in a hostel which was supported by the public. Though he does not say explicitly that the municipality of Gadara subsidized the hostel, this is quite possible, particularly if we assume that the city profited in some way from the baths situated on its territory. This tradition of the healing of lepers is apparently connected with the appellation of the bathing complex as *Thermae Heliae* [= Elijah's Baths]. This name is a reference to the Biblical story about the healing in the Jordan waters of Na'aman, the commander of the Aramaean army, who had leprosy, in the waters of the Jordan River following the advice of Elisha, the disciple of Elijah (*II Kings* 5, 1–16). If so, at the time of Antoninus the people of Hammat-Gader adopted the Biblical tradition of Elijah of Gilead, and gave his name to the therapeutic baths. The method of treatment of the lepers, as depicted in this detailed account, was very strange. They used a special bath in the spa (*solium*) only at night. When they went into the bath, which was opposite the opening of the *clibanus*, they used candles and incense, and practised a mysterious ritual. As a result they saw visions which, according to Dechent, were relics of ancient superstitions.[111] The liturgy described by this eyewitness notes that the lepers bathed and were treated by incubation, as was practised in ancient therapeutic centres, *Asclepeia*, in a great bath opposite the *clibanus*. This recalls the pagan rite of incubation as executed in the cults of Aesculapius or other healing gods in the Graeco-Roman world.[112] It seems that

---

[109] Hieronymus, *Onomastikon* 23.

[110] Antoninus Placentinus, *Itinerarium* 7; See also Abel (1938): II: 459; Green and Tsafrir (1982): 84–85; Wilkinson (1977): 81; Hirschfeld and Solar (1981): 202; Hirschfeld (1987): 105–106; Dvorjetski (1988): 95–96; idem, (1992a): 107–108; Yegül (1992): 124.

[111] Dechent (1884): 194; See also Vincent and Abel (1932): 277–285.

[112] Hirschfeld and Solar (1981): 202; Hirschfeld (1987): 105; Weber (1997): 336.

Hammat-Gader was a medical centre specializing in the treatment of leprosy, and, in general, of serious skin ailments, as early as the time of the Emperor Hadrian.[113]

The eighth-century CE Byzantine chronographer Syncellus lists the towns and regions in which King Jannaeus the Hasmonean won victories, including Pella, Abila, Hippos [= Sussita], Philoteria [= Beit Yerah], the Bashan, and Gadara—and, in connection with the latter, the baths of Hammat-Gader.[114] In this text the existence of hot water springs or baths, and the fact that they are in the territory of Gadara, is emphasized. Syncellus adds to our information from classical historical sources the fact that the hot baths were in, or adjacent to, the city of Gadara, or immediately below it. Thus, we have unimpeachable evidence from ancient sources in Syriac, Greek and Latin that the therapeutic baths in Hammat-Gader were a dominant and inseparable part of the district (χώρα) of Gadara.

We have no knowledge of what happened to the baths towards the end of the Byzantine period, but it may be assumed that the site was damaged in one of the earthquakes which occurred in the area during this period.[115] Hirschfeld considers that the baths were apparently destroyed in the eighth or ninth century CE.[116] It seems that according to Syncellus's evidence it have to be postponed it to the ninth century CE.

Later Muslim sources refer to the baths in the past tense. In the tenth century the Muslim geographer al-Muqaddasi, wrote of the hot springs of al-Ḥammah.[117] According to him those who suffered from boils, swellings, abscesses, or similar afflictions came to this place to bathe for three days. After this they immerse themselves in another, cold spring, and then, by the grace of God, they were cured. There were buildings round these springs, and each of them devoted to the cure of a specific disease. The sufferers bathed and were cured at this site since the time

[113] For further details see chapter 5 on *The Healing Properties of the Spas in the Eastern Mediterranean in Ancient Times.*
[114] Syncellus, *Chronographia* 5.235.
[115] For the several earthquakes see, for instance, Willis (1928): 73–103; Shalem (1941): 117; Amiran-Kallner (1950–1951): 225–226; Croke (1981): 122–147; Russell (1985): 37–59; Karcz and Lom (1987): 4–17; Tsafrir and Foerster (1992): 231–235; Gil (1994): 29–58; Tsafrir and Foerster (1995): 179–180; See also the discussion in chapter 2 on *Geological, Hydrological and Medicinal Aspects of Hot Springs in the Eastern Mediterranean—Past and Present.*
[116] Hirschfeld (1987): 107.
[117] Al-Muqaddasi, *Ahsan al-taqasim fi ma'rifat al-aqalim* 185.

of Aristotle. Aristotle asked the ruler to destroy the buildings, so that men should not think that doctors were unnecessary. Al-Muqaddasi added that he verified this story: 'there are to be found here waters of various qualities, and with various therapeutic characteristics; anybody who comes here today has to bathe in them all, in order to make sure that he receives treatment suitable to his condition'.[118]

As a result of the destruction of the bathhouses and the lack of supervision by the government, the site returned to the condition it had been in at the time of Strabo. The hot springs continued to attract bathers, as is attested by the Arabic geographer al-Yāqūt and the cosmographer ad-Dimašqī, but they were drawn only from among the local population. The latter one says as follows:[119]

> From the hot springs [= el-Ḥamme], too, that rise at a village called Jadar [= Gadara] and where there are waters for healing every sort of disease that men suffer from—there comes down a great river [= the Yarmuk] that joins the Jordan.

The name of Hammat-Gader and its baths was preserved in the Arabic name of the site, Tel el-Hammeh, and in the name of the mound within which was discovered the ancient synagogue—Tel Bānī, from the Greek βαλανεῖον, 'the mound of the bath'.[120] Geographers and travelers, such as Buckingham, Burckhardt, Seetzen, Oliphant, and Schumacher, who visited the spot in the nineteenth century and the beginning of the twentieth found the site deserted, with only the very top of the building projecting above ground.[121] Anybody who visits the Hammat-Gader thermo-mineral baths today cannot but marvel at the remnants of the glory and elegance of the culture of those who lived there during the Roman period.

The Roman thermal baths of Hammat-Gader constitute an imposing architectural complex, of exceptional size and intricacy. They are situated at the southern end of the site, between the Roman theatre and the channel of the Yarmuk, and cover an area of about 5,000 square

---

[118] Le Strange (1965): 335–336; Sukenik (1935a): 21–22; idem, (1935b): 111–112.

[119] al-Yāqūt, *Muʿjam al-buldan* 113; ad-Dimašqī, *Nuhbat ad-dahr fi agaʾib al-bahr wa-l-bahr* 107; See also Le Strange (1965): 54; Mershen and Knauf (1988): 132.

[120] Avi-Yonah (1993): 565; Gichon (1978: 46) indicates that the βαλανεύς is the inspector, who collected money for the entrance to the baths. According to his report there are some sided rooms that were uncovered in excavations in Palestine and were used for baths' workers.

[121] Buckingham (1821): 145, 153–158; Burckhardt (1822): 148–149; Seetzen (1854): 188–189; Oliphant (1880): 131–139; Schumacher (1888a): 149–160.

metres. The baths were built round a spring of mineral water, *'Ain el-Maqle*, which emerges with a temperature of 51°C in the southern part of the site. On its bank was built the 'hill pool' from which the water was diverted into a series of bathing pools. So far seven pools have been uncovered, each of them in a separate hall of distinctive size and design. The pools, in each of the halls, enabled the bathers to become accustomed gradually to the differing degrees of heat of the water, as they went from hall to hall in a progression which came to an end in a pool built by the side of the spring. The huge, splendid halls and the extensive pools display a distinct similarity between the baths of Hammat-Gader and other imperial baths elsewhere in the world. Since they are therapeutic baths with hot mineral waters they do not have the usual features of a bathhouse, such as the *caledarium* or the *hypocaust*. In other words, the thermal complex lacks artificial heating installations. Their principal feature is the pools of hot, luke-warm, and cold water which were made to flow from the nearby springs. As has been noted, the bathing complex of Hammat-Gader is very similar to that of the city of Bath, in south-west Britain and Terme Taurine in Italy.[122] (See Fig. 10).

The evidence of Origenes of the third century CE, the first writer to refer explicitly to these baths, tallies with the findings of the archaeological excavations. The baths were built at two main periods: the Roman-Byzantine period, during which most of the parts of the complex were built gradually, and the early Muslim period, during which far-reaching alterations were executed in a relatively short time.[123] On the basis of architectural and archaeological considerations, these two scholars maintain that the Hall of the Niches (*Area D*) was planned and built in the earlier period, at the beginning of third century CE or the end of the second CE, while the oval bathing-hall (*Area A*) and the other parts of the building were constructed in the course of the third century CE or at the beginning of the fourth CE. In their view, comparison with

---

[122] See the final report of the excavation at Hammat-Gader: Hirschfeld (1997); See also idem, and Solar (1979): 230–231; idem, (1981): 199–219; Hirschfeld (1987): 101–116; Hirschfeld and Cohen (1992): 283–306; Avi-Yonah and Hirschfeld (1993): 565–573; Dvorjetski (1988): 98–113; idem, (1992a): 110–115; For Bath Spa see, for instance, Cunliffe (1995): 129, Fig. 31; For Terme Taurine see Köhler (2002): 295–305; See also the descriptions in chapter 3 on *The Medicinal Hot Springs and Healing Spas in the Graeco-Roman World*.

[123] Hirschfeld and Solar (1981): 198–199; idem, (1984): 33; On the presence of the Roman army at the region of Hammat-Gader, see the details in chapter 8.4.3.

similar complexes which have been excavated—one in Tunisia, dated at the end of the second century CE, and one in Alexandria, dated at the third century CE—may be of assistance in fixing the date of the construction of the Hammat-Gader spa.[124]

During the fourth century CE a magnificent colonnade was added, in order to decorate the internal space of the hall of the columns (*Area C*). Some alterations in this area and repairs to the buildings can be discerned. They may be linked with the evidence of Cyril, the fourth-century CE Bishop of Jerusalem. As remarked above, he stated that there was a devastating earthquake in Palestine in 363 CE, and that, among other places, *Aina de Gader* was damaged. According to Hirschfeld and Solar, this may explain a number of repairs to the complex: limestone patches in the longitudinal walls of the oval hall (*Area A*), and strange joins in the magnificent colonnade between the tops of the monumental columns and the pillars on both its sides (*Area C*). These two scholars conjecture that the people of Gadara and Hammat-Gader exploited the repair work executed as a result of the earthquake in order to improve the appearance of the baths.[125] One cannot ignore the fact that at the end of the fourth century CE Eunapius claimed that the Hammat-Gader baths were second only in their beauty to those of Baiae, which were, in his view, the most beautiful in the whole of the Roman world.[126] (See Figs. 11, 12, and 15).

The therapeutic baths of Hammat-Gader reached the height of their fame and entered a phase of intensive construction in the fifth century CE. The imperial building inscriptions found in the hall of the fountain are evidence of this. These dedicatory inscriptions attest to the baths' reputation, and to the fact that many of those who flocked to the site from far and wide in the empire, and made it a focus of interest on the part of wealthy and powerful men, were cured, and wished to perpetuate their memory in its magnificent halls. This was a very common phenomenon in all the cities of the Roman Empire, and was a major factor in forming the character of the Roman-Byzantine city.[127]

Three dedicatory inscriptions from the fifth to the seventh century CE are of prime importance in reconstructing the history of the

---

[124] Krencker and Kruger (1929): 224–225; Kolataj (1976): 218–229; idem, (1983): 186–194.

[125] Hirschfeld and Solar (1981): 201; idem, (1984): 33.

[126] Eunapius, *Vitae Sophistarum* 459.

[127] Hirschfeld (1987): 106; For all inscriptions found at Hammat-Gader, see Di Segni (1997): 185–266 and Amitai-Preiss (1997): 267–278.

Hammat-Gader thermal baths.[128] The earliest is an inscription in the
spirit of classical culture, created by Eudocia, the wife of the Emperor
Theodosius II, which adorns the hot springs and baths. The inscription
contains a list of personal names, pagan and Christian titles, mythological figures, and prominent parts of the bath: pools, fountains, the *clibanus*,
and more. Two Greek mythological figures—Hygieia and Galatea, both
of them appropriate to therapeutic baths—are also named. As noted
above, Hygieia was the patron of therapeutic springs, and Galatea was a
nymph, associated with springs and water sources as were all nymphs.[129]
Eudocia compares the *clibanus* to *Paean*, the physician of the Olympian
gods in Greek mythology—an allusion to the special therapeutic
powers of the Hammat-Gader baths. We do not know whether Eudocia
visited the Hammat-Gader baths for medical treatment, nor whether
she built, renovated or decorated any of its buildings.[130] Hirschfeld and
Solar maintain that the inscription was carved in the floor after the
hall had been built. In their view, the decorative marble fountains on
the edge of the central pool in the hall of the fountains were added
at the time of Eudocia.[131] A poem of praise composed by Eudocia in
honour of the baths, written in Homeric metre, has many references
to the Iliad, and, even more, to the Odyssey. Greek intellectuals born
in Gadara—the epigrammatic poet Meleager mentioned above, the
Epicurean Philodemus, a contemporary of Cicero, and the Cynic
Oenomaus—also wrote about Homer; Meleager claimed that Homer
was of Syrian origin.[132] Green and Tsafrir point out that, in addition
to expressions taken from the works of Homer, the influence of other

---

[128] Green and Tsafrir (1982): 77–82; Hirschfeld and Solar (1981): 203; idem, (1984):
37, 39; Hirschfeld (1987): 106; Dan (1984): 54–55, 227; Ovadiah (1977): 445–446;
idem, (1998): 17.

[129] Green and Tsafrir (1982): 77–96; Meïmaris (1983): 388–398; Dvorjetski (1988):
102–107; idem, (1992a): 111–112; Dunbabin (1989): 13; Di Segni (1997): 228–233;
Belayche (2001): 272–273; On Eudocia the Empress, see Gregorovius (1892); Abel
(1952): II: 331–337; Holum (1976): 280–292; Cameron (1982): 217–291; Holum
(1984): 112–146, 175–225; On Eudocia the poetess, see Ludwich (1882): 206–222;
idem, (1897): 24–114; Schreiber (1984): 180–181.

[130] On various options of Eudocia's visit to Hammat-Gader, see the discussion
in chapter 5 on *The Healing Properties of the Spas in the Eastern Mediterranean in Ancient
Times*.

[131] Hirschfeld and Solar (1981): 203.

[132] Geiger (1985): 3–16; Luz (1988): 222–231; Schürer (1991): II: 49–50; Geiger
(1994): 221–230; See also Dilts and Kennedy 1997, s.v. 'Homer'; On the Greek Cynic
in the Talmud, see Dvorjetski (1988): 36–42; Luz (1989): 49–54; Dvorjetski (1992a):
111; Luz (1992): 42–80; idem, (2003): 97–107.

classical authors—Aeschylus, Sophocles and Euripides—is also apparent. They conclude that this constitutes evidence that admiration for the culture of classical Greece was widespread in intellectual circles in the fifth century CE. This poetical inscription, like the bathing complex of Hammat-Gader itself, was a relic of the classical culture which was in the process of disappearing under the influence of the Christian faith and religious fanaticism.[133] The architecture and sculpture which the Empress found at this site aroused in her strong echoes of the cultural ambiance of her youth. In addition to the two ladies, Indian and Matrona, mention may be made here of the statue of the Three Graces, referred to in the *Jerusalem Talmud* when two Rabbis met while bathing at the site (*Shabbat* 3, 4 [6a]).[134] A marble statue of a man all of whose left shoulder is covered in a loose-flowing *toga* has been discovered in *area E*. Hirschfeld and Solar conjecture that this statue, whose head is missing, is of Aesculapius, the god of healing.[135] In this connection it is important to recall that in the classical world round buildings known as *tholoi*, in which were kept sacred snakes, were dedicated to the god of healing. Such a *tholos* was named after the donor Alexandros of Caesarea; it was built in the *tepidarium*, which was undoubtedly one of the two luke-warm pools mentioned in Eudocia's inscription.[136] (See Figs. 13, 14, and 19).

In view of the mention of Saint Elias, 'Ηλίας ἀγνός, the famous and well-beloved Biblical figure adopted by the Christians, scholars have surmised that part of the bathhouse was named after the prophet Elijah.[137] As has been noted above, in Antoninus' *Itinerarium* the *Termae Heliae* baths are called 'the baths of Elijah'.[138] Scholarly opinion holds that Empress Eudocia learnt about the Roman Emperor Antoninus Pius (138–161 CE) from a statue or inscription at this site. It is believed that the mention of his name is not accidental, and that the foundations of the bath were laid in his time, perhaps even with his support. This is believed to be evidence that the Hammat-Gader bath was already in use in the second century CE.[139]

---

[133] Green and Tsafrir (1982): 77–80.
[134] For more details see chapter 6.2 on *The Sages at the Therapeutic Sites.*
[135] Hirschfeld and Solar (1981): 218; idem, (1984): 28–29; cf. idem, (1997): 148–152, Pl. VI.
[136] Avi-Yonah and Shatzman (1981): 89; Green and Tsafrir (1982): 87–88.
[137] Green and Tsafrir (1982): 88.
[138] Antoninus Placentinus, *Itinerarium* 7.
[139] Green and Tsafrir (1982): 88; Hirschfeld and Solar (1984): 38.

The Emperor Anastasius (491–518 CE) is mentioned in four other inscriptions. They show that the donor Alexandros was the governor (*hegemon*) of Palestina Prima and its capital, Caesarea. Di Segni and Hirschfeld believe that Alexandros' epithet περίφρων—reasonable, thoughtful—indicates that hot baths were considered at that time to be therapeutic site, and not only places for holidays and entertainment, as had been the case in the fourth century CE.[140] Alexandros initiated repairs and construction at the site, and scholars comment that this tallies with the Emperor Anastasius' dynamic activities, described by Malalas—massive construction of various sorts of buildings, such as fortifications, harbours, aqueducts and public baths.[141] (See, for instance, Fig. 19).

Antoninus Placentinus, who visited the Hammat-Gader thermal baths in the second half of the sixth century CE, tells us of the tradition of healing lepers. The infected with leprosy bathed and were treated by incubation, as was done in the ancient centres of Aesculapius, in a large bath, opposite the entrance to the *clibanus*. The details of his description of the process undergone by the lepers is confirmed by the design of the double-sloped bathing pool which has been excavated in its entirety in *area A*.[142] Green and Tsafrir conjecture that this bath was separate from the entire complex which served the majority of the bathers; but it is impossible to know whether the term *clibanus* refers to part of the complex, or to the main building.[143] Avi-Yonah comments that from the fourth century CE onwards the law concerning lepers became more stringent. They were forbidden to enter the forum or the public baths; they were, therefore, allotted a special pool, as, for instance, that in Beth Shean-Nysa-Scythopolis, which is outside the town. It was renewed by Bishop Theodore in 558/559 CE.[144]

In the Hammat-Gader baths there is a bathing-pool in a separate architectonic space, whose entries and exits can all be locked. In this isolated pool dozens of clay lamps of a type characteristic of the third and fourth century CE, have been found. They are quite uniform, and none of them contain the soot which is usually found on the lip of

---

[140] Di Segni and Hirschfeld (1986): 251–268; See especially idem, (1986): 256.
[141] Malalas, *Chronographia* (1831): 139–140; See also Di Segni and Hirschfeld (1986): 263.
[142] Hirschfeld and Solar (1981): 209–211; Hirschfeld (1997): 132–134.
[143] Green and Tsafrir (1982): 85.
[144] Avi-Yonah (1963): 325–326.

a lamp that has been used. Hirschfeld and Solar conjecture that they were thrown into the pool during the performance of some ritual; but it may also be that they were set down on the edge of the pool, and fell into it. If this bath was used by the lepers, as in Antoninus of Placentia's account, these two scholars believe that the healing of the lepers began when the pool in *area B* was inaugurated. It should be added that the pool and the hall have been dated, on archaeological grounds, to the third and fourth centuries CE.[145] This is a reasonable assumption, since the promotion of the Hammat-Gader baths as a cure for leprosy was an important method of advertising the site and increasing the profitability of the baths.

At the end of the Byzantine period the site was damaged by an earthquake, which affected the whole region. The damage to the monumental baths influenced the Mu'āwiya Inscription, a Byzantine Greek inscription of the seventh century CE. This dedicatory inscription was found in the hall of the fountains, and celebrates the reopening of the baths at the beginning of the reign of the Caliph Abdullah Mu'āwiya, the founder of the Umayyad dynasty, on December 5, 662 CE. The fact that the inscription is in Greek, the cross at its head, and the use of Byzantine dating, prove that in the early days of the Umayyad dynasty the Arab administration did not change the administrative arrangements or the religious and cultural character of the Greek towns. The restoration of the baths, which was one of the first building projects of the Caliph Mu'āwiya, reveals the interest of the Umayyad Caliphs in Palestine, and their contribution to its development, and particularly to that of the Jordan Valley. In the course of the excavations it became clear that the Umayyad construction was massive: some of the pools in *Areas B, C*, and *E* were filled in and paved over, and the longitudinal walls of the oval hall (*Area A*) were repaired and rebuilt. The ceramic material which was found over the oval pool is all from the early Muslim period. This, like the ceramic findings in other areas of the excavation, bears out the accuracy of the Mu'āwiya Inscription, which tells of the repair and reconstruction of the bath in 662/663 CE. The inscription refers to the function of the baths: 'for the health of the sick'; it appears that this completes the phrase which appears in Eudocia's inscription: 'who are born to suffering'.[146] (See Fig. 21).

---

[145] Hirschfeld and Solar (1981): 209–211; See also Rosental and Sivan (1978): 11, nos. 450–451.

[146] Hirschfeld and Solar (1981): 203–204; Hasson (1982): 97–101; Blau (1982): 102;

Engravings discovered in the floor of the hall of the fountains (*Area D*) tell of the end of the Hammat-Gader baths. These engravings, in Kufic script, were made after the building was abandoned, but before the walls collapsed and completely covered the floor of the hall. In one of them there appears the phrase *Allahumā*, a common form of address to God, which was in use in Palestine only in the early Muslim period, until the middle of the ninth century. Thus, these engravings indicate the ninth century, at the latest, as the final period at which the building was in use.[147]

Three components of the above account can fix the chronological framework of the baths: the inscription from the period of Muʾāwiya written in Byzantine Greek inscription, the engravings in Kufic script, and the Corinthian pillars of the columned gate. (See Fig. 11). Scholarly opinion is that the bathing complex was built in the Roman period (second to third century CE), and the monumental columned gate was added at this time, or at the beginning of the Byzantine period (fourth to fifth century CE). The building, which was in continual use, was repaired and rebuilt in the year 662/663, and was in continuous use thereafter until the ninth century at the latest.[148]

We shall now turn to some other finds, and to the nature of the construction, which will complete the chronological framework of this magnificent complex. (See Fig. 10).

The most impressive find is a row of 32 marble fountains along the border of the pool (*Area D*), which were set up at a late stage in the baths' existence. They fed water into the pool through lead pipes, of varying sizes, but with a standard pattern: a sort of altar, with the head of an animal from whose mouth the water gushed forth on the side towards the lake. Fountains in the shape of men or animals from which the water flowed forth were common, as can be seen from the discussion in *Tosefta, Avodah Zarah* 6, 6 (Tsukermandel ed., p. 469): 'No man should put his mouth to the face which provides water for the town and drink from it, lest he appear to be kissing an idol; he should take the water in his hand and drink'. On archaeological grounds the system of fountains was erected at the time of the Empress Eudocia,

Green and Tsafrir (1982): 94–96; Di Segni and Hirschfeld (1986): 265–266; Hirschfeld (1987): 107; Dvorjetski (1988): 109–110; idem, (1992a): 113; Di Segni (1992): 315–317; Zeyadeh (1994): 124; Di Segni (1997): 237–240.

[147] Hirschfeld and Solar (1984): 36–37; Amitai-Preiss (1997): 267–269.

[148] Hirschfeld and Solar (1979): 230–234; Hirschfeld and Cohen (1992): 283.

in the middle of the fifth century CE. The hall of the fountains is one of the biggest architectural spaces which has been discovered in Palestine. The central section measures 29.6 × 13.9 metres, and with the addition of the two wings it is 53.5 metres long. It is surmised that this hall was open to the heavens, and constituted a sort of *natatio*, a feature common in large baths of the Roman period. The walls of the hall of the fountains are made of big limestone rocks, meticulously dressed, in contrast to the other walls of the complex, which were made of basalt and bonded with cement. This method of building is typical of monumental construction in the eastern Roman provinces in the second and third centuries CE. In the course of the excavations it came to light that this hall was earlier than the other parts of the complex. There were five recesses leading from the longitudinal walls of the hall, which had been preserved to a height of 5.3 metres: a semi-circular recess in the centre and on both sides of it rectangular recesses, two on each side. The central recesses were roofed with beams in the shape of half-domes, only the first course of which has survived. A similar system of recesses is to be found in the central bathing hall of the baths of Bath Spa, which were built in the first and second centuries CE. The overall similarity between the two bathing complexes is an indication of an architectural model according to which the Hammat-Gader fountains were built.[149] (See Fig. 12).

The remains of the arch above *Area E* which have survived indicate that it reached a height of 13.9 metres above the bottom of the pool. Fragments of a glass mosaic which were found on the floor of the hall bear witness to the splendour of the decorations of the upper parts and ceiling of the hall. The arch was cruciform, of the type found in the imperial baths built in Rome at the time of the Emperors Caracalla and Diocletian, in the third century CE.[150]

Close to the frontal wall on the west in *Area F* the main water-pipe was discovered. It is made of stone links. In one section, 8.8 metres long, 17 links survived *in situ*. Joined together, they formed a pipe with an inner radius of 0.5 metres. Similar pipes have been found in the

---

[149] Hirschfeld and Solar (1981): 212, 215; idem, (1984): 28, 36–37; Hirschfeld and Cohen (1992): 287–288; Hirschfeld (1997): 102–116, 135–139 (*Area D*), 148–152 (*Area E*); See also Robertson (1971): 255–261; cf. the Hadrianic bath at Leptis Magna and see Caffarelli, Bandinelli and Caputo (1967): 99–100, Fig. 242; Scarborough (1969): 78–80, Fig. 6.
[150] Hirschfeld and Solar (1981): 212–213; Robertson (1971): 255–261.

water supply systems of the Roman period (second and third centuries CE) in Tiberias, Sussita and Jerusalem. The purpose of the pipe was to supply cold water from the springs in the north of the site. In the Umayyad period the character of *Area F* was altered. A system of new installations turned it into an additional bathing area. Its area was reduced by a basalt wall supporting a ceiling; below the roofed area were installed several baths and small bathing rooms, entered from the north by a basalt staircase. This area was used for bathing until the destruction of the baths in the ninth century CE.[151]

The bathing hall next to the spring in *Area G* was undoubtedly the crowning glory of the bathing route in the site. Excavations round the spring are of the greatest importance, since the spring was the focal point of the baths, and by understanding it we can reach an understanding of the workings of the whole complex. Moreover, as is well known, in ancient times it was usual to consider that such natural phenomena as the Hammat-Gader springs were holy. It was to be expected that a sanctified construction, like the altar facing the hot spring at Bath Spa, would be found near the spring.[152] Bathing in the pool close to the spring was, therefore, both a religious and a therapeutic experience. This spring was presumably the hottest in the complex. In the centre of the hall an oval pool was constructed, and in the centre of the floor was a dedicatory inscription in Greek, celebrating the completion of a work of construction by a high-ranking official called Petrus Romanus. The inscription may have been written to celebrate the building of the pool, or it may have had a less important purpose. Apparently the pool was in constant use until the destruction of the complex.[153]

In the northern concourse (*Area H*) there is a group of marble faces in one of the corners of the entrance hall. These were apparently cut off from the various fountains (mainly in *Area D*) in the iconoclastic period of the 'Abbāsid dynasty.[154] (See Fig. 10).

By virtue of its location and massive dimensions, the *Thermae* was clearly the dominant feature of the layout of Hammat-Gader. Apart from the bathing complex the spa of Gadara comprised cultic structures, residential quarters, Byzantine houses, hospices, shops and various

---

[151] Hirschfeld and Solar (1981): 217–218; Hirschfeld (1997): 119–123 (*Area F*), 155–156.
[152] Hirschfeld and Solar (1981): 215; Hirschfeld and Cohen (1992): 287; Hirschfeld (1997): 94–102; Cunliffe (1986): 16–43; idem, (1995): 35–38.
[153] Di Segni (1992): 312; idem, (1997): 241, 243.
[154] Hirschfeld and Cohen (1992): 285; Hirschfeld (1997): 54–62.

provisions for amusement. To the north of the bathing complex, a portion of the paved street leading toward the theatre has been uncovered. The width of the street was about 12 metres. The small size of the theatre is evidence of its ritual character, for the ten stepped rows of seats could accommodate only about 2000 spectators. The total length of the theatre 29.6 metres, which is 100 feet, is identical to that of the Hall of Fountains (*Area D*), the largest of the bathing halls in the Hammat-Gader *thermae*. This raises the possibility that the bathing complex, the theatre, and the colonnaded streets connecting them were planned together and erected simultaneously.[155] (See Map 3). Vestiges of a Byzantine church have been located east of the eastern sector of Hammat-Gader. Hirschfeld assumes that on or adjacent to the spot where the church stood there may have originally been a pagan sanctuary. He reminds us that the purification of pagan ritual sites and their conversion into Christian places of worship was very common during the Byzantine period. The most famous example being the Church of the Holy Sepulchre in Jerusalem, built in the reign of Constantine on the ruins of a pagan sanctuary of Aphrodite.[156] Weber rejects this idea that this spot was formerly occupied by a pagan shrine, and from his point of view it remains a vague hypothesis.[157] In the area near the western mound, Tel Bānī, a synagogue was built at the beginning of the fifth century CE. The original floor had been paved with tiles arranged in geometric patterns (*opus sectile*). Later, the prayer hall (13 × 13.9 metres) was covered with colorful mosaics laid in figurative patterns. Four mosaic inscriptions dedicated in the names of donors, who contributed to the synagogue building, was found embedded in this floor. These donors might have been cured at Hammat-Gader spa and commemorated their recovery by contributing to the development of the thermo-mineral site as many others according to historical and archaeological evidences throughout the ages.[158]

---

[155] Sukenik (1935a): 27–30, Fig. 7; Avi-Yonah (1993: II: 569) thinks that the seating capacity was of 1500 to 2000, while Segal (1995a: 45–46) assumes that it was of 1000; According to Frézouls (1952: 79–81) the theatre must be understood as an Odeon connected to the Bathhouse; Hirschfeld (1987: 111–112) adds that this suggestion was confirmed by recent archaeological excavation; For the amusement evidence see chapter 8.5 on *Kefar Agon, the Domain of Gadara and Its Affinity to Leisure and Amusement Culture.*

[156] Hirschfeld (1987): 113; See also Zeyadeh (1994): 123; For the Church of the Holy Sepulchre in Jerusalem see Wilkinson (1981): 164–165.

[157] Weber (1997): 336.

[158] Sukenik (1935a); idem, (1935b): 41–61; Klein (1939): 45–47; Naveh (1978): 54–64; Foerster (1983): 11–12; Dvorjetski (1988): 114–125; Avi-Yonah (1993): II:

To conclude our discussion of Hammat-Gader, we shall only note that the archaeologycal investigation of this important and interesting site is not complete. In the future it behooves us to continue to clarify fully the excavations of the baths complex. It is also fitting to uncover in the areas between Tel Bānī and the Roman theatre, with the purpose of uncovering more remains of houses of the town's residents—where we look forward to further Christian, Jewish, Syriac and Muslim finds.

4.3   Hammat-Pella

There were also hot springs close to the city of Pella. Tel Paḥel (Greek, Πέλλα; Arabic, Fâḥil) was situated on the slopes of Gilead, east of the Jordan Valley, about 12 kilometres south-east of Beth Shean-Nysa-Scythopolis. (See Map 1). In antiquity, from the Canaanite period until the Middle Ages, there was an important town there.[159]

Pella was one of the towns of the Decapolis. In the town, which was fortified, and very famous from its earliest days, there have been found remnants of an acropolis, two temples and a basilica. Many graves have been discovered in the vicinity. Within the borders of Paḥel were Arbel [= Irbid], which had an acropolis of its own and several tombs, Jabesh Gilead, and Efron, which is mentioned in the account of Judas Maccabaeus' retreat. It may be that the territory of Paḥel extended as far as Rammatha, the fortress to which the Jews of Gilead fled, and from which Judas Maccabaeus rescued them.[160]

Many historical sources attest to its identity: among them are epigraphical documents, archaeological surveys and pilot excavations, and the similarity of the ancient name to the Arabic name.[161] The earliest

---

566–569; Urman (1995): 595–605; For people who commemorated their recovery, see the discussions in chapter 5.4.2 and in chapter 9.3.3 on *The Epigraphical Material from Hammat-Gader.*

[159] Yāqūt remarks, 'I think that Fâḥil is a foreign name, for I find no meaning for it in the Arabic tongue' (III: 853); Le Strange (1890): 439; See also Guérin (1868): 288–292; Merrill (1881): 442–447; Albright (1926): 39–42; Steuernagel (1927): 404–405; Richmond (1934): 18–31; Patai (1936): 223; Abel (1938): II: 405–406; Glueck (1951): 254–257; Richardson (1960): 242–243; Smith (1968): 13; Bourke (1997): 94–115; Hennessy (1997): 256–259; Negev and Gibson (2001): 383; da Costa, O'Hea, Mairs, Sparks and Boland (2002): 503–533.

[160] Avi-Yonah (1984): 160–161.

[161] Smith (1993): III: 1174; Smith (1968): 134–137; idem, (1973): 250–256; Excavations in the site were undertaken in 1958 by Richardson and Funk, in 1967 by Smith and since 1979 and into the 1990s by Smith, McNicoll and Hennessey; See also Vogel and Holtzclaw (1981): 66; Geraty and Herr (1986): 47–49; Khouri (1988): 21–27;

mention of Pella is in the Execration Texts. In the Late Bronze Age it appears in other Egyptian texts, such as the lists of Thutmosis III and Seti I. Two of the El-Amarna letters mention Mut-Balu, ruler of Pella. The Egyptian Anastasi Papyrus mentions Pella, together with Rehov, as a centre where certain parts of chariots were made for Egypt.[162] It is not mentioned in the Bible but reappears in the Hellenistic-Roman period. Presumably, Fâḥil is the original Semitic name; 'Pella' may have been chosen by the Greeks because of the similarity of sound.[163] The name Pella was in any case borrowed from the well-known Macedonian town of the same name. Since the latter was the birth-place of Alexander the Great, it has been suggested that this Pella, like the neighbouring Dium, was founded by Alexander himself, as a gloss on the text of Stephanus Byzantinus reports.[164] But in view of the uncertainty of this notice, it remains possible that Pella was founded by one of the *Diadochoi*, perhaps Antigonus, who kept a firm hold of Palestine for some ten years (311–301 BCE).[165]

Pella is mentioned in connection with the conquest of Palestine by Antiochus the Great in 218 BCE.[166] By the time of Alexander Jannaeus it was a centre of Hellenistic culture. He made several attempts to conquer it and succeeded in about 80 BCE, when its habitants chose to leave rather than accept the Jewish faith.[167] It was detached from the Jewish realm by Pompey, and was rebuilt by Gabinius, governor of Syria.[168] That it was part of the Decapolis is attested by Pliny, Eusebius, as well as Epiphanius.[169] It seems to have been destroyed by the Jews in 66 CE, in revenge for the murder of the Jews of Caesarea, but Eusebius

---

Walmsley (1988): 142–159; Edwards, Bourke, Da Costa et al. (1990): 58–93; Walmsley (1992): 539–541; Walmsley, Macumber, Edwards et al. (1993): 165–231; Watson and Tidmarsh (1996): 293–313.

[162] Negev and Gibson (2001): 383; These authors have made a mistake by writing that Pella was in alliance with Hammat-Gader instead of Hammatu, commonly identified with Tel el-Hammah on the southern edge of the Beth Shean Valley. See Ahituv (1984): 112–113; On other remains, see Bourke (1993): 61–163; Knapp (1993).

[163] Nöldeke (1885): 336.

[164] Stephanus Byzantinus, *Ethnika*, s.v. 'Πέλλα'; Stephanus is the only source that Pella was called 'Berenike', a name which it will have acquired in the Ptolemaic period; See Schürer (1991): II: 147.

[165] Schürer (1991): II: 146–147.

[166] Polybius, *Historiae* 5.70.12; See also Avi-Yonah (1984): 160; Walbank (1992): 123–140.

[167] Josephus, *Bellum Judaicum* 1.104; idem, *Antiquitates Judaicae* 13.397.

[168] Josephus, *Bellum Judaicum* 1.156; idem, *Antiquitates Judaicae* 14.75.

[169] Pliny, *Historia Naturalis* 5.74; Eusebius, *Onomastikon* 80; Epiphanius, *Panarion, Adversus Haereses* 29.7.

relates that the Christians of Jerusalem fled to Pella when Vespasian prepared his attack. In the later Roman and Byzantine periods it was one of the centres of the Christians community and its bishops in the fifth and sixth century CE are known.[170]

According to Eusebius the Biblical Jabesh lay only six Roman miles away, on the road from Pella to Gerasa. He also notes that Ammathus lay 21 Roman miles south of Pella, which corresponds to the distance between modern Amatha and Fâhil.[171] The mound is on the terraces of Fâhil (Arabic: Tabaqât Fâhil)—a level plain, about 2.5 by 1.5 kilometres in area, a little higher than the Jordan Valley. Heaps of ruins to a height of 22.5 metres have accumulated. On the east the mound is joined to the mountains by a ridge, but it rises steeply above the valley to the north and above Wadi Jirm al-Mawz in the south. In this valley flow the many springs from which Pahel derived its fame. On the southern side of the valley is Tel el-Hutzan, a natural hill on which the acropolis of the town was situated.[172]

Pliny the Elder calls the springs '...Pellam aquis divitem...' [= Pella with the springs of salvation].[173] This Hammtha was apparently well known for its high quality, and is mentioned in connection with the visit of Rabbi Ze'ira, one of the greatest of the Palestinian *halakhic* Rabbis, who went there from Tiberias for medicinal problems:[174]

> Rabbi Ze'ira [= who was a priest] went to Hammtha de Pahel, and found himself outside [= that is, to the east] of a field of Babylonian palms. [= Fearing that he had inadvertently left the Israelite territory of Trans-Jordan and had rendered himself unclean], he sent to Rabbi Hiyya bar Va, who asked the two sons of Rabbi Ebythar from Damma. They said to him, 'Priests are accustomed to going that far.
>
> (*Jerusalem Talmud, Shevi'it* 6, 1 [36c]).

---

[170] Josephus, *Bellum Judaicum* 2.156; cf. Eusebius, *Historia Ecclesiastica* 3.5.2–3; See also Brandon (1951): 168–171; Sowers (1970): 305–320; Avi-Yonah (1970): 118, 121; Schürer (1991): II: 147–148; Walmsley (1995): 321–324; Negev and Gibson (2001): 383.

[171] Eusebius, *Onomastikon* 22, 32; See also Schürer (1991): II: 145, 147; Issac and Roll (1976: 15–19) assumed that the road from Scythopolis to Pella and from the latter to Gerasa was paved at the intermission in the fights before the Romans' attack on Jerusalem in 70 CE. It was designated to connect Caesarea, the main Roman camp, not only with Scythopolis but even with the Hellenistic cities in the Trans-Jordan.

[172] Smith (1993): III: 1174.

[173] Pliny, *Historia Naturalis* 5.74.

[174] Neubauer (1848): 274; Dechent (1884): 179; Klein (1925): 59; idem, (1939): 35–36; Horowitz (1923): 276; Avi-Yonah (1976): 63; Levine (1985): 160; Dvorjetski (1992a): 62; Weber (1997): 334; For the purpose of using the hot springs of Pella by Rabbi Ze'ira, see the discussion on *The Healing Properties of the Spas in Ancient Times* in chapter 5 and on *The Sages at the Therapeutic Sites—Aims and Deeds* in chapter 6.2.

Hammtha itself, according to the text, was considered one of the towns of the Land of Israel, but the vicinity was considered to be foreign, and priests did not go beyond the place where the 'Babylonian palms' grew. Beyond them, all the population was non-Jewish.[175] The palms were known for their medicinal properties especially for digestive disturbances.[176]

There are several sources, which bear the names 'Ammatho' (with the letter *alef*), or 'Hammthan', or 'Amatho' (with the letter *ayin*) as a located probably in the eastern Jordan, opposite Jericho. It might be identified with Hammtha de Paḥel, but this theory is only hypothesis. The *Midrash* tells of a palm tree, which grew in Hammthan; a branch from a Jericho palm was grafted on to it, and bore fruit:

> Rabbi Tanhuma said: "There was once a palm tree in Ammatho that did not yield fruit. A palm-gardener passed and saw it; said he: 'This engrafted tree looks to [= a male palm] from Jericho'. As soon as they grafted it, it yielded fruit".
>
> (*Genesis Rabbah* 41, 1, Theodor-Albek ed., p. 387)

and in the parallel version in *Numbers Rabbah* 3, 1, it is written:

> Rabbi Tanhuma said: "There was once a palm-tree in Hammthan which would not bear fruit. They grafted it and still it would bear no fruit. A palm-gardener said to them: 'She [= The barren palm-tree in question] sees a palm-tree at Jericho and longs for it'. So they brought a portion of it and grafted it and forthwith it bore fruit".

In *Midrash Psalems* 92, 11 (Buber ed., p. 410), is related:

> Our Masters related: 'It happened that a female palm which was in (Ammito) [stood in Hammthan] yielded no fruit, even though a scion of a male palm had been grafted upon it. Then a palm-grower said: "It gazes upon a male palm above Jericho and has a desire for it", and they went and got a scion of that palm and grafted it on, and the female yielded fruit forthwith'.

Klein emphasizes that the original version of Ammatho was Hammathan or Hammtha; in the Greek version, 'Αμμαθοῦς.[177] The different versions of this story show that the Semitic name was altered as a result of the influence of the Greek environment; instead of the name

---

[175] Ne'eman (1971): I: 410–411.
[176] For the palm-trees and dates syrup see Krauss (1910): 245; Klein (1933): 4; Vohalman (1939): 68; Dvojetski (1992a): 148; Dalby (2003): 113–114.
[177] Klein (1939): 6–7.

Hammthan Ammthan is also found, and in another place Amtho (with *ayin*) (*Jerusalem Talmud, Shvi'it* 9, 2 [38d]), and in the above quotations the names Ammatho or Ommatha, which should be read Ammatha, also appear:[178]

> 'And all the cities of Sihon king of the Amorites, which reigned in Heshbon' (*Joshua* 13, 10) Beth Haram [= refers to] Beth Ramtha. Beth Nimrah [= refers to] Beth Nimrin. Succoth [= refers to] Direla. Zaphon [= refers to] Amm'tu.

According to the *Jerusalem Talmud* tradition (*ibid.*) Zaphon (*Joshua* 13, 27) is = Ammatho, in other words, Ammatho stood in place of Zaphon.[179]

Under the entry 'Hammtha de Pehal' Neubauer writes: 'We shall not hesitate to identify Pehal with the town of Pella in Trans-Jordan, today called Tabaqât Fâhil'. He assume that the thermal spring was Pella rather than within the city's territory itself.[180] If so, claims Weber, 'the present hot spring of Hammat ad Dāble is a possibility although the scarce ruins at the spot are insufficient to conclude the existence of monumental buildings'. Moreover, Weber emphasizes that it is not convincing to locate the famous *Nymphaeum* of Pella here. This well-known monument was shown on numerous autonomous coins of the late second-early third century CE.[181] (See Fig. 23). Avi-Yonah places Hammtha de Pahel 25 kilometres south-west of Hammat-Gader, about 5 kilometres east of the Jordan.[182] Klein, followed by Press, considers Hammtha de Pahel to be identical with Tel el-Hamma, about 2 kilometres north-east of Hirbet Pahel.[183] 'There is, in fact, no contradiction between these two identifications', maintains Ne'eman, 'since the former apparently refers only to the town of Pahel, while the latter refers to the place of the hot springs, Hammtha de Pahel'.[184] Schumacher supposed that the spring should be located at downtown Pella.[185] This locality,

---

[178] Klein (1924): 43; idem, (1939): 122.
[179] Klein (1939): 7.
[180] Neubauer (1868): 274.
[181] Weber (1997): 334; For the *Nymphaeum* on Pella's coins, see Seyrig (1959): 69; Price and Trell (1977): 44, Fig. 72; Spijekerman (1978): 211, 215; Nicolet (1981): 51; Meshorer (1985): 92, no. 251; Schürer (1991): II: 147; Weber (1993): 31–34; Dvorjetski (1992a): 197–199; idem, (1994a): 14–15; idem, (1996a): 40*, 44*; See the discussion in chapter 8.2 about *The Numismatic Expression of the Medicinal Hot Springs of Pella*.
[182] Avi-Yonah (1984): 160.
[183] Klein (1925): 59; See also Press (1955): II: 264–265.
[184] Ne'eman (1971): I: 411.
[185] Schumacher (1888b): 88–89.

nowadays known as mentioned Wadi Jirm al-Mawz, was renowned in antiquity for its abundance of water and several sources still today grant outstanding fertility to this place.[186] Traces of a pagan shrine transformed later into Christian church were uncovered at the site of the so-called civic complex. Two columns of dark chloritic limestone were reused in the atrium of the Byzantine sanctuary to flank the central portal. In the fill beneath the wide stairway of the west side of the Civic Complex church, a fragment of a life-size statue of dark blue schist of apparent Egyptian provenance was found. It features an enthroned deity draped with a thick garment covering the legs up to the hip. The dark stone and the characteristic drapery indicate that it belonged to a copy of the famous Alexanderine cult statue of Serapis, created by the Greek sculptor Bryaxis in the late fourth century BCE. Thus, it is possible that a *Serapion* was located in the vicinity of Pella's Roman-period forum in Wadi Jirm al-Mawz.[187]

In short, Hammtha de Paḥel, like other *Hammoth* [= thermo-mineral baths] mentioned above, is characterized by its name, which is evidence of its connection with hot springs. The suburb of Pella = Paḥel was not only an integral part of the district (χώρα) of the *polis* of Pella, but also part of the history and life of Pella, its mother town.

4.4 KALLIRRHOE

Close to the eastern shore of the Dead Sea, 4–5 kilometres south of the outflow of the river Zarqa Maʾin several more hot springs flow out of the cliff which runs along the sea shore. The best known is Hammam Ez-Zara, a group of hot springs next to which are cold springs; the waters of both types are drinkable. This site is usually identified as Tseret HaShahar, Hirbet Zara, a town in the territory of the tribe of Reuben (*Joshua* 13, 19), known in the Second Temple period as Kallirrhoe.[188] (See Map 1 and Fig. 24).

---

[186] Weber (1997): 334.

[187] Smith and Day (1989): II: 56–57; Smith (1992): 204–205; Weber (1993): 47–49; idem, (1997): 334–335.

[188] Thomsen (1907): 76; Smith (1922): 480; Abel (1933): I: 461; (1938): II: 457; Press (1955): IV: 828; Avi-Yonah (1976): 45; idem, (1984): 167; Vilnaey (1985): 6645; Strobel and Clamer (1986): 381–384; Reeg (1989): 569–570; Strobel (1990): 81–85; Dvorjetski (1992a): 71; idem, (1995b): 306–308; Clamer (1997a); The identification proposed for Tseret HaShahar with Kallirrhoe, because of the general name commonly used by the Arabs for the hot springs located there Ez-Zāra or Zārāt, is unfounded; See Kallai (1986): 441; Oded (1972): 779–780.

Kallirrhoe—Καλλιρρόη—is 'the good, pleasant, water (stream)',[189] or 'beautiful springs' in the words of the author of the *Aruch Completum*.[190] In the ancient world this term was applied to hot springs and medical facilities in the Mediterranean region, of which the most famous was the Καλλιρρόη spring, close to the Acropolis in Athens, under the Olympus, the temple of Zeus Olympius. According to Smith it may have been what Pliny the Elder calls the Well in the Garden of Jupiter, and what Pausanias calls a cavity into which the waters of the flood of Deucalion drained.[191]

Etymologically, the meaning of the name Καλλιερέω is the appearance of signs and omens presaging desirable occurrences while making sacrifices.[192] Kallirrhoe appears in Greek mythology as a nymph, the daughter of Oceanus. It is also common as a woman's name: for instance, granddaughter of Argos, the daughters of Accalos, Scamander, Nestos, Maeandros, Tethys, Lycus the King of Lycia, Oeneus the King of Calydon, and the second wife of Alcmaeon. It is spelled in Latin— Callirrohe.[193] In our view this nymph also personifies the relationship between therapeutic springs in the classical world and the cults which were practised in them.[194]

Klein points out that the original Hebrew name of the 'bathing place' in Kallirrhoe was *Ayin Tova*—the Good Spring.[195] Theodor and Albeck add that the meaning of the word is Good Spring, like the Greek name Kallirrhoe, since in the *Genesis Rabbah* 33, 4, these springs are classified, like those of eddy, gulf, of Gader [= Hammat-Gader] as boiling hot springs:[196]

---

[189] Liddell and Scott (1985): 396; See also Dvorjetski (1994a): 16.

[190] Kohut (1926): VII: 115.

[191] Pauly-Wissowa (1919): 1669; Dechent (1884): 198; Donner (1963): 60, note 2; See also Smith (1904): 144; Smith (1922): 147–149; Smith and Lockwood (1988): 81; Other sites which were named Callirrhöe are in the city of Calydon Ætolia and Carrhae in the north-west part of Mesopotamia; See Smith (1922): 244–248, 486; See also Dvorjetski (1994a): 16.

[192] Liddell and Scott (1985): 396.

[193] Pauly-Wissowa (1919): 1668–1669; Aldington and Ames (1989): 193; Harvey (1986): 18, 88; Reeg (1989): 570; Dvorjetski (1992a): 71.

[194] See the discussion in chapter 3.3 on *The Ritual Worship at the Medicinal Hot Springs in the Graeco-Roman World*.

[195] Klein (1925): 21; idem, (1929): 9.

[196] Theodor and Albeck (1965: 308–309) think that Hammei-Tiberias is omitted, since the only powerful springs are mentioned. The cavern spring of Paneas was introduced for the reason that the Jordan River exits there; On Paneas-Caesarea Philippi, modern Baneas see Wilson (2004); cf. *Babylonian Talmud, Shabbat* 108a.

'The fountains also of the deep and the windows of heaven were stopped' (*Genesis* 8, 2). Rabbi Leazer said: In connection with punishment it is written, 'On the same day were all the fountains of the great deep broken up' (*ibid.*, 7, 11); but in connection with good it is written, 'The fountains also of the deep…were stopped', but not 'all' the fountains, the exceptions being the great spring [= of Biram], the eddy [= of Gader], and the cavern spring of Paneas.

It may be pointed out that Rabbi Yohanan mentions Aina Rabbati de Biram' [= the great spring of Biram instead of Ayin Tova; as has been mentioned above, this was Hammei-Ba'arah [= hot springs]:[197]

> Rabbi Yohanan said: 'three of them remained: the eddy of Gader, Hammei-Tiberias, and Aina Rabbati de Biram' [= the great spring of Biram = Baaras, Ba'arah].
>
> (*Babylonian Talmud, Sanhedrin* 108a).

The *Midrash* identifies Kallirrhoe with Lasha.[198] The toponym Lasha is found only in *Genesis* 10, 19, which reads: 'And the border of the Canaanites was from Sidon, as thou comest to Gerar, unto Gaza; as thou goest unto Sodom, and Gomorrah, and Admah, and Zeboiim, even unto Lasha'. The Aramaic translation of the Torah, attributed to Jonathan ben Uzziel (also known as Targum Eretz-Israel A, or Pseudo-Jonathan) reads in this passage 'unto Kaldahi', instead of the town of Lasha, which was on the border of the land of Canaan. *Deuteronomy* 1, 7, says: 'Turn you, and take your journey, and go to the land of the Amorites…in the plain, in the hills, and in the vale, and in the south, and by the sea side, to the land of the Canaanites, and unto Lebanon'. The Aramaic translation reads to *Deuteronomy* 1, 7: 'to Canaan, as far as Kalduhi'.[199] Kohut maintains that Kaldahi and Kalduhi should be translated 'Kallirrhoe'.[200] Since Lasha probably comes from the Semitic root *lsʿ* meaning 'bore', 'drill', 'perforate', the name does not help identify its location.[201]

---

[197] On Aina Rabbati de Biram see the discussions in chapter 4.5 on *The Historical-Archaeological Analysis and Healing Cults of Hammei-Ba'arah* and in chapter 6 on *The Daily Life at the Thermo-Mineral Baths according to Rabbinic Literature.*

[198] See below and see also Neubauer (1868): 254; Krauss (1907–1908): 107; Steinberger (1964): 423; Ginzberg (1963): IV: 532; Schürer (1991): I: 325; For the development of the Arabic pronunciation, see Schwartz (1906): 262.

[199] Ginzburger (1903): 18, 301.

[200] Kohut (1926): VII: 115.

[201] Borée (1930): 26.

The name of the site appears in different versions, with minor variations: 'And the border of Canaan was from Sidon...as far as Lasha, which is Kalada' (*Sifrei on Deuteronomy*, 6); 'As far as Lasha. Rabbi Leazer said as far as Kalara' (*Jerusalem Talmud, Megilla* 1, 11 [71b]); 'And the border of the Canaanite was...as far as Lasha, as far as Kalhrai' (*Genesis Rabbah* 37, 6, Theodor-Albeck ed., p. 348).[202]

The correct transliteration of the name Kallirrhoe is to be found in Hieronymus' Latin translation of *Genesis* 10, 19, which was apparently derived from the above sources:[203]

> Quod Lasa sit, quae nunc Callirrhoe, ubi aquae calidae prorumpentes in mare mortuum defluunt [= since Lasha was situated where Callirrhoe is now, at the place where hot springs which flow into the Dead Sea erupt].

Hieronymus identifies Lasha with the hot springs of Callirrhoe [= Ez-Zara Oasis] on the east coast of the Dead Sea below Zarqa Ma'in. Supposedly Hieronymus is following Pseudo-Jonathan which has 'as far as Callirrhoe' completing the quotation of *Genesis* 10, 19, and substituting Callirrhoe for Biblical Lasha.[204] There is, however, no archaeological support for such a location.[205]

By emending the toponym, Welhausen equated Lasha with Laish, that is, Dan of *Judges* 18, 27,[206] a convincing identification since the boundary description of *Genesis* 10, 19. However, it is not located in the Hashemite Kingdom of Jordan.[207]

The springs of Kallirrhoe are closely linked to the life of Herod the Great, and particularly to his final years (37–4 CE). His illness became ever more severe, and was plainly incurable. The doctors laboured in vain to ease his sufferings, and thought he might find relief in the springs of Kallirrhoe (*Bellum Judaicum* 1.656–658; *Antiquitates Judaicae* 17.171–172). The account of Herod's last illness attests to the importance he

---

[202] 'Kalada' in London manuscript; In Oxford and Vatican manuscripts 'Kaladhi'; In *Yalkut Shimoni to Deuoteronomy* 801: 'Kadlahi'; See Krauss (1899): 550; Klein (1925): 143; In a manuscript from the *Geniza to Siferi Zuta* the site and the properties of the water appear as 'Klraha'. See for that Epstein (1930): 76, lines 10–12; See also Deines (1993): 159–160.

[203] Hieronymus, *Liber Hebraicarum Quaestionum in Genesim* 955.

[204] Simons (1959): 94–96; McNamara (1972): 193; Alexander (1974): 181–182, 185; MacDonald (2000): 59.

[205] Donner (1963): 60–62; Westermann (1984): 524; Strobel (1989): 663–639; idem, (1997): 271–272.

[206] Wellhausen (1876): 403–404.

[207] MacDonald (2000): 59; See also Abel (1938): II: 368.

attached to this thermo-mineral site. Despite his acute pains and his stubborn attachment to life, he agreed to be moved from Jericho to Trans-Jordan. It was not enough for the doctors that he bathed in the hot springs; they made one last attempt to save the tyrant's life, by immersing him in a bath of hot oil—a common treatment in the Imperial period. But he suddenly sank into a deep coma. When he recovered, he agreed to be taken back to Jericho. The hope for his recovery was thwarted. Immediately afterwards he died of his illness, though not before arranging for the execution of his son Antipater (*Bellum Judaicum* 1.664; *Antiquitates Judaicae* 17.187). In both sources Josephus gives a similar description of the attempts to cure him, mentions Kallirrhoe, and adds that the spring waters, as well as having unique healing qualities, had a therapeutic affect when drunk.[208]

Dechent surmises that, considering the ruler's mental instability and his fondness for Greek customs, it was logical that he should build a new independent medical facility, and even give the site a new name.[209] According to him, Herod the Great made administrative arrangements for the site, since in other places in Palestine, such as Ascalon, Caesarea and Machaerus he founded splendid artificial baths. Dechent believes that after Herod's death his son Herod Antipas stayed in Machaerus several times, and that he and his courtiers made use of the therapeutic springs of Kallirrhoe.

The details given by Josephus enable us to establish with absolute certainty the location of Kallirrhoe on the eastern side of the Dead Sea, and also to presume that the spa was closer to the northern tip of the sea than to its southern end. This is confirmed even more exactly by Pliny the Elder, who was a contemporary of Josephus, and mentions Kallirrhoe, with its hot spring and its therapeutic qualities, in conjunction with his description of the Dead Sea:[210]

> Eodem latere est calidus fons medicae salubritatis Callirrhoe, aquarum gloriam ipso nomine praeferens [= On the same side <of Machaerus> there is a hot spring with healing qualities, Callirrhoe, whose very name bears witness to the reputation of its waters].

---

[208] Scholars differ as to whether Herod suffered from intestinal cancer, diabetes or venereal disease. Others find in Josephus' descriptions indications of a serious liver complaint and other possibilities; For the intensive discussion see chapter 5 on *The Healing Properties of the Spas in the Eastern Mediterranean in Ancient Times.*

[209] Dechent (1884): 197–198; See also Neuburger (1919): 71.

[210] Pliny the Elder, *Naturalis Historia* 5.72; See also Stern (1974): I: 469–470; For Machaerus excavations, see for example, Donner (1982): 175, note 7.

Solinus, of the third century CE, also writes of the medicinal value
of Kallirrhoe:[211]

> Callirhoe Hierusolymis proxima, fons calore medico probatissimus et
> ex ipso aquarum praeconio sic vocatus [= Callirrhoe, which is close to
> Jerusalem, is a source of benefit, as is proved by its therapeutic heat, and
> its name is derived from its famous waters].

Our sources say nothing whatsoever about any settlement at this spot.
We can, however, deduce from the Greek treatise of Ptolemaeus, an
Alexandrian geographer of the second century CE, that there was a
Jewish settlement in Kallirrhoe as early as the second century CE. He
specifically states that Kallirrhoe was one of the Jewish settlements in
Trans-Jordan, and fixes its geographical position exactly:[212]

> Καλλιρρόη...ξϛ ιβ′ λᾱ ϛ′ [= Kallirrhoe: 67° 5' longitude; 31° 10'
> latitude].

Braslavsky gives several political, strategic and economic reasons for
believing that the Jewish settlement in Kallirrhoe existed at least from
the first quarter of the first century BCE.[213] In the first quarter of the
first century BCE the Hasmonean King Jannaeus waged war on the
borders of the Nabataeans in Trans-Jordan, conquered the land of
Moab from them, and imposed taxes on its inhabitants (*Bellum Judaicum*
1.164); thereafter he built the fortress of Machaerus on the peak of
one of the mountains in the region (*ibid.*, 7.164–179). 'The fortress'
says Josephus 'was close to the borders of Arabia, and looked down
from on high like an observation tower over the land of Arabia' (*ibid.*),
or 'opposite the mountains of Arabia' (*ibid.*, 1.171). But the citadel
also looked down on 'the valley which cuts off Machaerus from the
west'—the valley of Kallirrhoe. The citadel of Machaerus was destroyed
by Gabinius, but was rebuilt and strengthened by King Herod the Great
(*ibid.*, 7.174–177). According to Pliny, it was a most important citadel,
second only to Jerusalem.[214] Beneath the peak of Machaerus, 'Herod
took a great stretch of land, surrounded it with a wall, and founded a
city' (*ibid.*, 7.176). The city doubtless strengthened and revivified the
Jewish garrison in Machaerus, where John the Baptist was beheaded. It

---

[211] Solinus, *Collectanea Rerum Memorabilium* 35.4; See also Stern (1974): II: 418.
[212] Ptolemaeus, *Geographia* 5.15.6; See also Stern (1974): II: 168.
[213] Braslavsky (1956): III: 374.
[214] Pliny the Elder, *Naturalis Historia* 5.72; Stern (1974: I: 479) remarks that Pliny
locates Machaerus and Kallirrhoe southern to the Dead Sea, and this is a mistake.

took part in the great Jewish revolt against the Romans, helped to keep the Roman expeditionary force away from Machaerus, and defended the fortress until the time when, together with Herodium and Masada, it was one of the last three Jewish fortresses to survive after the fall of Jerusalem (*ibid.*, 7.190–209).

There are also echoes of the existence of a Jewish settlement in Machaerus [= Michvar] in the Rabbinic literature:

A. Rabbi Eliezer ben Diglai said, 'My father's household had goats on the Mountain of Michvar, and they used to sneeze from the odour of the compounding of the incense' (*Mishnah, Tamid* 3, 8; See also *Jerusalem Talmud, Sukka* 5, 3 [55b]; *Babylonian Talmud, Yoma* 39b).

B. In the mountains of Michvar beacons were lit in order to signal the beginning of the Jewish months (*Jerusalem Talmud, Rosh Hashana* 2, 3 [58a]). This custom was abolished at the time of Rabbi Judah the Patriarch (*ibid.*, 2, 1 [58a]).

C. The mountains of Michvar are included in the 'three regions' of Trans-Jordan in relation to the *halakhic* precepts concerning purification by burning: 'What area in Trans-Jordan is [= referred to as] mountains? Rabbi Simeon ben Eleazar says: '[= An area] such as the mountains of Michvar and Gedor, and other areas like these'. And its lowlands? 'Heshbon and all of its towns which are in the tableland...And its valley? [= An area such as] Beth Haran, Beth Nimrah and other areas like these'. (*ibid., Shevi'it* 9, 2 [38d]; cf. *Tosefta, ibid.*, 7, 10–11).

D. The translation attributed to Jonathan ben Uzziel identifies Michvar with Jazer (*Numbers* 32, 3). Klein comments: 'This is not a real comparison, but a homiletic interpretation; the name Jazer was said to be derived from the root *a-z-r* (to help), and the name in the Torah was transferred to Michvar, which helped the people of Israel at the time of their wars with the Romans'.[215] Barslavsky's view, which is more probable, is that 'the Jews of Michvar, like the Jews of neighbouring Kallirrhoe, needed a Biblical name in order to add the lustre of holy writ to their place of residence'.[216]

The fortress of Michvar, today el-Mukawer, and the town below it, which were 1220 metres above the level of the Dead Sea, needed

---

[215] Klein (1925): 78.
[216] Braslavsky (1956): III: 375.

an outlet to the Dead Sea in order to ensure unbroken contact with Judaea. The only place which could fulfil this vital strategic function was the Kallirrhoe valley; only there was it possible to construct a small town with a harbour for the Jewish mountain settlements.[217] True, the descent from the heights of Michvar to the Kallirrhoe valley was steep and difficult, but it seems that the path created by Herod the Great at this period made transport much less difficult. Abel wrote in his report that it was still possible to discern sections of the road with border-stones, and that they were disappearing under the falls of basalt round the hill of Taf-Ez-Zara, which dominates the Kallirrhoe valley from a height of 280 metres.[218] From all this, we may deduce that there was a Jewish settlement in Kallirrhoe as long as the Michvar fortress was in Jewish hands. Barslavsky comments that, since it was the harbour of Michvar, the site of hot baths, and a well-watered valley, Kallirrhoe was capable of sustaining a substantial population on the shores of the Dead Sea; and it is most probable that it was one of the towns 'like them' in the *halakhic* precepts concerning purifycation by burning.[219] Ptolemaeus's notes on the Jewish settlement at Kallirrhoe in the second century CE are, therefore, probably correct. Jewish Kallirrhoe of the second century CE was the continuation of the settlement which existed during the hundred and forty years of the existence of the Michvar fortress.

The Kallirrhoe valley was not inferior to Ein Gedi, which is situated opposite it, as a tropical enclave. As in Ein Gedi, palm-trees and persimmons were no doubt grown. The two palm-trees depicted in the Madaba mosaic map at the right-hand end of the valley and south of the main hot spring are evidence of the cultivation of palms in Kallirrhoe. Similar palm-trees are included in the areas round Jericho and Zoar.[220] According to the Arab geographer al-Edrīsī of the eleventh century CE, in the middle ages cereals and dates were still being transported by ship from Ez-Zara and Zoar to Jericho and the other settlements of the Jordan Valley.[221]

The mosaic map of Madaba allots a considerable area to Kallirrhoe. (See Fig. 25). It is bordered by a narrow river on the left, and a broader

---

[217] Braslavsky (1956): III: 375; See especially Schult (1966): 144–148.
[218] Abel (1909): 213–242.
[219] Braslavsky (1956): III: 376.
[220] Avi-Yonah (1954): 25; Hepper and Taylor (2004): 35–44.
[221] al-Idrīsī, *Kitāb nuzhat al-mushtāq fī ikhtirāq al-'afāq* 3; See also Abel (1933): I: 505; Almog and Eshel (1956): 48; Raz (1993): 196.

one on the right. The left-hand river is doubtless the Nahli'el, and the right-hand the Arnon. The white space left between the rivers by the artist seems to indicate the Kallirrhoe valley, even though it is no more than 4 kilometres long. At the top of the white space appear the words θερμὰ Καλλιρόης—'the hot baths of Kallirrhoe'. Avi-Yonah points out that the inscription is placed over three springs, adding that the northern-most is depicted as a round pool from which a stream flows to the sea. The central pool is square, and above it is an arc (a so-called *nymphaeum*); the waters of this pool also flow into the sea. The southern pool is shaped like a stream, which comes down from the mountains and broadens out in its central section to a sort of lake, divided by a black dam. It might be probably a bathing reservoir with flowing hot water which could be mixed, when required, with cooler water or minerals. Above this stream are depicted two palm-trees, which indicate the abundance of water and the fecundity of this area. South of the springs of Kallirrhoe is depicted the valley of Arnon with its steep banks. The precipitous effect is created by blue cubes on a black background; the part of the river closest to the Dead Sea is lighter, since the light penetrates between the rocks there more.[222] Braslavsky sees the big pool as a two-roomed bath; in the centre of the room with the apse is a bath, surrounded by a broad floor for the bather to sit, to lie and sweat, or to rest. He maintains that the second room served as a dressing-room and cloakroom, and that the small round building is most probably also a pool surrounded by a floor, like the ancient baths of Tiberias.[223] The archaeological remains at the site are rather poor. Remnants of these constructions can be seen there even now, although they are difficult to interpret. Only the third installation might perhaps be identical with a rectangular depression, which local people call *al-Madās* [= bath-place, shower], chiselled into the rock.[224]

Avi-Yonah believes that the creator of the Madaba map obtained his information from Hieronymus, where waters of the hot springs are described as following to the Dead Sea: 'ubi aquae calidae prorumpentes in mare mortuum defluunt'.[225] But the reasons for his depicting

---

[222] Avi-Yonah (1954): 40; Donner (1992): 39–40; Weber (1997): 333–334; Clamer (1999): 222; For pools and Palm Groves represented in mosaics see Blázquez (1999): 251–252; On the affinity of the baths to the ships' load in the Dead Sea according to the Madaba Map see Dvorjetski (1996): 82–88 and the discussion in chapter 5.4 on *The Medicinal Properties in Light of Archaeological Finds*.

[223] Braslavsky (1956): III: 374.

[224] Donner (1992): 19, 39–40; Weber (1997): 334; Clamer (1999): 224.

[225] Avi-Yonah (1954): 4.

Kallirrhoe are unknown. According to Donner, the mosaicist must have had an excellent knowledge of the region, because he probably came from Madaba or lived in or around Madaba. Only with such a familiarity of the region could he have depicted the run of the Wadi Zarqa Ma'in realistically from a north-south to an east-west direction and placed the site's name at the beginning of its lower course, where the hot springs are situated.[226] Donner emphasizes that Kallirrhoe was chosen because of its proximity to Madaba. He raises another important question in his research on Kallirrhoe: did the mosaicist depict all the therapeutic facilities in Kallirrhoe, or only some of them? On this question Donner accepts Heidet's conjecture, that Kallirrhoe's therapeutic facilities, which are depicted in the Madaba mosaic, were situated on the sea-coast, but in the course of time were engulfed by the rising waters of the sea. The therapeutic buildings of Kallirrhoe were flooded several times by the seasonal overflow of the sea, and were finally abandoned. Earthquakes and the effect of the salt water completed their destruction. Donner's view, that the mosaicist did not think it necessary to depict all of Kallirrhoe's bathing and therapeutic facilities, but only a representative selection which was characteristic of the place, seems most probable. Such a selection would include both the enclosed circular bath and the *nymphaeum*. He maintains that we may assume that there were several such enclosed baths in the vicinity of 'Ain Ez-Zara, but that all traces of them have disappeared as a result of the water, the saline air, and earthquakes.

In the sixth century CE Christian writers mention the 'springs of Moses', which are often confused with those of Kallirrhoe. In Dechent's view, they should be looked for north of the Dead Sea.[227]

Since no remains of Kallirrhoe had been found near the Dead Sea by the 1960s, and since neither Eusebius nor Hieronymus translates or identifies Lasha as Kallirrhoe, Barth[228] and, following him, Bar-Droma,[229] claim that these are significant reasons for believing that Lasha should not be placed at Kallirrhoe, close to the Dead Sea in Eastern Trans-Jordan, but in the northern regions of Syria. This hypothesis is very extreme, as is attested by the reports of historians, geographers and

---

[226] Donner (1963): 62–64; See also Weber (1997): 334.
[227] Dechent (1884): 201; See also the discussion in this chapter about *Hammei-Livias*.
[228] Barth (1909): 10–11.
[229] Bar-Droma (1958): 25–28.

travellers on the topographical position of Kallirrhoe and the quality of its springs—and, of course, by the archaeological evidence which has recently come to light and will described below.

On the eastern side of the Dead Sea, between its northern tip and the Arnon valley, there are many hot springs containing sulphuric minerals.[230] During the nineteenth century many scientists and travellers, such as Irby and Mangles,[231] Robinson and Smith,[232] Lynch,[233] Tristram,[234] Kersten,[235] Buhl,[236] Brunnow and Domaszewski[237] identified the hot springs of Wadi Zarqa Ma'in with Kallirrhoe. They claimed that they found four large springs and a number of small ones in Kallirrhoe; that sulphuric vapours rose from them; that the temperature of the water was very high; and that there was much vegetation—in particular, wild date palms—in the vicinity.

Even before the unique Madaba map was published, Conder and Dechent surmised that the Kallirrhoe baths should be identified as the hot springs of 'Ain Ez-Zara, which are situated about two kilometres south of the outfall of Wadi Zarqa Ma'in.[238] Over the years their view has been affirmed by Manfredi,[239] Musil,[240] Heidet,[241] Abel,[242] Scarötter,[243] Seetzen,[244] Neubauer,[245] and Donner.[246]

Remains of the ancient settlement of Kallirrhoe have been found close to 'Ain-Wafiya [= 'the perfect, or satisfactory, well'] and in other places in the Jordan Valley. Opposite the well, which measures 31 × 20 metres, there are the remains of a tower known as Hirbet Ez-Zara. West of the tower are the remains of buildings and elongated fences. A few minutes away, north of the bathing or irrigation pool, close to the

---

[230] Donner (1963): 63.
[231] Irby and Mangles (1823): 466–467.
[232] Robinson and Smith (1838): II: 455; See also Robinson (1865): 162–164.
[233] Lynch (1854): 229–232.
[234] Tristram (1873): 230–252.
[235] Kersten (1879): 208–209.
[236] Buhl (1896): 123.
[237] Brünnow and Domaszewski (1905): II: 326.
[238] Conder (1889): 280: Dechent (1884): 196–201.
[239] Manfredi (1903): 266–271.
[240] Musil (1907): I: 98–100, 240.
[241] Heidet (1909): 121–135.
[242] Abel (1909): 213–242.
[243] Schrötter (1924): 45–46.
[244] Seetzen (1854): 366–371.
[245] Neubauer (1868): 36–37.
[246] Donner (1963): 63–65.

edge of Wadi Ez-Zara, is another ruin, measuring 15.60 × 6.30 metres due to the reports in the mid-50s of the 20th century by Braslavsky.[247] There was a Roman road from the Jordan River to this site, and Ilan maintained that it was not impossible that Josephus was referring to this road when he wrote that Herod 'crossed the Jordan to be treated in the baths of Kallirrhoe'.[248]

Excavations in the mid-80 and 90s of the 20th century on the lower rock terrace have provided evidence of two periods of occupation: the Early Roman and the Early Byzantine. The earliest occupation dates from the reign of Herod the Great, end of the first century BCE to the end of the first century CE. The second, the Early Byzantine period, dates from the middle of the fourth century to the end of the fifth century CE. A large villa was excavated in Area I that can be compared with the residences of the last Hasmonaeans on the western side of the Dead Sea and Herod's palaces in Jericho, which served as pleasant country houses during the cold season. The Early Roman date was confirmed by further excavations of two other building complexes that seem to represent either private country houses or larger farmsteads, situated beside perennial streams and surrounded by small estates or farmland. More building complexes and farming installations have been recorded by recent surveys. The most extensive ruins however are situated on the shore (Site I). Because it is situated close to the waterfront, it seems logical to speak of an ancient harbour or anchorage place at Kallirrhoe. Other harbor installations are on the Dead Sea, Rujm el-Bahr and Qasr el-Yahud, both of which are sites which seem less important than Ez-Zara.[249]

Clamer assumes that Kallirrhoe was planned in connection with Herod's building activities at Jericho and the rebuilding of the palace-fortress of Machaerus.[250] It may have been primarily designed as country site with thermal baths and a small harbour or anchorage place, which offered the connecting link between Jericho and Machaerus. While the recreation centers were dose to the seashore where the hot springs gushed into the Dead Sea and access was easy for convalescent and

---

[247] Braslavsky (1956): III: 136–139, 344; See also Strobel (1966): 149–162; Negev (1976): 187.

[248] Ilan (1971): 149; See Clamer (1989): 225.

[249] Clamer (1999): 223–224; idem, (1997a); See also 'Amr and Hamdan (1996): 434–445.

[250] Clamer (1999): 224.

sick people arriving by boat, villas and farmhouses were situated on the lower terraces and within the oasis, dose to watercourses and surrounded by a small private domain planted with trees and vegetables. According to archaeological evidence, Kallirrhoe was abandoned and destroyed, like Machaerus, at the end of the First Jewish Revolt. With the spreading of unrest and open rebellion against the Romans and the Roman army controlling the area of the Dead Sea, Kallirrhoe was probably cut off from the west some time before the stronghold of Machaerus fell into the hands of the Romans in 72 CE. The inhabitants of the villas and country houses may have left the village before the arrival of the Roman army in the Moabite highlands.

The hot springs of ʿAin Ez-Zara are well known today to all picnickers and visitors from Amman and its surroundings, who come down the modern highway connected to the asphalt road along the Dead Sea shore. On weekends they invade the oasis by the thousands, enjoying swimming in the Dead Sea and bathing in the natural rock-cut pools created by the hot springs. With regard to the uniqueness of this area with its rich natural flora and fauna and important archaeological remains, new proposals have been launched to preserve the oasis as a natural and archaeological park and as a tourist attraction with the facilities of a modern spa nearby.[251]

Since no permanent settlement of the sixth century CE has left substantial remains in the oasis, there was no permanent occupation at Kallirrhoe during the later Byzantine period. However, this does not exclude the possibility that the people living in the region paid occasional visits to the area in order to enjoy the curative waters even in their natural pools and waterfalls on the shore, as it occurs today. Alternatively, they may have been engaged in seasonal farming and harvesting. A few jars found in surface soil and dated to the beginning of the sixth century CE may stem from such occasional visits or seasonal cultivation. The descent from the Moabite hinterland to Kallirrhoe/Ez-Zara was difficult. From Mishnaqa a long downward climb of more than 1000 metres passed through the desolate and in part steep mountain cliffs. During Roman times a main road connected the site of ʿAin Ez-Zara with inland Zarqa Maʾin and the palace-fortress of Machaerus, segments of which zigzagging along the slopes were observed by early travellers and can be discerned today. We may assume

---

[251] Clamer (1997b): 10, 12.

that the roads were not maintained after the destruction of Machaerus and Kallirrhoe. Although during the fifth–sixth centuries CE the village of el-Mukawer close to Mishnaqa developed into a pilgrim's site with churches dedicated to John the Baptist, it is difficult to imagine pilgrims venturing down from Mishnaqa to Ez-Zara to take a curative bath in the hot springs. They probably preferred Hammei-Ba'arah, as did Petrus the Iberian, and used the road branching off halfway down from the path to Ez-Zara.[252] Let's examine now the historical-archaeological analysis of this particular fascinating spa.

4.5   HAMMEI-BA'ARAH

Ba'arah is a bathing site with very hot potable thermo-mineral springs east of the Dead Sea and close to Wadi Zarqa Ma'in, whose waters flow into the Dead Sea together with the river water. Today it is known by the Arabic name of Hammam Ez-Zarqa or Hammamat Ma'in, from the Ez-Zarqa (Nahli'el) river on whose northern edge it is situated. Its water flows in the channel of the Zarqa valley which descends from the mountains of Moab to the Dead Sea, about 4 kilometres from its eastern shore. The spring is named after the river, and the meaning of the name is 'blue', because of its blue waters. The temperatures of the springs are 61.8°C, 54.4°C, and 43.3°C. The Roman roads leading to these springs prove that it was an important bathing site.[253] (See Map 1 and Fig. 26).

According to the Rabbinic literature, its waters survived from the time of the Flood:[254]

> Rabbi Yohanan said: 'three of them remained: the eddy of Gader, Hammei-Tiberias, and Aina Rabbati de Biram' [= the great spring of Biram].
>
> (*Babylonian Talmud, Sanhedrin* 108a).

---

[252] Donner (1999): 225.

[253] Manfredi (1903): 266–271; Thomsen (1907): 30; Klein (1910b): 28–29; Sapir (1911): 10; Abel (1911): 26–29; Smith (1920): 571, note 2; Horowitz (1923): 118; Abel (1933): I: 460–461; Patai (1936): 224; Press (1948): I: 69, 116; Ilan (1971): 148; Avi-Yonah (1976): 34–36; Donner (1982): 175–180; Avi-Yonah (1984): 167; Reeg (1989): 418–419; Schürer (1991): I: 326; Dvorjetski (1992a): 64–70; Weber (1997): 332–333; Clamer (1999): 221–225.

[254] For more details see the discussion in chapter 6.1 on *The Halakhic Stance of the Sages towards Curative Hot Springs and Baths*.

Josephus provides in his *Bellum Judaicum* (7.186–189) a very picturesquely description of the site of the springs, called by him Βαάρας:[255]

> In this same region [= northern to Machaerus] flow hot springs, in taste widely differing from each other, some being bitter, while other have no lack of sweetness. Many springs of cold water also gush up, nor are these confined to the low-lying ground where all are on one level; but—what is still more remarkable—hard by may be seen a cave, of no great depth and screened by a projecting rock, above which protrude, as it were, two breasts, a little distance apart, one yielding extremely cold water, and the other extremely hot. These when mixed provide a most delightful bath, possessing general medicinal properties, but particularly restorative to the sinews. There are also Sulphur and Alum mines in the district.

Josephus gives a detailed description of the springs—hot and cold, sweet and saline—which pour out profusely on the site. The most wonderful feature of the site is, in his view, the cave. It seems that this account confirms the statement of the *Jerusalem Talmud* (*Shabbat* 3, 1 [6a]) that there were two baths there, one of sweet and one of salt water. Those who frequented the baths were afraid to lift the planks which covered the cold water and bathe in the sweet water. Although they claimed that they used only the salt water for therapeutic purposes, they were forbidden to bathe on the Sabbath. He tells also about a wild plant in the ravine, of an amazing size, which produces a root bearing the same name 'Baaras'. It is 'Flame-coloured and towards evening emitting a brilliant light, it eludes the grasp of persons who approach with the intention of plucking it, as it shrinks up and can only be made to stand still by pouring upon it certain secretions of the human body'. To touch it is fatal, 'unless one succeeds in carrying off the root itself, suspended from the hand'. Even though people used to dig all round it, then tie a dog to it and dies instantly after that as a vicarious victim (*Bellum Judaicum* 7.180–184). Despite all these dangers it is in great demand, since it enables one to kill demons and spirits, which enter living men's bodies, and they can be driven out by means of this root. Thus, the 'Baaras' is not only a deadly poison; it is also a wonderful elixir of life, a proven cure—again, only by the power of touch—for all those whom the evil spirit that has entered their body and soul threatens with certain death.

---

[255] *Bellum Judaicum* 7.186–189; See also Kottek (1994): 130–131, 136–137; For the site's healing qualities see chapter 5.

The Church Father Eusebius, bishop of Caesarea in the fourth century
CE, writes of the site in his *Onomastikon*, under he heading 'Beelmeon
(*Numbers* 32, 38)' that it is 'beyond the Jordan, which the sons of Reuven
built. And to this day there is a large village by the name of Beelmaus
near Baaru in Arabia, where the ground spontaneaously sends forth
hot waters, at a distance of nine miles from Heshbon. And the prophet
Elisha was from this place'.[256]

Baalmaon or Beelmeon was a city in the land of Moab, in the vicinity of Madaba (*ibid.; Ezekiel* 25, 9), also known as Beon (*Numbers* 32, 3),
Bethmeon (*Jeremiah* 48, 23), and Beit-baal-meon (*Joshua* 13, 17). In the
opinion of most scholars, the name Beon is a phonetic corruption of
the name Maon. Baal was the principal Canaanite deity, who caused
the wind to blow and the rain to fall, made men be fruitful and multiply,
and ruled over the animal and vegetable kingdoms, the desert and the
gods who were associated with him. Temples of Baal, with altars to
perform his cult, were erected in the cities. The prophets and priests of
Baal served in his temples. The inhabitants of Palestine often ascribed
special characteristics to the Baal who was worshipped in a particular
place, and called him by a distinctive name which included the name
of the place (Baal Hazor, Baal Hermon, Baal Peor, Baal Tsafon, Baal
Pratzim, etc.) or some other element (Baal Zevuv, Baal Brith, etc.)
After the death of Gideon a special temple of Baal, known as 'Beth
Baal Brith' [= the House of the Baal of the Covenant] was built in
Shechem (*Judges* 9, 4). His worship also spread beyond the Jordan.
The name 'Beit Baal Maon' testifies to the existence of a temple of
this god, whom the Moabites called 'Baal Maon', as does the name
'Bamoth Baal' which was also a centre of worship for his devotees.
Baalmaon is mentioned in the monument which Mesha the King of
Moab raised to celebrate his victory over Omri, King of the northern
kingdom of Israel, conquered the whole region and annexing the land
of Madaba to his country (*II Kings* 1, 1; 3, 1–5). In the early days of
Hasmonaean rule a number of actions were taken to ease the lot of the
Jews of Trans-Jordan. The Jewish colony there continued to exist after
the destruction of the Temple, and flourished again under the aegis of
the House of Tobias. Their principal enemies were the people of 'Baal
Baon'. They were nomads (Bedouins) who ambushed on the roads and
looted merchant caravans (*I Maccabees* 5, 4). The people of Baon laid

---

[256] Eusebius, *Onomastikon* 44; See also Melamed (1966): 22.

ambushes for the Jews, perhaps in order to cut off their links with the Nabataeans. Judas Maccabaeus invaded their country, and surrounded them and burnt them down in their towers (*I Maccabees* 5, 4–5; II, *ibid.*, 8, 30; 10, 24–38; 12, 2). In his *Onomastikon* Eusebius emphasizes that 'to this very day' the site was known as Beelmaus, which was undoubtedly a derogatory change of name.[257]

In the Latin translation of the *Onomastikon* by the Church Father Hieronymus, of the late fourth and early fifth century CE, the site is called Baaru.[258] Dechent surmises that the name Βαάρας was given to a part of the valley, and possibly to the mountain, alongside of which springs gush forth.[259] This suggestion may be confirmed by a comparison between the words of Eusebius and Hieronymus' version. Eusebius said that Beelmeon lies close to the mountain of the hot waters, whereas Hieronymus states: 'iuxta Baaru in Arabia, ubi aquas calidas sponte humus effert' [= close to Baaru in Arabia, in a place that the ground brings forth hot water spontaneously].[260] It has been made clear to us, therefore, that there is a mountain that bears this name. In the *Onomastikon* under the entry 'Kariataim', Eusebius also mentions Ba'arah, spelt Βαρη,[261] and Hieronymus translates this as Bare.[262] Furthermore, in the Latin translation of *Genesis* 36, 24, where Anah is described as having found *HaYamim* in the desert, Hieronymus explains that *HaYamim* were *aquae calidae* [= hot waters].[263] Some scholars have surmised that this is a reference to the existence of hot springs; and this accord with the spirit of the story, which extols the discovery of the springs. But it is hard to establish which springs the text alludes to. It may be assumed that these were the hottest springs in the region, and were well known in the Byzantine period; it may well be, therefore, that the reference is to the springs of Ba'arah.[264]

There is a description of the Ba'arah baths in the biography of the monk Petrus of Iberia, of the fifth century CE, who had been appointed Episcopus of Maioumas-Gaza. The hagiographic *Life of Petrus Ibericus* was originally written in Greek by his student, companion and heir

---

[257] Posner, Paul and Stern (1987): I: 115–116; Anonymous (1965): II: 68–69.
[258] Hieronymus, *Onomastikon* 45.
[259] Dechent (1884): 200.
[260] Hieronymus, *Onomastikon* 45.
[261] Eusebius, *Onomastikon* 112.
[262] Hieronymus, *Onomastikon* 113.
[263] Hieronymus, *Liber Hebraicarum Quaestionum in Genesim* 1043.
[264] See, for instance, Dechent (1884): 173; Krauss (1907–1908): 105.

Johannes Rufus, but, like many other Monophysite texts, has survived only in a Syriac translation. Petrus and Johannes did not only visit the holy places in Jerusalem and its vicinity. They travelled to Trans-Jordan accompanied by another monk, in order to visit holy places, particularly the tomb of Moses on Mount Nebo. From the biography it appears that before this he visited Ba'arah (in Syriac—Ba'ar) where, he says, there were hot fountains in which he could heal his body, which had become weakened by his deprivations. The site was far from human habitation, and there was a risk of an attack by bandits, so he could not reach it alone; he was, therefore, accompanied by many soldiers and civilians. His companions hoped to be able to bathe in the hot springs, since they were in an isolated spot which few had the courage to reach. When they reached the spot they saw a wondrous sight: a deep, narrow valley surrounded by high mountains, in which streams of hot water issued forth both from the depths of the earth and from the spurs of the black mountains, which absorbed the hot mists with which they were covered. They increased the temperature, and covered the whole site with clouds of thick vapour, like smoke from a chimney. Because of the unbearable heat, the people of the region refrained from bathing in the springs, and did so, though with difficulty, only during the winter. Then, after bathing at the site, they hurried home, since they could not stand the oppressive heat. Petrus' disciple wrote that when Petrus visited the site the weather was mild and there was a pleasant breeze. Those who joined him on his excursion said: 'We have never undergone such a miraculous experience'. In this place there is a wondrous sight: a cave, in one wall of which there are two holes, one *amah* apart, from each of which water flows. One stream is very cold, while the other is composed of very hot boiling water. Both streams, the hot and the cold, flow together into the centre of the cave, and when they mingle they create a luke-warm bath, pleasant and healthy to bathe in.[265]

The evidence of Petrus of Iberia accords with the information provided by the sources quoted above as to the geographical and topographical position of the site, its characteristics, its therapeutic powers, and its name, which was undoubtedly given it because of the unique cave situated there.

---

[265] Petrus the Iberian, 82, 87.

One can clearly see on the sixth century CE Madaba mosaic map four Greek letters, αρου, adjoining the inscription θερμὰ Καλλιρόης, thermal waters of Kallirrohoe. Avi-Yonah completes the name as follows [Βα]άρου, and adds that the very mention of Ba'arah in the Madaba map testifies to the importance of the springs.[266] (See Fig. 25).

The coincidence of the mention of the name by Eusebius, Hieronymus, and the Madaba map led Klein to assume that the name was derived from the Semitic root *beit-ayin-resh*; and since the *ayin* is not pronounced in Greek, it is called Βάρις.[267] In his opinion, therefore, the version of the name in the *Babylonian Talmud, Sanhedrin* 108b, Aina Rabbati de Biram', should be corrected from Biram to Biraas; that is, the great spring of Biraas; i.e., of the place Ba'arah. Hirschberg gives Hamburger's opinion that Biram is a shortened word, corrupted from the Hebrew word *bar*; in other words, *be'er ham* [= hot-water well]; thus the Biram version, and not Biraas, is to be maintained.[268] Neubauer,[269] Kohut,[270] Press,[271] and Yankelevitz[272] are convinced that the preferred version is Biraas. A completely different opinion of the Talmudic expression for the great spring of Biram is presented by Braslavsky, who is of the opinion that it should be Aina Rabbati de Bei-Ram', the great spring of Bi-Ram. This is a small lake, Birket Ram that is found in a volcanic crater on the Golan. In his opinion, the original Semitic name is preserved in the Arabic name of Birket Ram.[273]

Dechent states that the name Ba'arah is related to the word *baar*, 'burning', because traces of an underground fire are noticeable at the location.[274] Neubauer completes the picture of the location of the site in light of the contexts of the expressions *Har HaBarzel* [= iron mountain], 'strong smoke', 'gate or opening to hell' both in Josephus and in the Talmudic literature.[275]

On the dispute in regard to the kinds of palm trees whose fronds may be used as a *lulav* on the *Sukkot* [= Tabernacles] Feast, it is written:[276]

---

[266] Avi-Yonah (1954): 39.
[267] Klein (1925): 21, note 8.
[268] Hirschberg (1920): 219.
[269] Neubauer (1868): 36.
[270] Kohut (1926): II: 59.
[271] Press (1948): I: 116.
[272] Yankelevitz (1988): 15.
[273] Braslavsky (1958): III: 339.
[274] Dechent (1884): 200.
[275] Neubauer (1868): 36–37.
[276] Neubauer (1868): 37, note 2.

> Rabbi Joshua ben Levi said and some say that Rabba bar Mari said it
> in the name of Raban Yohanan ben Zakki: 'There are two date trees
> in the valley of Hinom and smoke rises from between them, and that is
> what we have learned, the palms of *Har Habarzel* are kosher and this is
> the opening of Hell'.
>
> (*Babylonian Talmud, Sukka* 32b).

Josephus mentions that HaBarzel mountain is in Trans-Jordan and
spreads out 'up to the land of Moab': (*Bellum Judaicum* 4.46). Baaras,
Baaris, or Ba'arah is found, therefore, in this region, and it is possible
that, as Neubauer had it, it is the site mentioned in the Talmud as 'the
gate of Hell', for this appellation means 'the underground fire' in the
Talmudic literature (*Babylonian Talmud, Shabbat* 39a).[277] In his description of Baaras, Josephus relates the following in the *Bellum Judaicum*
(4.180–181) about a root that grew there and that is similar to a fire.

One should notice that the remains of the name [Βα]άρου are
inserted inside the black hilly background in the Madaba map. It may
be assumed, then, that the mosaic artists' inclination was to describe
the huge outpourings of lava on the heights of the mountains of Moab,
especially *Har Habarzel*, north of Baaras.[278]

The Prophet Isaiah wrote (30, 3): 'For *Tophet* is ordained of old; yea,
for the king it is prepared; he hath made it deep and large; the pile
thereof is fire and much wood; the breath of the Lord, like a stream
of brimstone, doth kindle it'. In other words, his fire-pit has been
made both wide and deep, with plenty of fire and firewood, and with
the breath of the Lord burning in it like a stream of sulfur. It may be
surmised that Isaiah was influenced by the name Ba'arah, which was
already current during the First Temple period, because the springs of
Baaras mentioned for the first time by Josephus, are the hottest sulphuric
springs in the whole Dead Sea region, and do indeed 'burn'. As is well
known, sulphuric deposits collect through a process of intense volcanic
crystallization. It can be assumed that the 'streams of brimstone' are
springs and streams of hot water which emit sulphur throughout the
vicinity and spread the powerful odour of Hydrogen Sulphide in the
atmosphere.[279]

---

[277] For the view of the Sages that the source of the 'heat of the thermal springs'
is 'the subterranean fire of Gehenna', see in chapter 6.1 on *The Halakhic Stance of the
Sages towards Curative Hot Springs and Baths*.

[278] Braslavsky (1958): III: 339; Avi-Yonah (1954): 24.

[279] See also *Isaiah* 34, 9–10 and the discussion in chapter 1.3 on *The Semitic Origin
and Biblical Survey of the Thermo-Mineral Springs*.

In several places in the Rabbinic literature, the name *Mei Ba'arah* [= the waters of Ba'arah] was corrupted to *Mei Me'arah* [= the waters of the cave]. Moreover, in various places in the *Mishnah*, the *Jerusalem* and *Babylonian Talmuds*—the expression *Mei Me'arah* appears in parallel to *Mei Tiberias* [= the waters of Tiberias; the letter *heit* is omitted in the word *Mei*, thereupon it transfer to be the word *Hammei*], or 'the hot springs of Tiberias', or 'the baths of Tiberias' [= Hammei-Tiberias], in various contexts. Here are a number of examples:

> One who bathes [= on the Sabbath] in the water of the cave [= *Me'arah*] or in the water of Tiberias [= Hammei-Tiberias] and dries himself, even though with ten towels, may not carry them away in his hands; but ten men may with one towel dry [= or wipe] their faces, their hands and their feet and bring it away in their hands.
>
> (*Mishnah, Shabbat* 22, 5)

> He who washes in the cave or in the water of Tiberias and dries himself, even with ten towels, should not bring them along in his hand.
>
> (*Tosefta, Shabbat* 16, 15)

> But when the people observed the secondary prohibitions [= 'fences'] imposed by the Sages, the Sages gradually permitted them the entire apparatus once again, [= having made their point], progressing to the point at which they permitted them to use cave water [= *Me'arah*] and even the hot springs of Tiberias.
>
> (*Jerusalem Talmud, Shabbat* 3, 3 [6a])

> There we have learned: He who bathes in cave water [= *Me'arah*] or in the water of Tiberias [= Hammei-Tiberias] dried himself, even with ten towels, may not then carry them in his hand.
>
> (*ibid., ibid.*)

> We bathed in salt water and they forbade us to bathe altogether. Because they entreated they allowed them more and more latitude...to bathe in *Mei Me'arah* and Hammei-Tiberias...but did not allow them to carry towels. Who permitted them to carry towels? Rabbi Hanania ben Akavia...He who bathes in the cave or in the water of Tiberias...on himself, but others may not splash him.
>
> (*Yerushalmi Fragments from the Genizah, Shabbat* 3, Ginzberg ed., p. 75).

Of all the hot springs in the eastern Mediterranean basin, only the heat of the springs of Ba'arah are compared to the thermal springs of Tiberias; and even the *Babylonian Talmud* (*Shabbat* 147a) insists: 'the waters of the cave [= *Me'arah*] are like the waters of Tiberias. Just as the waters of Tiberias are hot, so, too, the waters of *Mearah* are hot'.

In *Midrash Genesis Rabbah* (76, 5, collection 149 in the Paris Manuscript) we find a version which does not appear in the other *Midrashim*,

which comments on the Biblical verse 'And Jacob went forth from Be'er
Sheba in order to escape from his brother Esau', explains where the
incident took place, and how Jacob was able to endure the intense heat
of the site. According to Epstein, it is clear that the phrase 'When you
pass through the water I am with you' is interpreted as referring to the
parting of the Jordan, and the conclusion 'When you go through the
fire' to mean that Jacob went into a place whose waters were boiling
hot, 'like those of Tiberias', and was not scalded. In order to resolve
the question of how Jacob could withstand the intense heat, Rabbi Levi
claimed that there was a cool place whose heat was only moderate.
Therefore, Rabbi Levi's words are followed immediately by the phrase
'Jacob went in there'—that is to say, to that cool spot. This *Midrash*
speaks of Ba'arah, boiling-hot springs, and 'a place similar to the Tiberias baths'; and Rabbi Levi's reference to a 'cool spot in Ba'arah' is a
good definition of a site where hot and cold waters mingle. Epstein
adds that this story demonstrates that those who told it were aware
of the existence of thermal springs in eastern Trans-Jordan, and that
in one of them, the hot springs were cooled by the intermingling of
cool water.[280] In the light of all this, it is clear that this was the place
in which Jacob was saved from scalding and from the 'injury of heat',
as is said in the 'prayer of the bath', which is found in our sources
(*Tosefta, Berakhot* 7, 17; *Jerusalem Talmud, ibid.*, 9, 4 [14b]; *Babylonian
Talmud, ibid.*, 60a).

Hirschberg emphasizes that the designation of Ba'arah in the *Babylonian Talmud* (*Sanhedrin* 108a) as *Rabbati* [= great] shows that this site
enjoyed great publicity in ancient times; so much so that miraculous
legends, of which Josephus tells at great length, grew up. These are
connected with the red plant, mentioned above, which grows there,
emits rays of light at eventide, and kills anybody who touches it; the
contrivances for uprooting it; the use of its roots for expelling spirits and
demons from human beings; and, even more, his picturesque description
of the site.[281] Press clarifies that the Roman roads leading to the hot
springs of Ba'arah prove that here was an important bathing place.[282]

---

[280] Klein (1925); 22; idem, (1929): 1–8; Lieberman (1935): I/1: 82; Epstein (1957):
98–99; Braslavsky (1958): III: 333–339; Rosental (1991): 325–353; I presented a paper,
entitled 'The contribution of the Term "Mei Me'arah" to the Study of the Thermo-
Mineral Baths in Eretz-Israel', in the 13th World Congress of Jewish Studies, which
was held in the Hebrew University of Jerusalem, 12–17 August 2001.
[281] Hirschberg (1920): 219.
[282] Press (1948): I: 116.

Dechent adds that the coins found there accidentally come from the Roman period demonstrate that many people used these springs and perhaps Herod the Great himself used to bathe at this healing site.[283]

Hirschberg and in his footsteps Yankelevitz state that the hot waters of Baʾarah are not mentioned in the sources after the destruction of the Second Temple. It may be assumed that this healing place, and like it, Kallirrhoe, too, were destroyed or that the Jewish settlement ceased there altogether, since they were not close to any large city.[284] This determination by the two researchers indicates that they were unaware of the possibility of identifying Hammei-Baʾarah with Kefar Baru on an Aramaic bills of sale from the mid of the second century CE; of the description of Petrus the Iberian; of the importance of the recording of the location of Baaru in a cartography document, the Madaba map; of a dedicatory of a Greek inscription; and of the testimonies of geographers and travelers.[285]

The site has never been investigated archaeologically. But papyrological, cartographic and epigraphic evidence cast light, some of it new, on the name of the site and its cultic and therapeutic characteristics.

A. The Aramaic bills of sale from the village of Baru, from the days of Bar Kochba revolt, are living proof of the fact that during the revolt life carried on normally in certain places.[286] Houses and fields were bought and sold with no suspicion of the coming disaster; the use of both Aramaic and Hebrew indicates that in the wave of national emotion sparked off by the revolt the status of Hebrew was enhanced, although it was already used as a living language, though less common than Aramaic, at the time; the inhabitants of the south of the Dead Sea fled from their homes at the outbreak of the revolt, whereas the Jews, who lived in the more northerly region of Trans-Jordan, stayed in their villages until the third year of the revolt. This is important since

---

[283] Dechent (1884): 201.

[284] Hirschberg (1920): 219; Yankelevitz (1988): 16.

[285] On the archaeological evidence see the discussion below; For testimonies of geographers and travellers in the nineteenth century, see for example Tristram (1866): 507–562; idem, (1871): 334–355; Kersten (1879): 208–209; Buhl (1896): 128; Donner (1963): 63–64 stresses that these scholars identified wrongly the site and their mistake derived from misunderstanding of Josephus, *Bellum Judaicum* 7.186–189; See also Seetzen (1859): 383–385; Musil (1907): 89–99.

[286] Milik (1954): 182–190; idem, (1955): 253–254; idem, (1957): 264–268; See also Abramson and Ginsberg (1954): 17–19; Birnbaum (1957): 108–132; idem, (1958): 12–18; Puech (1977–1978): 213–221; Beyer (1984): 320–321.

it shows that villages east of the Dead Sea formed part of the area controlled by Bar Kochba. No caves of refuge have yet been found east of the Dead Sea, but it seems that two documents in our possession originated in a cave of refuge not far from the hot baths in the valley of Zarqa Ma'in.[287] In the view of Broshi and Qimron, 'It may well be that this is a settlement on the east of the Dead Sea; apparently Meniat Umm Hassan, above the springs of Hammam Ez-Zarqa, close to Wadi Zarqa Ma'in (triangulation point 207113).[288] The site is about five kilometres north-west of Michvar, and more or less opposite Mitzpeh Shalem and the caves of Muraba'at. The editors add that scholars generally agree that the Greek form of the name Βααρου corresponds to a place-name originating in a Semitic language and derived from the root *beit-ayin-resh*, which described the hot springs. This etymological interpretation is quite uncertain, but if it is correct it is hard to explain the absence of the letter *ayin* in the name 'Kefar Baro'. Nonetheless, the ending *-o* is frequent in Nabataean nouns such as the name of the king *Malko*, or of the queen, *Hagaro*.[289]

B. The mention of the name [Βα]άρου in the Madaba map is evidence of the importance of its baths. As noted above the traces of the name appear in the map against a black mountainous background. It may be surmised, therefore, that the artist intended to portray the huge outcrops of lava on the heights of the mountains of Moab, and, in particular, the 'HaBarzel Mountain' north of Ba'arah.[290] Donner adds several confirmatory details from various sources relating to the portrayal of the site on the Madaba map. Under the second *alpha* in the name BAAPOY the valley changes course from a north-south to an east-west direction, and is bordered by black stones. According to Donner, the artist wanted to show the marked change in direction of the Zarqa Ma'in Valley, about 5.5 kilometres from the Ez-Zarqa fountain. This is quite a remarkable

---

[287] Eshel (1998): 52–56; See also Gulak (1994): 215; Cotton and Yardeni (1997): 123–129.

[288] Broshi and Qimron (1986): 208–212.

[289] Kutsher (1959): 8–11; idem, (1962): 21–22; Naveh (1991: 234–231) claimed that the correct reading of Milik's document was 'Kfar Brio'. Since the final syllable of the village's name in both documents in question was o, it is hard to say whether Kfar Bero/Berio refers to the Baaras of Eusebius' *Onomastikon*, as Broshi and Qimron (1986: 207) believed, or to a settlement such as Be'erot. It is, therefore, impossible to decide whether Kefar Baro or Kefar Bero is the correct reading. Naveh's decision was accepted by Cotton and Yardeni (1997).

[290] Donner (1982): 176–177; idem (1992): 39; See also Schürer (1991): I: 326; Clamer (1999): 222; Piccirillo and Alliata (1999): 56.

fact. This depiction seems to show that the hills at the mouth of the Zarqa Ma'in valley are at a significant distance from the sea-shore, like those on the eastern shore of the Dead Sea, and that they form a broad coastal plain through which the water flows, with the accession of a stream flowing into the sea from the north-west. This, says Donner, is a geographical error, which requires explanation. Moreover, the map gives the impression that Ba'arah baths are to be found in the part of the valley where the water emerges, while the literary sources indicate the baths of Hammamat Zarqa Ma'in. He believes that in ancient times there were hot springs and bathing facilities east of the spot where the Ma'in Zarqa baths are located today. An expedition promoted by the German Evangelical Institution for the Exploration of the Holy Land visited the site in 1963, in order to test this hypothesis.[291] In Donner's view, in the course of time the hot waterfalls changed their direction and the places where they flowed over the rocks, and this can be seen in the mineral deposits, which take the form of stalactites, stalagmites, and other shapes. In the first investigation on the ground there were found remains from the Chalcolithic and Early and Late Bronze ages, and a few from the Roman-Byzantine period, but none from the Muslim period. Donner assumes that the name Baaru was moved far to the east on the map, not because the hot baths were on the upper mouth of the Zarqa Ma'in valley, but because the artist could not find a sufficient space on its western side. The portrayal of the site in the map is cartographically inexact, and this calls for an explanation, since the other details relating to eastern Trans-Jordan are exact. The Zarqa Ma'in valley does not flow through a broad coastal strip, but descends directly from the mountain into the Dead Sea. The mountain descends steeply. If we assume that the map-maker was from Madaba, he must have seen the baths of Zarqa Ma'in himself, and have used the ancient path from Madaba, which is still in use today, to reach the spring. It may be that what looks like a stream which flows from the north-east and descends to the valley of Zarqa Ma'in is in fact only a depiction of the path, since there is no other stream in the vicinity which could have influenced the artist. From this path the place where the spring of the Wadi Zarqa valley emerges can be seen from below. Viewed from above, the region looks as the artist depicted it; it is very doubtful whether at his time he could have seen and noted all the details, because

---

[291] Donner (1982): 177–179.

of the difficulty in reaching the spot. In short, Donner concludes that the mosaicist went no further than do travellers and tourists in our own day. None the less, he intended to emphasize the importance of Hammei-Ba'arah and Hammei-Kallirrhoe in his time.

C. A dedicatory inscription in Greek, dated to the first century CE, the Roman period, was discovered in al-Harra (Euthymia?) in southern Syria, close to the Roman road from Damascus to Dera'a. It was first published in 1952 by Sordel, and is today in the National Museum in Damascus. Its connection with the thermo-mineral baths of Ba'arah has not been discussed by scholars until recently,[292] when Hübner pointed out the connection of a votive inscription to the local cult of the Baaras springs, Hammei-Ba'arah, which is a very rare and unique finding in the Levant. In his view, it can provide information about the healing art practised there.[293] The inscription is in five lines, adorning a basalt altar, devoted by Diomedes Charetos, a Roman official of Bataneae in the rank of a governor (*eparches*) and military commander (*strategos*), who appealed to the local god, Zeus Beelbaaros.

It appears that this person was healed as a result of the therapeutic properties of the Ba'arah baths, and in thanks for this he made a contribution or a vow to Zeus Beelbaaros, the local Baal of Ba'arah. It may be that this was one of the gods of the Trans-Jordanian heights parallel to the Moabite god Kemosh.[294] It may seem strange that the Roman governor and general of Bataneae should have offered up thanks in Ba'arah in Trans-Jordan, of all places. Hübner's explanation is that he came there as a result of health problems, and, after successful treatment, felt the need to give thanks and raise an altar to the local Baal of Ba'arah. Had he had different medical advice, he could have bathed in Hammat-Gader or the Hammei-Tiberias. Diomedes gave thanks to a god who did not exist in Bataneae or the Hauran, because he had visited the baths of Ba'arah. Appeals to the local Baal with the addition of the name Zeus are also found in Gerasa for Baalbosoros, Jupiter Optimus Baaltzeida, and Zeus Baalpeor. The mention of the principal god of Gaza, Zeus Maranas, in the city of al-Karak, and of Zeus Damascanus, Zeus Patanus and Zeus Heliopolites in Bosra furnish

---

[292] Sordel (1952): 45–46, Pl. 4:1; Dittenberger (1977), *OGIS* no. 422; See also Lifshitz (1977): 20.
[293] Hübner (1995): 252–255.
[294] Worschech (1992): 393–401.

evidence of the worship of gods of localities other than the place where the inscription was found. Zeus Beelbaaros in the inscription before us is a local version of the Moabite god Kemosh; in his view, the name Kemosh—able to revive—indicates the god's therapeutic capabilities.[295] Kemosh was the god of the Moabites, and in the Bible they are given the poetic name 'the people of Kemosh' (*Numbers* 21, 29; *Jeremiah* 48, 46). In the Mesha inscription a deity by the name of *Ashtar Kamash* is mentioned (line 17). Some scholars claim that the name Ashtar refers to Kamosh's female partner, while others believe that *Ashtar Kamash* is a composite name, and that Kemash is identified with the male god Ashtar. In addition to the worship of Baalpeor in the land of Moab (*Numbers* 25, 1 et seq.) there was also a site known as Baalmaon (see above), which indicates the existence of a shrine. In *Numbers* 22, 41, a place in Moab known as Bamoth Baal, doubtless a site, at which Baal was worshipped, is mentioned. It may be that these names indicate the worship of local Baals, in addition to the major gods with Kemosh at their head. But it is also possible that Kemosh was worshipped in these places, and that the Baal element in their names denotes Kemosh the god of Moab.[296] None the less, it seems that the local god Zeus-Beelbaaros is not Kemosh, but the god who was worshipped on the site; and his name—apparently Baalmaon—is confirmation of this. In the light of Eusebius' evidence, it seems that because of the cult practised on the site the name Baalmaon was changed to Beelmaus.[297] The Talmudic name Ein Bechi (*Babylonian Talmud, Pesahim* 117a), which refers to the town of Baalbek, is reminiscent of its earlier name: Baalbechi. It may be that the former name of the site was Baalmaon, and that its name was changed, as appears from the words of the prophet *Hosea* (2, 17): 'For I will take away the names of *Baalim* out of her mouth, and they shall no more be remembered by their name'. Later it was known as Aina Rabbati of Biram [= Biraas, Ba'aras]: the baths of Ba'arah.

In the Byzantine period there was a hospice (Ξένεον) near the church in Baalmaon, which accommodated both sick and healthy on their way to and from Ba'arah. There is evidence of this in a Greek mosaic inscription in the 'Church of the West', which was discovered in 1934

---

[295] Hübner (1995): 253–254.
[296] Cassuto (1962): 186–188; Timm (1989): 162–165; Worschech (1992): 393–401; Weber (1997): 333.
[297] Eusebius, *Onomastikon* 44.

and deciphered by de Vaux and Piccerrilo.[298] In the mosaic floor were depicted twenty four towns in Palestine and Trans-Jordan. Only eleven towns have survived. Each of them is represented by a single church, and they are in the main in geographical order. The geographical order is disturbed only in the case of the local town, Beelmounim: Ma'in.

The style of the dedicatory inscription to Zeus Beelbaaros is, to a considerable extent, reminiscent of the style and content of dedicatory inscriptions which have been discovered in curative baths of the Classical World. (See Fig. 27). Within the Roman Empire a deity with local or wider signficance is joined to a parallel deity in the Graeco-Roman world, in accordance with their powers and the extent of their influence.[299] Thus, as we have already seen, the therapeutic deities both of Gaul and of Germany were often identified with Apollo the healer; for instance, in the shrines of Essarois, near Dijon, and of Hochscheid, near Bernkastel.[300] In Aachen Apollo was linked to the local deity, Grannus, as the principal god of a group of therapeutic baths. In one of the suburbs of Aachen an altar dated to the beginning of the second century CE, which may indicate the nature of the cult of Apollo Grannus, has been discovered. The god sits on a royal throne, holds a lyre and a plectrum in his hand, and carries a quiver of arrows on his right shoulder. The inscription states that the altar was dedicated 'in fulfillment of a vow' by Latinus Macer, a native of the city of Verona, the *praefectus castrorum* of the Legion IX *Hispania*, who underwent medical treatment in the spa.[301] (See Fig. 4). Jackson surmises that this distinguished personage visited the therapeutic site because Apollo Grannus was one of the best-known therapeutic deities, and the ailing Emperor Caracalla visited the sites sacred to him on the 'tour of the shrines' which, according to Cassius Dio, he made in the years 211–217 CE.[302] The inscription to Zeus Beelbaaros is the

---

[298] de Vaux (1938): 227–258, especially pp. 250–255; Piccerrilo (1989): 237; idem, (1995): 251–253.

[299] See the survey in chapter 3 about *The Medicinal Hot Springs and Healing Spas in the Graeco-Roman World.*

[300] Hatt (1985): 205–238; Dehn (1941): 104–111, Pl. 14; Krug (1993): 176–177; Cüppers (1982); Hugot (1963): 188–197.

[301] Dehn (1941): 104–111, Pl. 14; Jackson (1988): 163; Nesselhauf and Petrikovits (1967): 268–279.

[302] Jackson (1990a): 8; idem, (1988): 163; See also Cassius Dio, *Historia Romana* 78.15.3–7; Engelmann (1980): no. 802; Jackson (1990a): 8; idem, (1988): 163; Krug (1993): 175; See also in chapter 7 about *The Roman Emperors at the Spas in the Eastern Mediterranean.*

only evidence of the cult practised in the curative baths in the eastern Mediterranean, apart from historical and numismatic evidence from the city of Tiberias about its suburb, Hammei-Tiberias, and from the city of Gadara about its suburb, Hammat-Gader.[303]

Just as the Roman governor Diomedes Charetos was treated in the Hammei-Ba'arah baths, so was 'Amr Ibn Luhayy in the first half of the fourth century CE, as we learn from the *Kitab al-Asnam* of Hisham Ibn al-Kalbī.[304] Ibn al-Kalbī, an Iraqi scholar of the eight–ninth century CE, says that, after forcibly gaining control of the Ka'ba, the holy site in Mecca, 'Amr ibn Luhayy became seriously ill, and the doctors recommended that he should visit a hot spring (*hamme*) in Trans-Jordan (*al-Balqa*). On arriving at the hot spring he bathed in its waters and was healed. During his stay at the site he noted that its inhabitants were idol-worshippers. They told him that they prayed to their gods for rain and for victory over their enemies. He asked them to give him the idols, took them to Mecca, and erected them round the Ka'ba.[305] This is not the place to discuss the historical authenticity of his special visit and his cure. None the less, Ibn Luhayy is credited with instituting the tradition of introducing various statues of Greek and Roman gods and goddesses to Mecca, which was customary in pre-Christian times. In the pre-Islamic period many dozens of idols were worshipped in Mecca. The most important were the goddesses al-'Uzza, Allat, Manat, and Hubal, a male god whose name was a synonym for the god (Allah) of Mecca. In the *Koran* (*Sura* 53) these three goddesses are mentioned: on the conquest of Mecca in 630 CE, Muhammed, who has declared his intention to cleanse the city of idolatry, harangues the believers: 'These goddesses are nothing but names, which you and your forefathers invented with no authority from Allah'. The names of these gods are mentioned in *Bilād ash-Shām*, and appear in Nabataean inscriptions some centuries earlier.[306]

Muslim historians and geographers mention the tradition that Ibn Luhayy brought the statue of Hubal to Mecca, and emphasize the idol-worship which was rife among the local inhabitants, and particularly at

---

[303] See *The Historical-Archaeological Survey of Hammei-Tiberias* in 4.1 *and of Hammat-Gader* in 4.2 above and in chapter 8.1 and 8.3 on *The Numismatic Expression of the Medicinal Hot Springs of Tiberias and Gadara.*

[304] Hisham Ibn al-Kalbī, *Kitab al-Ansnam* 5.13.

[305] Faris (1952): 7; Teixidor (1977): 73.

[306] Sordel (1952): 67–74; Gawlikowski (1990): 2666–2667; Donner (1995): 7; Weber (1997): 338.

the Ka'ba, in the pre-Islamic period. Instances of this are to be found in Ahmad al-Baladhuri's *Kitāb futuh al-buldān* [= Book of Conquests of Lands] (869), Ibn Wadiah al-Ya'qubi's *Kitab al-buldān* (891) [= Book of the Lands], and others.[307] At an earlier date the Arabic historian Ibn Hisham 'Abd al-Malik (ob. 834) added an important detail in his book *Kitab Sirat Rasul Allah* [= The Life of Muhammed]. Amr Ibn Luhayy asked the people of Moab, who worshipped gods which brought down rain, to give him an idol; they gave him Hubal, and he took him to Mecca. Hubal was the most famous deity in the Ka'ba; he had the form of a man, with seven arrows before him.[308] Scholars have suggested a number of etymological sources for the name Hubal: either from the Accadian *habalu*—to destroy, to devastate, to damage; or from the Arabic *habila*—in modern usage, bereavement, thus linking him to the subject of death; or from the Arabic word *hibil*—the Ancient One. This interpretation derives from the fact that in the Ka'ba Hubal was linked with Abraham, who was described as an old man.[309] A further possibility, which accords with the concept discussed here, is that the name Hubal was derived from *HaBaal*—the Baal. Since neither Biblical Hebrew nor Arabic possessed vowel signs, Hubal could have been derived from *HaBaal*, just as there are many versions of the name Muhammed (Mohamed, Muhamad, and Mahomet).

The tradition that the idol Hubal [= HaBaal] was taken from the peoples who dwelt close by the hot spring in Moab to the Ka'ba in Mecca may well indicate that Zeus Beelbaaros was a local variant of Baalmaon, who may have been the Hubal of the Muslim sources.

Returning to the anecdote of Hisham Ibn al-Kalbī about 'Amr Ibn Luhayy, who was treated in Hammei-Ba'arah—it seems to Weber that it is able to draw some conclusions on the nature and iconography of those pre-Islamic idols that were introduced to the shrine of Mecca by 'Amr Ibn Luhayy after his visit to the thermal springs east of the Jordan River.[310] According to archaeological evidence, predominately male divinities were venerated there. Greek god of medicine, Asklepios coincided with Zeus and could easily be identified with older local gods such as Baal or Kemosh. Hygieia, the daughter of Asklepios and the personification of health, as well as the Egyptian Sarapis or Serapis

---

[307] Al-Baladhuri, *Kitāb futūh al-buldān* 119; al-Ya'qubi, *Kitāb al-buldān* 10.
[308] Ibn Hisham 'Abd al-Malik, *Kitāb Sirat Rasul Allah* 50–51.
[309] Fahd (1958): 55–79; idem, (1971): 536–537.
[310] Weber (1997): 338.

played an important role in the Levant especially at the thermo-mineral baths as a healing and fertility gods. It was most likely that about these idols the visitors mentioned in Ibl al-Kalbī's story: 'to them we pray for rain'. Another aspect of these idols can be confirmed by the reliefs like those from Kufr Ma or Umm Qais [= Gadara]—showing the armed healing god provide firm evidence for those of the idols with military character: 'For them we seek victory over the enemy'.[311]

4.6   HAMMEI-LIVIAS

On the eastern side of the Jordan Valley was the large town of Livias (Λιβιάς) or Julias, opposite Jericho. (See Map 1). The Bible mentions a town called Beth Haram or Beth Haran east of the Jordan, in the territory of the Amorite king of Heshbon named Sihon (*Joshua* 13, 27). The toponym appears first as the name of a possession of the Gadites who are said to have rebuilt Beth Haran along with several other sites (*Numbers* 32, 36). It occurs again as one of these cities, this time located in the valley in association with Beth Nimrah, Succoth, and Zaphon (*Joshua* 13, 27). The Hebrew *Beth Haran(m)* may be translated as 'house of the summit place', and may provide geographic information about the site's location. In the *Jerusalem Talmud, Shevi'it* 9, 2 [38d]), Beth Ramtha is given a more recent name of this Beth Haram.[312] Eusebius states that the Beth Haram of *Joshua* 13, 27 is a Gadite city, and places it near the Jordan. He reports that it was called Bethramtha in Aramaic and later called Livias.[313] Like Eusebius, the Talmud locates Beth Ramtha on the Jordan and belonging to the Gadites. Hieronymus likewise identify the Biblical

---

[311] For the relief from Umm Qais see Sourdel (1952): 47; Künzl and Weber (1991): 82, note 5; On the relief from Kufr Ma see Schumacher (1886a): 81, Figs. 33–34; idem, (1886b): 337, Fig. 118; Abdul-Hak (1951): 66, no. 31.

[312] Neubauer (1868): 247; Thomsen (1907): 38; Smith (1920): 314; Abel (1931): 217–223; idem, (1938): II: 273; Glueck (1943): 20–21; Press (1948): I: 82; Van Zyl (1960): 93; Harder (1962): 60–63; Borée (1968): 76; Ottosson (1969): 86; Avi-Yonah (1976): 28; Aharoni (1979): 432; MacDonald (2000): 120; Donner and Cüppers (1967: 22–23) suggest that this region is portrayed in the Madaba mosaic map; In *Tosefta, Shevi'it* 7, 11, both towns Beth Haran and Beth Nimrah (today Shuneh-Nimrin) situated in the Jordan Valley are called Beth Nimrah Ramtha. Schürer (1991: II: 176) has doubts whether Beit [= Beth] has been omitted here before Ramtha or if it was known simply as Ramtha.

[313] Eusebius, *Onomastikon* 48, 13–15; See also idem, *ibid.*, 12, 16; On Tel er-Râmeh see Conder (1889): I: 238–239; Smith (1920): 314; Kelin (1925): 12–13; Starr (1935): 290; Schürer (1991): II: 176, note 500.

Beth Haram with the place known by them as Βηθραμφά or Bethramtha and adds: 'by Herod in honour of Augustus'.[314] The evidence accords with the site of Tel er-Râmeh on the south side of the Wadi Hesban, almost exactly midway between Jericho and Heshbon.

Bethramtha is in any case identical with Βηθαράματος, where Herod the Great possessed a palace that was destroyed during the insurrection after his death.[315] This Bethramphtha was then rebuilt and fortified by Herod Antipas, and named Julias in honour of the wife of Augustus. Josephus alone uses the official designation Julias. It served as an administrative centre for several nearby villages, including Beit Hayesimot (Hirbet Suweimeh), at the northern end of the Dead Sea, opposite Jericho. Josephus still writes of the town as Julias during the time of the Jewish war, when it was occupied by Placidus, one of Vespasian's generals. Emperor Nero gave it with its fourteen villages to Agrippa II, King of Judaea.[316]

Pliny the Elder, Ptolemy, Hierocles, Eusebius, Hieronymus, Syncellus and others give the name as Livias instead of Julias, and the town is also frequently referred to elsewhere as Livias.[317] Since the wife of Augustus was really called Livia, and was only admitted into the *gens* Iulia in virtue of her husband's will, and therefore bore the name Julia only after his death—it seems that Livias was the older of the two names.[318] The early Roman remains at the site were fairly poor, a fact that weighs against its identification as Bethsaida.[319]

The most accurate description of the location of the city with its *aquae calidae* is given by Christian pilgrims: Egeria of the end of the

---

[314] Hieronymus, *Onomastikon* 49, 13.

[315] Josephus, *Bellum Judaicum* 2.59; In the parallel passage, *Antiquitates Judaicae* 17.277, the name is corrupt; See Schürer (1991): II: 177, note 503; Press (1948): I: 82; Avi-Yonah (1976): 28; Stern (1983a): 87; Levine (1984): 52; Dvorjetski (1992a): 92.

[316] Josephus, *Bellum Judaicum* 2.168, 4.438.454; idem, *Antiquitates Judaicae* 18.27; 20.8; Eusebius, *Chronicle* 149–150; Syncellus, *Chronographia* 605; The identity of Livias with Josephus' Betharamphtha-Julias is beyond reasonable doubt; *Bellum Judaicum* 2.252 and *Antiquitates Judaicae* 20.159 certainly have Julias = Bethsaida in mind. See Schalit (1951): 117; Hoehner (1972): 87–91; Avi-Yonah (1984): 166; Schürer (1991): II: 177–178, notes 504 and 507; Isaac (2000): 341; Negev and Gibson (2001): 80–81.

[317] Pliny the Elder, *Naturalis Historia* 13.44; Ptolemy, *Geographia* 5.15.6, 5.16.9; Hierocles, *Synecdemus* 44; Eusebius, *Onomastikon* 48; Hieronymus, *Onomastikon* 49; Syncellus, *Chronographia* 605.

[318] Smith (1920): 314; Schürer (1991): II: 177.

[319] Negev and Gibson (2001): 81; Waterhouse and Ibach (1975): 227–228.

fourth century CE, Petrus of Iberia of the fifth century CE, Theodosius and Antoninus from Placentia the sixth century CE Palestinian pilgrims and after them Gregory of Tours, according to whom Livias lay beyond the Jordan, in the neighbourhood of warm springs. In all likelihood it was placed in the class of hallowed waters endowed with supernatural healing powers.[320]

Egeria's description of her pilgrimage furnishes a penetrating glimpse into the devotion of the Christian traveller. The pilgrim road in general continues via Livias (Tel er-Râmeh) towards Esbus (Heshbon) on the plateau, turning off to the Springs of Moses and Mount Nebo. It can be illustrated from her movements in the desert of Sinai, around the sites associated with the experiences of Moses and the children of Israel. One of these sites was Libiada [= Libias = Livias], with the remains of the dwellings of the children of Israel. It seems that after having crossed the Jordan on her way from Jerusalem, she had stayed at Livias and then taken the road to Heshbon. At the sixth mile Egeria took a deviation to the hot springs of Moses and from there climbed to the summit of Mount Nebo.[321]

Petrus of Iberia Bishop of Maioumas-Gaza became weakened from self mortification, left his monastery and went to take a cure at the thermal waters of Ba'ar and Hammei-Livias in order to heal his body. Since his youth Petrus had bruised his body and tormented it by various forms of ascetic discipline, so that his flesh had wasted away and only his skin and a thin one at that—was stretched over his dried up bones.[322] Petrus took the same road as Egeria in search of a cure for his afflictions. After bathing in the hot springs of Moses, with a little benefit, because the springs were not very hot, the party continued his way to the hot springs of Baaru, Hammei-Ba'arah, where the waters were much hotter and more curative. The journey offered bishop Petrus and his companion, the opportunity to stop at the sanctuary of Moses where he had been as a youth before his conversion to monasticism.

---

[320] See the discussions below and in chapters 5 on *The Healing Properties of the Spas* and in 9.1 on *The Perspective of the Church Fathers and Pilgrims to the Therapeutic Sites*.

[321] Egeria, *Itinerarium* 10; See Donner (1979): 104; Starowieyski (1979): 297–318; Hunt (1982): 86; Maraval (1982): 167–168; Limor (1983): 49–68; idem, (1998): 67; Wilkinson (1981): 104–106; MacDonald, Adams and Bienkowski (2001): 495; For the exploration in the site, see Abel (1931): 380–388.

[322] Petrus of Iberia, 82–85.

Two other descriptions have much in common, and can be assumed
to speak of the same place. One is by Theodosius, author of the *De Situ
Terrae Sanctae*, which describes the Land of Israel and its neighbours:[323]

> In ipsa Liviada Moyses lapidem de uirga percussit et; fluxerunt aquae
> inde abundantius totam terram irrigant; dactylorum incolatum majorem
> habent. Ibi et Moyses migravit a seculo. Et ibi aquis calide sunt, ubi
> Moyses lavit et in ipsis aquis calidis leprosy mundantur [= In this Livias
> Moses struck the rock with his rod, and the waters flowed out. Thence
> emerges a rather large steam which irrigates the whole of Livias. There
> are found the large dates of Nicolaus. There Moses departed this life,
> and there are the warm waters where Moses bathed, and in these warm
> waters lepers are cleansed].

In other words, Theodosius relates with great precision that Livias, is
beyond the Jordan River, twelve Roman miles from Jericho and pilgrims
could visit the water made to flow from the rock [= The Springs of
Moses], the place of Moses's death and the hot springs of Moses where
lepers come to be cured.

The other description is by Antoninus of Placentia, one of the earliest
Italian pilgrims, who visited the Levant in 570 CE, and wrote:[324]

> Ibi in proximo est ciuitas quae uocatur Liuiada, ubi remanserunt duo
> semis tribus Israhel, antequam Iordanem transirent, in quo loco sunt
> termae ex lauantes, quae uocantur Moysi, ibi etiam et leprosy mundantur.
> Est ibi fons, aqua dulcissima, quae pro catarticum bibitur et sanat multos
> languores, non longe a mare salinarum, in qua etiam et Iordanis ingreditur
> subtus Sodoma et Gomurra, ad cuius litus sulphur et bitumen colligitur.
> In qua mare mense Iulio et Augusto et medio Septembrio tota die iacent
> leprosy; ad uesperum lauant in illas termas Moysi et aliquotiens, quem
> uult dues, mundatur. Nam et generalitati est aliqua paramitia [= Nearby
> is a city called Livias, where the two half-tribes of Israel remained before
> crossing the Jordan, and in that place are natural hot springs which are
> called *termae of Moses* <Baths of Moses>. In these also lepers are cleansed.
> A spring there has very sweet water which they drink as a cathartic, and
> it heals many diseases. This is not far from the Salt Sea, into which the
> Jordan flows, below Sodom and Gomorrha. Sulphur and pitch are col-
> lected on that shore. Lepers lie in the sea there all through the day in
> July, August, and the early part of September. In the evening they wash
> in these Baths of Moses. From time to time bythe will of God one of
> them is cleansed, but for most of them it brings some relief].

---

[323] Theodosius, *De Situ Terrae Sanctae* 19; See Bernard (1893): 14.
[324] Antoninus, *Itinerarium* 10; Willkinson (1977): 82; See also Stewart (1896): 9–10;
Berger (1982): 72.

Dechent maintains that according to Theodosius the springs of Moses are to befound close to Livias, that is to say some miles from the Dead Sea, whereas Antoninus places it close to the Dead Sea. According to Dechent, these two descriptions should be conflated, and the springs of Moses should be sought on the north-west shore of the Dead Sea.[325] Moreover, Theodosius mentions briefly that lepers are also treated in the hot springs, while Antoninus describes the method of treatment in greater detail. First of all, he says that there are very sweet waters in the spring, and they are drunk as a purgative and cure many illnesses. In some ways Antoninus's words recall Josephus' words of praise concerning the baths of Kallirrhoe. Next, Antoninus says that the spring is not far from the Dead Sea, and that the lepers lie in it all day in the months of July, August, and half of September; in the evening they bathe in the springs of Moses themselves (*in ipsis termis*), and find relief there by the grace of the Lord.[326]

It is astonishing that we have no other information about a spring with such signal therapeutic qualities, particularly since it was so close to Jericho. Dechent's explanation is that in the sixth century CE therapeutic properties over and above their real merits were attributed to many springs, and they became sanctified either because of Biblical allusions or because of the spread of legends about them.[327] It may be, therefore, that at that period the importance of the springs of Moses was overstated. It may also be that the spring dried up, as happened with several other sulphurous springs to the west of the Jordan in the vicinity of Jericho, according to Fraas.[328]

A cotemporary of Antoninus of Placentia, the bishop and historian Gregory of Tours in France, points out briefly and laconically in his *De Gloria martyrum* the contribution of the curative site to the lepers:[329]

> Sunt autem et ad Levidam civitatem aquae calidae,...ubi similiter leprosy mundatur; est autem ab Hiericho duodecim millia.

Pliny the Elder wrote that the dates of Jericho were especially good but also good were those from Archelais, Phasaelis, and Livias. The

[325] Dechent (1884): 202–203.
[326] See above chapter 4.4 on *The Historical-Archaeological Analysis and Healing Cults of Kallirrhoe*.
[327] Dechent (1884): 203.
[328] Fraas (1879): 113–119.
[329] Gregory of Tours, *De Gloria Martyrum* 1.18; 'Levidam' [al. Leviadem]; See also Schürer (1991): II: 178.

outstanding qualities of these dates, wrote Pliny, were their juiciness
and their sweetness.[330] The dates of Livias are praised by Theodosius:
'ibi habet dactalum Nicolaum maiorem'.[331] The Madaba Map also
pictures date palms still growing in the area of Livias-Betharamtha in
the sixth century CE.[332]

From the Byzantine administrative lists one can learn about three
Bishops from Livias: Letoius, who was at Ephesus in 431 CE; Pancratius,
at Chalcedon in 451 CE; and Zacharias, at Jerusalem in 536 CE.[333]

Today most archaeologists identify the ruin of the unexcavated Tel
er-Râmeh as the site of the ancient town Livias-Betharamtha. Tel er-
Râmeh is a hill rising in the plain beyond Jordan, about 12 miles from
Jericho. It has surface evidence of pottery or mosaic stone cubes from
the Byzantine and early Islamic eras.

4.7   THE WATERS OF ASIA

'The waters of Asia' is another thermal spring in Palestine mentioned
in the *Babylonian Talmud Shabbat* 109a, in the following words:

> The Rabbis taught: 'One may bathe in the waters of Gerar,[334] in the
> waters of Hammthan, in the waters of Asia, and in the waters of Tiberias
> but not in the Great Sea [= the Mediterranean] nor of steeping pools
> nor of the Dead Sea'.

Scholars' opinions about the identity of Asia, and its exact location,
have been many and various. The generally accepted view rests on
the similarity between Asia (first letter: *ayin*) and Asia (first letter: *aleph*).
Therefore, they tried to locate it in the continent of Asia. Asia Minor
in general and the cities Lydda [= Laodicea], Apamaea [= Aspamia],
and the province of Cappadocia in particular were known to the Sages
(*Jerusalem Talmud, Kil'aim* 9, 3 [32c]; *Babylonian Talmud, Baba Bathra* 56a;
ibid., Baba Mezia 84a; *ibid., Yevamoth* 121a; *ibid., Avoda Zarah* 8b; *ibid.,
Pesahim* 50a). Rappoport, for instance, identifies Asia with the city of

---

[330] Pliny the Elder, *Naturalis Historia* 13.44.
[331] Theodosius, *De Situ Terrae Sanctae* 19.
[332] Avi-Yonah (1954): 25; Hepper and Taylor (2004): 35.
[333] Schürer (1991): II: 177, note 505.
[334] Assimilation of the letters *dalet* and *reis* in Hebrew caused the fault Gerar instead
of Gader; See München manuscript to *Babylonian Talmud, Shabbat* 109a; See also Rabbinovicz (1839): II: 240; Klein (1939): 74; Ne'eman (1971): I: 112; Neusner (1991):
167–168; Dvorjetski (1992a): 56–57; idem, (2002a): 43; idem, (2003): 27.

Hierapolis in the province of Phrygia in Asia Minor, which was a famous spa; he also claimed that it was known as *Maia de* [= water of] *diomeset*.[335]

Obviously, the 'waters of Asia' which the Sages compared to the waters of Hammat-han and Tiberias cannot be located in the continent of Asia. Neubauer points out that since each of the other three places mentioned in the *baraitha* are in Palestine, it is clear that Asia must also be there: 'Why should the Talmud mention here only hot springs in Asia, and not those in Mesopotamia or Persia'?[336] Ish-Shalom also emphasizes that the Rabbis intended to refer to places close by, known to all the people; thus, they spoke of the waters of Gader, Hammthan and Tiberias together with those of Asia. Therefore, he maintains, the Sages meant neither the city of Sardis nor the city of Asia in Lydia, nor Hierapolis, but another town called Asia (with *aleph* or *ayin*). He concluded that they meant Lydia in northern Syria.[337] Bar-Droma, who found it difficult to locate this Asia in Asia Minor, interpreted the word rather than giving it its straightforward meaning: 'Perhaps Asia here is not a proper name, viz. the name of a particular place, but rather the name for a particular type of water—mineral water used for medicinal purposes, from the root *a-s-a* (as in *issi*—an Essene, *asia*—a doctor), meaning to strengthen, to heal'.[338] This hypothesis is not acceptable, since it cannot be that in this Talmudic context the name Asia appears in a different sense from that which it has everywhere else in the Rabbinical writings. Moreover, Bar-Droma quotes Weinstein, who claims that here Kallirrhoe, on the eastern shore of the Dead Sea, is meant.[339] Thus, Bar-Droma himself is not completely satisfied with his daring suggestion to interpret the name differently. It should be added that Jastrow and Krauss also identify Asia with Kallirrhoe and its vicinity east of the Jordan and close to the Dead Sea.[340] Hirschberg maintains that the claim that the waters of Asia are the springs of Kallirrhoe is too far-fetched. He also rejects Krauss's idea, that the waters of Asia are called after the Essenes, who lived in this area and used these waters not only for baptism and bathing, which were done only in cold water,

---

[335] Rapoport (1857): 154–155.
[336] Neubauer (1868): 309.
[337] Ish-Shalom (1901): 46–47.
[338] Bar-Droma (1958): 638.
[339] Bar-Droma (1958): 638, note 74d.
[340] Jastrow (1950): 1098; See Horowitz (1923): 63–64; Press (1955): IV: 744; Schmitt (1975): 61.

but also for healing the sick. If this were so, they would be called the waters of Issaim, and not Asia; Asia is a place-name, like the names of the other springs, none of which is named after a sect. Similarly, says Hirschberg, the name *Assai* [or *Issaim*] does not occur anywhere in Talmudic literature.[341] Schwartz claimed that the Palestinian city referred to was Assiot. He based this view on a passage in the *Babylonian Talmud, Gittin* 4b: 'Rabbi Yitzhak said: there was one city in the Land of Israel, and its name was Assiot'. He maintained that the city of Assiot was situated south-west of the Baneas, about half an hour's journey from the village of Asias, and that it was also mentioned in other passages of the Rabbinic literature, such as 'a story of Asia': 'It once happened at Asia that a man [= a diver] was lowered in to the sea and only his leg was brought up, and the Sages ruled: [If the recovered leg contained the part] above the knee [the man's wife] may marry again' (*Babylonian Talmud, Yevamoth* 120b); 'Said Rabbi Abbahu: "Karina is a sweet wine which comes from Asia". Raid Rava: "In its own place, however, it is rendered unfit if left uncovered, the reason being that it is the "local wine"'' (*ibid., Avoda Zarah* 30a). The sea which is mentioned as being next to Asia is 'the sea of Huli' [= the Huleh Lake].[342]

Because of the association of the place-name Asia (with *aleph* or *ayin*) to water in the Talmudic literature, some scholars suggest that an ancient settlement on the sea-coast is intended:[343]

> If a man had fallen into the water, whether or not within sight of shore, his wife is forbidden [= to marry him]...Again it once happened in Asia that a man was let down by a rope into the sea and they drew up again naught save his leg. The Sages said: 'If [= the part of the leg recovered] included the part above the knee his wife may marry again; but if only the part below the knee she may not marry again.
>
> (*Mishnah, Yevamoth* 16, 4)

> A *castellum* which distributes its waters into [= separate] reservoirs, if it has a hole the size of a wine-skin stopper does not disqualify [= its waters for serving for ritual ablution]. But if [= there is] not [= such a hole, it does] disqualify the *miqweh*. This issue on three separate occasions

---

[341] Hirschberg (1920): 225; There is no hint in the ancient sources that the Essenes used thermo-mineral waters, springs or baths. See Kottek (1983): 96–97.

[342] Schwartz (1900): 9–10, note 2, 228, note 2; cf. Klein (1930): 21–23.

[343] Such as Etzion Gaver, on the Red Sea coast, modern Eilat; The phonetic explanation is as follows Etzion> Ezia> Asia (with the letter *ayin* > Asia (with the letter *aleph*); Most of the references below are based on Klein (1939): 122–123; see also Vilnaey: (1970): I: 5937; Reeg (1989): 51.

was brought by the inhabitants of Asia before [= the members of the Academy of] Jabneh, and on the third [= occasion] they permitted it, even if the hole was [= only] the size of a needle.

(*Tosefta, Miqvaot* 4, 6, Tsukermandel ed., p. 656)[344]

Someone who leads a rope to the owners. If it is conducted usually it is lawfulness. But if it is conducted irregularly it is disqualified. Concerning this law did the men of Asia go up for the three successive festivals to Jabneh, and on the third festival they [= the authorities of Jabneh] declared it valid for them.

(*Tosefta, Parah* 7, 4, Tsukermandel ed., p. 636)[345]

Theses are the valid lawfulness in among cattle... [If] its liver decayed, it is valid. Concerning this law did the men of Asia go up for the three successive festivals to Jabneh, and on the third festival they [= the authorities of Jabneh] declared it valid for them.

(*Tosefta, Hullin* 3, 10, Tsukermandel ed., p. 504)

Said Rabbi Simeon ben Eleazer: 'Rabbi Meir went to Asia to intercalate the year and he did not find there a Scroll of Esther written in Hebrew, so he wrote one out from memory, and then he went and read [= the Scroll of Esther] from it.

(*Tosefta, Megilla* 2, 5, Lieberman ed., p. 349)

And it has been taught that Rabbi Meir was in Asia.

(*Jerusalem Talmud, Megilla* 4, 1 [74d])

Rabbi Meir was dying in Asia. He said: 'Go and tell the people of the Land of Israel, Your Messiah is coming', [= so that they would be sure to bury him in the Land of Israel]. Even so, he said to them, 'Place my bier on the seashore, as it is written, 'For he has founded [= the Land of Israel] upon the seas, and established it upon the rivers' (*Psalms* 24, 2).

(*ibid., Kil'aim* 9, 3 [32c])

Rabbi Meir lay dying in Asia. He said: 'Tell the sons of the Land of Israel that is your Messiah is coming [= home, for burial]'. And even so, he said to them, 'Place my bier at the seashore, for it is written, He has founded it upon the seas, and established it upon the rivers' (*Psalms* 24, 2).

(*ibid., Ketuboth* 12, 3 [35b])

Rabbi Meir once went to intercalate the year in Asia.

(*Babylonian Talmud, Megilla* 18b)

---

[344] Cf. Lieberman (1939b): IV: 16–17; Following Sperber's translation and explanation: (1998): 131; The *castellum* was frequently built on pillars, like a modern water tower, and was situated close to the city walls; Safari (1969: 330) claims that this event definitely proves that it was done in Asia, which is identified with Etzion Gaver since there is no purified water in Asia Minor as it certainly was according to the *halahka* on non-Jewish land.

[345] Cf. Lieberman (1939b): III: 242.

Behold Rabbi Judah declared that Samuel said in the name of Rabban
Simeon ben Gamaliel, 'What means that which is written: Mine eye
affecteth my soul, because of all the daughters of my city?' (*Lamentations*
3, 51). There were a thousand pupils in my father's house; five hundred
studied Torah and five hundred studied Greek wisdom, and of these there
remained only I here and the son of my father's brother in Asia.

(*Babylonian Talmud, Sotah* 49b)[346]

Rabbi Hiyya bar Zarnuki and Rabbi Simeon ben Yehozadak once went
to Asia to intercalate the year.

(*ibid., Sanhedrin* 26a)

The elements that all these sources have in common are: first, Asia
is not a state, but a particular city. Secondly, it is a place in which the
year was intercalated. Thirdly, Asia is not particularly far from the
Land of Israel. Fourthly, it may be that it was a non-Jewish city, but
its inhabitants included both observant Jews and priests who dealt with
purification by sin-offering water. In addition to these criteria, Klein
bases the location of Asia on Eusebius' identification of Etzion Gaver:
'Close to the desert, a stopping-place of the children of Israel, as is
related in the Book of *Numbers*, and in the Book of *Deuteronomy*—the
city of Esau; and it is said that it is today Ασία, near the Dead Sea,
Eilat'.[347] Hieronymus, the translator of Eusebius' *Onomastikon*, writes the
name Asia as Essia: 'quam nunc Essiam nuncupari putant' [= which
they now believe to be called Essia].[348]

It can be deduced from one of the *halakhot* (*Tosafta, Miqvaot* 4, 6) that
Asia (with *alef* or *ayin*) was a city in which its inhabitants and those who
came there to trade found an arrangement for the distribution of water
and baths; according to Klein these were not simply baths, but natural
therapeutic hot water baths. He relies on the *baraitha* to the *Babylonian
Talmud* (*Shabbat* 109a) with which we introduced this discussion. He
maintains, therefore, that there were therapeutic springs close to the
town of Asia, which flowed out of the copper mines in the vicinity of

---

[346] Safari (1969: 330) indicates that there is no decision to which Asia the source
is meant.

[347] Klein (1937): 121; Eusebius *Onomastikon* 62: λέγουσι δὲ ταύτην εἶναι τήν Ασίαν;
See also Klein (1967): 205; Braslavsky (1954): 366; idem, (1965): 452–453; Sperber
(1998): 131; Taylor (2003): 115; cf. Reeg (1989): 52; Tokatzinski (1970): 33; The original place of the inhabitants who were buried at Beth Shearim is fairly documented in
inscription no. 17: ΗΣΙΤΩΝ [= of the inhabitants of Asia (with *ayin*)].

[348] Hieronymus, *Onomastikon* 62; Melamed (1966: 30) translates: 'Etzion Gaver (*Numbers*
33, 35)...it is said that this is עציא nearby the Red Sea and Αϊλα [= Aeila =
Eilat]'.

Etzion Gaver. He adds: 'Everywhere where this metal is to be found it can be assumed that there are also therapeutic springs'.[349]

Neubauer,[350] following Ryland, puts forward the most convincing theory: that Asia should be identified with the town of Essa, east of Lake Kinneret. This city is mentioned by Josephus (*Antiquitates Judaicae* 13.393) in his description of the wars of Alexander Jannaeus east of the Jordan:[351]

> Thereupon Alexander once more marched on the city of Dium and captured it, and then led his army against Essa, where Zenon's most valuable possessions were, and surrounded the place with three walls; and after taking the city without a battle, he set out against Gaulana in the Bashan and Seleucia. After taking these cities as well, he captured in addition the Valley of Antiochus, as it is called, and the fortress of Gamala.

Kohut,[352] Sapir,[353] Hirschberg,[354] and Patai[355] accept Ryland's and Neubauer's hypothesis, that in Essa (with *alef*) = Assa (with *ayin*) = Asia (with *ayin*) there were undoubtedly medicinal hot springs. Hirschberg considers that in that period Essa was a therapeutic site of hot springs, but that in the course of time its sources dried up or were blocked up. He adduces the example of Rabbi Joshua ben Levi, 'went from Lydda to Beth Guvrin because of bathing' (*Jerusalem Talmud, Shevi'it* 8, 11 [38d]), and emphasizes that today no remnant of a spring used for bathing in Beth Guvrin-Eleutheropolis survives.[356] This particular example is erroneous, since a baths complex was uncovered in Beth

---

[349] Klein (1934): 126–127.
[350] Neubauer (1868): 38; Reland (1714): 776.
[351] Zenon was the ruler of nearby Philadelphia; See *Antiquitates Judaicae* 13.325 and *Bellum Judaicum* 1.104; In contrast with the version Ἔσσαν in *Antiquitates Judaicae* 13.393 there is a version in *Bellum Judaicum* 1.104 which bears the word Γερασαν. Accordingly, some scholars tend to emend like as written in *Antiquitates Judaicae* 13.393. Ἔσσα appears in the German translation of Heinrich Klementz, Berlin (1925), but in the Hebrew translation of Schalit (1973: 108)—the name Gerasa [= Γεράσα] is replaced. In Schürer's opinion (1907: II: 179, note 357) Ἔσσα is an error made by the copier and Γαράσα (not Γεράσα) is the preferred one; See also Feldman ed., (1965): 424, note d; Press (1955: IV: 774) comments that due to the other cities mentioned in Alexander Jannaeus's conquest, Essa is located in the Golan and adjacent to Lake Kinneret. Therefore he identifies Asia (with the letter *ayin*) = Ἔσσα with the village Hamma on the eastern shore of Lake Kinneret with its thermo-mineral waters; cf. Mittmann's idea to identify Essa with Hammthan castle (1987: 56–60).
[352] Kohut (1926): VI: 229.
[353] Sapir (1911): 102.
[354] Hirschberg (1920): 225.
[355] Patai (1936): 25.
[356] Hirschberg (1920): 225.

Guvrin lately.[357] Hirschberg points out that there were also hot springs
which had been therapeutic sites but were not described as such in
the Rabbinic literature—for instance, Beth Haram or Beth Haran 'on
the other side of Jordan, east-wards', and later called Ramata (*Tosefta,
Shevi'it* 7, 11), or Beth Ramatha (*Jerusalem Talmud, ibid.*, 9, 2 [38d]). Beth
Ramatha (Βηθαραμφθᾶ) was later renamed Livias (Λιβιάς) in honour
of the wife of Augustus.[358] Close to the city were hot springs and date
groves, according to the reports of Petrus of Iberia of the fifth century
CE and Antoninus of Placentia of the sixth century CE.[359]

4.8   EMMAUS-NICOPOLIS

There were hot springs in several places in Palestine known as Emmaus.
The name was derived from the Hebrew Hammat, Aramaic Ham-
mata or Hammat, transliterated into Greek as Ἀμμαοῦς or Ἐμμαοῦς,
and Latin as Ammaus or Emmaus. As has been mentioned, Josephus
himself interpreted the word Emmaus as 'hot baths', and wrote of
Ἐμμαοῦς of Tiberias, or Ἀμμαθοῦς of Tiberias.[360] Apparently at a later
date other sites of cold therapeutic springs were also called Emmaus;
so this widespread name is of no help in determining whether there
were hot springs at a particular site.[361] The evidence of the fourth
century author Ammianus Marcellinus illustrates this point. He says
that in Mesopotamia a single place in which there are springs is called
in Syriac both *Maia Kariri* and Emmaus.[362]

The city of Emmaus is situated on the edge of the coastal plain,
at the foot of the mountains of Judaea, on the route from Jerusalem

---

[357] Cohen (2002): 187–194.

[358] Hirschberg (1920): 225.

[359] Petrus of Iberia 81; Antonius of Placentia, *Itinerarium* 10; Klein (1925): 65; Abel
(1933): I: 459; Avi-Yonah (1984): 166; Schürer (1991): II: 171–172; See also the discussions in this chapter and on *The Healing Properties of the Spas in the Eastern Mediterranean
in Ancient Times* in chapter 5.

[360] Josephus, *Bellum Judaicum* 4.11; idem, *Antiquitates Judaicae* 18.36; See, for instance,
Grätz (1853): 112; Neubauer (1868): 100; Krauss (1899): 58–59; Taylor (2003): 53,
109, 128: Ἐμμαοῦς (in Greek) and Emmaus (in Latin); See the extensive discussion in
chapter 1.4 on *Terminology*.

[361] Hirschberg (1920): 224.

[362] Ammianus Marcellinus, *Res Gestae* 18.6.16; Rolfe notes in his translation (1963:
443, note 2) that the original name is Emmaus; See also Rapoport (1857): 111; Horowitz
(1923): 51, note 1; Dvorjetski (1992a): 81, 115, note 225.

to the sea. (See Map 1).[363] The historical survey of Emmaus which appears below reveals an intriguing phenomenon: the name of the spot was Emmaus at a period when it had only cold therapeutic springs, or perhaps only one spring with therapeutic characteristics, and no hot springs at all. Towards the end of the Byzantine period certain Greek authors called the site Ἐμμαοῦς πηγὴ. Greek and Roman authors used a more or less standard formula to describe other sites in Palestine in which there were therapeutic springs, such as Tiberias and Hammat-Gader, since such springs were a dominant and inseparable part of these districts and their chief cities. Thus, for instance, we find τὰ τῶν ὑδάτων θερμῶν λουτρὰ (the baths of hot water), or θερμῶν ὑδατῶν θερμὰ λουτρὰ (the hot baths of hot water), or τὰ θερμὰ ὑδάτα (the hot waters), or an expression which clearly and unambiguously points up the connection between one or more specific springs and hot water: θερμῶν ὑδάτων πηγαί (springs of hot water).[364]

By contrast, although the various references in the Talmudic literature to Emmaus indicate that both in its natural characteristics and in the daily life of its people it was strikingly similar to the better known therapeutic sites of Tiberias and Hammat-Gader, Emmaus was known primarily as a 'beautiful spot' with 'lovely and pleasant waters', referring to its public bathhouse, the *demosin*, a name which became a synonym for the original name of Emmaus (*Avot de Rabbi Nathan*, Version A, 14, Schechter ed. p. 59). Certain well-known events took place in the *demosin* of Tiberias. In Emmaus, too, there is mention of a pleasure-seeking and profligate way of life, which was exemplified in the matter of those disqualified to marry, in the butcher's shop within its bounds which was associated with idol-worship, in the special sorts of food which were eaten there, and, in addition, in the presence of Roman soldiers who apparently lived there and were an important factor in the development of the town, just as in similar sites throughout the Roman Empire which we have discussed above.[365]

---

[363] Thomsen (1907): 21; Sapir (1911): 100; Horowitz (1923): 51–52; Beyer (1933): 218–246; Abel (1938): II: 314–316; Avi-Yonah (1936): 155; Press (1948): I: 23; Avi-Yonah (1976): 55; idem, (1984): 105–106; Schürer (1991): I: 512–513; Lemaire (1975: 15–23) suggests that the name Emmaus is a late version for the name 'Mamst', which appears on the handles of the 'king jars', dated to the seventh-eighth centuries BCE, and are abundant in Judaea.

[364] See the discussion below and in chapter 1.4 on the *Terminology*; See also Dvorjetski (1992a): 115; idem, (1999): 122.

[365] See the discussions below and in chapter 6.2 on *The Sages at the Therapeutic Sites—Aims and Deeds.*

Close to Emmaus there were what the geologist Avnimelech describes as 'hot sediments';[366] and, as we have shown, hot springs are side effects of the activity of extinct volcanoes. In the course of our survey of the history of the Emmaus baths we shall try to explain why no trace of hot springs has ever been discovered there, and why this site is different from all the therapeutic baths of the Levant.

The history of Emmaus-Nicopolis is inseparably connected with its position on the edge of the Ayalon Valley, at the border between the plain and the mountains. On the east it is closed in by the steep wooded slopes of the Judaean hills, which emphasize its position as the final station on the way from the mountain passes on the way to Jerusalem, while to its west there stretches a broad level plain. In addition, there was another important factor which afforded it the status of a centre of pilgrimage, not only for the Christian world: the healing properties of its waters.

Until the Hasmonean revolt there apparently existed at this location a small, unimportant Jewish village, whose original Hebrew name was Hammat; it was also called Hammat of Judaea (*Midrash Aggadah to Song of Songs* 6, 9, Schechter ed., p. 41) in order to distinguish it from other places in Palestine with the name Hammat. According to ancient historical sources this name was generally given to settlements close to hot springs. In this case, however, there are clear indications that the name Hamma in Hebrew, Hammatha or Hammtha in Aramaic, Emmaus—Ἐμμαοῦς or Ἀμμαθοῦς in Greek—was given to a settlement close to springs which had therapeutic properties but were not hot.[367] The strategic importance of Emmaus is expressed in its earliest mentions in our sources, in *Maccabees I*, 3, 40, 57; 4, 3: the Seleucid army camped there during its third campaign against Judas Maccabaeus; they were defeated and their camp was captured. The battle of Emmaus (161 BCE), in which Judas exploited his topographical advantage to defeat the Seleucid king, proved to the authorities that this was a site of strategic importance, and a few years later Bacchides, the representative of the regime in Judaea, fortified the town (*Maccabees I*, 9, 50–51). Josephus also tells of this in his *Antiquitates Judaicae* (13.15–16).

---

[366] Avnimelech (1935): 59–63; See the discussion in chapter 2 on *Geological, Hydrological and Medicinal Aspects of Hot springs in the Eastern Mediterranean—Past and Present.*

[367] See the discussions below and in chapter 1.4 on *Terminology*; See Grätz (1853): 112; Neubauer (1868): 100; Krauss (1899): 58–59; Klein (1915): 157–158; Hirschfeld (1988): 9; Levine (1984): 168.

The region of Judaea was encircled by fortresses of the Hellenistic army: the northern border was closed in by the fortresses of Jericho, Beit Horon and Emmaus, a royal castle in Gezer barred the way to the west, and there was a similar castle in Beit Tzur, on the southern border of Judaea. The Hellenistic fortress of Emmaus has been located at Hirbet 'Eqed, east of Emmaus, a place which commands the surrounding country. The results of recent excavations have underlined the strength of the fortress. The location of the castle, close to the civilian settlement of Emmaus, brought development and prosperity to the town. Towards the end of the first century BCE Emmaus surpassed Gezer, and it is mentioned as being a big city. This is clear from the activities of Gaius Cassius, one of the conspirators against Julius Caesar, in Judaea. He came to Judaea in order to organize his forces against Caesar's successors, and for this purpose levied a heavy tax on its various regions. When his demands were not acceded to he took vengeance on the towns of Judaea, including Emmaus.[368] In the list of the *toparchies* of Judaea in the time of Herod Emmaus is listed as a regional capital (*Bellum Judaicum* 3.55). Pliny the Elder describes it as the capital of a *toparchy*, and says that it was close to Lydda-Diospolis.[369] Varus, the Roman legate in Syria, also punished the town by setting fire to it in the year 4 BCE, since it was a centre of the revolt against Herod's dynasty and the Roman army (*ibid.*, 2.71).[370]

It appears that the tragic event of the destruction of the city and the flight of its Jewish inhabitants was a significant turning-point in the life of the city. Samaritans and pagans replaced the Jewish population. From the sources quoted below it is apparent that the town lost its Jewish character, and the Jews constituted a minority of the population.

At the beginning of the Great Revolt against the Romans, Emmaus surrendered to Vespasian, as did the other non-Jewish towns in the region—Antipatris, Lydda and Jabneh. Stationing a unit of the Roman army, the Legion V *Macedonia*, in Emmaus, was one of the operations intended to cut off rebel Judaea in preparation for Vespasian's

---

[368] Avi-Yonah (1962): III: 847; Hirschfeld (1976): 3; Stern (1981): 171–173; Hirschfeld (1988): 13–14; Bar-Kochva (1980): 184–185; Kasher (1988a): 60–61; For the unconsistent usage of the site in Josephus, see the difference spelling between Ἐμμαοῦς (*Bellum Judaicum* 1.222) and Ἀμμαοῦς (*Antiquitates Judaicae* 14.275).

[369] Pliny, *Naturalis Historia* 5.14.70; See Stern (1974): I: 476; Schwartz (1990): 56; Alon (1996): 145; Later on the *toparchy* was Nicopolis territory. See Beyer (1933): 242–243.

[370] Stern (1983a): 86–90; idem, (1983b): 181; Horowitz (1923): 51.

advance on Jerusalem (*Bellum Judaicum* 4.444–445). A number of inscriptions and gravestones of soldiers belonging to this legion, as well as
to the Legion X *Fretensis*, have been found in the area. They generally
bear the name of the soldier, his rank, his place of origin, his unit, his
age, and his years of service. A statue of an eagle from the Roman
period also attests to the presence of the Roman army in the area.
Emmaus was integrated into the network of roads which the Romans
began to construct from the year 70 CE or since the days of Emperor
Hadrian onwards. There are traces of the presence of the Roman army
in the area in the Rabbinic literature and likewise afflictions and persecutions of the Jews after the defeat of the Great Revolt (*Lamentations Rabbah*
1, 16; *Mekhilta de Rabbi Ishmael, Masechta behodesh*, 1, Horovitz-Rabin ed.,
pp. 203–204). Apparently corvees were also employed for the erection
of bathhouses for the use of Roman soldiers and officials.[371]

Documentary and archaeological evidence both attest to the recovery of the Jewish community in Emmaus after the destruction of the
Temple, and the inhabitants' feeling of securiety under the Roman
regime. In the Rabbinic and Christian literature Emmaus is described
as a flourishing and dynamic town.

Emmaus was chiefly known as a 'beautiful place' with 'beautiful and
delightful waters'. This view was based mainly on its public bathhouse,
which also served as a popular place of entertainment.[372] There are
various versions of the story of Rabbi Eleazar ben Arakh, one of the
outstanding disciples of Rabban Yohanan ben Zakkai, who left his
Rabbi and went to Emmaus, where 'his reputation as a Torah scholar
diminished', and it was even said that 'his learning was uprooted'. This
deed, which as has been remarked, is described in many ways in the
Rabbinic literature, repeatedly demonstrates the dangers inherent in
visiting therapeutic sites, particularly for the sake of engaging in the
frivolous occupations of this world and the pursuit of pleasure.[373] It

---

[371] Vincent and Abel (1932): 316–355; Bar-Kochva (1980): 188: Hirschfeld (1988):
13–14; Avi-Yonah (1993): II: 385; Schürer (1991): I: 512–513; Issac (2000): 428–429;
See also Michon (1898): 269–271; Landau (1976): 89–91; Fischer (1989): 187; 70 CE
is Roll's own opinion (1976): 41–42; cf. Avi-Yonah (1950–1951): 54–60; Issac (1978):
49; For the military presence, see Klein (1915): 158; Lieberman (1932b): 454–455;
Alon (1967): I: 42; Büchler (1967): 147; Shatzman (1983): 26; Keppie (1986): 420;
Oppenheimer (1991): 40, 94–95; Fischer, Issac and Roll (1996): 327–328.

[372] Hirschberg (1920): 224; Hirschfeld (1988): 14–15; idem, (1976): 4; Schwartz
(1986): 120; On the water supply system of the city, see Hirschfeld (1978): 86–92;
idem, (2002): 187–198.

[373] For the various versions of Rabbi Eleazar ben Arakh leaving for Emmaus, see

is important to note that in some versions of this literature the term *demosin* became a synonym for the name Emmaus; for example, 'The reputation as a Torah scholar of him who went to *demusit*, to a beautiful place with beautiful waters, was diminished' (*Avot de Rabbi Nathan*, Version A, 14, Schechter ed., p. 59). The term *demosin or demusit* is a corruption of the Greek word δημόσιον, which is apparently a shortened version of the expression δημόσιον λουτρόν, or δημόσιον βαλανεῖον, which is also used to describe the baths of Tiberias. It means 'public baths', or, more exactly, 'public therapeutic baths'.[374] It is related of Rabban Yohanan ben Zakkai, who went to Emmaus and cured there his bulimia (*Ecclesiastes Babbah* 7, 11).[375]

Emmaus had a rich agricultural hinterland and was close to commercial routes, and its markets were famous. This can be deduced from the words of Rabbi Akiva, who met Rabban Gamaliel and Rabbi Joshua in 'the *itliz* of Emmaus' when they went there to buy a cow for the wedding feast of the son of Judah the Patriarch (*Mishnah, Kritut* 3, 7; *Babylonian Talmud, ibid.*, 15a; *ibid., Makkot* 14a; *ibid., Hullin* 91b). The original meaning of the word *itliz* was a fair, and its connotation in Greek is exemption from tax. It is known that there was a special combination of a market and an amusement centre in Hammat-Gader. This quarter was an important spa, well known in the East, and in the open period for bathing, which was relatively short, a fair was held there. In any case, our informant, the Church Father Epiphanius, indicates that the fair took place once every year, since people came to bathe at the site.[376] We cannot know for certain whether the *itliz* was a purely Jewish market, but Safrai claims that the impression given by the sources is that it was not a non-Jewish pagan affair, like the fair (*yarid*). Moreover, he emphasizes, there is no unambiguous evidence as to whether the

---

Babylonian Talmud, Shabbat 147b; *Midrash Ecclesiastes Babbah* 7, 7 (His visit was accomplished after Rabban Yohanan ben Zakkai's death); *Avot de Rabbi Nathan*, Version A, 14, Schechter ed., p. 59 (According to the Oxford manuscript the version is 'Maus'); *ibid.*, Version B, 29 (Schechter ed., p. 59); See also Finkelstein (1950): 187; Goldin (1955): 77–78; Alon (1967): I: 63; Urbach (1953): 63–64; Herr (1982): 334; Dvorjetski (1992a): 85; Goshen-Gottstein (1993): 186; See chapter 6.2 on *The Sages at the Therapeutic Sites—Aims and Deeds.*

[374] Horowitz (1923): 53; Gichon (1979): 102; idem, (1986–1987): 55; idem, (1993): II: 387; Bar-Kochva (1980): 185; Krauss (1929): I/1: 73) notes that *demosit* means a bath and Emmaus = Hammtha = hot water.

[375] Rosner (2000): 43; Dvorjetski (1992a): 84, 118, 141–142; On the Bulimia, see in chapter 5 on *The Healing Properties of the Spas in the Eastern Mediterranean in Ancient Times.*

[376] Epiphanius, *Panarion, Adversus Haereses* 416–417.

Palestinian *itliz* was clearly connected to idol worship.[377] But it is impossible to ignore the evidence of a connection between idol worship and the *itliz*, as attested by a number of texts: 'The place of the *itlin* is a place of their idol worship' (*Mekhilta de Rabbi Ishmael, Beshalach*, 1, Horovitz-Rabin ed., p. 83), or the hint that the *itliz* was a place of sexual profligacy: 'Rabbi Abba bar Kahana said: "*Pathruthim* and *Casluhim* set up bazaars where they stole [= interchanged] each other's wives"' (*Genesis Rabbah* 37, 5, Theodor and Albek ed., p. 348). The *Mishnah, Arachin* 2, 4, provides more evidence of this, since the families of Emmaus, *Beit Hapegarim* and *Beit Sepphoriya*, were consider unfit for marriage by reason of their place of domicile, unless there was evidence that they were legitimate. Hirschberg deduces from this text that the profligacy and dissipation at the therapeutic sites 'impaired the purity of family and race among the Jews, and their inhabitants were considered unfit for marriage'.[378] It appears that at Emmaus where visible evidences of the practice of Graeco-Roman religion have survived there.[379]

The history of Emmaus constantly underlines its strategic importance. The improvement of the network of Roman roads, which was executed for military and administrative reasons, made an important contribution to the rapidity of urbanization and to the commercial, economic and municipal prosperity of the town, both in the later Roman period and, even more, in the Byzantine period.

Evidence of the presence of rebels in the region of Emmaus at the time of the revolt of Bar Kochba has been found in a cave on the heights of Hirbet 'Eqed. It includes pottery shards and four coins. A 15 metre long tunnel has also been discovered, leading to a large plastered water tank. Hirschfeld notes that the layout and the findings indicate a smaller version of the concealed caves found near Ein Arub, and the many secret caves found in the vicinity of Beth Guvrin. He adds that it is not clear whether this cave, which is about 2.5 kilometres from the town of Emmaus, was prepared specially in view of the coming revolt by the Jews of Emmaus.[380] The names of the key sites on the

---

[377] Safrai (1984): 143, 155; See also Klein (1910c): 106; Lieberman (1959): 75–78; Dvorjetski (1992a): 86, 118, 160, 169–170; For the term *itliz* see the discussion in chapter 6.2 on *The Sages at the Therapeutic Sites—Aims and Deeds.*

[378] Hirschberg (1920): 236.

[379] Goshen-Gottstein (1993): 186, note 59; Alon (1996): 645; See the discussion in chapter 6 on *Daily Life at the Thermo-Mineral Baths according to the Rabbinic Literature.*

[380] Hirschfeld (1988): 16; See also Gichon (1982): 35–42; Kloner (1982): 16–20; Kloner and Tepper (1987): 242.

road to Jerusalem on which the Romans set up check-points show that Emmaus was one of the foci of the fighting, and Hadrian set up a guardpost there in order to trap those who wished to join the war: 'Hadrian...positioned three guard forces, one at Hammtha and one at Kefar Lekitia and one at Beit el D'Yahud. He said: who ever escapes from here, will be caught from there, and whoever escapes from there, will be caught from here' (*Midrash Lamentations Rabbah* 1, 45).[381]

It should be pointed out that it was not only the small Jewish community which had existed in Emmaus from before the Bar Kochba revolt that continued to live there; its location, between Judaea and the Samaritan region, influenced its character, and a Samaritan community, which in time turned into a majority, grew up alongside the Jewish one. We may, therefore, surmise that these hiding-places served the Samaritans as well as the Jews of the area. Incidental remarks about local customs indicate the Samaritan character of Emmaus. Various Sages, including the southerner Rabbi Aha, are said to have visited the town and eaten different sorts of Samaritan food there (*Jerusalem Talmud, Avoda Zarah* 5, 4 [44d]).[382] The Samaritan inscriptions found in the site show that the majority of its inhabitants were Samaritans.[383] Further, according to Kutscher the changes of the name, which began as Hammat and evolved into the Arabic ʿImwās (initial *ayin*), show a shift from *chet* to *ayin* which took place as the result of the linguistic influence of the Samaritans.[384] There is, however, evidence of the existence of a small Jewish community in the town until the end of the Byzantine period.[385]

---

[381] Oppenheimer (1991): 40; idem, (1982b): 25–26, note 4; In *Midrash Lamentations Rabbah*, 1, 392, according to the Romi manuscript, the version differs: 'Hadrian... positioned three guard forces, one at Hammat-Gader, and one at Bethlehem and one at Kefar Lekitia'; See the discussion in chapter 7.2 on *Hadrian*; For other identifications, see Mor (1991): 165–166.

[382] For the Samaritans' participation in the Bar Kochba revolt, see Alon (1971): II: 24–26; Büchler (1980): 115–121; Mor (2003: 172–183) remarks that the Samaritans did not fight on the Jews' side, but separately in their own region; For the local Samaritan food at Emmaus, see Schwartz (1982): 188; Dvorjetski (1992a): 86, 119, 172.

[383] Ben Zvi (1976): 82–183; Safrai (1977): 107; Schwartz (1982): 188; idem, (1986): 121; Hüttenmeister and Reeg (1977): II: 603–609; Dvorjetski (1992a): 119; Avi-Yonah (1993): II: 386; Alon (1996): 742–746; The monk Joannes Moschus (*Pratum Spirituale* 3032), of the end of the sixth and the beginning of the seventh century CE, tells of a band of robbers, who attacked families who lived in Nicopolis—Christians, Samaritans and Jews—on their return from Jerusalem, where they had celebrated the Easter festival.

[384] Kutscher (1976): 93–96.

[385] Klein (1920): no. 116; Sukenik (1935a): 32–39; Klein (1939): 46, 80, no. 5; Naveh (1978): 59; Schwartz (1982): 188; Dvorjetski (1992a): 86–87, 119.

According to the Church Father Eusebius, there was a severe earthquake in 131 CE, which destroyed the town, but nothing about a
therapeutic spring there.[386] At the beginning of the third century, in
223 CE, as part of the process of urbanization which took place at the
time, Emmaus was granted the full rights of a town and was renamed
Nicopolis.[387] In a work entitled *Chronicon Paschale*, an anonymous writer
of the seventh century CE, writes that the city was rebuilt in 223 CE,
thanks to the efforts and prayers of the historian Julius Africanus, who
was appointed governor of Emmaus and travelled on a mission to the
Emperor Elagabal to receive his permission for the rebuilding of the
city, which was thereafter known as Nicopolis.[388]

As a result of its elevation to the status of a Roman city Nicopolis
was granted certain municipal rights: administration of an area equivalent to that of the former toparchy; partial exemption from taxes; the
right to mint coins; and the Roman name Nicopolis (Νικόπολις, the
city of victory)—that is to say, the victory of Rome over Judaea—which
was added to its former name.[389] Sozomenus and Nicephorus Klistos
state that the new name was given immediately after the conquest of
Jerusalem, in memory of the Roman victory over the Jews.[390] According to Meshorer, the town struck coins for the first time in the reign
of the Emperor Lucius Verus (161 CE); they bore the figure of Zeus
seated and holding by the hand a small figure of Nike, the goddess of
victory, who is presenting him with a wreath.[391] We may assume that
its municipal rights were expanded mainly during the reign of the
Emperor Elagabal; and, indeed, in 219 CE three types of coin were
struck. The town's rights also included the additional territory which
it had been granted; and we may now understand why a therapeutic
spring frequently appears from now on in the historical, particularly
the Christian, sources.

---

[386] Eusebius, *Chronicorum Libri Duo* 2237; See also Guerin (1982): 198.

[387] Cassiodorus Aurelius, *Chronicon* 1236; See also Bazzocchini (1905): 38; Guérin
(1982): 198.

[388] *Chronicon Paschale* 657; See also Guérin (1982): 198; Hieronymus (*De Viris Illustribus* 673) corroborates these details; See also Guérin (1982): 198; Wallack-Samuels,
Rynearson and Meshorer (2000): 115.

[389] Jones (1931): 82; Hirschfeld (1988): 17.

[390] Sozomenus, *Historia Ecclesiastica* 1280; Walford (1855): 239; Nicephorus Klistos,
Historia Ecclesiastica 536.

[391] Meshorer (1985): 56; There is no mention of this numismatic evidence in the
historical sources; See also Hirschfeld (1988): 30; Schürer (1991: I: 512, note 142)
remarks that the coins seem to show that the name 'Nicopolis' was in use in 70–221
CE; de Saulcy (1874): 172–175, 406.

From the entry 'Emmaus' in the *Onomastikon* of Eusebius it appears that the status of Emmaus-Nicopolis was confirmed during the Byzantine period:[392]

> Emmaus (*Luke* 24,13). Whence came Cleopas in [= who came out] Luke's Gospel. The same is now Nikopolis, a famous city of Palestine.

Emmaus is mentioned in the New Testament as the place where Jesus appeared to his disciples after his crucifixion. There, it is said that two men, Cleopas and his friend, went from Jerusalem to the village of Ἐμμαοῦς three days after the crucifixion,[393] speaking of the crucifixion and resurrection of Jesus. Jesus joined the two, who did not recognize him, and asked them what they were discussing. They told him of the crucifixion and of the women who came to the tomb and found it empty. Jesus explained the words of the prophets, saying 'Ought not the saviour to have suffered these things, and to enter into his glory?' When Cleopas and his friend drew near the village, they asked Jesus to come to their house. He did so, and when they ate he broke the bread and blessed it. They then recognized him, but he vanished from their sight. (*Luke* 24, 13–35). In the version of this story which is accepted today in the Christian world Emmaus was 'about sixty furlongs (*stadia*) from Jerusalem'—some 11 kilometres.[394] The Greek manuscripts Codex Vindobonensis, Codex Cyprius and Codex Sinaiticus, which is the oldest and most reliable, state that the distance was 160 *stadia*. It has been conjectured that this difference stems from the visit of the third century CE Christian commentator Origenes, who visited Emmaus-Nicopolis and, when he realized that it was more than sixty *stadia* from Jerusalem, corrected the manuscripts of the New Testament accordingly.[395]

Apparently traditions about Jesus, that after his death he met two of his disciples in Emmaus, drew Christians to the place. It is doubtful, however, if this is the Emmaus mentioned in the Gospel according to *Luke* 24, 13–35.[396] Many Christian sources mentioned traditions about

---

[392] Eusebius, *Onomastikon* 90; Taylor (2003): 53; The revisor Melamed (1966: 44) adds 'from that day 'Imwās near Latrun'.

[393] Re'emi (1974): III: 474; See also Dalman (1935): 228–231; Safrai (1965): 116.

[394] *Stadia* is 184.36 metres.

[395] Manor (1979): 21–22.

[396] According to widely accepted opinion, Emmaus, the site of Christ's appearance before two of his disciples after his resurrection, has been identified during the Crusader period with three different locations: ʿAmwās, in the foothills of the mountains of Judaea; el-Qubēbe, ca. 15 kilometres to the north-west of Jerusalem; and Abū Ġōš, ca. 15 kilometres to the west of Jerusalem. Churches were erected at all three sites

Jesus in connection with Emmaus-Nicopolis, and it appears that many Christians were influenced by these contentions. The fact is that its former status was now accompanied by another factor—the place had become a focus of pilgrimage in the Christian world.

It seems that Hieronymus accepted Eusebius' opinion, which identifies Emmaus in the Gospels with the important city that in his day was called Nicopolis. Indeed, this Church Father left behind more detailed testimony on this subject in the eulogy he delivered for one of his apprentices, Paula, who had founded the nunnery in Bethlehem: 'She came to Nicopolis, which had previously been called Emmaus and in which our Lord is recognized as having broken bread, and therefore the house of Cleopas was turned into a church. From there, she continued on her way and climbed up to Lower and Upper Beit Horon'.[397]

Sozomenus, the fifth century CE Christian historian, brings testimony of great value to clarify why Emmaous-Nicopolis became a famous city in Palestine:[398]

> There is a city in Palestine now called Nicopolis. The holy Gospels mention a village (because that is what it was then) by the name of Emmaus. However, the Romans, who controlled Jerusalem and had been victorious over the Jews, called this settlement Nicopolis to commemorate their great victory. In front of this city, close to an intersection of three roads—there was the place where Jesus walked in the company of Cleopas and his retinue after his resurrection. There is the spring of Jesus, whose waters give a cure not only to the illnesses of people who bathe in it, but also to various animal diseases. They say that when the Messiah stayed with his disciples, he deviated from the path one day to wash his feet in this spring, and from then on its waters had a special quality of removing all types of illnesses and suffering from humans and animals.

Theophanes, a ninth century CE monk and chronicler, also makes mention of the well-known spring in Emmaus-Nicopolis for all kinds

---

during the 12th century; See Vincent and Abel (1932): 5–67, 356–371; Bagatti (1947): 1–3, 47–48; de Vaux and Steve (1950): 92–96; Figueras (1978): 132–134; de Sandoli (1980); Pringle (1993): I: 7–17; Ehrlich (1996): 165–169; Another site called Ἀμμαοῦς by Josephus (*Bellum Judaicum* 7.217) was Motza (Qolonia) 5–6 kilometres from Jerusalem. It was identified with the veteran settlement established by Vespasian after the Jewish war; See Issac (2000): 428; Dvorjetski (1992a): 89–92; Press (1948): I: 24, (1955): IV: 825; Bazzocchini (1905): 32–33.

[397] Hieronymus, *Paulae et Eustochii ad Marcellam, Epistola* XLVI (A), 883; For the archaeological remains of the church and the cartographical evidence, see the discussion below.

[398] Sozomenus, *Historia Ecclesiastica* 5.21; Walford (1855): 239; Bidez and Hanson (1960): 228–229; See also Vincent and Abel (1932): 414; Dvorjetski (1992a): 121–122.

of illnesses of human beings and animals. 'It is told that the divine Messiah washed his feet in it at the end of his travels'. He adds that the Emperor Julian the Apostate ordered the spring to be blocked because of the wonders that were associated with it, including the wonders of healing that were generated in it.[399]

Dechent states that Sozomenus' information that other creatures, too, besides human beings, were cured of various illnesses, and Theophanes' statement, which expanded talk on the subject in regard to the use of the waters, too, for the needs of animals in Emmaus-Nicopolis, do not have to surprise us. In his view, healing waters of the spring were frequently used for such purposes; by way of example, he points to Sipuntium, a spring in Italy used for similar needs.[400]

Despite the damming of the spring, its location was well known in the years that followed, for its existence in Emmaus-Nicopolis is mentioned in the journey of the monk Saint Willibald, who visited the Holy Land in the eighth century CE. The story of his travels were anonymously publicized in the ninth century CE:[401]

> He [= Willibald] came to Emmaous, a village in Palestine that the Romans called by the name of Nicopolis after their victory and after the destruction of Jerusalem. There, in the house of Cleopas, which now became a church, they glorified him, he who had broken bread in this house; and when he desired a well of living water, he saw a spring on the main road, where he went with two of hid disciples, Luke and Cleopas, after his resurrection. This is the spring in which when the Messiah was alive, he washed his legs after his journey; from that time one, those waters were made effective by God for various ways of healing; and when they are drunk, they instill health and prevent illnesses both of human beings and of animals.

Cedrenus, too, reports in his *Historiarum Compendium* on the spring of Emmaus-Nicopolis in 1057. He also mentions, as did his predecessors, that the spring provides a cure for sicknesses, and that the Emperor Julian dammed it because of the wonders that it was said to produce:[402]

---

[399] Theophanes, *Chronographia* 5854; Vincent and Abel (1932): 414; Dvorjetski (1992a): 122; For Emperor Julian's deed, see Reland (1714): 759–760; Abel (1938): II: 315; Horowitz (1923): 52.

[400] Dechent (1884): 209–211.

[401] Willibald, *Itinera Hierosolymitana* 293; Vincent and Abel (1932): 419; Dvorjetski (1992a): 123.

[402] Cedrenus, *Historiarum Compendium* 582; See also Vincent and Abel (1932): 416; Dvorjetski (1992a): 123.

In Nicopolis in Palestine, in Emmaus, there is a spring that heals all
kinds of suffering of humans and animals. They relate that our divine
Lord washed his feet at the conclusion of his travels...and he [= Julian]
dammed up the spring after he had become jealous of it, and the tree
fell.

Like him, Michael the Syrian, twelfth century Patriarch of the Jacobites
of Antioch, also relates the story, again mentioning the other name of
the city, Nicopolis.[403] The last documentation in regard to the spring
with the special healing qualities is brought by Nicephorus Klistos in
1320.[404] In his description of the essentials, which were already known
in Christian writings, he is very much influenced by Sozomenus. He
does not, however, state anything in regard to the action of the Emperor
Julian against the 'spring of salvation' in Emmaus-Nicopolis, not even
the reasons motivating the emperor to do so.

The special qualities of the waters of Emmaus, as presented above,
are clearly legendary in every way. Apparently this assumption is somewhat invalidated because of the epigraphic find of a magic charm,
whose content and illustrations are fascinating, that was discovered
inside an Emmaus grave in 1896. It is a Jewish-Aramaic charm, dating
to the third century CE. It was made, in Vincent's opinion, by a Jewish
artisan at the request of a Christian.[405] (See Fig. 28).

Cartographic evidence from the Byzantine period sheds some light
on the strategic importance and status of Emmaus-Nicopolis. In the
Peutinger map, which charts the roads of the Roman Empire, and
dates from the fourth century CE, Emmaus appears under its original
name, corrupted by the transliteration to Latin: Amavente. Emmaus-
Amavente also appears on the map between Gophna, on the height
of the mountain, and Lod, in the plain. The distances ascribed to the
various routes—19 miles from Gophana to Emmaus, and 12 miles from
Emmaus to Lydda—correspond to the distances Jerusalem-Emmaus-
Lydda.[406] In the Madaba map, of the sixth century CE, Emmaus
appears under its new name: Νικόπολις (Nicopolis). Avi-Yonah finds it

---

[403] Michael the Syrian, *Chronique* 187; See also Vincent and Abel (1932): 416;
Dvorjetski (1992a): 123.
[404] Nicephorus Klistos, *Historia Ecclesiastica* 10.31; See also Vincent and Abel (1932):
Bazzocchini (1905): 36; Dvorjetski (1992a): 124.
[405] Vincent (1908): 382–394; See also Goodenough (1958): 71–80; idem, (1964):
X: 154; Naveh and Shaked (1985): 60–63; Vilnaey (1976): I: 210; See the discussions
in chapter 5 on *The Healing Properties of the Spas* and in chapter 9.3.1 on *The Thermal
Baths of Emmaus-Nicopolis*.
[406] Finkelstein (1978): 71–79; idem, (1979): 27–34.

strange that the map-maker completely ignored the former name, and did not identify Nicopolis as the Emmaus which appears in *Luke* 24, 13 even though this identification was to be found in the *Onomastikon*.[407] In the portrayal of the town a Greek basilica with triangular pediment and domed apse appears. The prominence given to the city of Emmaus-Nicopolis is evidence of its importance as a station on the pilgrim route to Jerusalem and its environs. Nicopolis appears on the border of a sixth century mosaic floor of a church in Ma'in, which is the Moabite settlement Baalmaon. Since this is one of the cities in Palestine and Trans-Jordan with churches, the church is portrayed as having a pediment and a dome—the symbol of the city of Nicopolis.[408]

Remains of the church found at Emmaus, called el-Kenisah, attracted the attention of explorers as early as 1875. The main work, however, was carried out by the Dominican Fathers, Vincent and Abel.[409] The excavators distinguished the remains of five structures: recesses hewn out of the rock and foundations of walls. They assigned to the second and first centuries BCE; Remains of a Roman villa (18 × 17 metres), dated to the second century CE. The mosaic pavement was composed of a pattern of circles and octagons combing into squares and lozenges filled with various kinds of guilloche motifs; A Christian basilica (46.4 × 24.4 metres) dated to the third century CE, was divided into a nave and two aisles by two rows of thirteen columns each; A basilica (18 × 10 metres) with two rows of six columns each, and behind it a baptistery supported by four columns; And a twelfth century Crusader church built in the prevailing Romansque style.[410]

In the course of the many archeological excavations that took place at the site over the years, researchers attempted to establish the essential of Ἐμμαοῦς πηγή, more precisely πηγή σωτήριος [= the spring of salvation]. Gichon stresses that the excavations conducted by him at Emmaus 'did not reveal an explanation of the hot water that is thought to have burst forth there from deep underground in those days

---

[407] Avi-Yonah (1954): 64, Pl. VII; See also Monteagudo (1999): 256; Duval (1999): 139–140.

[408] De Vaux (1938): 227–258, Pl. XII; Tsafrir (1984): 423, 425; Vilnaey (1976): I: 84, 807.

[409] Vincent and Abel (1932); See also Guillemot (1882): 103–106; Vincent (1936): 403–415; idem, (1948): 348–375; Ovadiah and Gomez-de Silva (1982): 122.

[410] Avi-Yonah (1993): I: 385–387; Crowfoot (1941: 71, 125, 145) observed that the dates suggested by the excavators were unacceptable.

and that imparted its name to the place'.[411] Nevertheless, a bathhouse discovered at the site consists of a series of adjoining rooms arranged in a row. (See Figs. 29 and 30). The visitor progressed through the *caldarium, tepidarium,* and *frigidarium* along a straight line. The courtyard and *apodyterium* were destroyed in one of the many earthquakes that wreaked havoc on the area recorded in 498, 502, and 507 CE. In fact, the original bathhouse, apparently built in the third century CE, was damaged during an earthquake and rebuilt along smaller lines with some of the rooms taking on new or different functions. For example, the original *tepidarium* became the *caldarium.* It is possible that there was also an additional room that served as an *unctorium,* or oiling room, or *sudatorium,* or sweating room.[412] The fourth room in the row of rooms appears, in Hirschfeld's opinion, as a later addition to the original bathhouse. He speculates from similar parallels of Roman bathhouses in the region of Syria, that this was an original bathing room. The closest example apparently is the bathhouse in Barad in northern Syria, which is dated to the second or beginning of the third century CE. Its plan is almost identical to that of Emmaus both in style and in building technique: massive hewn stone, vaulted walls system, semi-cupolas, and others. The building of the bathhouse in Emmaus according to a model imported from the region of Antioch testifies to the influence that the centre had on a relatively distant place like Emmaus, in Hirschfeld's opinion.[413] Following the Arab conquest in 639 CE, Emmaus was struck by a plague that claimed thousands of lives.[414]

In the Crusader period, the *frigidarium* of the bathhouse was devided into a lower and an upper room by a wooden ceiling installed 2.2 metres above the pavement. This ceiling was carried by horizontal beams set in sockets in the walls. It became the pavement of the upper room. The

---

[411] Gichon (1980): 20; Gichon (1979: 102) assumes that the hot springs were blocked during an earthquake at Emmaus in 1546 or on a specific day in the eleventh or twelfth century; Figuers (1978: 134) notes that the spring at Emmaus may have been extinct as a result of seismic activity, but he ignores the information in the Classical sources; Anyway, Gichon's idea is not accepted since the sources themselves emphasis the term 'spring' and under no circumstances not 'hot springs', or 'hot baths'.

[412] Gichon (1979a): 101–110 idem, (1979b): 125–126; idem, (1980): 228–234; idem, (1986–1987): 54–57; idem, (1993): I: 386–388; See also Nielsen (1990): II: 41, C.338; Tsafrir (1984): 107; Schwartz (1998b): 165.

[413] Hirschfeld (1988): 21–22; See also Butler (1908): II: 300–303.

[414] al Yâqût, *Mu'jam al-buldān*, III: 729; Le Strange (1890): 393–394; Marmardji (1951): 150; See also van Kasteren (1892): 80–99; Horowitz (1923): 52; Press (1948): I: 24; Avi-Yonah (1993): II: 385.

ceiling was dismantled after the Crusaders were driven out, and the building was turned into a Muslim holy place. The belivers turned the wall sockets into niches for oil lamps. Fragments of these lamps were found in abundance in the upper strata.[415]

In short, the name Emmaus is simply the Greek version of the Hebrew name Hammat, and of the Aramaic name Hammtha, which indicate the hot springs situated on the site. Today there is no trace of hot baths there, but basalt formations, which are evidence of volcanic activity in the region, have been found in the vicinity of the Ayalon Valley. There can be no doubt that the Emmaus which figured in the wars of the Maccabees and was known as Nicopolis in the Roman and Byzantine periods is indeed Emmaus in the Ayalon Valley, close to the Arab village 'Imwās, near Latrun.

To sum up, according to historical-archaeological analysis of the spas, they served not only for medical proposes but for leisure and recreation. Certain places gained great fame because of their healing qualities and their effectiveness in curing health ailments and were used as sacred cult locations. Hammat-Gader was indeed a special combination of a festival, an entertainment centre and a place of social gathering. It was famous both for the medicinal water springs and for the life of debauchery. The ritual worship is expressed in interesting types of Hygieia, Aesculapius, the Three Graces and more. Besides the Graeco-Roman gods, Egyptian Sarapis and the local Zeus Baalbaaros played an important role in the nature of the spas as healing and fertility local gods. An approach placed the thermal springs in the class of hallowed waters endowed with supernatural healing powers. This frame of mind is reflected in the tradition of bestowing holy names on the therapeutic baths such as the *Baths of Moses* to Hammei-Livias and *Thermae Heliae* to Hammat-Gader. The historical-archaeological surveys with the ritual characteristics of the curative sites like-wise shed light and add unique information about variegated use of medicine in antiquity, the maladies, and the relationship between Jews and Gentiles in the eastern Mediterranean basin as will be lightened in the following chapters.

---

[415] Gichon (1993): I: 388; idem, and Linden (1984): 156–169; During the Crusaders a garrison of Knights Templar was stationed at Emmaus-Nicopolis.

CHAPTER FIVE

THE HEALING PROPERTIES OF THE THERMO-MINERAL BATHS IN THE EASTERN MEDITERRANEAN IN ANCIENT TIMES

Since antiquity people have felt the beneficial and soothing effect on their pains and diseases of bathing in medicinal hot springs.[1] From sources dating to the Second Temple period it emerges that the ancients knew the healing properties of these waters. The book of Enoch I (67, 8), which hints at the source of the thermal springs—'they give off a smell of Sulphur from the hell-fire', mentions who used them and for what purposes:[2]

> For the kings and the mighty and the exalted and those who dwell on the earth for the healing on the flesh and the spirit.

Public baths generally and medicinal baths in particular were considered by the Romans as centres of culture, education, sport and therapy. In Roman times sizable military resources were diverted to building facilities at the thermae, not out of concern for others but to promote their own interests. Among others, sick and wounded soldiers were sent to these places, which served as rest and recreation centres for healthy soldiers too. Most of the Sages approved of the Romans' enterprise in introducing the baths into Palestine, because cleanliness and care of the body were greatly valued in their eyes. Many of the Sages used the baths, and Hillel the Elder was reported to have had a ready answer to the question, 'Where are you going?'—'To perform a religious duty, to fulfill the commandment of washing in the bathhouse' (*Leviticus Rabbah* 34, 3). Despite the usual attitude that 'the pleasure of human beings are pool and bathhouses' (*Ecclesiastes Rabbah* 2, 8), rules for bathing were established. For example, when engaged in it one should not reflect on words of Torah (*Babylonian Talmud, Berakhot* 24b);

---

[1] See, for instance, Jackson (1990a); idem, (1999); This overview is based on Dvorjetski (1992a); idem, (1992b); idem, (1993a); idem, (1994a); idem, (1994b); idem, (1994c); idem, (1997a); idem, (1999a); idem, (2001–2002); idem, (2003); idem, (2004); idem, (2006–2007); idem, forthcoming [a].

[2] *Enoch, I*, 67, 8.

one should not pray when at the baths, nor even ask after a person's health (*ibid.*, *Shabbat* 10b); if one's father was old or ailing one entered and bathed him as this concerned his dignity (*ibid.*, *Pesahim* 44b); a special prayer was composed for recital before going into the baths and a prayer of thanksgiving was offered after leaving (*Jerusalem Talmud*, *Berakhot* 9, 4 [14b]). In the world of the Sages hygiene was a matter of principle and of such importance that it was made a rule that a Torah scholars may not live in a city without a bathhouse (*Babylonian Talmud*, *Sanhedrin* 17b).[3]

5.1 The Nature of Therapeutic Baths in Light of the Classical Literature

Classical writers too were acquainted with the healing baths of the Levant. Pliny the Elder in the first century CE writes in his masterpiece *Historia Naturalis* of Tiberias and the town's unique feature:[4]

> ab occidente Tiberiade, aquis calidis salubri [= and Tiberias with its salubrious hot springs on the west].

The thermal springs of Hammat-Pella in Trans-Jordan—he calls:[5]

> Pellam aquis divitem [= Pella rich with its waters].

Pliny also mentions the remedial value of the Kallirrhoe thermal springs also in Trans-Jordan, and notes that,[6]

> prospicit eum ab oriente Arabia Nomadum, a meridie Machaerus, secunda quondam arx Iudaeae ab Hierosolymis. eodem latere est calidus fons medicae salubritatis Callirrhoe aquarum gloriam ipso nomine praeferens [= On the east it is faced by Arabia of the Nomands, and on the south by Machaerus, at one time next to Jerusalem the most important fortress in Judaea. On the same side there is a hot spring possessing medicinal value, the name of which Callirrhoe, itself proclaims the celebrity of its waters].

---

[3] See especially the discussions in chapter 3 on *The Healing Qualities and Spa Therapy* and in chapter 6 on *Daily Life at the Thermo-Mineral Baths according to Rabbinic Literature.*

[4] Pliny, *Historia Naturalis* 5.71; See also Smith (1922): 482; Stern (1974): I: 469.

[5] Pliny, *Historia Naturalis* 5.74.

[6] Idem, *ibid.*, 5.74; Dvorjetski (1992a): 73; Weber (1997): 333; Dvorjetski (2001–2002): 491; It seems that the name Kallirrhoe spelt with *K* instead of *C*, is more accurate; On this particular thing, see the explanation and the significance of the name in chapter 4.4 on *The Historical-Archaeological Analysis and Healing Cults of the Therapeutic Site of Kallirrhoe.*

A contemporary of Pliny, Josephus, adds in his composition *Bellum Judaicum* that the waters of Kallirrhoe, which pouring into the Asphaltitis Lake [= the Dead Sea], are sweet and also good for drink, and in his treatise *Antiquitates Judaicae* he repeats again that 'the waters of which beside all their other virtues are also good to drink'.[7] He also gives in his essay *Bellum Judaicum* a picturesque description of Hammei-Ba'arah, emphasizing that the Ba'arah springs are good for every ailment, especially nervous disease: 'These when mixed provide a most delightful bath, possessing general medicinal properties, but particularly restorative to the sinews.[8]

Solinus in the third century CE reiterates in his treatise *Collectanea Rerum Memorabilium* that Kallirrhoe is:[9]

> Callirrhoe Hierusolymis proxima, fons calore Medico probatissimus et ex ipso aquarum praeconio sic vocatus [= Callirrhoe in the vicinity of Jerusalem is a source of approved goodness owing to its curative heat and it derives its name from the fame of the water].

From the literary account *Vitae Sophistarum* of the fourth century CE Greek biographer Eunapius it transpires that people in search of a cure flocked from Athens to Hammat-Gader, as the group following his venerated teacher the neo-Platonist Iamblichus and his disciples.[10]

Emerging from the descriptions of the Church Father Epiphanius—bishop of Salamis and a contemporary of Eunapius—is a colorful atmosphere that prevailed at the site, which attracted people seeking healing from throughout the Empire. A regional ritual celebration was conducted there, as was a kind of annual fair, πανήγυρις, during which men and women bathed together.[11]

In the fourth century CE Ammianus Marcellinus remarks in his *Res Gestae* that in Palestine there were many hot springs that were used for medicinal purposes, but he does not give their names:[12]

---

[7] Josephus, *Bellum Judaicum* 1.656–657; idem, *Antiquitates Judaicae* 17.171.

[8] *Bellum Judaicum* 7.186–189; See also Kottek (1994): 136–137; νεύρων is translated by H. Thackeray as 'sinews', which may be acceptable, but 'nerves' could be better—or at least not less acceptable—rendering. See for this, Simchoni (1968): 386; Kottek (1994): 137.

[9] Solinus, *Collectanea Rerum Memorabilium* 35, 4; See also Stern (1980): II: 4 (18).

[10] Eunapius, *Vitae Sophistarum* 459; Sukenik (1935a): 21; Lieberman (1946): 354; Hirschfeld and Solar (1981): 202; Dvorjetski (1988): 92; Yegül (1992): 121.

[11] Epiphanius, *Adversus Haereses* 30, 7; See also Sukenik (1935a): 21; Hirschfeld and Solar (1984): 30; Dvorjetski (1988): 93–94; idem, (1992a): 106–107.

[12] Ammianus Marcellinus, *Res Gestae* 14.8.12; See also Stern (1980): II: 604–605; Dvorjetski (1996a); idem, (1996b).

in locis plurimis aquae suapte natura calentes emergent, ad usus aptae
multiplicium medellarum [= in numerous places warm springs gush forth,
adapted to many medicinal uses].

'A desolate place with very hot and curative springs'—is the description found in the biography of the fifth century CE monk Petrus of
Iberia for Hammei-Ba'arah. He left his monastery at Maioumas-Gaza
and went to the thermal waters of Ba'ar in order to heal his body, which
had become weakened from self-mortification. He also went to take a
cure by bathing in the thermal waters of Livias, which were called at
those days *the Springs of Moses*. Since his youth Petrus had bruised his
body and tormented it by various forms of ascetic discipline, so that his
flesh had wasted away and only his skin and a thin one at that—was
stretched over his dried-up bones. In his old age, indeed, he became
so weak that he threw up with bloody 'omit even what little food he
swallowed'. Undoubtedly, this was his motive for going to the site.[13]

The Christian historian Sozomenus a contemporary of Petrus of
Iberia brings testimony of great value to clarify why Emmaus-Nicopolis
became a famous city in Palestine in his *Historia Ecclesiastica* emphasizing that:[14]

> There is the spring of Jesus, whose waters give a cure not only to the
> illnesses of people who bathe in it, but also to various animal diseases.
> They say that when the Messiah stayed with his disciples, he deviated
> from the path one day to wash his feet in this spring, and from then on
> its waters had a special quality of removing all types of illnesses and
> suffering from humans and animals.

Due to Saint Willibald, who visited the Holy Land in the eight century,
to the ninth century chronicler Theophanes, the chronographer George
Cedrenus, who reported in his *Historiarum Compendium* on the spring of
Emmaus-Nicopolis in 1057 and to Michael the Syrian, twelfth century
Patriarch of Antioch—it was a well known therapeutic site. The last
documentation in regard to the spring with the special healing qualities
is brought by Nicephorus Klistos in 1320. In his essay of the essentials,
which were already known in Christian writings, he is very much influenced by Sozomenos. However, he notes that when the waters of the

---

[13] Petrus of Iberia, 81–82, 87.
[14] Sozomenus, *Historia Ecclesiastica* 5.21; Dechent (1884): 209–210; Walford (1855):
239; Vincent and Abel (1932): 414; Dalman (1935): 229; Williams (1987): 125; Dvorjetski (1992a): 122.

site are drunk, they instill health and prevent illnesses both of human beings and of animals.[15]

The most interesting literary references appear in the travelogue of the pilgrim Antoninus from Placentia in northern Italy, who visited the region in 570 CE. He spoke in his *Itinerarium* about the traditions and methods of healing the lepers:[16]

> ciuitate ad milia tria sunt aquas calidas, quae appellantur termas Heliae, ubi leprosi mundantur, qui e xenodochio habent de publicum delicias. Hora uespertina inundantur termae. Ante ipsumclibanum aquae est solius [sic] grandis, qui dum impletus fuerit, clauduntur omnia ostia, et per posticum mittuntur intus cum luminaria et incensum et sedent in illo solio tota nocte, et dum soporati fuerint, uidet ille, qui curandus est, aliquam uisionem, et dum eam recitarit, abstinentur ipsae termae septem diebus et intra septem dies mundatur [= three miles from the city, are warm springs, which are called the Baths of Helias (*Thermae Heliae* = Elijah), in which lepers are cleansed. There is also a hospice. The baths are cleaned in the evening for the enjoyment of the public. In front of the furnace for heating the water is a large bench, and while it is full all the doors are closed. Sick persons are brought through the portico into the bath with lamps and incense, and sit upon that bench all night. While they are asleep they see a vision concerning one of them that is to be cured, and until he has repeated it to them the baths are shut up for seven days. Within the seven days they are cleansed].

According to this testimony, a public hospice was built in order to provide therapeutic services and entertainment for the visitors. It does not say, however, that the city financed its upkeep, although it may be assumed that this was so, for the city benefited from the large income from the healing springs. The origin of the name, *Baths of Elijah* (*Thermae Heliae*) derives from the Biblical story of the cure of Na'aman, commander of the Aramaean army, who had leprosy, in the waters of the Jordan River following the advice of Elisha, the disciple of Elijah (*II Kings* 5, 27). In the Byzantine period, the residents of Hammat-Gader adopted the Biblical traditions about Elijah, and called the medicinal baths after him *Thermae Heliae*. His grave is identified as being in the

---

[15] Willibald, *Itinera Hierosolymitana* 293; Theophanes, *Chronographia* 160; George Cedrenus, *Historiarum Compendium* 583; Michael the Syrian, *Chronicles* 187; Nicephorus Klistos, *Ecclesiastica Historia* 10, 31; See also Vincent and Abel (1932): 414–419; Dvorjetski (1992a): 88, 121–124.

[16] Antoninus Placentinus, *Itinerarium* 7; Dechent (1884): 194; Wilkinson (1977): 81; Hirschfeld and Solar (1984): 30; Dvorjetski (1992a): 107–108; Weber (1997): 336; Hirschfeld (1997): 5–6; Dvorjetski (2006–2007): 16.

Gilead, not far from Gadara. Elijah's selection as patron of the bath of the lepers accords with his special quality as a healer. In light of the mention of Holy Elijah, the famous Biblical figure that Christianity adopted in the Eudocia inscription that will be discussed later, it seems that some of the thermo-mineral baths were named for him.[17]

The description of the bathing of the lepers is painted in a very strange light. The ill could use a certain bathtub in the baths only at night. Their passageway to the bathtub, which was opposite the *clibanus* opening, caused them hallucinations as they held candles and incense in a strange ritual. The lepers were cured by way of incubation, as was customary in the ancient medical centres of Aesculapius, in a large bathtub opposite the *clibanus* opening. This bathtub might be separated from the overall complex that served all the bathers. The lepers used these lamps as an element of some ritual ceremony conducted at the therapeutic bath.[18]

The special inn built and maintained by the local inhabitants for the lepers testifies to the fame of Hammat-Gader as a place of healing for leprosy. The place certainly served as a centre for curing leprosy in particular and skin diseases in general already at the time of Hadrian. Its mention in the Talmudic literature is not by chance; during his reign, and perhaps even with his aid, the foundations were laid for the edifice of the spa in Hammat-Gader, whose publicity as a place of healing assisted its reputation and its profits.[19]

Lepers used also the *aquae calidae*, the hot springs dedicated to Moses, situated north of the Dead Sea at Livias, across the Jordan River from Jericho. The most accurate description of the city is given by the Christian pilgrim Theodosius, who visited the region in 530 CE, and emphasizes as follows:[20]

> In this Livias Moses struck the rock with his rod, and the waters flowed out. Thence emerges a rather large stream which irrigates the whole of Livias...There Moses departed this life, and there are the warm waters where Moses bathed, and in these warm waters lepers are cleansed.

---

[17] Hirschfeld (1987): 103–104; See also Green and Tsafrir (1982): 32.
[18] Hirschfeld and Solar (1981): 202, 206; For the lamps, see also the discussion below.
[19] Dvorjetski (1997b); idem, (2004); idem, (2006–2007).
[20] Theodosius, *De Situ Terrae Sanctae* 10, 8; See also Dechent (1884): 202–203; Dvorjetski (1992a): 135; Schürer (1991): II: 178; Dvorjetski (2006–2007): 17.

Antoninus of Placentia reports mainly about the Baths of Moses and their properties:[21]

> Nearby is a city called Livias, where the two half-tribes of Israel remained before crossing the Jordan, and in that place are natural hot springs which are called the Baths of Moses. In these also lepers are cleansed. A spring there has very sweet water, which they drink as a cathartic, and it heals many diseases. This is not far from the Dead Sea, into which the Jordan flows, below Sodom and Gomorrah. Sulphur and Bitumen are collected on that shore. Lepers lie in the sea there all through the day in July and August, and the early part of September. In the evening they wash in these Baths of Moses. From time to time by the will of God one of them is cleansed, but for most of them it brings some relief.

Another example for Antoninus's contribution to the study of the thermo-mineral baths is while extols the salty water and the sweets of the Tiberias thermal springs for its therapeutic properties.[22] The French traveller Arculfus (670 CE) also tells of Tiberias and its thermal springs.[23] Saint and historian Bede Venerabilis, known as the 'Father of English History', documented the holy places in 729 and mentions: 'Tiberias thermal and salubrious springs.'[24]

The special nature of Hammei-Tiberias as a healing potion is attested in the *Chronicles* of the twelfth century historian Michael the Syrian, head of the Christian community of Antioch who wrote in Syriac that there was a systematic therapy by draughts of it:[25]

> For the use of those wishing for a cure, there were also earthenware pitchers, which were artistically arranged. On each of them was inscribed the frequency with which it activated the stomach of a person who drinks from it. And everyone would choose a jar according to the quantity that he wants.

His unique testimony provides an unequivocal demonstration for the important role of drinking the thermo-mineral baths. It completes and correlates closely the authenticity of the Rabbinic literature, which will be shown later in this chapter.

---

[21] Antoninus Placentinus, *Itinerarium* 7; Dvorjetski (1992a): 135.
[22] Idem, *Itinerarium* 7; Stewart (1896): 6; Dvorjetski (1992a): 101; idem, (2001b): 89–90.
[23] Arculfus, *De Locis Sanctis* 26–27; Dvorjetski (1992a): 101.
[24] Bede Venerabilis, *De Locis Sanctis* 316; Dvorjetski (1992a): 101.
[25] Michael the Syrian, *Chronicles* 4; Assaf and Meir (1944): 10; Buchmann (1957): 24; Meiri (1973): 32; Dvorjetski (1992a): 102; idem, (1999a): 119–120.

People of all kinds bathed at the thermo-mineral baths. Josephus relates that when King Herod's illness became more and more acute 'though he was suffering greater misery than could well be endured, he still had hopes of recovering, and so he summoned his physicians and made up his mind to use whatever remedies they might suggest. He therefore crossed the Jordan River and took baths in the warm springs at Kallirrhoe'.[26]

In his autobiography, Josephus writes that his rival John of Gischala of Upper Galilee wrote to him and asked for his permission to take Hammei-Tiberias 'for the good of his health'. According to Josephus, Yohanan used the baths only for two days, and then began to organize sedition against him.[27]

Rabbi Judah the Patriarch, for example, customarily visited the therapeutic baths at Hammat-Gader and at Hammei-Tiberias at set times and also dealt with people's needs, as will be illustrated later on (*Babylonian Talmud, Shabbat* 40b; *Ecclesiastes Rabbah* 5, 14). There are some intents and actions of some of the Roman Emperors at the thermo-mineral baths in the eastern Mediterranean basin either for treating their maladies or for visiting their legions not merely for military reasons, such as Vespasian, Hadrian and Caracalla.[28]

5.2 KNOWLEDGE AND RECOMMENDATIONS ACCORDING TO THE RABBINIC LITERATURE

Except in isolated cases it is not expressly stated in the Rabbinic literature that the Sages took the baths. The paucity of material on this

[26] Josephus, *Antiquitates Judaicae* 17.168–171; See also Josephus, *Bellum Judaicum* 1.656–657; Smith (1922): 480; Kottek (1994): 61–62; On Herod and his historical background see Kokkinos (1998); On the symptoms that Josephus reports Herod as suffering from as well as the different diagnoses that have been proposed in modern times see for example, Neuburger (1919): 51–58, 71; Muntner (1953): 134–136; Perowne (1956): 185–186; Meyshan (1957): 154–155; Sandison (1967): 381–388; Shalit (1978): 319, 501; Ladouceur (1981): 25–34; Dvorjetski (1992a): 143; Macdonald (1995): 286; Litchfield (1998): 283–284; Mader (2001): 56; Kokkinos (2002): 28–35; See also chapter 4.4 on *The Historical-Archaeological Analysis and Healing Cults of Kallirrhoe*.
[27] Josephus, *Vita* 17.85–86; See also idem, *Antiquitates Judaicae* 2.614; Kottek (1994): 61; Mason (2003): 127; On John of Gischala, see Rappaport (1982): 479–493; idem, (1992): 98–99; See the discussion in chapter 4.1 on *The Historical-Archaeological Analysis and Healing Cults of Hammei-Tiberias*.
[28] See the intensive discussions in chapter 6 on *The Daily Life at the Thermo-Mineral Baths according to Rabbinic Literature* and in chapter 7 on *The Roman Emperors at the Spas in the Eastern Mediterranean Basin*.

subject stems from the tendency of Talmudic corpus to play down the private concerns of central personalities in national life, and possibly also from the low level of medical knowledge.[29]

Rabbi Simeon ben Yohai and his son, Elazar, went to the thermal bath of Hammei-Tiberias, and were cured after they remained for a lengthy period in the cavern and their body produced a skin disease according to the *Jerusalem Talmud, Shevi'it* 9, 1 [38d]:[30]

> For thirteen years Rabbi Simeon ben Yohai lived hidden in a cave. The cave [= was next to] a carob tree. [= He stayed there] until his body became afflicted with [= a skin disease that looked like] rust spots. At the end of thirteen years he said, 'Shouldn't I go out to see what has happened in the world?'...When he saw that the [= political] difficulties [= that had led him to hide in the cave] had diminished, he said, 'Let us go down and visit the *demosin* in Tiberias.' [= After enjoying the baths, Simeon] said, 'I should enact an ordinance [= to benefit the city], just as our patriarchs did...' [= Simeon said], 'Let us purify Tiberias [= from corpse uncleanness]'.

Rabbi Judah the Patriarch went to the thermal baths at Tiberias and stayed there for remedial purposes amongst others. The texts do not elucidate the medical condition for which he went there. His disciple describes his actions, the mode of his bathing and his drinking:[31]

> Rabbi Yitzhak ben Abdimi said: 'I once followed Rabbi into the baths, and wished to place a cruse of oil for him in the bath. Whereupon he said to me, 'Take [= some water] in a second vessel and put [= the cruse of oil in it].
>
> *(Babylonian Talmud, Shabbat* 40b)

In *Ecclesiastes Rabbah* 5, 11, it is related that,

---

[29] See the discussion in chapter 6.2 on *The Sages at the Therapeutic Sites—Aims and Deeds* and the test case of Rabbi Judah the Patriarch in chapter 5.5 below; See also Buchmann (1968): 199; Simon (1978a): 35–38; Dvorjetski (1992a): 128–133; idem, (1994b); idem, (1996a).

[30] On the analysis of several versions of this story [(*Jerusalem Talmud, Shevi'it* 9, 1 [38d]; *Genesis Rabbah*, 79 (Theodor-Albek ed., pp. 941–945); *Esther Rabbah*, 3, 3; *Psikta de Rav Kahana*, 16 (Mandelbaum ed., pp. 191–194); *Ecclesiastes Rabbah*, 10, 8; *Babylonian Talmud Shabbat* 33b–34a; *Midrash Psalms*, 17, 13 (Buber ed., p. 134)]—see Levine (1978): 143–185; See also Shiponi (1963): 18–23; Hirschberg (1920): 237–238; For this kind of skin disease, see Muntner (1938): 51; On the term *demosin*, see the discussion on *Terminology* in chapter 1.4.

[31] See Rashi explanation to *Babylonian Talmud Shabbat* 40b; Epstein, *Babylonian Talmud, Shabbat* (1957): 188, note 5; See the version in *Ecclesiastes Rabbah* 5, 11; For the reasons of Rabbi Judah for going to various spas, see Dvorjetski (2001a); idem, (2002).

Rabbi came out of the bath, wrapped himself in his garments and sat
down to attend to the people [= who brought to him their difficulties].
His servant mixed for him a cup; but being busy with attending to the
people, he had no leisure to receive it from him, and the servant became
drowsy and fell asleep. Rabbi turned, and gazing at him exclaimed,
'Rightly did Solomon say, Sweet is the sleep of a labouring man, whether
he eat little or much; but the satiety of the rich will not suffer him to
sleep—like me who am busy attending to needs of the people; I am not
even allowed to sleep'.

Those references apparently seem to be of secondary importance.
However, it reflects the authenticity that Hammei-Tiberias spa was also
known for the medicinal value of their water when drunk. It transpires
from the *Mishnah* (*Machshirin* 6, 7) that the spa at Hammei-Tiberias
possessed the natural property of a purgative:[32]

One drinks of the water of Tiberias even though it issues clean [= from
the anus].

For this purpose water of palm-trees were used: 'The first cup [= thereof]
loosens, the second causes motions, and the third passes out just as it
enters' (*Babylonian Talmud, Shabbat* 110a).[33]

Special glasses were used for drinking this water, which were called
Kasaia Tiberiah [= the glasses of Tiberias] (*ibid., Nida* 21a). They were
large at the base, constricted at the rim, transparent and very thin
(*Jerusalem Talmud, Nida* 2, 7 [50b]).[34]

Systematic therapy by draughts of Hammei-Tiberias is cited by the
twelfth century chronicler Michael the Syrian as mentioned before.[35]
It seems that the daily use of the term *fahortha* [= earthenware pitch-
ers] is now more understandable in connection with Tiberias and its
suburb Hammei-Tiberias (*ibid., Eruvin* 5, 1 [22b]).[36]

A contemporary of Michael the Syrian, Moses Maimonides, the
most prominent Jewish Medieval physician, states in his explanation
to *Mishnah* (*Machshirin* 6, 7), that the quality of Hammei-Tiberias is
that it is a purgative when drunk.[37] Rabbi Moshe ben Nachman, the

---

[32] Buchmann (1968): 200; Kohut (1926): IV: 13; Horowitz (1923): 86.
[33] Löw (1924): 346; Klein (1929): 8–11.
[34] On glass trade and industry in Tiberias, see for instance, Lieberman (1932a):
207–208; Schwartz (1988): 104; Dvorjetski (1994b): 40, note 18.
[35] Michael the Syrian, *Chronicles* 4.
[36] Vohalman (1939): 208.
[37] Maimonides to *Mishnah, Machshirin* 6, 7.

thirteenth century Jewish scholar known as HaRamban, and one of Judaism's primary Torah commentators, notes that the water is bitter, and it is drunk by rheumatics and epileptics.[38] An important and basic activity became a way of life in the *halakhic* rules of bathing: 'One may bath in Mediterranean Sea and in Hammei-Tiberias [= on the Shabbat] even if it is intended as a cure, but not in the stepping pool or in the Dead Sea when it is intended as a cure' (*Jerusalem Talmud, Shabbat* 14, 3 [14c]).

Not only is the best time for bathing as a cure expressed in the Talmud but so is the season recommended for taking medicinal potions. This was from the Passover festival to Pentecost (*Babylonian Talmud, Shabbat* 147b):[39]

> Rav Judah said in the Rav's name: 'The complete period of *demosith* is twenty one days, and Pentecost is included'.

Apart from therapy by drinking, *demosith* ground and the mud bath were also used. This transpires from the prohibition against standing on the muddy sediment of the medicinal bath on the Shabbat, since it served for physical exercise and a cure, even if one did not wash in it or exercise (*Babylonian Talmud, Shabbat* 147b):[40]

> Rabbi Hiyya bar Abba said in Rabbi Yohanan's name: 'One may not stand on the mud of *demosith*, because it stimulates [= the body] and loosens [= the bowels]'.

Furthermore, the Sages also used medical products when they visited therapeutic baths. This also applies to the pebbles, which were used for therapeutic purposes, in addition to spreading *Peloma* on the body or on particular parts of it (*Jerusalem Talmud, ibid.*, 4, 6 [7a]; *ibid.*, 18, 1 [16c].[41] The word *Peloma* has been adopted as the Hebrew term for mud or *pelose* as used in Balneology. It is, in fact, a derivative of the Greek πηλός. The international term, *peloid*, from the same Greek root, forms a generic name which includes all clinical media such as muds, peat moss, fanghi, schalmm, which are used in Peloidtherapy.[42]

---

[38] The *Babylonian Talmud* with Rav Elfas, *Shabbat* 18a.
[39] On the term *demosith*, see the discussion on *Terminology* in chapter 1.4; See also Krauss (1929): 73; Bar-Kochva (1980): 185.
[40] Goldstein and Schecter (1956): I: 713; Lieberman (1963): 71–73.
[41] Dvorjetski (1995a).
[42] Buchmann (1955): 287–292.

The healing qualities of the therapeutic springs were known to the
Sages. A long and distinguished list of Sages and ordinary folks visited
the therapeutic baths for healing among them some of the greatest
Sages of the generation. There are knowledge and recommendations
on thermo-mineral waters in the Talmudic literature.[43]

The thermo-mineral waters were active against general debilitation.
This property is perhaps manifested through in the account by Rabbi
Abbahu, head of the academy in Caesarea in the third century CE,
who required the help of two slaves on his journey to Hammei-Tiberias
and his vigour returned to him only after he had immersed himself in
the water (*Jerusalem Talmud, Betza* 1, 6 [60b]). There is also the anecdote of Rabbi Joshua ben Levi, who leaned on the shoulder of Rabbi
Hiyya bar Abba when he entered the *demosin* of Tiberias (*ibid., Shabbat*
1, 2 [3a]) suffering from weakness.[44]

Sufferers from various skin ailments used the thermal springs. This
may be inferred from a question asked of Rabbi Yose, that he permitted
Rabbi Samuel bar Abba to bathe on the Shabbat as a rash had erupted
on his body, and he replied angrily, 'Even on Ninth of Ab and even on
the Day of Atonement' (*ibid., Berakhot* 2, 7 [8c]). Or, 'For it was taught:
'One may bathe in Hammei-Tiberias and in the water of stepping in
the Lake of Sodom, even if he has scabs on his head' (*Babylonian Talmud,
Shabbat* 109b); and the report of meeting of Rabban Simeon ben
Gamaliel with those afflicted by boils on the way to Tiberias:

> Once when I was walking on the road from Tiberias to Sepphoris, a
> scholar met me and said to me: "There are twenty four kinds of skin
> disease, but there is none that is harmful to sexual intercourse except
> *Ra'athan*[45] alone."
>
> (*Leviticus Rabbah* 16, 1)

Apparently it seems that the connection to his walking from Tiberias
to Sepphoris and to the words of that scholar about twenty four kinds
of skin disease is not comprehended. It can be assumed that Rabban
Simeon ben Gamaliel met on his way people who were afflicted with
boils and they were going to be cured at Tiberias. Another text emphasizes that an old man afflicted with boils met him (*Jerusalem Talmud,
Ketuboth* 7, 11 [31d]).

---

[43] Dvorjetski (1992a): 130–132; idem, (1994b); idem, (1996a).
[44] Jackson (1990a): 1–2.
[45] On *Ra'athan*, a kind of skin disease, see Katzenelson (1928): 303–343; Muntner
(1938): 141–143; Preuss (1993): 323–347.

The Tiberias Sages used to warn the inhabitants against becoming infected by sufferers from leprosy and from *ra'athan*, as appears in *Leviticus Rabbah* 16, 3:[46]

> Rabbi Yohanan and Rabbi Simeon ben Lakish [= gave rulings]. Rabbi Yohanan said: It is prohibited to go four cubits to the east of a leper [= since the wind in Palestine is mostly from the west, and is thus liable to carry the disease germs to a person east of the leper]. Rabbi Simeon ben Lakish said: Even a hundred cubits. They did not really differ; the one who said four cubits referred to a time when there is no wind blowing, whereas the one who said [= not even] a hundred cubits, referred to a time when a wind is blowing. Rabbi Meir would not eat eggs that came from an alley of lepers. Rabbi Ami and Rabbi Assi would not enter a leper's alley. Resh Lakish, when he saw one of them in the city, threw stones towards him [= to attract his attention without going too close to him, and remind him to remain in the quarantine area], and said: 'Go to your place, and do not defile other people'.

These lepers may not have been residents of Tiberias, but had gone there from various places for a cure at the therapeutic baths in the town. Sufferers from various skin diseases were also helped by Hammat-Gader: 'When Emperor Hadrian climbed the slop from Hammat-Gader to Gadara city he found there a little Jewish girl covered with sore boil' (*Midrash HaGadol to Deuteronomy* 26, 19, ed. Fish, p. 603). Rabbi Ze'ira used probably the spas of Hammat-Gader and Hammtha de Paḥel [= Hammat-Pella] for his dermatological disease (*Jerusalem Talmud, Terumot* 2, 1 [41b]; *ibid., Shevi'it* 6, 1 [36c]).[47]

The Sages ascribe to the 'Well of Miriam' a virtue of curing sick persons (*Mishna, Avot* 5, 6; *Babylonian Talmud, Ta'anit* 9a). After the Israelites had crossed the Red Sea Miriam sang a song of triumph, in which all the women joined (*Exodus* 15, 20–21). Miriam and Aaron spoke against Moses on account of the *Cushite* woman whom he had married, whereupon God summoned Moses, Aaron, and Miriam to the tabernacle of the congregation, reproved her, and punished her with leprosy. She was healed through the prayers of Moses, but was obliged to remain without the camp of the Israelites for seven days, although the people did not proceed until she had returned (*Numbers* 12). Miriam died in the desert at Kadesh, where she was buried (*ibid.,*

---

[46] Yudelevitz (1950): 20–21.
[47] For more details about Rabbi Ze'ira, see chapter 4.3 on *The Historical-Archaeological Analysis and Healing Cults of the Therapeutic Site of Hammat-Pella* and chapter 6.2 on *The Sages at the Therapeutic Sites—Aims and Deeds*.

20, 1). When Miriam talked against Moses, she did not intend to slander him; she wished him to live with his wife and raise children (*Deuteronomy Rabbah* 4, 6). But when she was punished with leprosy, and had to remain without the camp, God honored Miriam by officiating as priest Himself (*Babylonian Talmud, Zevahim* 102a). The Israelites waited for her seven days (*ibid., Sotah* 9b), for she had once waited for Moses by the river (*Exodus* 2, 4). She is regarded as leader and the savior of Israel (*Micah* 6, 4; *Exodus Rabbah* 24, 1). For her sake a marvelous well accompanied the Israelites, a rock from which water flowed. This well was in the shape of a sieve-like rock, out of which water gushes forth as from a spout. It followed them on all their wanderings, and it settled opposite the Tabernacle. Upon the entrance to the Holy Land this well disappeared (*Babylonian Talmud, Ta'anit* 9a), and was hidden in a certain spot of the Sea of Tiberias. Standing upon Mount Carmel, and looking over the sea, one can notice there a sieve-like rock, and that is the Well of Miriam (*ibid., Shabbat* 38a). Once upon a time it happened that a leper bathed at this place of the Sea of Tiberias and hardly had he come in contact with the waters of Miriam's Well, when he was instantly healed. *Leviticus Rabbah* 22, 4, reports:[48]

> An incident id related of a certain man suffering from boils who went down to bathe in Tiberias. It so happened that he floated into Miriam's well, and he bashed there and was healed. Where is Miriam's well? Rabbi Hiyya bar Abba answered: It is written, *It is seen upon the face of Yeshimon* (*Numbers* 21, 20). If anyone ascends to the top of Mount Yeshimon he will see a kind of small sieve in the sea of Tiberias. This is the well of Miriam. Rabbi Yohanan ben Nuri says: 'Our Rabbis have calculated its position, which is directly opposite the middle gate of the ancient synagogue of Tiberias'.

In *Numbers Rabbah* 18, 22, there is another description:[49]

> An incident is related of a certain blind man at Shihin, who went down into the water to bathe. He came across Miriam's well and bathed in it and was healed.

In the region of the Sea of Galilee, between Tabgha spring and el-Hasal spring, a spring named Job's spring or Job's oven spouts. According to

[48] Krauss (1909–1910): 178–179; Horowitz (1923): 106–107; Avisar (1973): 463–464; Bennahum (1985): 87–88; On the connection between thermo-mineral wells in lakes or in the sea shore, see the discussion in chapter 2.2 on *The Geothermal Energy Utilisation in the Jordan Valley.*
[49] Horowitz (1923): 106–107; Halevi (1963): 778.

the Arabic tradition, Job washed himself in this spring and was cured from leprosy. Since this incident, the spring was named after Job. Up to date there is a prevalent idea by those who live in the area that it has medicinal properties and as in the past, people come to immerse in its waters. Probably this spring has radioactivity virtues.[50] A legend in the *Babylonian Talmud, Baba Bathra* 15b, indicates that:

> Rabbi Yohanan and Rabbi Eleazar both stated that Job was among those who returned from the [= Babylonian] Exile, and that his house of study was in Tiberias.

The origin of such a story is presumably inserted in the Biblical tradition (*Job* 2, 7) since the Satan 'smote Job with sore boils from the sole of his foot unto his crown'.

The therapeutic baths were also deemed an effective cure for nervous conditions. In addition to Josephus and Petrus the Iberian knowledge about Hammei-Ba'arah—the *Tosefta* in tractate *Teharot* 6, 7, also cites the deed of 'a certain dangerous man', possibly ill with a nervous disease, taken to Hammei-Tiberias. To Emmaus-Nicopolis went Rabban Yohanan ben Zakkai, in the grip of manic condition suffering from the illness of Bulimia:[51]

> It is related of Rabbi Yohanan that he was once seized with faintness through hunger. He went to Emmaus and sat down to the east of a fig-tree and was cured. He was asked 'Whence have you [= that the fig is a remedy?] He replied, 'From David, as it is written, "And they gave him a piece of a cake of figs... and when he had eaten, his spirit came back to him (*I Samuel* 30, 12)"; and they applied to him the text, The excellency of knowledge is, that wisdom preserveth the life of him that hath it.
>
> (*Ecclesiastes Rabbah* 7, 12, 1)

It might be that David is mentioned here since the site Emmaus was well known by its immoral character of debauchery.[52] It might be that this therapeutic place was also renowned for the same property as that at Hammei-Ba'arah.

From an examination of the names of the Sages accompanying the Patriarchs who came to the sites, it is possible to show that Rabbi Judah

---

[50] Nun (1953): 389.

[51] Rosner (2001): 43; On the Bulimia, see for example, Liberman (1962): 125; Goldstein and Schecter (1956): I: 95; Kohut (1926): II: 98–99.

[52] Epstein, *Babylonian Talmud, Shabbat* (1957): 193; On the social and cultural aspects of Emmaus and Hammat-Gader, see chapter 6; See also Dvorjetski (1999a); idem, (2003).

the Patriarch and his grandson Rabbi Judah Nes'iah arrived with their attending physicians. They customarily visited the therapeutic places at set times and also dealt with people's needs.[53] Rabbi Judah the Patriarch also resorted to the help and advice of doctors; and as he was such an eminent person, he would have had access to the best Jewish physicians available in the country at the time. Thanks to his friendship with Emperor Caracalla, he might also have consulted Roman physicians, although this is not recorded anywhere in the Talmudic literature.

Rabbi Judah's personal physician was Mar Samuel the astronomer. The Talmud calls him Assia, 'the physician' in Aramaic—a title that was given to only very few of the Sages (*Babylonian Talmud, Baba Metzia* 85b). Mar Samuel was born in Nehardea in Babylonia and studied in his youth at the academy of Rabbi Judah ben Betheira in Nisibis, capital city of the Armenian kings. Nisibis was endowed with a medical school, and it is probably here that Mar Samuel obtained his medical instruction. There, he acquired his knowledge of Greek medical terms and practices.[54] His medical notes, advices, even experiments are numerous. He studied anatomy extensively, and was also a versatile medical researcher who maintained high ethical standards: when anyone objected to experiments being performed on them, he experimented on himself, for example passing a sound into his stomach (*ibid., Shabbat* 41a). He strongly advocated cleanliness: 'Cold ablutions in the morning, and washing the hands and feet in warm water in the evening are better than all the medicines in the world' (*ibid., Shabbat* 108b). He had expert knowledge in epidemiology and preventive medicine (*ibid., Berakhot* 45a; *ibid., Hullin* 46a; *ibid., Shabbat* 107a). In clinical practice, he was first and foremost a famous ophthalmologist (*ibid., Avoda Zarah* 28b) and invented a remedy for eye inflammation that was named after him 'Collyrium of Mar Samuel' (*ibid., Shabbat* 108b). He also excelled in cardiology (*ibid., Gittin* 67b), and was an expert embryologist and paediatrician (*ibid., Nidda* 26b; *ibid., Mo'ed Qatan* 14a). Based on the teachings of Galen, whose contemporary he was, he advocated homeopathic therapies, on the principle of *similia similibus*. Thus, for example, he recommended laxative foods for the treatment of diarrhea, and the administration

---

[53] See, for example, chapter 6.2 on *The Sages at the Therapeutic Sites—Aims and Deeds*.
[54] See, for example, Hoffmann (1873): 34–35; Funk (1914): 99; Margalit (1962): 62; idem, (1970): 31; Zeide (1951): 42.

of red wine after bloodletting: 'Red wine to replace red blood' (*ibid.*, *Shabbat* 129a). Similarly, he advised to open the mouth in a hot bath, because 'heat expels heat' (*ibid.*, *Shabbat* 41a).[55]

Examining the Rabbinic sources it is substantial that the Patriarch had a group of permanent escorts who were familiar with the field of medicine. Most of the Sages, who accompanied the Patriarchs to the thermo-mineral baths were from a Babylonian origin, such as Rabbi Hanina, Rabbi Hama bar Hanina, Rabbi Hiyya, Rabbi Ami and Rabbi Zeiʾra.[56] It is not inconceivable that those sages received their guidance from Mar Samuel and under his supervision.[57]

In conclusion, all literary sources—Greek and Roman writers, of Church Fathers and Christian pilgrims and of Rabbinic literature—show several common denominators. Firstly, the thermo-mineral baths were considered also as centres of therapy; secondly, people of all kinds bathed there; thirdly, certain thermo-mineral places in the eastern Mediterranean basin gained great fame because of their healing qualities and their effectiveness in curing health ailments and disturbances, such as dermatological conditions, urinary and digestive tracts, general debilitation, rheumatism, weakness, and nervous diseases. Moreover, the properties of the therapeutic thermo-mineral baths in the Roman and Byzantine periods may be classified as follows: The Tiberias hot springs—treatment of conditions of the urinary and digestive tracts, general debilitation, various skin diseases and rheumatism; Hammat-Gader—treatment of various skin diseases, digestive tract conditions, rheumatism; the Baʾarah hot springs: great value for every condition, especially nervous diseases; the Kallirrhoe springs—treatment of various skin diseases, digestive tract conditions and rheumatism; Hammat-Pella—treatment of skin diseases; Emmaus-Nicopolis—treatment of nervous diseases, venereal diseases and also the treatment of animals. (See Tab. 2).

---

[55] Krauss (1911): 241; Kagan (1952): 58; Zeide (1954): 57–59; Margalit (1962): 68–69, 78–79; Muntner (1972): 4; Simon (1978): 57; Preuss (1993): 536; Newmyer (1996a): 2906.

[56] On their medicinal occupation, see for example, Margulis [n.d.]: 57; Bacher (1925): 5; Zeide (1951): 38–39; Tzuri (1931): 329; Greenvald (1936): 152; Rosner (1977a): 154; Beer (1982): 284; Ayli (1987): 143; Rosner (1996): 2883–2887.

[57] Dvorjetski (1992a): 139–140; See especially Rosner (1996): 2883.

5.3   THE CAIRO *GENIZA* FRAGMENTS AS
HISTORICAL-MEDICINAL EVIDENCE

The special healing qualities of the thermo-mineral springs in the
eastern Mediterranean gained a great reputation both in the country
and outside it in the course of the Roman and Byzantine periods, just
like the licentiousness that was carried on then. Various circles in the
Levant population, and even outside the country, used to come to the
thermal waters for vacation, enjoyment, and above all for healing.[58]
The Cairo *Geniza* fragments shed light on and complement our knowledge of different subjects dealing with the everyday life experiences at
the spas as shown in the above chapters. Due to the *Geniza*, a difficult
human chapter has been revealed to us—that of Jewish 'boil sufferers'
(leprosy) in the city of Tiberias'. A total of 17 documents have been
published that directly pertain to this matter; these date to the second
quarter of the eleventh century CE, except for several in which lepers
are mentioned incidentally.

Many came to the thermal baths at Hammei-Tiberias in order to find
balm for their illnesses. The lepers called themselves 'the tormented';
some wrote rhymed descriptions of their condition and their unbearable
diseases 'We are tormented with boils and we absent ourselves with bad
eczema, locked up in our houses, as though in cages incarcerated. We
go deaf from it, blind from it; we are stunted from it, encircled with
every contagious kind of boil.'[59] In this and other documents, emphasis
is placed on 'We, the afflicted young,' or 'your brothers, the tormented
young in Tiberias.'[60] Among the lepers were women: 'And limb after
limb, we fell, men and women.'[61] Among the sick were also those who
were the leaders of the communities: 'Heads of states [= cities] and
heads of families.'[62] The description of the great suffering of the lepers was sent in a letter to the city of Jerusalem from 'your tormented
brothers in the state of Tiberias,' with a plea for help: 'We are smitten
with boils, open wounds, a fresh plague; pieces of our flesh are cast to

---

[58] Dechent (1884): 173–210; Krauss (1909–1910): 32–50; Hirschberg (1920): 215–
246; Dvorjetski (1988); idem, (1992a); idem, (1992b); idem, (1994a); idem, (1994b);
idem, (1995a); idem, (1996a); idem, (1996b); idem, (1997b); idem, (1999a); idem, (2003);
idem, (2004); idem, forthcoming [a]; idem, forthcoming [b].
[59] TS 13 J 19, f. 19; Mann (1969): II: 197; Gil (1983): II: 457.
[60] TS 12.213; TS 6 J 4, f. 17.
[61] Bodl. MS Heb. c 13, f. 15.
[62] TS 16.248.

the ground, and the worms swarm about our flesh; and we are alive and our wounds are incurable.'[63] The expressions are taken from *Isaiah* 1, 5–6, in which there is a graphic description of the people of Israel covered with wounds and contusions. A similar version is conveyed in another letter, signed by 'the afflicted, battered by the affliction of Job, in Tiberias.' Details of it recall what is written in *Deuteronomy* 28, 35: 'The Lord will smite thee in the knees, and in the legs, with a sore boil, whereof thou canst not be healed, from the sole of thy foot unto the crown of thy head.' And in *Job* 2, 7: 'and smote Job with sore boils from the sole of his foot even unto his crown.'[64] The letter went on: 'Men and women, children and the aged are afflicted with sore boils, poxes from the sole of the foot to the head, wounds and contusions and fresh affliction, wormy flesh, melted away over the bone, and we are living, and our affliction is mortal.'[65] Is there really something to all these descriptions, or was it all perhaps a great exaggeration?

Small pox is a contagious, dangerous illness. The skin rash attacks the face, arms, hands, chest, and sometimes even the mucous membrane in the mouth, the nose, and throat. In addition to a high fever and a burning sensation of the skin, heart defects and blood-circulation disorders can appear. Weakness of the circulation might cause death, even in the absence of special complications. The most frequent dangerous complications are general toxemia owing to the penetration deep into the body of pus from the pox; also pneumonia, blindness, and deafness.[66] At another point in the letter signed by the lepers, it is written: 'Boils are transmitted to my right hand'.[67] Boils are a broad concept in dermatology. It is a difficult inflammation of the skin, a contagious and cancerous leprosy. Sometimes, though, the term boil symbolizes a difficult illness in general.[68]

Shocking descriptions appear in a letter to Fostat [= ancient Cairo] in which a sense of the terrible end of those afflicted by fate is indicated: 'Our fingers are falling off, our limbs are dropping, our hands are getting smaller, our legs are becoming shorter, our knees are failing us, our eyes are growing dimmer, and it is said about us that we are

[63] TS 16.18; Mann (1969): II: 196–197; Gil (1983): II: 467–469.
[64] See also *Babylonian Talmud, Baba Bathra* 15b.
[65] TS AS 147.10; Isaacs (1994): 79; Mann (1969): I: 168; II: 196–197.
[66] Goldstein and Schecter (1956): I: 9–10; Leibivitz and Draifus (1960): 255–256.
[67] Bodl. MS Heb. C 13, f. 15; Neubauer and Cowley (1906): II: 224; Mann (1969): II: 198; Gil (1983): II: 463–464.
[68] Leibowitz (1976a): 422.

like those awaiting death and are no more...every day limbs, limbs
are buried'.[69] We have here an authentic, illustrative description of
a chronic, contagious illness—leprosy—which manifests itself in skin
changes, in alterations of the nerves and mucous. The cause of the
illness is *Mycobacterium leprae*, which was identified for the first time by
the Norwegian scientist Gerhard Hansen in 1872. Its characteristic
signs are the thickening of the skin to the extent of that of a lion's
face, blindness, loss of the sense of the peripheral nerves, paralysis,
distortion of the shape of the arms and legs, and the falling off of
fingertips, toes, or nose.[70]

Because of the nature of the contagious sickness, a building was
placed at the disposal of the sick, and the letter to Fostat stresses that
'from the time their place was destroyed, they remain in the streets.'[71]
There are those who are of the opinion that the building was destroyed
in the earthquake that struck the city of Tiberias in 1033.[72] The
assumption that the building was destroyed because of the Bedouin
wars that were waged in this area in 1028–1029 is more convincing.[73]
These wars also brought about a disruption of letter communication
and the aid that had been received from Egypt. With the Fatimids'
victory over the Bedouins, calm prevailed and requests for aid were
renewed. Typical of the relative quiet that then prevailed are the opening words and flowery passages at the start of letters from this period,
such as a letter of recommendation carried by an envoy of the lepers
of Tiberias: 'We reside quietly and ensconced in peace.'[74] It is possible that Michael the Syrian, who lived in the twelfth century, meant
this building in his composition, *Chronicles*: 'A wonderful building was
destroyed, collapsed...and on it were wonderful edifices, and inns on
every side of it.' It is even possible to learn from his report about the
special nature of the Tiberias therapeutic springs as medicinal potions,
mentioned above. Those who were in need of healing also had clay
jugs, artistically arranged. 'All these buildings were destroyed.'[75]

[69] TS 16.248; Mann (1969): II: 193; Shaked (1964): 69; Gil (1983): II: 472–473.
[70] Browne (1975): 485–493; Leibowitz (1976b): 888; See also Goldstein and Schecter
(1956): II: 1005–1008.
[71] Westminster Coll., Fragm. Heb. Cair. Misc., f. 25; Assaf (1946): 39; Mann (1969):
II: 356; Gil (1983): II: 462.
[72] Assaf and Meir (1944): 11.
[73] Gil (1983): I: 152.
[74] TS 13 J 23, f. 13; Mann (1969): II: 193–195; Gil (1983): I: 152, 329.
[75] Michel the Syrien, *Chronicles* 466; Assaf and Meir (1944): 10.

A compulsory tax was levied on the sick in Tiberias for the service people; these people laundered their clothes from the infection: 'We have a heavy burden for those who service us, washing out our clothes from the stench and the blood and the rot, and all of us are tossed about like stones, we have no feet and no hands.'[76]

The poor sick organized themselves and send emissaries to Fostat to raise funds. In several of the letters of recommendation of the lepers' messengers, which were written by Hillel son of Yeshua the Cantor, places remained empty for recording the names of emissaries who were not yet known to him. The Tiberias community possibly had prepared forms for the specific matter, and messengers would often be sent to obtain aid for those whom fate had struck. The money was collected by 'a clerk of the merchants' in Tiberias, Sa'adia the Levi son of Moshe, who divided it 'in front of the comrades and the elderly.'[77] It can even be inferred from the language of the letter that the money was collected in a special appeal in Fostat.[78] Two letters show that two messengers were dispatched: one was a leper, Calef son of Yeshua the HaZubi of Haleb; the other, the healthy—Ovadia.[79] Calef's death-bed will has been preserved, and we learn from it that the man was a person of means, dealt in the linen trade and spices, and bought a rooming house in Tiberias.[80] Mention of the death of the suffering leper, Calef HaZubi, testifies to the fact that people sick with leprosy were not prevented from travelling and coming into contact with the public. It should be noted that in Islamic ritual law, leprosy and the leper have no connection with defilement and purity. The illness is mentioned only rarely in travel literature, though it seems that special neighborhoods were allotted to lepers in the Muslim east, too; for instance, in Damascus. The sickness was less widespread in the East than in the West, and so did not preoccupy the legal sages of Islam.[81]

---

[76] TS AS 147.10; Gil (1991): 285, 322.

[77] Westminster Coll., Fragm. Heb. Cair. Misc., f. 2; Mann (1969): II: 356; Gil (1983): II: 462–463.

[78] Gil (1983): I: 151–152.

[79] TS 10 J 12, f. 22; TS 16.18; Mann (1969): II: 356; Assaf and Meir (1944): 11; Goitein (1967): 476, note 17; Gil (1983): II: 460.

[80] TS 13 J 1, f. 8; Goitein (1967): 387, no. 85; Mann (1969): I: 166–167; See also Goitein (1980): 112; Gil (1983): II: 458.

[81] Ullman (1970): 243–244; Lazarus-Jaffe (1982): 215; Katzenelson (1928): 304–353.

The purpose of the lepers' coming to Tiberias was—in the words of one of the letters sent to Fostat—'to seek healing from the waters and the air.'[82] The healing tradition of the warm springs of Tiberias, known already in the Second Temple period, was for disorders of the urinary and digestive systems, skin illnesses, general weakness, and rheumatism.[83] One notices in letters asking for assistance a separation between 'the sufferers who are residents of Rakkath' or 'who live in Rakkath'—in the letters of Hillel son of Yeshua, who writes in the name of the lepers—and 'the sufferers living outside Rakkath' or 'sufferers, who outside Rakkath reside.'[84] It may be assumed the residence of the ill was outside the city.[85] In the mid-fourth century CE, the law relating to lepers became more severe. They were forbidden to enter the forum or the public bath houses, and therefore a special pool was allotted to them, like that in Beth Shean-Nysa-Scythopolis, which was actually located outside the city.[86]

Rakkat was a fortified city in the domain of the tribe of Naphtali (*Joshua* 19, 35), located between Hammat and Kinneret, identified as Tel Akeltya, two kilometres northwest of Tiberias.[87] Talmudic sources identify Rakkat with Tiberias. If we interpret the words literally, the intention is to those ill people who live outside Tiberias and used to heal themselves in the springs of Hammat-Gader;[88] they had had a medicinal tradition for leprosy since the days of the Emperor Hadrian.[89] An impressive documentation of the tradition—that within seven days, lepers are cured of their illness in the baths of Hammat-Gader, *Thermae Heliae*, which are the 'Baths of Elijah'—is presented by the sixth century CE pilgrim Antoninus of Placentinus. He tells of the lepers' pool and the bathing processes, accompanied by a ritual with candles and incense, which were like an incubation—just as people used to go for healing in the ancient centres of Aesculapius, the god of medicine—in

---

[82] TS 13 J 23, f. 13; Assaf and Meir (1944): 12; Mann (1969): II: 194–195; Gil (1983): II: 469.
[83] Dvorjetski (1994b); idem, (1996a).
[84] TS 8 J 14, f. 20; Bodl. MS Heb. C 13, f. 17; ibid., f. 18; TS 16.248; TS NS 325.81 a; Mann (1969): II: 193, 197; Gil (1983): II: 463–467; See also Schwab (1912): 127.
[85] Assaf and Meir (1944): 12.
[86] Avi-Yonah (1963): 325–326; Mazor and Bar-Nathan (1995): 129; Zias (1997): 55–56.
[87] *Jerusalem Talmud*, *Megila* 1, 1 [70a]; *Babylonian Talmud*, *Sanhedrin* 12a; cf. *ibid.*, *Megila* 6a; Amir (1976): 437.
[88] Gil (1983): I: 153.
[89] Dvorjetski (1997b); idem, forthcoming [b].

a large bathtub that was placed opposite the entrance of the *clibanus*.[90] The fame of Hammat-Gader as a medicinal place for leprosy was an important means of propaganda for residents of the site, whose concern was the profitability of the baths. In the words of Antoninus, the sick people who came to the healing thermal springs of Hammat-Gader were accommodated in a hostel that was publicly supported. It was not explicitly stated, though, that the mother city Gadara financed the hostel. This was possible, however, if we assume that the city benefited from any of the profits of the medicinal springs in its jurisdiction.[91]

Muslim historians and geographers provide a very important detail for the history of Hammei-Tiberias that aids us in clarifying why it is stated in the *Geniza* that the sufferers came to be healed in the city of Tiberias itself, rather than in its suburban hot springs. It seems that in the period of the Umayyad Caliphs, new bath houses were constructed, not where there were springs, but at the conduit to the city of Tiberias. The Egyptian-Muslim al-Ya'qubi (891) relates that the hot springs 'bubble up and never fail summer or winter. They carry the hot water into the baths by conduits, and thus people have no need of fuel for heating their water'.[92] The Persian Muslim al-Istahrī (951) added: 'There are hot springs which flow out near the city, rising about two leagues away; but even when the water reaches the town—although from the length of the conduit it has somewhat cooled—it is still so hot that skins thrown into it have the hair removed, and it is impossible to use the water (for bathing) until (cold water) has been mixed with it. This water is what is generally employed in the hot baths and the (mosque) tanks (for ablution).'[93]

al-Muqaddasi wrote a very important and detailed description:[94]

> Near Tiberias are boiling springs, which supply most of the hot baths of that town. A conduit goes to each bath from the springs, and the steam the water heats the whole building, whereby they have no need of artificial firing. In an outer building they set cold water, which, in certain proportion, has to be mixed with the hot by those who wish to bathe; and this same also serves in the (mosques) for the ablution. Within this

---

[90] Antoninus Placentinus, *Itinerarium* 7; Green and Tsafrir (1982): 32; Hirschfeld (1987): 105–106.
[91] Dan (1984): 117.
[92] al-Ya'qubi, *Kitab al-buldān* 115.
[93] al-Istahrī, *Suwar al-aklim* 58; Le Strange (1890): 334.
[94] al-Muqaddasi, *Ahsan al-taqasim fi ma'rifat al-aqalim* 185; Le Strange (1890): 335–336; Sukenik (1935a): 21–22; Buchmann (1968): 200; Meiri (1973): 32–33.

district are other hot springs, as at the place called al-Ḥammah [= the
thermal waters].[95] Those who suffer from the scab, or ulcers, or sores,
and other such-like diseases, come to bathe here during three days, and
then afterwards they dip in the water of another spring, which is cold,
whereupon—if Allah vouchsafes it to them—they become cured. I have
heard the people of Tiberias relate that all around these springs, down
to the time of Aristotle, there were bathhouses, each establishment being
for the cure of a specific disease, and those who were afflicted thereby
sojourned here and bathed for their cure. Aristotle, however, demanded
of the king of that time that these bathhouses should be pulled down,
lest thereby men should become expert from recourse to physicians. That
there are here several different waters, with various medicinal properties,
would appear to be a certain fact; for every sick person who comes here
now is obliged each one to immerse himself completely in the (mixed)
waters, in order to insure that he shall get to that which, in particular,
may heal his special disorder.

The Spanish Muslim geographer al-Idrīsī wrote in 1154 about
the many sufferers who apparently lived in a separate camp near the
thermal springs outside the city of Tiberias and on other sick people:
'and sick people from all neighboring countries stream to these springs,
especially those who are exhausted, lame, paralyzed, wounded, rheumatoid, and those with boils and eczema. They stay in the waters for
three days and become well with Allah's help.[96] To this list of healing
indications, one should add what Rabbi Moses ben Nahman, known
as HaRamban, said that those with *falaj* [= Podagra, gout] and those
who have the falling sickness [= epileptics] drink the waters of Hammei-
Tiberias.[97]

The special healing qualities of the thermal waters of Tiberias, as
manifested in the letters of the sufferers of this fate that were found in
the Cairo *Geniza*, are authentic and realistic and receive reinforcement
in the reports of pilgrims, historians and geographers of the period.
Hammei-Tiberias are good for curing many illnesses, their utility in
calming and soothing pains and diseases being among the most famous.[98]
(See Tab. 2).

---

[95] The springs named al-Ḥammah must be those of Gadara, or Ἐμμαθᾶ or
Ἀμμαθᾶ, in the Yarmuk Valley, near the present town of Umm Qais; See Le Strange
(1890): 336.

[96] al-Idrīsī, *Kitāb nuzhat al-mushtāq fī ikhtirāq al-ʿafāq* 10; Le Strange (1890): 339.

[97] *The Babylonian Talmud with Rav Elfas, Shabbat* 18a; *Maimonides to Mishnah Machshirin*
6, 7; See also Le Strange (1890): 339.

[98] Dechent (1884): 73–210; Robinson and Smith (1841): 258–260; Buchmann (1933):
299–300; idem, (1947): 90–106; Meiri (1973): 29–34; Simon (1978): 57–62; Dvorjetski
(1994b); idem, (1996a); idem, (2004): 16–21.

5.4   MEDICINAL PROPERTIES IN LIGHT OF ARCHAEOLOGICAL FINDS

From the archaeological finds at the thermo-mineral baths in the
Graeco-Roman world it is possible to learn about the variegated use
of medicine in antiquity, the maladies, the curative methods, ritual
worship in the sites, and the relationship between various classes. At
this stage they are quite sparse in the eastern Mediterranean basin,
and it is difficult to indicate finds of medical instruments at the healing places. However, certain finds may point to the properties of the
therapeutic baths.[99]

5.4.1   *Numismatic Evidence*

The medicinal qualities of the thermo-mineral baths in the eastern
Mediterranean may be inferred from the coins of the cities of Tiberias,
Gadara and Pella, within whose municipal boundaries were remedial
thermae.[100]

The Tiberias coins served to publicize the Tiberias hot springs in
the form of the goddess of health Hygieia, alone or together with
her father Aesculapius, god of medicine; He was identified with the
oriental and local deity of Sarapis, who is represented on the coins of
Tiberias, the city of the thermo-mineral waters. The administrators
of the city were well aware of the value of the curative springs and
coins were issued bearing the effigy and Sarapis in his quality as god
of health;[101] Hammat-Gader promoted its baths with the image of
the Three Graces; and on its coins Pella showed off Athena and the
nymphaeum. It is possible that statues of Hygieia and Aesculapius, of the

---

[99] For general survey on the medicinal hot springs and spas in the Graeco-Roman
world, see Jackson (1990a); Dvorjetski (1997a); Jackson (1999); See especially the discussion in chapter 3 on *The Medicinal Hot Springs and Healing Spas in the Graeco-Roman
World*; This overview is based on Dvorjetski (1992b); idem, (1993a); idem, (1994a);
idem, (1994b); idem, (1994c).

[100] For Tiberias coins, see de Saulcy (1874): 335; Kindler (1961): 54, 58; Rosenberger
(1977): 67; Meshorer (1985): 34–35; Dvorjetski (1990); For Gadara coins, see Spijkerman
(1978): 137–155; Meshorer (1985): 80, 83; Henig and Whiting (1987): 18–19, 27–28;
Dvorjetski (1990); idem, (1993a); idem, (1994c); On Pella coins see Smith (1973): 58–59;
Spijkerman (1978): 215; Meshorer (1985): 92; Price and Trell (1977): 44; Bowsher
(1987): 63; Dvorjetski (1992a): 197–199; idem, (1994a): 14; idem, (1994c).

[101] McCasland (1939): 221–227; Kindler (1961): 30, 40; Dvorjetski (1992a): 187–189;
idem, (1994a): 11–12; idem, (2001–2002): 500–501; Compton (2002): 312–329; Dvorjetski (2004): 21, 26; See the discussion in chapter 8.1 on *The Numismatic Expression of
the Medicinal Hot Springs of Tiberias*.

Three Graces, of Athena, and Hercules were set up in temples in the vicinity of the therapeutic baths, as was customary at remedial sites in the Graeco-Roman world. The purpose of all this was to attract people to come to these spas for the cure, and so to stimulate the towns' economies.[102] (See Figs. 8, 22, 23, and 33).

5.4.2   *The Epigraphical Material*

Inscriptions in general faithfully tell the history and daily life of the thermo-mineral baths. Most of them were from private persons on the occasion of their visit at the sites—a visit that inspired wonder and gratitude in the presence of the healing powers of the baths.

A magic amulet was discovered in a tomb at Emmaus-Nicopolis and dated to the third century CE, inscribed with an incantation in Aramaic to clear up the afflictions of the patient from his head, muscles, testicles, and ears.[103] The description of the snake, the attribute of Aesculapius and Hygieia, on the amulet seems to hint at the therapeutic qualities, which are documented by Church Fathers as good not only for human beings but also for animals.[104] (See Fig. 28).

The epigraphic material from the bathhouse at Hammat-Gader consists of about seventy Greek inscriptions and some engraving in Kufic script in situ from the ninth century CE. Except for the small group of building inscriptions, most texts open with the words Ἐν τῷ ἁγίῳ or (ἱερῷ) τόπῳ μνησθῇ, which means 'in this holy place may someone be remembered'. The formula is very common throughout the eastern Mediterranean basin in Late Roman and Byzantine inscriptions. It generally appears in connection with holy places, such as temples, synagogues, churches, monasteries, and pilgrimage sites. The use of this kind of formula indicates that the *thermae* were regarded not as a pleasure resort or a sporting place consecrated to hygiene and body care, but as a healing site endowed with a God-given power of restoring health. The texts were dictated to local artisans, and permission to have the commission carried out was paid for by the visitor by means of an offering to the ἅγιος τοπός—*Holy place*.[105] (See Figs. 17 and 18).

---

[102] Spijkerman (1978): 82–83, 91–92, 97–98; Meshorer (1985): 82–83; Dvorjetski (1992a): 190–193; idem, (1993); idem, (1994c); idem (2001–2002): 501–502; idem (2004): 20–21, 26; See chapter 8.3 on *The Numismatic Expression of the Medicinal Hot Springs of Gadara*; See there Fig. 33 on the image of the ring from Gadara.

[103] Vincent (1908); cf. Naveh and Shaked (1985): 60–63.

[104] Vincent and Abel (1932): 416–418; Dvorjetski (1996a): 44.

[105] Di Segni (1999): 185–186.

Some of the visitors mentioned their homeland, among them an *agens in rebus* from Gaza, a notary from Damascus, a lawyer from Tyre, a family from Bosra; an acclamation in honour in Pamphylia shows that some of its citizens came here as well. Several visitors indicated their title, rank or profession: among them army officers, public servants and an aristocratic family, composed of a count, his wife the *comitissa* and another woman, illustris by rank. The stage professions represent the largest group: a dancer, a piper, an actress, a juggler, and perhaps a strolling actor. These performers were permanent or visiting members of its staff in the Roman theatre of Hammat-Gader, which was still active in the Byzantine period.[106] Two engravers (of precious stones and seals), two marble workers, a scriber and public weighers are also mentioned;[107] Governors are mentioned as responsible for construction works in several inscriptions in the bathhouse. Such is the case of the building inscription in the small elliptical pool in the time of Flavius Petrus Romanus. Alexander and Leon from Caesarea built the *tholos* of the warm pool. Three metric inscriptions mentioning the governor of Palestina Secunda Mucius Alexander bear witness to restoration and reconstruction works during the reign of Emperor Anastasius (491–518 CE).[108] (See Figs. 14, 15, 16, 17, 18, 19, and 20).

The most important inscription bears the name and title of Byzantine Empress Eudocia, Emperor Theodosius II's wife (408–450 CE). The poetic inscription in Homeric style glorifies the hot springs 'for those in pain', and extols the marvels of the architectural complex—the *clibanus*—erected around them.[109] Meïmaris suggests that Eudocia's visit to the famous baths could be associated with a medical reason.[110] The *Vita Melaniae Junioris* written by Gerontius, abbot on Mount of Olives, recounts that during the inauguration of Saint Stephen Protomartyer church in Jerusalem on May 15, 439 CE, an accident caused her severe pain in her left leg and Empress came to Hammat-Gader to cure it.[111] (See Fig. 13).

---

[106] Segal (1990): 100.
[107] Di Segni (1992): 309–310.
[108] Di Segni and Hirschfeld (1986): 265–267.
[109] Hirschefeld (1981): 203; Green and Tsafrir (1982): 77–91; Dvorjetski (1988): 101–107; idem, (1992a): 111–112; Di Segni (1997): 228–233.
[110] Meïmaris (1983): 394.
[111] Gerontius, *Vita Melaniae Junioris* 59, 244; See Habas-Rubin (1996): 112–113; Di Segni (1997): 232.

Other parts of Hammat-Gader were referred to by names and titles of various people, such as 'Elijah the Holy', whose honor the thermae were later said to have been named *Thermae Heliae*.[112] The inscription comprises a list of first names, pagan and Christian titles, mythological figures and things that are clearly part of the baths, such as pools and fountains. Two figures of Greek mythology are also mentioned in the inscription: Hygieia and Galatea. Both suit the spas. Hygieia was goddess of health and the patroness of spas, and Galatea was a nymph associated in springs and water-sources. The *clibanus*, the source of the hot stream, is called Paean, the physician of the gods, because of the healing powers of its waters.[113]

At Hammat-Gader no less than 24 inscriptions are decorated with one or more crosses, and all are later than 455 CE. The Church viewed with suspicion the habit of mixed bathing—not only for the sake of modesty, but also because of the dictates of ascetic behavior.[114] (See, for instance, Figs. 13, 14, 16, 18 and 21).

On a slab of grey marble from Hammat-Gader there is a depiction of feet as well as two hands pointing to the southeast. Below the left foot and hand there is a Greek inscription, which bears the name Asklepios and the repeatedly formula Ἐν τῷ ἀγίῳ or (ἱερῷ) τόπῳ μνησθῇ Ασκ[λή]πιος [= in this holy place may Asklepios be remembered]. Asklepios [= Aesculapius] was the god of medicine, but is also well known as a man's name.[115] They may reflect the old pagan custom of presenting votive legs, symbolizing the legs of Serapis, as thanks offered for being cured. Votive feet were often dedicated to pagan gods, especially by pilgrims who had reached the end of their journey; in this case, however, the late date and the orientation of the drawing—toward Mecca—are a clear indication of its Islamic origin and significance in the Umayyad or 'Abbāsid period. According to Islamic law, every Muslim who attains his majority has to pray five times a day. He need

---

[112] See the unique evidence of Antoninus from Placentia below and his report in chapter 4.2 about *The Historical-Archaeological Analysis and Healing Cults of Hammat-Gader.*

[113] Hirschefeld (1981): 203; Green and Tsafrir (1982): 77–91; Di Segni (1997): 228–233.

[114] Di Segni (1997): 186; Dvorjetski (2006–2007): 19–22; See also the discussion in chapter 9.3.3 on *The Epigraphical Material from Hammat-Gader Thermal Baths.*

[115] Roozenbeek (1990): 26; Di Segni (1997): 193, Fig. 8; Amitai-Preiss (1997): 274–275; On stone slabs with imprints of feet, in some cases with a few pairs of feet on each slab, see Cante (1984): 193.

not go to a mosque but may perform the prayers (*salāt*) in a dwelling room or any other place. It is thus possible that this slab served as an indication of the correct direction to be adopted by Muslims when they prayed within the precincts of the thermae.[116] The right foot and the left hand depicted on the slab have six digits. The phenomenon of six fingers or toes (polydactylism) is not uncommon and is an inherited genetic abnormality, especially in closely-interbred communities. The appearance of polydactylism in ancient art and archaeology is not widespread. Barnett recorded ten cases, all of a divine or semi-divine nature, which cover a wide chronological and geographical range.[117] It seems that this giant or the person who inscribed the inscription in Greek prayed to god, who watched over and safeguarded all aspects of everyday life. He had presumably wrought a cure to some affliction on his hands and feet, which caused him pains.

Toward the end of the Byzantine period, the location was hit by an earthquake. The destruction caused the baths is documented in a Greek-Byzantine inscription from the seventh century. The dedicatory Greek inscription, discovered in the Fountain Hall, cites the reopening and renovation of the baths in the early days of the Caliph Abdallah Mu'āwiya, founder of the Umayyad dynasty, on 5 December 662 CE. The goal of this work is emphasized very clearly: εἰς ἴασην τῶν νοσούντων [= for the healing of the sick].[118] (See Fig. 21).

Likewise, the donors' inscriptions in the synagogues at Hammat-Tiberias, dated to the fourth century CE and Hammat-Gader of the fifth-sixth century CE, contribute information on Jews and gentiles, who went there.[119] The mosaic inscriptions from both sites were dedicated in the names of donors who contributed to the synagogues' buildings. These donors might have been cured at the spas of Hammat-Gader and Hammei-Tiberias and commemorated their recovery by contributing to the development of the sites. The formula of the blessing in the inscription from Hammat-Tiberias 'May he be alive', or 'to survive safely' (ζήσῃ or σωζέστω) repeated five times, is unusual, and such a

---

[116] Gibb and Kramers (1974): 493, s.v. 'salāt'; Amitai-Preiss (1997): 275.

[117] Barnett (1986–1987): 5–6; idem, (1990): 46–51; See also Amitai-Preiss (1997): 276.

[118] Hirschfeld and Solar (1981): 203–204; Hasson (1982): 97–101; Blau (1982): 102; Green and Tsafrir (1982): 94–96; Di Segni and Hirschfeld (1986): 265–266; Dvorjetski (1988): 109–110; idem, and Last (1991): 162; Dvorjetski (1992a): 113; Di Segni (1992): 315–317; idem, (1997): 237–240.

[119] Dothan (1983); See also Sukenik (1935b); Avi-Yonah (1993): 566–569.

blessing, wishing the donors life, is apt for sick people who have come to the place for a cure.[120] (See Fig. 31). The Aramaic name *Meinuk* which means baby and appears several times in the dedicatory inscription from the synagogue at Hammat-Gader, attests that their parents brought their children to be cured there.[121]

The sixth century CE Madaba mosaic map, which laid in a Byzantine church at Madaba in Jordan, allots considerable space to the thermomineral waters of Kallirrhoe and Ba'arah, including the inscriptions [Βα]άρου and θερμὰ καλλιρόης.[122] (See Fig. 25). The mosaicists of the Madaba map represented along the eastern shore of the Dead Sea three constructions: a round pool from which water flows, a square reservoir with a semi-circular construction probably a *nymphaeum* and a channel widening in the plain, barraged by a wall or a dam, pouring water into the lake. This construction was a basin for bathing filled with flowing hot water, which could be mixed with cooler waters or with minerals. The archaeological remains at Kallirrhoe, 'Ain Ez-Zara, are rather poor. All the constructions vanished entirely except the third installation. Traces of ancient harbour have been destroyed by road works. Roman villa compounds with rooms aligned along a central peristyle courtyard are suggested that the remains of the ancient buildings there were originally baths built by King Herod the Great.[123]

We know of boats in the Roman Empire that carried various cargoes from the healing sites. Among them were glass vessels, simple and decorated bottles; and ceramic vessels that contained liquids for healing purposes. For examples, the healing site in northern Spain, Salus Umeritana, gained fame from its waters, which were exported to distant locations. (See Fig. 6). Glass bottles from the thermal medicinal waters in the Bay of Naples, Baiae and neighboring Puteoli, arrived in North Africa and other countries; engraved on them were schematic scenes of the thermal baths where the bottles were manufactured and marketed.[124] (See Fig. 5).

The two boats described on the Madaba map carried, apparently, cargoes relating to the medicinal materials of the healing sites. These

---

[120] Roth-Gerson (1987): 67.
[121] Naveh (1978): 11: 58.
[122] Avi-Yonah (1954): 39–40; Donner (1982): 175–180; Piccirillo (1993): 206.
[123] Donner (1963); Clamer (1989); idem, (1993): 221–225; Dvorjetski (1995b); Clamer (1996); Weber (1997): 333–334.
[124] Painter (1975): 54–67; Jackson (1990a): 7.

were probably ceramic and glass containers, medical instruments and consumer items for the patients. The various colors of the boats' cargo may indicate their essence. It is known that the color of small ceramic vessels, jars and little flasks, was diverse, depending on the type of clay and the nature of the refining process. Most had a 'natural' clay color, reddish-brown; there were also bright and dark-grey vessels. The glass vessels that were most prevalent were colorless translucent ones; however, not a few vessels were made of a colorful brown, green, or blue color. Ceramic and glass vessels and other items were placed in piles in a bulk, and not inside a container. One may surmise that the cargoes were covered with sheets of cloth to preserve and protect them. It seems that the ships' load in the Dead Sea according to the Madaba map was connected to the thermo-mineral baths of Ba'arah and Kallirrhoe, which can be any kind of glass vessels, pottery assemblages, and medical instruments to the very many populace who came to the sites to be cured. Moreover, the Madaba map served, among other things, as a guide for those wishing specifically to visit particular spas, presumably with the intent of taking advantage of the healing benefits of the spring waters.[125]

5.4.3   *Little Finds*

The discovery of an unusual hoard of glass fragments at Hammat-Tiberias and at Hammat-Gader may indicate healing by means of potions, as was mentioned above from the Talmudic corpus, especially for the unique *Kasaia Tiberiah*, The glasses of Tiberias. As no glassworks was revealed in the baths complex of Hammat-Gader, most probably that the factory existed either at the neighboring site Hammat-Tiberias, or the city of Gadara supplied such vessels, glasses and other things to the thermal baths. In the garden area of the Ganei-Hammat Hotel on the west coast of Lake Kinneret an excavation was conducted by Oren, but only a brief report on the early Islamic material has been published. A large building of circa 250 metres was uncovered comprising nine spacious rooms and underground reservoirs and latrines. The building was provided with a water system for drinking water and for drainage. A workshop where pottery was glazed was found in one of the rooms with pots *in situ* reflecting the different stages of production. A number

---

[125] Dvorjetski (1996c); For the voyages for health and cures, see Chevallier (1988): 322–325.

of artefacts including iron ploughs, chisels, drills and other tools were
found in another room and in yet another jewellery, rings, and other
cosmetic articles were found. The building was first constructed in the
Umayyad period, und destroyed in the mid-eighth century CE, after
which it was rebuilt and used in later times. The nature of the finds
suggests that the building was a significant industrial complex. Other
evidence of industrial activity at the site suggests the existence of a
glass factory at the site.[126]

Comparing to all other therapeutic sites, from a quantitative examination, it appears that most of the glass vessels found in the excavation
at Hammat-Gader are closed vessels, such as bottles, juglets, *amphoriskoi*,
tubes, and jars dated from the third-fourth century CE to seventh-eighth
century. Also noteworthy is the relatively large number of glass lamps
and drinking vessels—cups and goblets, plates and bowels.[127] This fact
is indeed indicative of the use in the baths of various perfumes, oils,
and creams that were stored in closed vessels as well as other medicinal
ointments and materials. Additionally, vessel stamps were revealed at
the site below the debris resulting from the 749 CE earthquake. Thus,
it can be assumed that they were in use until the destruction of the site.
All five pieces bear devout phrases; four features the expression *alwafā
lillah* [= Honesty to God], and the fifth, *Bismillah* [= In the Name of
God].[128] Miles suggested that vessel stamps used for labeling pharmaceutical containers and measuring cups for liquids, semi-liquids, various
substances and seeds which were all part of the Arab pharmacopoeia.[129]
Balog reaffirmed this thesis that the vessels were for substances used
in the every day medical practice of the eighth and ninth centuries.[130]
Morton holds that there was no need to indicate a special qist stamp for
olive oil, as the term 'qist' of the glass weights, was a general reference
measure for olive oil and was most universally known.[131]

The use of olive oil in baths was undoubtedly continued from the
Roman period, as the Roman tradition of baths and bathing was
adapted by Islam.[132] Several utensils containing ampullae and flasks for

---

[126] Oren (1971): 234–235; Zeyadeh (1994): 126; See also Dvorjetski (2001–2002):
506.
[127] Cohen (1997): 396–431; See also Rabbi Judah the Patriarch's deeds at Hammei-
Tiberias.
[128] Lester (1997): 432–441.
[129] Miles (1960): 384; cf. Morton (1985): 33–35.
[130] Balog (1976): 29; See also Lester (1997): 432.
[131] Morton (1987): 32–33.
[132] Yegül (1992): 341–349.

perfumes and oils and bronze vessels for holding oils, were known from various spas' sites throughout the Roman Empire for digestive disorders, internal ailments as well as dermatological treatments.[133]

The majority of the lamps were found concentrated in two areas in Hammat-Gader and approaches 350, In *Area B* they were found in groups on the bottom of the small rectangular pool. Another concentration of lamps was found in an alcove, in the southern wing of the Hall of Fountains in *Area D*. They uncovered also in groups and apparently had been stored there. It is interesting to note that many of the Hammat-Gader lamps lack the soot marks which are characteristic of oil lamps even after single use. The large quantity of such lamps suggests the possibility that they were linked to certain cults or traditions practised in the baths complex. It might also correlate to Hammat-Gader numerous dedicatory inscriptions and formulas 'in this holy place' considered to be a 'holy place'.[134]

Hirschfeld and Solar are convinced that Antoninus Placentius' description regarding the bathing procedures, which the lepers underwent at Hammat-Gader, correlate closely both with the characteristics of the double-sloped pool in Area B and with the oil lamps found in it. They are all very similar in style and all lack the soot. The lepers used these lamps as an element of some ritual ceremony conducted at the pool. On the basis of archaeological appraisals, the pool and its hall have been dated to the third-fourth centuries CE.[135] It is already been seen that the use of ritual lamps has been found in several cult places in Palestine. This originally west-Semitic practice had become a universal form of tribute, above all in private and domestic rituals. However, these lamps might have fallen accidentally to the pool. The special inn built and maintained by the local inhabitants for the leper testifies to the fame of Hammat-Gader as a place of healing for leprosy.[136]

---

[133] Heinz (1983): Fig. 15; Yegül (1992): Fig. 33; Nenova-Merdjanova (1997): 30–37; See the survey of *The Spas in the Graeco-Roman World* in chapter 3; Lester's (1997: 433) comments that 'oils were applied to protect the skin from direct contact with various minerals and salts'—is partial; and that 'very little has been written about the use of thermo-mineral baths'—is baseless and very superficial; See also Ben-Arieh (1997): 347–381.

[134] Uzzielli (1997): 319.

[135] Hirschfeld (1981): 209–211; idem, (1984): 30, 33.

[136] Belayche (2001: 272) is convinced that the mention of the lamps supports her hypothesis that it taken over by the Christian community as well as the inn there. Unfortunately, there are no unequivocal Christian epigraphical or literary evidences for that; See Dvorjetski (1988): 10; idem, (1994b); idem, (1996a).

There were certainly cults of Serapis and Aesculapius practiced at
the city of Gadara. A bearded marble mask found there, is most likely
a pilgrim's souvenir from the Alexandrian Serapion.[137] Aesculapius is
shown on a lost altar in a military attitude, wearing an armour and
holding the spear with the serpent in the hand. The military attitude
of the healing god seems to be a local feature. A similar representation of the same warrior healing god comes from Kufr Ma on the
Golan Heights.[138] It is important to point out that the Sa'd collection
of engraved gems from Gadara includes some intaglios and cameos,
which devoted to Serapis, Hygieia, and Aesculapius as well, dated to
the first-second century CE.[139] (See Fig. 32).

According to the archaeological finds in the Graeco-Roman world,
Gadara must have been the place where specialized surgeons and
physicians provided a reliable treatment of various diseases. A tomb
within the Early Byzantine crypt of the great mausoleum in the western suburb of Gadara city was found. Besides various glass vessels it
produced a set of cosmetic instruments made of metal. A pair of iron
forceps evidences that one of the individuals buried in the grave was
a dentist.[140]

At Hammam ad-Dable, in the fill beneath the wide stairway of the
west side of the Civic Complex church, a fragment of a life-size statue
of dark blue schist of apparent Egyptian provenance was found. It features an enthroned deity draped with a thick garment covering the legs
up to the hip. The dark stone and the characteristic drapery indicate
that it belonged to a copy of the famous Alexanderine cult statue of
Serapis, created by the sculptor Bryaxis in the late forth century BCE.
Thus, it is possible that a Serapion was located in the vicinity of Pella's
Roman-period forum in Wadi Jirm al-Mawz.[141]

The site of the thermal springs Ba'arah has never been investigated
archaeologically. There is a connection of a votive inscription found at
al-Harra in southern Syria to the local cult of the Hammei-Ba'arah.
The alter is dedicated by a Roman official of the Bataneae, named
Diomedes Charetos in the rank of a governor (*eparchos*) and military

---

[137] Weber (1997): 336.
[138] Sourdel (1952): 47; Künzl and Weber (1991): 82; Weber (1997): 336.
[139] Henig and Whiting (1987): 9–10, 21.
[140] Künzl and Weber (1991): 81–118.
[141] Smith and Day (1989): 56–57; Smith (1992): 204–205; Weber (1993): 47–49;
idem, (1997): 335.

commander (*strategos*).[142] For the sake of his recovery he donated the votive offering to Zeus Baalbaaros, the local god Baal of Ba'arah, who was identical with the Moabite god Kemosh.[143] (See Fig. 27).

In sum, then, according to the archaeological documents, the inscriptions described the history and daily life of the spas. Most of them were from private persons on the occasion of their visit at the sites—a visit that inspired wonder and gratitude in the presence of the healing powers of the baths; The ritual worship characteristics of Hammei-Tiberias, Hammat-Gader and Hammat-Pella are expressed in most interesting types of Hygieia, Aesculapius, Sarapis, the Three Graces, and the Nymphs. The coins of Tiberias, Gadara and Pella with their depiction and inscriptions enable us to understand the essence of the local worship and the identity of those who erected their baths. Greek Aesculapius could easily be identified with the local gods such as Baal. Besides the Graeco-Roman gods Egyptian Serapis and the local Baal played an important role in the nature of the spas as a healing and fertility local gods.[144]

5.5 A Test Case: The Medical History of Rabbi Judah the Patriarch

The Rabbinic literature contains more references to the maladies of Rabbi Judah the Patriarch than to the illnesses of any other of its Sages and personalities and provides an authentic and vivid picture of his illnesses. The numerous references to his own ailments and to other medical matters, such as spas, which were regarded highly for their ability to restore health, provide an authentic and vivid picture of medicine in the Roman period and of Rabbi Judah's medical history in particular. This information will be detailed and discussed.[145]

Rabbi Judah I (*HaNasi*) was the Patriarch of Judaea at the latter half of the second and beginning of the third century CE, and the redactor of the Mishnah, that vast volume of Jewish legal tradition. He is referred to also as *Rabbenu HaKadosh*, our holy teacher, or simply

---

[142] Sourdel (1952): 45–46, Pl. 4:1; Hübner (1995): 252–255.
[143] Worschech (1992): 393–394; Weber (1997): 333.
[144] Dvorjetski (1994a); idem, forthcoming [b].
[145] A primary abridged discussion is presented in Dvorjetski (1992a): 136–141; idem, (2001a): 232–236; See also idem, (2002).

as *Rabbi*. Judah was the son of Rabban Simeon ben Gamaliel and the
seventh or sixth generation descended from Hillel the Elder, having
been born, according to an *Aggadic* tradition, 'on the day that Rabbi
Akiva died,' during the Hadrianic persecutions (*Babylonian Talmud,
Qiddushin* 72b). He became the most eminent and powerful political
communal and religious leader of the Jewish people of his time. Both
his contemporaries and latter generations held him in veneration, and
regarded him as the saviour of Israel, as much as Simeon ben Setah,
Mattathias the Hashmonean, and Mordecai and Esther (*ibid., Megilla*
11a). The sages found in him all the qualities which they enumerated
as being to the righteous (*Mishna, Avot* 6, 8). They even associated his
name with messianic aspirations to the extent of applying to him the
verse (*Lamentations* 4, 20), 'The breath of our nostrils, the anointed of the
Lord' (*Jerusalem Talmud, Shabbat* 15, 1[15c]). His wisdom, sanctity, and
humility, as well as his wealth and close ties with the Roman Emperor,
became the subjects of numerous legends.[146] His mastery of the vast
volume of tradition, his great application to his studies (*ibid., Ketuboth*
104a), his humility (*Mishnah, Sota* 9, 15), coupled with self-confidence,
sound judgment, and a rule that was based on a strict discipline (*Babylonian Talmud, Ketuboth* 103b), combined to give authority to his leadership
and an undisputed status to the patriarchate.[147]

During his presidency, the Sanhedrin—the supreme religious and
political body of the Jews in the period of the Second Temple and
later—convened at different places from time to time. This would have
required its president to re-locate with it.[148] However, the *Babylonian
Talmud, Ketuboth* 103b–104a relates, that Rabbi Judah moved his domicile permanently from Beth Shearim to Sepphoris,[149] where he spent
the last seventeen years of his life. The move was said to be due to his
frail state of health:[150]

---

[146] Blidstein (1971): 366–372.
[147] For the period of Rabbi Judah I, see Graetz (1897): 192–219; Levine (1982):
93–118; Alon (1996): 709–717; Levine (1989): 33–37; idem, (2001): 103–137.
[148] Oppenheimer (1983): 258–260; Goodman (1992): 127–139; Büchler (1956):
235–236.
[149] Epstein (1936): 663; Oppenheimer (1991): 68; On Sepphoris, see Meshorer
(1979): 159–171; Kraay (1980): 53–57; Freyne (1980): 122–128; Meyers, Netzer and
Meyers (1992); Meyers (1992): 321–338; Ne'eman (1993); Weiss (1994); Weiss and
Netzer (1996).
[150] It is possible that number seventeen derives from the *Midrash*, which compares
Rabbi's years to those of Jacob spent in Egypt (*Jerusalem Talmud, Kil'aim*, 9, 3 [32b];
ibid., Ketuboth, 12, 3 [35a]; *Genesis Rabbah* 95, 28 (Theodor-Albek ed., p. 1234); *Tanhuma, Vayhi* 3 (Buber ed., p. 215); See Safrai (1982a): 150; Klein (1967): 90; Ne'eman
(1996): 38–42.

It was taught: Rabbi was lying [= on his sick bed] at Sepphoris but a [= burial] place was reserved for him at Beth Shearim. Was it not, however, taught: 'Justice, justice shalt thou follow' (*Deuteronomy* 16, 20): follow Rabbi to Beth Shearim. Rabbi was living at Beth Shearim, but when he fell ill, he was brought to Sepphoris because it was situated on higher ground and its air was salubrious.

He was buried in the famous necropolis used by the Jewish upper classes, at Beth Shearim.[151]

5.5.1 *Rabbi Judah's Bowel Disease*

According to the Talmudic sources, the most severe of Rabbi Judah's afflictions was his bowel disease. He suffered from it to the end of his days (*Babylonian Talmud, Ketuboth* 103b). It may be no coincidence that in *Ecclesiastes Rabbah* 7, 21—bowel disease is regarded as one of 'three complaints serious to the body, more serious than heart disease.' A compassionate and vivid description of Rabbi Judah's bowel symptoms is given in the following episode in the *Babylonian Talmud, Baba Metzia* 85a:[152]

> The stableman of Rabbi's house was wealthier than King Shavor [= Shapur of Persia]. When he would throw fodder to the animals, the noise the animals made was so loud it would be heard for three miles. [= The stableman] would schedule himself so that he threw the fodder at the same time that Rabbi entered his privy in order to drown out the noises made by him. Nevertheless, [= Rabbi's] voice lifted in pain was louder than theirs, and was heard even by seafarers.

In the Rabbinic literature, anal disorders are called *tachtoniot*, literally 'inferiors'.[153] The term referred primarily to hemorrhoids, but the non-medical compilers might well have used it to indicate any rectal or anal disorder that is accompanied by pain or bleeding. Piles are mentioned on numerous occasions in the Rabbinic literature. Thus, for example:[154]

---

[151] Blidstein (1971): 372; Guttmann (1954): 256–260; Safrai, (1958): 211; Shwabe and Lifshitz (1967); Avigad (1972); Levine (1989): 103; Weiss (1992): 357–371.

[152] Rabbinovicz (1887): 246; On Rabbi Judah's great wealth, see for instance, Krauss (1910): 17–26; Klein (1911–1912): 545–550; Alon (1971): 132–133; Levine (1989): 100–102; Oppenheimer (1991): 66–71; On Antoninus's traditions, see Jacobs (1995): 125–154; Cohen (1998): 141–171.

[153] Jastrow (1950): 1662; Perlman (1926): 103–104; Preuss (1993): 185–186; Goldstein and Shechter (1956): I: 440–441; See also Ben Horin (1933): 100.

[154] See also *Babylonian Talmud, Ketuboth* 10b–11a; *ibid., Nedarim* 22a; *ibid., Berachot* 55a.

Ten things that bring on *tachtoniot* include eating the leaves of reeds, the leaves or the sprouts of vines, and wiping oneself with lime, potters clay, or pebbles that have been used by another. Some add, to strain oneself unduly in a privy.

(ibid., Shabbat 81a)

Throughout antiquity small stones were used to cleanse the anus after defecation.[155] Rabbi Judah's striking preoccupation with this topic is demonstrated by the description of his visit to the thermo-mineral baths at Hammat-Gader in two parallel texts:[156]

Rabbi Hanina said, 'Once we were going up with Rabbi to Hammat-Gader, and he would say to us, "Choose for yourselves pieces of stones, and you will then be permitted to carry them about tomorrow."' [= on the Shabbat].

(Jerusalem Talmud, Shabbat 4, 6 [7a])

Rabbi Ze'ira in the name of Rabbi Hanina said, 'Once we were going up with Rabbi to Hammat-Gader. He would say to us, "Choose for yourselves smooth pebbles, and you will then be permitted to carry them about tomorrow."' [= on the Shabbat].

(ibid., Shabbat 18, 1 [16c])

On the occasion of his visits to the thermo-mineral baths of Hammat-Gader, Rabbi Judah is quoted to our utter astonishment, as giving just one single piece of Jewish ritual advice to his colleagues, 'Choose for yourselves smooth pebbles, and you will then be permitted to carry them about tomorrow.' Rabbi Judah the Patriarch presumably gave this instruction on the eve of Shabbat, when the carrying of any objects outside the home was prohibited on the following day. Therefore, he advised his disciples to make preparations beforehand, by choosing some pebbles for the following day. That made it permissible to carry them around on the Shabbat, for use after their likely bowel motion. It shows Rabbi Judah's enormous obsession with his bowels, if he stressed some trivial advice about the use of stones for cleansing after bowel motions on the Shabbat.[157]

[155] Preuss (1993): 547; Dvorjetski (1995a): 43–52; Buchmann (1955): 287–291.

[156] It is written wrongly and it must be Gader instead of Gerar; See Rabbinovicz (1887): 240; Klein (1939): 74; Neusner (1991): 167–168, 445.

[157] Hirschberg (1920): 232–233; On the use of smooth pebbles at the medicinal baths, see Dvorjetski (1995a): 43–52; idem, (1999): 117–129; On Rabbi Hanina's occupation in medicine, see Halov (1838): 27; Bacher (1925): 5; Beer (1982): 284; Kottek (1996): 2931.

As would be likely in a person suffering from bowel disease, there is evidence that Rabbi Judah was particularly fussy about his diet. He was concerned about the timing and frequency of his meals, possibly on the advice of his doctors and confidants: 'Rabbi was fastidious. When he ate by day, he would not eat in the evening' (*ibid., Pesahim* 9, 1 [37b]).[158]

We are informed about the diets of Rabbi Judah and the Roman Emperor, probably Caracalla, and the contemporary beliefs about different vegetables on the digestion:[159]

> Antoninus and Rabbi, from whose table neither lettuce, nor radish nor cucumber was ever absent either in summer or in winter; and as a master has said: radish helps the food to dissolve, lettuce helps the food to be digested, and cucumber makes the intestines expand.
> (*Babylonian Talmud, Avoda Zarah* 11a)

Rabbi Judah's bowel disease seems to have followed a fluctuating course. Some improvement, or at any rate a temporary remission, was achieved by means of a potion derived from a special apple-cider:[160]

> Our Rabbis taught: Rabbi once suffered from a disorder of the bowels and said, 'Does anyone know whether apple-cider of a heathen is prohibited or permitted?' Rabbi Ishmael ben Rabbi Yose replied, 'My father once had the same complaint and they brought him apple-cider of a heathen which was seventy years old. He drank it and recovered'. He said to him, 'You had this information all this time and you let me suffer!' They made inquiry and found a heathen who possessed three hundred jars of apple-cider seventy years old. [= Rabbi] drank some of it and recovered; whereupon he exclaimed, 'Blessed be the All-present who delivered His Universe into the keeping of guardians!'
> (*Babylonian Talmud, Avoda Zarah* 40b)

Rabbi Judah the Patriarch was forced to resort to this medication in the absence of alternative remedies because of his severe pains,

---

[158] *Jerusalem Talmud, Pesahim* 9, 1 [37b], Venice ed., 1523; For another example of Rabbi being fastidious, see *Babylonian Talmud, Sanhedrin* 11a.
[159] Ulmann (1950): 205; Feldman (1962): 216–219, 271–274; Kagen (1933): 91; Ben Horin (1937): 93–99; For the identification and conversations of the Roman Emperor, see Krauss (1910); Gutmann (1959): 422–424; Avi-Yonah (1970): 51–56; Herr (1971): 123–150; Safrai (1975): 52; Marmorstein (1971): 1116; Stern (1980): II: 626–627; Newmyer (1988): 108–113; Cohen (1998): 142–171; Millar (2001): 207.
[160] On apple-cider, see Krauss (1911): 245–246; Schocett (1933): 83; Rabin (1959): 149–152; Shapira (1962): 48; Steinfeld (1986): 125–143; On the connection between gout and drinking wine among the Roman aristocracy, see Nriagu (1983): 660–663.

despite the fact that it was the property of a gentile, and its origin was therefore ritually questionable. This recovery was neither complete nor permanent.

On one occasion, Rabbi Judah's illness must have been very severe indeed. The *Babylonian Talmud, Nedarim* 41a, describes an incident, when he was ill and 'forgot his learning'. He was helped to recall the texts by Rabbi Hiyya Rabba and by Katzra, his confidant, 'who never divulged this event' at the time.[161] While the nature of the illness that caused this temporary amnesia is not mentioned, his bowel disease is the likeliest cause of the episode.

Babylonian Talmud, Ketuboth 103b illuminates the arrogant attitude of Rabbi Judah to his bowel disease. During a discussion with Rabbi Hiyya, about the omens associated with the various causes of death, he declared, 'Dying of diarrhea is a good omen because most righteous men die of diarrhea'.[162]

> When Rabbi fell ill Rabbi Hiyya entered into his presence and found him weeping. 'Master,' he said to him, 'Why are you weeping?' Was it not taught: '[= If a man]…dying of diarrhea is a good omen because most righteous men die of diarrhea?'
>
> (*ibid., Ketuboth* 103b)

The fact that Rabbi Judah visited his privy several times on the day of his death is particularly mentioned in *Ketuboth* 104a: 'Rabbi's handmaid saw how often he resorted to his privy painfully taking off his *tefillin* and putting them on again, and he was sorry'.[163]

5.5.2   *Rabbi Judah's Other Illnesses*

Other descriptions of Rabbi Judah's diseases in the Talmudic sources do not lend themselves to a precise modern medical interpretation. A text in *Babylonian Talmud, Baba Mezi'a* 85a, describes that Rabbi Judah suffered torments for thirteen years:

> Rabbi said, 'How beloved is suffering'. He then accepted thirteen years of suffering upon himself: six [= years] of *Tzemirtha* and seven [= years] of *Tzafrana*.

---

[161] On Katzra [= laundryman], see Kohut (1926): VII: 178; Ayli (1987): 137–138; Efrati (1984): 19; Safrai (1995): 228–229; It is very interesting that some texts which deal with bowel diseases are reported by Rabbi Hiyya, such as remarked in the *Babylonian Talmud, Gittin* 70a and in *Midrash Deuteronomy Rabbah* 8, 4.

[162] *Babylonian Talmud, Ketuboth* 103b.

[163] *Babylonian Talmud, Ketuboth* 103b–104a; See Meir (1990): 147–177.

Talmudic scholars maintain that *Tzemirtha* refers to urinary calculi. However, as it was described in the Talmud by laypersons, it might have referred to pain from other urinary causes such as cystitis or urethritis.[164] Kook has claimed further support for Rabbi Judah's urinary disorder from a Talmudic text about 'Rabbi Judah' who boasted that there were twenty-four privies between his house and the house of study, to which he was able to resort every hour.[165] However, micturition in Talmudic times did not require the use of privies, as men passed water in the open without inhibitions. Moreover, the text does not refer to Rabbi Judah the Patriarch, but to another renowned Sage, Rabbi Judah bar Illai (*ibid.*, *Nedarim* 49b), who lived in the beginning of the second century CE. The Aramaic term *Tzafrana* or *Tzafdina*, from which Rabbi Judah was said to suffer, is said to refer to stomatitis, with bleeding gums and loosening of the teeth, including scorbutic stomatitis. But the term also might have been used for painful ulceration of the mouth from other causes.[166] That Rabbi Judah suffered from dental disease, possibly associated with the *Tzafdina* as mentioned above, is confirmed by a somewhat legendary description in three different texts:[167]

> Rabbi lived in Sepphoris for seventeen years and of that time he spent thirteen years suffering from a toothache... [= The Prophet] Elijah came to him [= to Rabbi] in the guise of Rabbi Hiyya Rabba. He said to him, "How does my lord do?" He said to him, "I have a tooth which is painful to me." He said to him, "Show me." And he showed it to him. [= Elijah] put his finger on the tooth and healed it. The next day Rabbi Hiyya Rabba came to him and said, 'How does my lord do? As to your teeth, how are they doing?' He said to him, 'From that moment at which you put your finger on it, it has been healed.'
>
> (*Jerusalem Talmud, Ketuboth* 12, 3 [35a])

Whereas the chronic toothache is not in doubt, it is difficult to explain the organic basis of the legendary cure, which is mentioned several times.[168]

---

[164] On *Tzemirtha*, see Preuss (1993): 228; Kohut (1926): VII: 26; Margalit (1962): 52; Goldstein (1968): 633; Sokoloff (1990): 466–467; On the *Tzafrana* = *Tzafdina*, see Kottek (1979): 71–72; idem, (1996): 2925–2926; Rosner (1996): 2877–2878.

[165] Kook (1968): 771–772.

[166] On *Tzafdina*, see Preuss (1993): 171–172; Mazia (1926): 152; Simon (1978): 37; See also Beeson and McDermott (1975): 154.

[167] Neusner (1985): 347–348; Freedman (1961): 261–262; Theodor and Albeck (1965): 305.

[168] Preuss (1993): 285; Shoshan (1977): 522–523; On the redaction of the legend in the *Babylonian Talmud*, see Friedman (1993): 132–133; Meir (1998): 300–337; See also Baumgarten (1981): 147–148.

The Rabbinic literature also includes references to Rabbi Judah's possible rheumatic problems.[169] It reports three times that:

> When Rabbi left [= the study of the Scroll of Lamentations on the eve of the Ninth of Ab] he suffered injury to his little finger, and applied to himself, 'Many are the sufferings of the wicked.' Said Rabbi Hiyya to him: 'For our sins has this happened to you, as it is written, "The breath of our nostrils, he anointed of the Lord, was caught for their corrupt deeds" (*Lamentations* 4, 20). Rabbi Ishmael ben Rabbi Yose said to him: 'Even had we not been engaged on this passage, I would have said so; now that we have been engaged thereon, there is so much the more reason to say so.' When he [= Rabbi] reached home, he put on it [= on his finger] a dry sponge and wrapped reed-grass round it, out-side the sponge. Said Rabbi Ishmael ben Rabbi Yose: 'From him we then learnt three things, a sponge does not heal, it only protects the wound; it is permitted to tie round it reed-grass which is in the house, since it is designedly kept in readiness [= for such purposes], and it is not permitted to read the Hagiographa [= on the Shabbat] except from *Minhah*-time onwards.
>
> (*Jerusalem Talmud, Shabbat* 16, 1 [15c])

The Hebrew terms do not in fact distinguish between an injury and any other painful lesion, nor is the term 'digit' specific for either a finger or a toe. However, a further text in *ibid., Besa* 5, 2 [63a], mentions the fact that 'Rabbi's digits were seen from his sandals'.[170] No explanation is given to the fact that his digits protruded from his sandals, but the unusual appearance, worthy of comment, might be due to swelling related to his joint problem. The repeated allusions to the same condition would indicate that this problem was of a recurring nature.

Rabbi Judah also suffered from unspecified ophthalmic pain. When he contracted an eye disease, his personal physician Mar Samuel offered to bathe it with a lotion. By far the most renowned of Samuel's remedies is his eye-salve, which is repeatedly mentioned in the Talmud. There follows one such passage in *Babylonian Talmud, Baba Metzia* 85a:

> Samuel Yarchina'ah was Rabbi's physician. One day Rabbi suffered from an eye ailment. [= Samuel] said to him, 'I will insert this medication into your eyes for you.' [= Rabbi] said to him, 'I cannot endure that treatment'. [= Samuel] said to him, 'I will gently salve the medicine for you on the surface of your eyes'. [= Rabbi] said to him, 'I cannot endure that either'. Faced with these circumstances, [= Samuel the physician]

---

[169] Neusner (1985): 410; Margulies (1993): 328–329; *Midrash Lamentations Rabbah* 4, 20 (Buber ed., p. 77); See also Sokoloff (1990): 72.

[170] *Jerusalem Talmud, Besa* 5, 2 [63a], Venice ed., p. 1523.

inserted a tube containing the medicine under [= Rabbi's] pillow and he was soon cured.

Apparently the vapour was sufficiently powerful to penetrate to the eye, though not applied directly. Elsewhere, when someone asked Mar Ukba to send some of Mar Samuel's eye-salve, he replied, 'Samuel also said that a drop of cold water in the morning, and bathing the hands and feet in hot water in the evening, is better than all the eye-slaves in the world' (*ibid., Shabbat* 108b). Rosner assumes that Samuel was recommending a prophylactic regimen to avoid eye infection. Samuel further stated that all liquids used for dissolving *collyrium* or eye-salves heal eye sicknesses but dim the eyesight, except water, which heals without dimming (*ibid., Shabbat* 78a).[171] However, presumably, the recovery of Rabbi Judah the Patriarch took place spontaneously, during this magic placebo treatment. A curious Talmudic juxtaposition of bowel disease and ophthalmic problems are relevant to our discussion of Rabbi's differential diagnosis. In the commentary on the Biblical curse in *Deuteronomy* 28, 65: 'Then the Lord will give you a trembling heart, failing eyes and sorrow of mind', *tachtoniot* are blamed for this combination of afflictions (*Babylonian Talmud, Nedarim* 22a). Another Talmudic text that links diseases of the bowels and of the eyes state: 'One must not visit those suffering with bowel trouble, or with eye disease, or from headaches' (*ibid.*, 41a).

Rabbinic literature describes Rabbi Judah's attitude to his distress, as well as his symptoms. On one occasion, he is quoted as 'welcoming his anguish', (*ibid., Baba Metzia* 85a), and in another text, he demonstrated his humble acceptance of his pain by exclaiming, 'many are the sufferings of the sinner'.[172] Shushan is the only scholar who claims that Rabbi Judah's oral, dental, and eye symptoms might have been psychosomatic, the result of a troubled conscience, as explained in the following episode: A calf being taken to the slaughter, broke away, hid its head under Rabbi's cloak, and lowed in terror. 'Go', said he, 'for this wast thou created'. 'Thereupon they said [= in heaven], 'Since he has no pity, let us bring suffering upon him'.[173] Rabbi Judah's suffering

---

[171] See also *Baba Mezia* 85b; On this kind of treatment, see Rosner (1977a): 161–162; On the use of *collyrium* as a medical powder for curing Rabbi Judah, see Ben Horin (1928): 126; Gordon (1938): 69–70; Majno (1991): 359.

[172] *Midrash Lamentations Rabbah* 4, 20 (Buber ed., p. 77); Margulies (1993): 328–329.

[173] Shushan (1977: 223–224) relies upon *The Babylonian Talmud, Baba Mezia* 85a; Rabbi Judah's deed is a well known example for the severity that the Sages regarded towards animals; See Rakover (1977): 206–207; Dvorjetski (2001): 24.

undoubtedly had an organic basis. Shushan's assumption can be entirely discounted. One should regard the Talmudic legend, of his lack of compassion for a calf destined for slaughter, as an anecdote that was prevalent among his entourage to rationalize the distressing and pro-longed suffering of this eminent Sage.

5.5.3   Illnesses in Rabbi Judah's Family

Rabbi Judah's illness may have had a familial component.[174] The Patriarch's grandson, Rabbi Judah Nesi'ah, who is more commonly known by the name Rabbi Judan,[175] is reported as also suffering from an affliction in a digit. The wording is virtually identical with that used for Rabbi Judah's own episodes: 'Rabbi Ami went up with Rabbi Judan Nesi'ah to Hammat-Gader. He injured his finger and put a plaster on it' (*Jerusalem Talmud, Avoda Zarah* 2, 2 [40d]). In this passage, too, the Talmudic terms in Aramaic do not distinguish between a finger and a toe, nor between an injury and some other lesion of the digit.

An obscure reference to *Tzara'at* in Rabbi's family occurs in the Talmud. Many scholars claim that *Tzara'at* in the Bible and the Talmudic literature refers not to leprosy but to Psoriasis—a condition that has a strong familial incidence.[176] During a lengthy discussion among the Sages, they speculated about the name of the Messiah:[177]

> The Rabbis said: 'His name is "the leper of the house of Rabbi" as it is written, 'Surely, he has borne our griefs, and carried our sorrows: yet we did esteem him a leper, smitten of God, and afflicted' (*Isaiah* 53, 4). Rabbi Nahman said: 'If he [= the Messiah] is of those living [= to day] it might be one like me, as it is written, "And their nobles shall be of themselves,

---

[174] *Midrash Lamentations Rabbah* 4, 20 (Buber ed., p. 77); Margulies (1993): 328–329; See also Yaretzky (1982): 427–432.

[175] See, for example, Ta-Shma (1971): 333; Levine (1989): 150–159.

[176] Most of the scholars assume that the *Tzara'at* mentioned in the Bible and in the Talmudic literature is not the chronic and infectious disease known as Lepra but the Psoriasis; Lepra was first introduced to the eastern Mediterranean from India by the soldiers of Alexander the Great. It has no paleopathological evidence before the Byzantine period. See Dauphin (1996–1997): 55; Mark (2002): 285–311; On the illness *Tzara'at* in general, see Münch (1893); von Bergmann (1897); Katzenelson (1928): 304–353; Cochrane (1961); Browne (1970); Hulse (1975): 87–105; Bennahum (1985): 86–89; Preuss (1993): 323–329; Zias (1989): 27–31.

[177] *Babylonian Talmud, Sanhedrin* 98b; On the hopes for salvation and the view about the Messianism of Rabbi, see, for example, Urbach (1988): 326; Oppenheimer (1991): 60–62.

and their governors shall proceed from the midst of them"' (*Jeremiah* 30, 21). Rav said: 'If he is of the living, it would be our holy Master.'

(*Babylonian Talmud, Sanhedrin* 98b)

However, there is no evidence that Rabbi Judah suffered from any skin disease. The Biblical laws of purity would have made an outcast of any person so afflicted. Nor is the 'leper of his house' identified anywhere else.[178] All that the redactor of the Talmudic corpus allowed to be published on leprosy in his own family was this one brief reference.

5.5.4   *Rabbi Judah's Physicians and Treatments*

In accordance with the contemporary doctrines of health care, Rabbi Judah took a number of active steps to alleviate his sufferings. He moved his residence from Beth Shearim, on the edge of the marshy Valley of Yizre'el, to Sepphoris in the healthier hilly region of the lower Galilee, took particular care with his diet, used remedies such as apple-cider, and also frequented the healing spas both at Hammei-Tiberias and at Hammat-Gader.[179] Apart from bathing there, he might also have drunk the waters.[180]

In addition to these measures, Rabbi Judah also resorted to the help and advice of doctors. As he was such an eminent person, he would have had access to the best Jewish physicians available in the country at the time. Thanks to his friendship with Emperor Caracalla, he might also have consulted Roman physicians, although this is not recorded anywhere in the Talmudic literature. His personal physician, Mar Samuel, was a famous ophthalmologist and invented a remedy for eye inflammation that was named 'Collyrium of Mar Samuel'. He also excelled in cardiology and was an expert embryologist and

---

[178] See the discussion on this theme in Epstein (1957): 109–111; Rapaport (1857): 77.

[179] See the discussion above; See also *Tosefta, Eruvin* 4, 16 (Lieberman ed., p. 110); *Jerusalem Talmud, Eruvin* 5, 7 [23d]; *ibid.*, (18, 11 [16c]; *Babylonian Talmud, Eruvin* 61a; On the reputation of Hammat-Gader, see Dvorjetski (1988); idem, (1992a): 53–61, 104–115; idem, (1992b): 445–449; idem, (1996): 39–45; idem, (1997): 567–581; Satlow (1995): 86–88; Dvorjetski (2003): 9–39.

[180] On Rabbi Judah's activities at Hammei-Tiberias, see *Babylonian Talmud, Shabbat* 40b and Rashi's explanation there; Epstein (1935): 189; On the unique healing qualities of its waters when drunk, see Blackman (1967): 688; *Mishnah, Machshirin* 6, 7; See Atlas (1951): 157–159; Buchmann (1957): 29; Dvorjetski (1994a): 39–42; idem, (1994b): 22–25.

paediatrician. Mar Samuel practiced according to the teachings of Galen, who was his contemporary.[181]

5.5.5 *Differential Diagnosis of the Patriarch's Illnesses*

Some of the medical information about Rabbi Judah the Patriarch does not help in the establishment of precise diagnosis. Thus, the identity of his personal physician merely attests to the prominence of the patient, and not to the conditions for which he consulted him. Likewise, his repeated attendance at the thermo-mineral baths at Hammat-Gader and at Hammei-Tiberias does not indicate the particular complaint for which he was seeking treatment. It merely suggests its severity and chronicity, and confirms the high repute of the resorts. He was past middle age at the time when his illnesses were documented. Therefore he might well have suffered from a number of different unrelated ailments.[182]

His most prominent and painful complaint was his bowel disease. Hemorrhoids cannot explain the entire picture. Usually, hemorrhoids do not give rise to distressing pains, except during episodes of acute thrombosis. Pronounced and long-term pain on defecation is more likely to be due to anal fissures or proctitis [= rectal inflammation]. Therefore, it is most likely that his chronic relapsing bowel disorder was due to inflammatory bowel disease.

The recurrent painful non-symmetrical digital lesions of Rabbi as well as of his grandson might be compatible with the diagnosis of familial gout.[183] *Tzemirtha* could then be due to uric acid stones. Ophthalmic

---

[181] Epstein (1935): 528–529, *The Babylonian Talmud, Shabbat* 108b; On Mar Samuel the physician, see Jost (1858): 136; Hoffmann: (1873); Schapiro (1901): 14–26; Mayer (1910): 190–195; Zeide (1954): 57–58; Margalit (1962): 62–85; Neusner (1966): 134–144; Preuss (1993), s.v. 'Samuel, Mar'; Rosner (1977a): 156–170; Beer (1982): 275; Kottek (1996): 2913; Rosner (1996): 2833–2887; On Galen's methods and influence, see for example, Nutton (1984): 315–324; Jackson (1988), s.v. 'Galen'; Newmyer (1996a): 2898–2906; Kottek (1996–1997): 80–89; Bar-Ilan (1999): 31–78; Nutton (2003); idem, (2004), s.v. 'Galen', 'Galenism'.

[182] For the differential diagnosis I owe many thanks to Dr. Y.W. Loebl (MD, FRCP), former consultant rheumatologist at Barnet Hospital at London and a Fellow of the Royal College of Physicians in London.

[183] *Babylonian Talmud, Sotah* 10a; The Talmud provides an uncannily accurate etiopathogenic description of an acute attack, many centuries before the morphology and pathology of uric acid crystals were elucidated: 'Rabbi Nachman was asked, "What is Podagra like?"—He answered, "Like a needle in the living flesh"'; See Wunderbar (1850): 21–22; Kohut (1926): VI: 297; Preuss (1993): 168; Rosner (1996): 2877; See also Rodnan and Benedek (1963): 317–340; Copeman (1964): 21–37; Rogers and Waldron (1995): 78–86; Kelley, Harris and Ruddy (1997): 1359–1396.

symptoms can occur in gout, although they are not common.[184] Gout, however, was very well recognized.[185] Had Rabbi's swollen foot resembled gout, this would have been perceived and mentioned as such. Moreover, the diagnosis of gout does not explain his bowel disease, which was his most prominently reported complaint. We therefore suggest that he must have suffered from a different arthropathy [= joint disease].

The diagnosis of inflammatory bowel disease and its known association with seronegative spondathritis and with the HLA B-27 tissue type would explain all the clinical and familial aspects of Rabbi Judah's diseases.[186] His digital lesions would be due to mild intermittent enteropathic arthropathy. The oral *Tzafdina* could be due to an associated stomatitis, and his painful eye involvement could well be due to uveitis. The urinary symptoms of the *Tzemirtha* might have been due in reality to non-specific urethritis or even to colitic abdominal pains, rather than to bladder stones. And finally, the *Tzara'at* 'in the house of Rabbi' and the familial digital lesions agree well with the established association between his presumed psoriasis, arthritis, and inflammatory bowel disease. Effective treatment was not available for the manifestations of inflammatory bowel disease in the days of Rabbi Judah the Patriarch. The Talmudic descriptions that he was 'cured' are probably just temporary remissions during the natural intermittent course of his unpleasant, but relatively benign conditions. Except for a single short episode, his ailments did not impair his eminence as a scholar or his power of leadership.

---

[184] Scharf, Nahir and Rubilovitch (1975): 251–252.
[185] Wunderbar (1850): 53; Brim (1936): 90–91; Preuss (1993): 168; Rosner (1977a): 58–59; idem, (1996): 2877; See also Scott (1988): 25–29; Jackson (1988), s.v. 'gout.'
[186] Dieppe, Doherty, Mcfarlane and Maddison (1985): 65–92.

CHAPTER SIX

DAILY LIFE AT THE THERMO-MINERAL BATHS ACCORDING TO RABBINIC LITERATURE

The medicinal Roman baths are mentioned in the genre of Rabbinic sources that deal with *Halakha* and *Aggadah* [= Tale] in different and varied contexts. We will deal in this chapter with the following issues: The special characteristics of the therapeutic baths; The *halakhic* stance of the Rabbis towards the baths in general and the medicinal hot springs in particular; *Halakhic* problems in daily life, which are involved in the nature of the hot springs and their solutions; The affinity between the Talmudic corpus and the Classical Literature regarding the features of these bathing places; and relationships between Jews and non-Jews in the thermal baths. There are several imminent problems raised while referring to the literature of the Sages, a treasure trove of information on social and economic history, daily life, and cultural, spiritual and literary history. By comparing parallel passages in Rabbinic literature does it emerge that the name of the therapeutic bath is not specifically mentioned in the texts; Why the failure to name Hammat-Gader is apparently tendentious? Did the Rabbis systematically refrain from revealing the name of the place where they were accustomed to stay, since they found the atmosphere of decadence and adultery there objectionable? What was the original name of Hammat-Gader baths according to a text in the Jerusalem Talmud? Furthermore, except in isolated cases it is not expressly stated in the Rabbinic literature that the Sages took the thermo-mineral baths. Why is there a paucity of material on this subject? Dealing with these essential and fundamental subjects, we will review the aims and deeds of the Sages at those sacred cult places and popular sites of healing.[1]

---

[1] This chapter is based on my following researches: Dvorjetski (1988): 50–76; idem, (1992a): 145–158; idem, (1994a): 22–27; idem, (1999a): 122–129; idem, (2001–2002): 494–500; idem, (2003); idem, (2004): 22–25; forthcoming [a].

6.1   THE *HALAKHIC* STANCE OF THE SAGES TOWARDS CURATIVE
HOT SPRINGS AND BATHS

The *Aggadot* of the Flood preserve the echo of the geological events in
which the Jordan Valley was also formed. The Sages of the Mishnah
and the Talmud attribute the origin of the therapeutic hot springs—as
does modern science—to volcanic processes during the Flood. The great
Palestinian *Amora*, Rabbi Yohanan bar Nafha said of them:[2]

> Three remained of the fountains of the great deep that burst apart at the
> time of the Flood (*Genesis* 7, 11): The eddy of Gader, Hammei-Tiberias,
> and the great spring of Biram.
>
> (*Babylonian Talmud, Sanhedrin* 108a)

According to him, the three regions containing the most famous hot
springs in the eastern Mediterranean basin—Gader, Tiberias and
Ba'arah[3]—are situated along the Syro-African Rift in the Jordan Valley.
Along with this, the legend links the healing springs with the sins of the
generation of the Flood. In one place it states that: 'The waters of the
public baths overwhelmed the Ten Tribes of Israel' (*ibid., Shabbat* 147b),
and the name of Rabbi Eleazar ben Arakh, one of Rabban Yohanan
ben Zakki's disciples, is connected with the baths at Emmaus-Nicopolis:
'He chanced there, was drawn by them, and forgot his learning' (*ibid.,*
147b).[4] All these attribute catastrophes in going to places with therapeutic springs.[5]

The cities with therapeutic springs were deprecated by the Sages for
the life of frivolity and licentiousness. The therapeutic actions of the
springs itself were interpreted negatively by the Sages. As far as they
were concerned, according to Rabbi Yose ben Halafta:[6]

> The springs received their heat from the nethermost fire of the under-
> world.
>
> (*ibid., Shabbat* 39a)

---

[2] See, for example, Kasher (1934): 8–9; Buchmann (1957): 26; idem, (1967): 195;
On Rabbi Yohanan bar Nafha, see Margalioth (1976): II: 481–494.

[3] On various names and identification of Hammei-Ba'arah, see chapter 4.5.

[4] On Rabbi Eleazar ben Arakh, see Margalioth (1976): I: 131–133; Goshen-Gottstein
(1993): 173–197; For several versions of Rabbi Eleazar ben Arakh's visit to Emmaus
and the descriptions of the site, see chapter 4.8 on *The Historical-Archaeological Analysis
of Emmaus-Nicopolis.*

[5] Hirschberg (1920); Leibovitz and Kurland (1972): 48–49; See also the discussion
in 6.2.

[6] Kasher (1934): 9; On Rabbi Yose ben Halafta, see Margalioth (1976): II:
521–527.

This idea about the source of their heat is apparently drawn from the Book of Enoch I (67, 1–13), which discusses it at great length and even demands that one learn a lesson from the burning springs about one's punishment in Gehenna [= by the fires of hell].[7] The names 'the eddy of Gader' and 'the fire of Tiberias' refer to their burning heat and perhaps to the fire of the underworld. The aura of mystery which enshrouded these therapeutic sites may perhaps be reflected in *Midrash Ecclesiastes Rabbah* 2, 8, which attributes to demons a central rôle in heating the springs: 'And the delights of the sons of men': i.e. public baths and lavatories. 'Women very many': i.e. numerous demons to heat them.[8]

Over the generations the Sages of the Mishnah and the Talmud wrestled with the various aspects of *halakhah* concerning the therapeutic hot springs. The nature of the hot springs has implications in law for daily life: cooking, drinking and danger of scalding; immersion; ritual washing of the hands, and bathing.[9] According to the *halakhah*, fire may not be used for cooking food on the Shabbat. On the other hand, the Rabbis did permit using the sun's heat for this purpose, but were divided about the permissibility of warming by means of the sun's by-products—that is to say, not via the direct heat of the sun but by things that were themselves warmed by the sun. Consequently, public baths heated by firing [= hypocaust] are considered by the *halakhah* as 'fire heated' and hence forbidden for use on the Shabbat. On the other hand, the Sages differ over whether the hot springs are the result of 'fire' or of 'sun'. Thus we learn in *Babylonian Talmud, Shabbat* 39a:

> It is the case that the men of Tiberias [= decided] that [= the hot springs were] the product of the sun, but the Rabbis forbade them [= their use] saying to them that they are the result of fire since they pass over the entrance to Gehenna.

As to the question of whether, in order to warm it, one may pass cold water through a pipe set in the hot springs of Tiberias, the *Babylonian Talmud, Shabbat* 39b, relates:

> Rav Hisda said: 'On account of the incident of what the people of Tiberias did and the Rabbis forbade them [= the practice of] putting

---

[7] Hirschberg (1920): 226–228; Buchmann (1947): 90; Kahana (1956): I: 61–62; Dvorjetski (1992a): 145–147; For the resemblance to the Classical sources that water passes over the fires and is heated, see Allen (1998): 23–25.

[8] Klein (1929): 10–11; Frazer (1951): 213–215; Dunbabin (1989): 33.

[9] Zevin (1980): 44–52; See also Shiponi (1962): 10–11; Yankelvitz (1988): 20.

away [= aught] in anything that add a heat, even by day [= i.e., before the Shabbat] has no sanction [= Lit., 'has ceased]. 'Ulla said: The *halakha* agrees with the inhabitants of Tiberias [= their action is permitted]. Said Rav Nahman to him, 'The Tiberians have broken their pipe long ago!' [= they themselves retracted. Thus all agree now that it is forbidden].

The Tiberians destroyed the aforementioned installation and thus determined that the waters of the hot springs may not be used for warming. Their intent was to obtain warmed sweet water for bathing and cooking. However, this again contradicted the laws of the Shabbat:[10]

> The men of Tiberias once passed a tube of cold water through a spring of hot water. The Sages said to them: 'If this is done on the Shabbat it is like water heated on the Shabbat and is forbidden both for washing and drinking; and if it is done on a Festival-day it is like water heated on a Festival-day and is forbidden for washing, but permitted for drinking.
>
> (*Mishnah, Shabbat* 3, 4)

Since there is no sweet water spring in the nearby vicinity, it is clear that pipes were installed to bring water from the springs in Wadi Fajas, 12 km south of the Sea of Galilee, to the baths of the hot springs of Tiberias. This theory was verified by the discovery of such a network to the bathhouse of Beit Yerah.[11]

The natural heat of the Tiberias hot springs was used for cooking, as evidenced by the *halakhah*:

> Who cooks [= food] with Hammei-Tiberias on the Shabbat is culpable.
>
> (*Babylonian Talmud, Sanhedrin* 40b).

And similarly by the words of Rav Hisda (*ibid., Pesahim* 41a):[12]

> Who cooks [= food with Hammei-Tiberias on the Shabbat is not culpable; [= who] cooks the Paschal offering with the Tiberias hot springs is culpable.

While in the *Jerusalem Talmud, Shabbat* 7, 5 [10b], the ideas differ:

> If he cooks in Hammei-Tiberias? Hezekiah said: 'It is forbidden'. Rabbi Yohanan said: 'It is allowed'. Said Rabbi Mana, 'I went to Caesarea, and I heard Rabbi Zeriqan in the name of Hezekiah [= state], 'So far as

---

[10] See also the *Jerusalem Talmud, Shabbat* 3, 4 [5c]; Epstein, *Babylonian Talmud, ibid.*, 36b: 181–183.

[11] Kalner (1947): 133–140.

[12] Shiponi (1962): 8–9; On Rav Hisda, see Margalioth (1976): I: 368–377.

Hezekiah is concerned, he has a question as to the status of an animal designated as a Passover offering which was cooked in Hammei-Tiberias'.

Another legal question is raised in the Talmudic version about the
use of the thermal springs of Tiberias for the ritual washing of the
hands and for required immersion:

> On Hammei-Tiberias, Hezekiah said: 'One does not use their waters
> for washing the hands but one may immerse the hand in them', and
> Rabbi Yohanan said: 'One may immerse the entire body but not one's
> face and feet'.
>
> (*Babylonian Talmud, Hullin* 106a)

In Hezekiah's opinion, the waters of Tiberias are invalid for ritually
washing the hands but valid for immersing the hands, whereas Rabbi
Yohanan allowed the immersion of the whole body except for the face,
hands, and feet. The reason flows from the nature of the waters, as in
Babylonian Talmud, Ta'anit 13a:[13]

> Said Rav Hana bar Ketina: It [= the discussion] was unnecessary but
> for Hammei-Tiberias [= which are hot and not drawn, and one may
> therefore immerse in them].

It is very important to point out that the term *Hammei-Tiberias* does
not signify that place specifically, but is a general term in Rabbinic
literature for thermo-mineral baths.[14]

Other legal questions discussed are: Is it permissible to bathe in the
Hammei-Tiberias on the Shabbat? And what of one who enters to
perspire in their heat? The replies varied:

> For Rabbi Simeon ben Pazzi said in the name of Rabbi Joshua ben Levi
> on the authority of Bar Kappara: At first people used to wash in pit
> water heated on the eve of the Shabbat; then bath attendants began to
> heat the water on the Shabbat, maintaining that it was done on the eve
> of the Shabbat. So [= the use of] hot water was forbidden, but sweating
> was permitted. Yet still they used to bathe in hot water and maintain.
> We were perspiring. So sweating was forbidden, yet the thermal springs
> of Tiberias were permitted. Yet they bathed in water heated by fire and
> maintained, We bathed in the thermal springs of Tiberias. So they forbade
> the hot springs of Tiberias but permitted cold water. But when they saw
> that this [= series of restriction] could not stand [= They could not be

---

[13] *Babylonian Talmud, Ta'anit* 13a, Epstein, *ibid.*, 56–58; On Rav Hana bar Rav Ketina,
see Margalioth (1976): I: 324.

[14] See the discussion on *Terminology* in chapter 1.4.

enforced, being regarded as too onerous for the masses], they permitted
the hot springs of Tiberias, whilst sweating remained in *status quo*.[15]

(Babylonian Talmud, Shabbat 40a)

The Rabbis taught: 'One may bathe in the waters of Gader, in the waters
of Hammthan, in the waters of Asia, and in the waters of Tiberias but not
in the Great Sea [= the Mediterranean] nor of steeping pools [= waters
in which flax is steeped] nor of the Dead Sea' [= in which one bathes
only for healing needs].[16]

(ibid., Shabbat 109a)

One may bathe in the waters of Tiberias, of a steeping pool, and in
the Dead Sea, even though there are wounds on his head [= which are
healed thereby].

(ibid., Shabbat 109b)

There we have learned that one who bathes in a cave[17] or in Hammei-
Tiberias may dry himself even with ten sheets but may not bring them
in his hand…for it is taught that one who bathes in Hammei-Tiberias
sprinkles himself but others may not sprinkle him.

(Jerusalem Talmud, Shabbat 3, 4 [5c])

And, parallel to this:

One who bathes in a cave or in the waters of Tiberias dries himself even
with ten sheets but may not bring them in his hand…one who bathes in
Hammei-Tiberias may not be sprinkled by others but does it himself.

(Tosefta, Shabbat 16, 15, Lieberman ed., p. 78)

In addition to the Sages' praises of the Hammei-Tiberias as 'good for
healing', their evaluation is also well reflected in the words of Rabbi
Dostai:[18]

Why are Hammei-Tiberias not in Jerusalem? So that the Festival pilgrims
should not say: if we made the pilgrimage only to bathe in Hammei-

---

[15] Forbidden. It is not clear whether these subterfuges were resorted to because the
Rabbis might punish non-observance, or because public opinion condemned the open
desecration of the Sabbath, even in respect of Rabbinical enactments; See Epstein,
Babylonian Talmud, Shabbat 40a: 186.

[16] On the names and sites Hammthan and The waters of Asia, see the discussion
on the *Terminology* in chapter 1.4, and *The Historical-Archaeological Analysis of The Waters
of Asia* in chapter 4.7.

[17] On the name Mei Me'arah and its affinity to Hammei-Ba'arah, see the discussions
on *Terminology* in chapter 1.4, and *The Historical-Archaeological Analysis and Healing Cults
of Hammei-Ba'arah* in chapter 4.5.

[18] Kasher (1934): 17, note 6; Buchmann (1967): 195.

Tiberias it would suffice us, and this would result in a pilgrimage not made for its own sake.

(*Babylonian Talmud, Pesahim* 8b)

The actions of the Romans, who introduced the culture of the baths to the eastern Mediterranean, earned differing and mixed reviews in the Rabbinic literature. On the one hand we read in a most intriguing passage:[19]

Rabbi Judah bar Ila'i said: 'How pleasant are the deeds of this nation [= the Romans]. They have made streets, they have built bridges, and they have erected baths'. Rabbi Yose was silent. Rabbi Simeon bar Yohai answered and said: 'All what they made they made for themselves; they built market places, to set harlots in them; baths, to rejuvenate themselves; bridges, to levy tools for them'.

(*ibid., Shabbat* 33b)

Rabbi Simeon bar Yohai sees the motivation for Rome's civic improvements, including the erection of bathhouses, in selfishness rather than in public spiritedness.

And, 'Public lavatories and bathhouses...that the evil kingdom makes...intended only for their own needs' (*Midrash HaGadol on Genesis* 44, 24, Margulies ed., p. 659).

And similar indications:[20]

None may help them [= the Gentiles] to build a basilica, scaffold, stadium or judges' tribunal; but one may help them to build public baths [= *demoseoth*; Varient: *bemoseoth*] or bathhouses; yet when they have reached the vaulting where they set up the idol it is forbidden [= to help them] to build.

(*Mishnah, Avoda Zarah* 1, 7)

People's pleasures are bathing ponds and bathhouses.[21]

(*Babylonian Talmud, Gittin* 68a)

What does the king do with that money? He builds..., and bathhouses... to cater to the needs of the poor.

(*Exodus Rabbah* 31, 11)

---

[19] On the authenticity of this dialogue of these Sages, see Ben-Shalom (1984): 9–24; On various evaluations of the Roman Empire, see, for example, Bacher (1896): 192–193; Hahn (1906); Friedläender (1922): 318–320; Bergman (1937): 150; Fuchs (1964); Herr (1970): 95–108; Newmyer (1996b): 89.

[20] On the terminology of public baths and spas, see chapter 1.4.

[21] See also *Babylonian Talmud, Shabbat* 12b; *Midrash Ecclesiastes Rabbah* 2, 19.

And, on the other,

> A government lives on four things general rates, bathhouses, theatres
> and taxes.
>
> (*Avot de Rabbi Nathan*, Version A, 28, Schechter ed., p. 85).

Further homilies preserved in later *Midrashim* teach that the deeds of
the Romans are well-intentioned and are reprehensible only because
of the accretions that adhere in them, such as the setting up of idol
worship in the bath houses, or attaching a house of prostitution to the
bathhouse:[22]

> It was a good thing they did in building public baths and bathhouses
> where rich and poor could bathe..., but while they were building them
> they said 'leave a place where we can practice idolatry and where we can
> hide the prostitutions'. The result is that their credit is their discredit.
>
> (*Batei-Midrashot, Midrash Hesed Leumim* 2, Wertheimer ed., p. 143)

Differing evaluations of the improvements and projects of the Roman
Empire are also found in the Classical sources, primarily in the Greek
literature. Even there one finds those who praised Rome and those who
maligned it, clearly paralleling the Talmudic texts cited above. While
Aeilius Aristides was shouting the praises of Rome in 143 CE, in the
early days of Antoninus Pius, we find his contemporary Lucianus of
Samosata's criticism and scorn for Rome, pouring contempt and derision
on the bathhouses as a symbol of the decadence of Roman society.[23]

Halahkhot [= Jewish religious laws] that deal with these springs and
whose concern was the Shabbat prohibitions, were adapted to take
account of the benefits of the therapeutic sites. At first the *halakhah*
clashed with the needs of life at the Hammei-Tiberias, and therefore
it is stated in the *Babylonian Talmud, Shabbat* 40a:

> When the Sages saw that they were not prevailing [= that the commu-
> nity could not accept the fact that they forbade them everything], they
> permitted them Hammei-Tiberias.

The *Jerusalem Talmud* (*Shabbat* 3, 4 [6a]) explains more completely:

---

[22] Herr (1970): 99–100; Dvorjetski (1992a): 154–155; idem, (1999a): 125.
[23] Aelius Aristide, Εἰς ʿΡώμην 97–101; Oliver (1953): 906; Lucian, *Nigrinus* 15–17,
20, 34; See also Herr (1970): 97–98.

Since they were fenced in [= restricted too much], they permitted them more and more until they permitted them the waters of the cave and Hammei-Tiberias.

Thereafter we find a definitive ruling in the *Babylonian Talmud* (*Shabbat* 109a):

Our Rabbis taught: 'One may bathe in the waters of Gader, in the waters of Hammthan, in the waters of Asia, and in the waters of Tiberias but not in the Great Sea [= the Mediterranean] nor in the waters of a steeping pool nor in the Dead Sea [= in which one bathes only for healing needs].

As we have seen, the *halakhah* did allow bathing in the therapeutic springs on the Shabbat, as opposed to bathing in ordinary water, in the sea, or even in the Dead Sea. The Sages had difficulty in finding *halakhic* authorization for this, since on the Shabbat it is specifically prohibited to treat an ill person whose life is not in danger. They were equally uncomfortable with the reason for giving permission to walk on the Shabbat from the cities of therapeutic springs to the springs themselves for a distance greater than the 'Shabbat limit', i.e., 2000 cubits (c. 1 km) from the edge of the city in any one direction only, e.g., from Tiberias to Hammei-Tiberias, and from Gader to Hammat-Gader.[24]

From the behavioural patterns at the baths and the *halakhot* connected with them, it is evident that the Sages did not prohibit the use of the baths *per se* but rather attempted to prevent the spread of the gentile practices in vogue there. The approach stems from the Sages' understanding that they would not be able to eliminate the phenomenon entirely; it sufficed to adapt it to their world-view. In any case, the use of the baths raised grave reservations because idolatrous statues were customarily displayed in them.[25]

6.2 The Sages at the Therapeutic Sites—Aims and Deeds

Thermal baths in Palestine were well known for their therapeutic qualities also throughout the Roman-Byzantine Empire. Specially celebrated

---

[24] See *Tosefta, Eruvin* 5, 16 (Lieberman ed.); *Jerusalem Talmud, ibid.*, 5, 7 [22d]; *Babylonian Talmud, ibid.*, 61a; See the discussion on these versions in chapter 6.2.
[25] See Elmslie (1911): 48–49; Lieberman (1939a): 54–58; idem, (1963): 248; Urbach (1988): 164–178.

were Hammei-Tiberias, Kallirrhoe, Hammei-Ba'arah, Hammat-Pella, Emmaus, and, above all, Hammat-Gader. (See Map 1 and Tab. 2). These places of healing served both as cultural centres and as meeting-places between Jews and non-Jews. In some of them there was a special combination of fairs, places of entertainment, and social gatherings. The aim of this chapter is to clarify the nature of these relationships by examining various *halakhic* questions discussed by the Sages as a result of confrontation with the requirements of daily life; to present evidence of everyday cooperation between Jews and non-Jews 'for the sake of peace', and its limitations; and to give examples of harassment by the Roman army in the baths of Palestine, a phenomenon well known throughout the Roman Empire.[26]

The process of development of therapeutic sites in Palestine, which bore a distinctly Hellenistic character, in a Semitic environment in general and in proximity to Jewish localities, may be illustrated by the deeds of illustrious *Tannaim* and *Amoraim*, among them the members of the family of the Patriarchs.

The earliest reference in the Rabbinic literature to the medicinal springs as an inhabited site is attributed to the era of Rabbi Meir, the most important disciple of Rabbi Akiva.[27] Only from his time onwards Hammat-Gader is frequently mentioned in Rabbinic literature, thus indicating that the development of the spa began in the second century CE. That was the period of prosperity for the cities of the Decapolis, to which Gadara belonged.[28] Plentiful provisions were made available at the hot springs by a large number of food merchants. Rabbi Meir is quoted in discussion with a Samaritan, who is trying to disprove the belief in the resurrection of the dead. The Samaritan questions Rabbi Meir ironically about the supply of sustenance to those who will come back to life in the days of the Messiah:[29]

---

[26] This section is based on the following researches: Dvorjetski (1992a): 159–179; idem, (1994): 22–27; idem, (1999a): 122–129; idem, (2001–2002): 494–500; idem, (2003); idem, (2004): 22–25; idem, forthcoming [a].

[27] On Rabbi Meir, see Bacher (1922): II/1: 18–23; Heiman (1964): III: 865–878; Margalioth (1976): II: 621–630.

[28] Josephus emphasizes that the city is Πόλις "Ελληνίς (*Bellum Judaicum* 2.97; *Antiquitates Judaicae* 17.320; On Gadara's importance and cultural distinction during the Hellenistic and Roman periods, see Dvorjetski (1988): 17–42; Schürer (1991): II: 132–136.

[29] Sukenik (1935a): 19–20; Dvorjetski (1988): 91; idem, (2004): 22; According to Ben-Arieh (1997: 380), a large amount of cooking and storage vessels revealed in the baths complex, and the structure was subdivided into small rooms, possibly stores,

'Since [= the dead] come back alive and clothed, who supplies them with food?' He [= Rabbi Meir] said to him, 'Have you ever been to Hammat-Gader?' 'Yes.' 'In the season or out of the season?' 'Both.' 'Were supplies of food obtainable there?' 'They were obtainable.' 'In the season or out of it?' 'Both in and out of the season, because crowds bring foodstuff there to buy and sell.' Rabbi Meir said to him, 'As He brings the crowds [= of the dead], so does He brings their sustenance'.

(*Midrash Ecclesiastes Rabbah* 5, 10)

This reply makes it clear that from the second century CE—the most prosperous period of the Decapolis, one of whose cities was Gadara, the mother city of Hammat-Gader—many food merchants would make their way to the spot in order to sell their goods to the visitors who came in great numbers during the bathing period, from the beginning of spring until the middle of the summer months, and throughout the year.

Rabbi Meir maintained friendly relations with the pagan philosopher of the school of younger Cynics, Oenomaus from Gadara, identified with Οἰνόμαος, one of very few Greek intellectuals mentioned in the Rabbinic literature. It is sometimes possible to hear Oenomaos' words echoed in those of Rabbi Meir. Oenomaos also conducted philosophical discussions with other Rabbis in Gadara or its outskirts, in the baths of Hammat-Gader, though he was mostly friendly with Rabbi Meir. They also discussed topics of daily life and matters concerning teaching and pupils.[30] Contacts between Jews and non-Jews in times of distress—for instance, visits to the sick, funeral orations, burials and visits of condolence—bear witness to deep and sincere friendship. There is evidence that Rabbi Meir was accustomed to pay condolences to non-Jews. When Oenomaos' parents died, Rabbi Meir came to his home in Gadara to console him. In *Ruth Rabbah* 2, 13, we read:

The mother of Abnimos of Gadara died, and Rabbi Meir went up to condole with him and found them sitting in mourning. Some time later his father died, and Rabbi Meir again went up to condole with him, and found them engaged in their normal occupations. He said to him,

---

food stands or even living quarters, similar to the 'row of shops' in the northern part of *Area C*. This might be as a reflection of the aforementioned text from *Midrash Ecclesiastes Rabbah* 5, 10.

[30] On Oenomaos see Margalioth (1976): I: 622–623; Sperber (1971): 1331–1332; Urbach (1971): 168, 185; Geiger (1985): 11–12; Luz (1986–1987): 191–195; idem, (1992): 42–80; Feldman (1993): 31; Hammerstaedt (1990): 2835–2865; See also Klein (1925): 39.

'It appears to me that your mother was dearer to you than your father!'
He answered him, 'Is it not then written, *To her mother's house*, but not 'to
her father's house'? Rabbi Meir answered him, 'Thou hast spoken well,
for a heathen indeed has no father'.[31]

A dispute between Rabbi Meir and other Sages, probably provides
further evidence for Rabbi Meir's visits to Gadara:[32]

> And Rabbi Meir agrees with Sages concerning a basilica, the two doors of
> which are not directly opposite one another. For example, the courtyard of
> Beth Gaddi and Hammatha... that all the same is the rule of the middle
> and the side. They are private domain for the Shabbat and public...
>
> (*Tosefta, Tohorot* 7, 14, Tsukermandel ed. p. 668)

A particular set of *halakhic* precepts dealing entirely with spiritual
solace, but also prescribing good deeds, is based on the principle of 'for
the sake of peace'; it is these which ordain relations of good neighbour-
ship between Jews and non-Jews:[33]

> One should visit the sick, both Jews and non-Jews... for the sake of
> peaceful relations.
>
> (*Jerusalem Talmud, Demai* 4, 6 [24a])

And moreover,

> They make a lament for, and bury, gentile deed for the sake of peace.
> They express condolences to gentile mourners, for the sake of peace.
>
> (*Tosefta, Gittin* 5, 5)

This expression appears again in contexts directly relevant to contacts
with non-Jews in the thermal baths on their festivals—contacts essentially different from the issue we are now discussing. Here, Rabbi Meir
acted in the spirit of the norm current in his day. The fact that hospitality was practised, whether in one's own home or at a meal given by
a non-Jew,[34] shows that both the leading *Tannaim* and, even more, the
common people, accepted the hospitality of non-Jews.

---

[31] 'No father'—in Jewish law, the child of a non-Jewish marriage has only mother-
right; See the variant versions in Lieberman (1939b): 80; See also Ne'eman (1990):
156–159.
[32] See also *Midrash Genesis Rabbah* 65, 22 (Theodor and Albeck ed., pp. 734–735);
Exodus Rabbah 13:1 (Shinan ed., pp. 254–255); *Babylonian Talmud, Hagigah* 15b.
[33] See also *Jerusalem Talmud Gittin* 6, 9 [47c]; *ibid., Avoda Zarah* 1, 3 [39c]; Urbach
(1958): 192; Cohen (1978): 56–58; On various deeds for Gentiles, see Dvorjetski
(2003): 12–13.
[34] As is said elsewhere of Rabbi Meir; see *Psikta de Rav Kahana* 59b (Mandelbaum

Rabbi Meir's aforementioned description that 'the masses bring their goods to buy and sell' is reminiscent of the description by the fourth century CE Church Father Epiphanius, concerning the annual fair, known as the Panegyris, which took place in Hammat-Gader.[35] The best-known names—πανήγυρις in Greek, *Nundinae* or *Mercatus* in Latin—do not appear in this form in the rabbinical literature; however, אטליז *itliz*, עטלים *atliz*, and יריד *yarid* do appear. *Itliz* is derived from the Greek ἀτελής, 'free from (customs) tax', and it appears that reduction of or exemption from tax was an essential part of the fair, which was devoted to the worship of idols.[36]

Emmaus, which was the headquarters of the Roman army at the time of the Great Revolt, and in which superannuated Roman soldiers may have lived, was well known for its high standard of living.[37] Its fame was due not only to the *itliz* which took place there, but also to the fact that it was 'a beautiful spot, with fair and pleasant waters' as was said of the *demosin*, the public baths, which served as a place of recreation.[38]

The term *etliz*, which originated, as has been said, as a synonym for *yarid*, bazaar, was used in Palestine to mean a fair without idols: in other words, it had no clear association with an idolatrous cult. It may be identified with the fairs 'given by the state and its great men'; but, as Safrai, following Epstein, points out, this is not necessarily so,

ed., p. 115); *Midrash Proverbs* 13, 25 (Buber ed., p. 74); cf. Visotzky ed., pp. 125–126; In *Psiqta Rabbati* 16 (Ish-Shalom ed., 82b) the opening version is corrupted.

[35] Epiphanius, *Adversus Haereses* 30.7.

[36] According to Liddel and Scott (1985: 590) the word ἡ πανήγυρις means a gathering, general assembly specially festivity for a deity; See also Kohut (1926): IV: 161; Jastrow (1950): 659; Lieberman (1959): 75–81; Safrai (1984): 139–140; Sperber (1998): 28; Cohn (1929: 11–44) suggests that the word derives from the Greek word ἱερίζω, which means to sanctify or to inaugurate; while Lévy (1901: 183–205) assumes that yarid might be κατάρασις, το go down to the sea shore or to the springs either for trade or for worship; Krauss (1937: 19–21) agrees with Lévy but emphasizes that such a walk or travel is the framework of commerce in the name of Heracles, patron of the merchants; See also Owens (1992): 3–4, 125–126; van Nijf (1997): 34–87; Rosenfeld and Menirav (2004): 161–163.

[37] As a central headquarters of the Roman army, see Josephus, *Bellum Judaicum* 2.567; 5.42.68; See also Vincent and Abel (1932): 316–355; Safrai (1982b): 21; Schürer (1991): I: 512–513; Isaac (2000): 428–429; For the history of Emmaus-Nicopolis, see chapter 4.8.

[38] *Midrash Ecclesiastes Rabbah* 7, 7; On the *demosin*, see Dvorjetski (1992a): 85; See the discussion on *Terminology* in chapter 1.4; On Emmaus and its abundant water, see Gichon (1979a): 101–110; Hirschfeld (1978): 86–92; idem, (1990): 197–204; idem, (1988): 9–30; See also *The Historical-Archaeological Analysis and Healing Cults of Emmaus-Nicopolis* in chapter 4.8.

since only one *Midrash* hints at the connection between the *etliz* and idolatry:[39]

> *Pe HaHirot*—there is no *Hirot* except the place of the Egyptians' freedom. The location of the *etlin* [= bazaars] is their place of idolatry.
> (*Mekhilta of Rabbi Ishmael, Besalach* 1, 9, Horovitz and Rabin ed., p. 83)

It is not clear whether the *itliz* was a Jewish market; but, as Safrai maintains, the impression from the sources is that it was not a pagan, non-Jewish affair as the *yarid* seems to have been.[40] However, the hint in *Midrash Genesis Rabbah* 37, 5 (Theodor and Albek ed., p. 348), that the *itliz* was a place of sexual licentiousness, should not be ignored:[41]

> Rabbi Abba bar Kahana said, 'The *Pathruthim* and *Casluhim* set up bazaars where they stole [= interchanged] each other's wives'.

It is true that this text speaks of adultery rather than ordinary prostitution, and that it is not necessarily connected with the situation which prevailed in the *yeridim*, the fairs; but it may be surmised that in every large-scale fair the question of adultery arose. Even so, this text bears a definite similarity to the remarks in the *Pesikta Rabbati* 21 (Ish-Shalom ed. p. 107), on the immorality of the people of Gadara and Susitha, who are represented by the figures of Gaius and Lucius, 'symbols of the peoples of the world', in the words of Lieberman, who embodied concepts of religion and morality widespread among non-Jews.[42]

> Gaius of Gadara and Lucius of Sussita [= Hippos] would sneak into each other's homes and cohabit with the wives of the others, the others with the wives of these. In time a quarrel fell out between them, and a man killed his father unaware that it was his father.

Hirschberg's conclusion from the *Mishnaic* tractate *Arachin* 2, 4, and the *Tosafta, ibid., 1*, 15 (Tsukermandel ed. p. 544) is that profligacy and immorality in the hot baths led to 'serious damage to the purity of family and race among the Jews, and their inhabitants were considered to be disqualified from marrying'. He maintains that families from Emmaus

---

[39] Safrai (1984): 143; Epstein (1957): 454–455; See also Safrai (1990): 118; According to Safrai, the people in Babylonia were not familiar with the *yarid* and could not understand precisely the *halakhic* issue; See also Beer (1982): s.v. 'shuk', 'sevakim'.

[40] Safrai (1984): 154–155.

[41] On the connection to licentiousness see *Genesis Rabbah* 79, 6 (Theodor and Albek ed., p. 940); Tal (1991): 157.

[42] Lieberman (1963): 67; See also Klein (1939): 28.

who could not produce evidence of their legitimacy—such as those of
Beit Hapegarim and *Beit Sepphoriya*—were considered unfit for marriage,
because of their place of residence.[43]

From all this we may conclude that the belief of the Rabbis that
spas were places of shame was not without foundation; it was even said
that their heat was derived from the infernal fires of Gehenna, and that
nothing but disasters resulted from visits to such places.[44]

The *halakha* forbade Jews to visit fairs, because of their idolatrous
nature. In the *Babylonian Talmud, Avoda Zarah* 12a, there are three reasons for this prohibition. The first, adduced in the name of Abbaye, is:
'because of the money paid for idolatry'; the second: 'Rava says...on
account of their festival'. The third reason is advanced in the name of
Rava bar Ulla: 'because of the period before the festival'. According
the latter two reasons, what is forbidden is not the fair, but doing business with non-Jews on the day of their festival, so that the Jew should
not appear to be taking part in their celebration, and in order to limit
social relationships with non-Jews. In another context the *Babylonian
Talmud, Avoda Zarah* 13a, explains that the prohibition stems from the
fear that one may enjoy the odour of fragrant plants in the shops which
sell them for idolatrous purposes. The *Jerusalem Talmud, Avoda Zarah* 1,
4 [39c], gives another explanation:

> When the idol is...inside [= the city], it is a case in which the [= idol]
> derives benefit from the imposts [= levied on the business done at the
> fair, and so it is] forbidden. [= But when the idol is] outside [= of the
> city], it is permitted [= to do business] because [= the temple of idolatry]
> does not derive benefit from the imposts [= levied in connection with
> the fair].

That is to say, the prohibition stems from the fact that at the fair reductions of customs duty are granted in honour of a particular god. A
Jew may not profit from the fruits of idolatry or from anything which
promotes it; therefore, he may take no part in the fair.[45] The *Jerusalem*

---

[43] Hirschberg (1920): 235–236; On these families, see also Dvorjetski (1992a): 86.

[44] *Babylonian Talmud, Shabbat* 39a; *ibid., Shabbat* 147b; *Avot de Rabbi Nathan*, Version
I, 14, (Schechter ed., p. 59); Enoch I, 67, 1–13 speaks on the hot springs in full details
and demands to take morale from the burnt springs on his sentence in the Gehenna
prospectively; See Dvorjetski (1994a): 19–22; idem (1999a): 123; See also the discussions in chapter 6.1 and in chapter 4.8 about *The Historical-Archaeological Analysis and
Healing Cults of Emmaus-Nicopolis*.

[45] Safrai (1984): 141, 147; See also Kohut (1926): IV: 161; Varhaftig (1987): 434;
Herman (1991): 220–222.

Talmud's explanation is a reflection of the practice prevalent in the
Roman Empire of dedicating fairs to the worship of different gods.[46]
The assertion that reductions in customs duty in the fairs are intended to
encourage purchases which contribute to the idolatrous cult is repeated
in different *halakhic* decisions, and in reference to various parts of the
country, including Acre, Dor, and Bothna.[47]

Among the most important deities in the pantheon of the town of
Gadara were Zeus, Athena, Heracles, and the goddess of the town,
Tyche. One of the most interesting designs in the coins of Gadara
is that of the τρεῖς χάριτες—The Three Graces—from the reigns of
the emperors Caracalla (211–217 CE), Elagabal (218–222 CE) and
Gordian III (238–244 CE). This is the only place in the region in
which the cult of these goddesses was practiced and minted on coins.
(See Figs. 22 and 33). This may be connected with the shrine erected
in their honour in the vicinity of the baths.[48] It is not impossible that
the fair at Hammat-Gader was in honour of Heracles, the patron of
merchants and peddlers, as Krauss has suggested,[49] of Zeus, or of the
Three Graces, as may be suggested by the story in the *baraitha* in the
Jerusalem Talmud, Shabbat 3, 4 [6a]:[50]

> Rabbi Aha bar Isaac went to bathe with Rabbi Abba bar Memel in
> [= the Bath of] the τρεῖς χάριτες. He saw a man sprinkling water on
> himself. He said to him, 'Doing it this way is forbidden on the Shabbat,
> because one thereby increases the mist and hardens the ground'.

Both Rabbis, Rabbi Aha bar Isaac and Rabbi Abba bar Memel, went
to bathe in the bath of the τρεῖς χάριτες, the Three Graces, and saw
a man sprinkling water on himself. According to Epstein's reading and
reconstruction, accepted by Lieberman,[51] we may learn from this about

---

[46] Safrai (1984): 141, 150–153; idem, (1994): 239–243; MacMullen (1970): 333–341;
Shaw (1995): 37–73; On the fairs and markets in the Roman Empire, see Frayn (1993);
DeLigt (1993).

[47] For Dor, see *Jerusalem Talmud, Avoda Zarah* 1, 4 [39d]; and Acre, *Babylonian Talmud,
ibid.*, 11b; and for Bothna, see *Sifre to Deuteronomy* 306 (Finkelstein ed., p. 339); See also
Ne'eman (1990): 155, 162; Oppenheimer (1991): 138–139; Safari (1994): 251–262.

[48] Meshorer (1985): 80–83; Meshorer's opinion refers only to the numismatic evidence; See also the epigraphical testimonies for the τρεῖς χάριτες in chapter 8.3 on
The Numismatic Expression of the Medicinal Hot Springs of Gadara.

[49] Krauss (1950): 19–21; and Safrai (1984: 144) follows him.

[50] Lieberman (1935): 83; On Rabbi Aha bar Isaac see Margalioth (1976): I: 75–76,
and for Rabbi Abba bar Memel, see Margalioth (1976): I: 12–13.

[51] Lieberman (1963): 249; Epstein (1930): 126; Sokoloff (1990): 269; See also Ginzberg (1909): 76; Dvorjetski (2000b): 91–93.

the cult of the Three Graces which was practised in the third century CE, and about the original name of the baths of Hammat-Gader: 'The Bath of the τρεῖς χάριτες', [= the Three Graces]. These Sages had close relationships with Rabbis, who were accustomed to frequent the baths—Rabbi Ze'ira, and, in particular, Rabbi Ami—and discussed matters of *halakha* with them.[52]

In Urbach's opinion, the state of affairs in the second and third centuries CE necessitated separation and dissociation from non-Jews and their society, and increasingly severe observance of the laws concerning the wine and cooked food of non-Jews, which were liable to serve as offerings to idols or to encourage the non-Jewish purchasers to overstep the bounds of morality.[53] Indeed, well-ordered public life in towns with mixed population depended on cooperation in various fields, 'for the sake of peace', or 'for fear of enmity'. In the words of the *Baraitha*: 'He went into the town, and found them celebrating; he celebrated with them, since he was only flattering them'.[54] For that very reason, however, they considered it necessary to fix bounds in this matter, and they did so.

This is one of three parallel versions in the *Jerusalem Talmud* of the answer to the question put to Rabbi Ami, at the initiative of the Gadaran Jews or Jews of Hammat-Gader:[55]

> Gadarans asked Rabbi Ami, 'As to the day on which gentiles make a feast, what is the law [= about doing business with them]?' He considered permitting it to them on the grounds of maintaining peace [= in relationships]. Said to him Rabbi Ba, 'And did not Rabbi Hiyya teach: 'The day of banquet of gentiles it is forbidden [= to do business with them]?' Said Rabbi Ami, 'Were it not for Rabbi Ba, we should have ended up permitting their idolatrous practices. So blessed is the Omni-present who has kept us distant from them!'
> (*Jerusalem Talmud, Avoda Zarah* 1, 3 [39c])

---

[52] See *Jerusalem Talmud, Shabbat* 6, 2 [8a]; *Babylonian Talmud, Hullin* 128b–129a; *ibid., Yevamot* 105a; *ibid., Baba Metzia* 36a; On Rabbi Ze'ira, see Heiman (1964): I: 386–398; Margalioth (1976): I: 259–266.

[53] Urbach (1988): 164; Urbach refers to *Mishnah, Avoda Zarah* 2, 1.

[54] *Jerusalem Talmud, Avoda Zarah* 1, 1 [39ba]; The idioms 'for the sake of peace' and 'for fear of enmity' might reflect different periods and not dissimilar implications. See Cohen (1975): 282–285; idem, (1978): 57–58.

[55] See the several parallel versions: *Jerusalem Talmud, Demai* 4, 6 [24a]; *ibid., Gittin* 6, 9 [47c]; The reading might be either *garda'ei* or *gadra'ei* [= weavers]; Schwartz (1998): 217; Levine (1986): 69; cf. idem, (1989): 102; See also Klein (1939): 28; On Rabbi Ami, see Margalioth (1976): I: 150–153, and on Rabbi Hiyya bar Abba, idem, (1976): 291–295.

The question under discussion was: is contact with gentiles in matters
permitted 'for the sake of peace' allowed on their festival day? Rabbi
Ami accepted the rigorous opinion of Rabbi Ba.[56] This text is also
evidence of the position of the Rabbi as an authority in the Jewish
community of Palestine, when a group of people laid their problems
before him.[57]

There is evidence of magic and idolatry in the public baths of
Tiberias as early as the period of the *Tannaim*. A polemic *Aggadah*
describes the greatest of the *Tannaim*, Rabbi Eliezer ben Hyrcanus,
Rabbi Joshua ben Hanaina, and Rabbi Akiva confronting a heretic.
Their struggle with him begins in the bathhouse:[58]

> When Rabbi Eliezer, Rabbi Joshua, and Rabbi Akiva went in to bathe
> in the baths of Tiberias, a *min* saw them. He said what he said, and the
> arched chamber in the bath [= where idolatrous statues were put up]
> held them fast, [= so that they could not move]. Said Rabbi Eliezer to
> Rabbi Joshua, 'Now Joshua ben Hanina, see what you can do.' When
> tat *min* tried to leave, Rabbi Joshua said what he said, and the doorway
> of the bath seized and held the *min* firm, so that whoever went in had
> to give him a knock [= to push by], and whoever went out had to give
> him a knock [= to push by]...
>
> (ibid., Sanhedrin 7, 13 [25d]).

Leisure culture in baths, and particularly in spas, also comprised
philosophical discussions and disputes between rival religions.[59] Here,
in the *baraitha* of the *Jerusalem Talmud*, the rivals are conducting their
dispute with the aids of supernatural forces. In the ancient world, rejection of a rival faith did not involve denial of the powers of the rival,
but, rather, interpretation of those powers as being derived from the
forces of darkness, the powers of Satan. Rabbi Joshua was victorious
even over the god of the sea. Hirshman conjectures that the heretic
was a follower of Jesus who returned to the place where Jesus himself
wrought a miracle when he walked on the water. This derogatory story
contrasts the power of Rabbi Joshua with the failure of the follower
of Jesus, who was drowned in the sea.[60]

---

[56] Urbach (1984): 145; Schwartz (2001): 174.
[57] Levine (1986): 67.
[58] Klein (1939): 59; Yudelevitz (1950): 64; Hirshman (1988): 121; Buchmann (1968):
198.
[59] Brown (1967): 141; Goodman (1983): 471; See also the discussion in chapter 3.5
on *Public Baths and Spas: The Roman Leisure Culture.*
[60] Hirshman (1988): 121; See Mark 6, 48; On the terminology of *min*, see Kimelman
(1981): 232–236.

This story enables us to reconstruct the architectural structure of Hammei-Tiberias to some extent. The text mentions a cupola. This was, in fact, a niche in which a statue would be set up. They were customarily built in public buildings, and particularly in therapeutic baths.[61] The statue of Hygieia, the goddess of health, or her father, Aesculapius, the god of medicine, may have been set up in such niches in the baths of Tiberias, as was usual in medicinal baths in the Roman and Byzantine periods.[62]

Another source from the *Jerusalem Talmud, Avoda Zarah* 4, 4 [43d] informs us that there were idols in the public baths of Tiberias, and that Rabbi Yohanan bar Nafha ordered that they should be smashed:[63]

> Rabbi Yohanan said to Bar Drosai, 'Go, break all the idols that are in the public baths [= of Tiberias]', and he went and broke all of them except for one. And why so? Said Rabbi Yose ben Rabbi Bun, 'Because a certain Israelite was suspected of going and offering incense on that one' [= and an idol worshiped by an Israelite is not subject to nullification at all].

The commentators consider that Bar Drosai was a gentile, and that Rabbi Yohanan apparently ordered him to shatter the idols in the public bath in order to use the fragments. He broke them all up apart from one statue, which it was suspected that a Jew had worshipped and could not be de sanctified. Urbach emphasizes that 'such a suspicion was most remote, and the tone of the story confirms this'. He rejects Lieberman's view, that 'the suspect Jew worshipped at the time of Hadrian's edicts, but it is hard to suppose that the memory of this act was preserved for more than a hundred years'.[64] Baer discusses Rabbi Yohanan's deed, and wonders why Rabbi Yohanan, who was known for his tolerance in matters of idolatry, should suddenly decide to commit a fanatical act, as had Mattathias the Hasmonean in his day when he smashed the idols in his town. His reply was that at that time there

---

[61] See especially *Mishnah, Avoda Zarah* 1, 7; See also Hirschberg (1920): 241; Buchmann (1956): 29; On some more explanation on the cupola, see Irshai (1984): 138–139.

[62] On statues which adorned baths, see Elmslie (1911): 48–49; The architecture and sculptures at Hammat-Gader were described in the poetic inscription of Empress Eudocia in the fifth century CE; See Green and Tsafrir (1982): 77–91; Di Segni (1997): 228–233; See also Yegül's (1992: 92–127) reconstruction plans of thermo-mineral baths; Dvorjetski (1988): 102–107.

[63] Baer (1961): 33; Safrai (1982a): 164; cf. Klein (1939): 60.

[64] Urbach (1988): 153; See also Lieberman (1946): 361–366; Friedman (1998): 77–92.

was an edict requiring the Jews to burn incense to idols.[65] Urbach
claims that 'in this story there is no hint of such an edict. Moreover,
Baer ignores the simple interpretation: here, the breaking-up of idols
is not an act of fanaticism, but, as appears from the context, and as
the commentators understood, this is a case of nullifying idol-worship
and using the material of which the broken idol was made'.[66]

This example emphasizes the *halakhic* standpoint of the Rabbis, who
were accustomed to bathe in therapeutic baths ornamented with statues.
Rabban Gamaliel of Jabneh used to do this in the baths of Acre, and
there he stated unambiguously: 'Aphrodite has become a decoration
of the bath' (*Mishnah Avoda Zarah* 3, 4; *Babylonian Talmud, ibid.*, 43b).
Later, Rabbi Judah the Patriarch permitted bathing in the Bath of the
Three Graces in Hammat-Gader. Nonetheless, when the Rabbis were
able to extirpate pagan elements from these places they did so, as in
the case of Rabbi Yohanan.[67]

'The place of the cupola', the niche of the statue, apparently served
as a reference-point for the townspeople. The *halakha* stated:[68]

> At first the people of Tiberias traverse the entire area of Hammthan,
> and the people of Hammthan reach only the bow. Now the people of
> Hammthan and Tiberias are one town.
>
> (*Tosefta, Eruvin* 5, 2, ed. Liberman, p. 111)

If Hammat was an integral part of the town of Tiberias, then the baths
of Tiberias were also within the town. In Klein's words, 'The Gentile
population and those whom it influenced made their mark on the
town of Tiberias, built temples and set up statues there'.[69] In front of
the municipal council-house stood a statue known as *Tsalma of the Bule*
(*Jerusalem Talmud, Avoda Zarah* 3, 13 [43b]. Another statue, the *Hadorei*

---

[65] Baer (1961): 33–34.

[66] Urbach (1988): 153, note 73.

[67] For Rabbi Judah's public activities at the spas, see below in 5.5 *The Medical History of
Rabbi Judah the Patriarch* and also Dvorjetski (1999a): 126–129; idem, (2003): 20–21; For
the case of Aphrodite in Acre and its interpretations, see Wasserstein (1980): 257–267;
Rosenthal (1980): II: 40–43; Zlotnick (1993): 49–52; Eliav (1995): 3–35; Halbertal (1998):
159–172; Schwartz (1998): 203–217; Jacobs (1998): 219–311; Eliav (2000): 416–454;
Schwartz (2001): 167–171; Eliav (2002): 411–433; Fridheim (2003): 7–32.

[68] See also *Jerusalem Talmud, Eruvin* 5, 1 [22d]; The indication 'at first' demonstrates
the possibility that this *halakha* was fixed at the Usha period, after the Bar Kochba
revolt. See Oppenheimer (1991): 58.

[69] Klein (1967): 99; On the sources' concentration in Tiberias and its suburb, see
idem, (1939): 56–57; Lieberman (1931): 113.

(Dorei) Tsalma (ibid., Berakhot 2, 1 [4d]; *ibid., Sheqalim* 2, 7 [47a], stood over one of the springs and served as an outlet for the water, *Dorei's penis.*[70] The *Jerusalem Talmud, Shabbat* 14, 4 [14d] says of Rabbi Yonah, who was known as 'forceful of the Land of Israel' and, together with Rabbi Yose, was head of the academy of Tiberias, that:[71]

> Rabbi Yonah had chills and fever. [= They brought him a medicinal] drink prepared of the phallus of *Hadorei* and he drank it.

Klein maintains that this statue stood in front of the entrance to the Ἀδριανεῖον, the pagan shrine within the hot baths in which the Emperor Hadrian was worshipped.[72]

The sources indicate that the Rabbis of Tiberias ordered that the statues be blinded. Rabbi Simeon ben Lakish ordered Gamaliel Zuga to blind the eyes of the statue *Tavnita* (*Jerusalem Talmud, Avoda Zarah* 3,11 [43b]; Rabbi Yohanan ordered Rabbi Yitzhak bar Matana to blind the eyes of the *Tsalma of the Bule* (*ibid.*, 3, 13 [43b]; and Rabbi Joshua ben Levi either ordered Rabbi Ya'akov bar Idi to blind the eyes of the *Adorei Tsalma*, or did the deed himself (*ibid.*).[73]

Another occasion mentioned by *Mishnah, Avoda Zarah* 1, 1–3, as one of the festivals of the Gentiles on which, and three days before which, there should be no dealings with them, was the day of a banquet:

> For three days before the idolatrous festivals of idolaters it is prohibited to have business dealings with them—neither to loan to them nor to borrow from them, neither to lend [= money] to them nor to borrow [= money] from them, neither to make payment to them nor to accept (re)payment from them...Rabbi Ishmael says, 'For three days before them and for three days after them it is forbidden'. But the Sages say, 'Before their idolatrous festivals it is prohibited, but after their idolatrous festivals it is permitted'.

The festivals included in the *Mishnah* the *Calendae*, the first of each month, and particularly the New Year; the *Saturnalia*, a Roman holiday

---

[70] Bacher (1927): 136; Klein (1967): 99; On the various ideas of the *Bule*, see Krauss (1922): 185.

[71] *Babylonian Talmud, Ta'anit* 23b; Lieberman (1935): 188; On Rabbi Yonah see Margalioth (1976): II: 512–513.

[72] Klein (1967): 99–100) relies upon Epiphanius's account, who reports that the Tiberians wished to convert the *Hadrianium* to a *demosin* because it stood in the vicinity of the baths; See above, note 35; See also Robinson and Smith (1841): 268–269; Sepp (1863): 152; Dechent (1884): 181; Vincent (1921): 440.

[73] Yudelevitz (1950): 18; See the discussion in Blidstein (1974): 158–159.

which fell on December 17th; the *Kratesis*, the Day of Sovereignty, August 1st, when Augustus conquered Alexandria; the *Genosia*, the Emperor's birthday or the day of his coronation; the days of birth and death of any Gentile are also festivals, on which the dead man's utensils are cremated.[74]

The *halakha* forbidding commerce on idolatrous festivals discussed an event which occurred in Decapolis. The Beth Shean fair took place inside the town, and only some of the shops took part in it: some shops were decorated, others were not. This was the situation in Beth Shean, and the Rabbis declared: with the decorated shops trade is forbidden; with those not decorated it is permitted.[75] The *Jerusalem Talmud, Avoda Zarah* 1, 2 [39c] gives authentic confirmation of the concurrence of festival and fair. Rabbi Ze'ira sent Rabbi Bibi to buy a small skein of wool during the *Saturnalia* in Beth Shean. The fair to which Rabbi Bibi was sent was one of the features of the festival.[76]

Roman fairs were seasonal events, as can be seen from rabbinical literature and from various patristic writings and chronicles, and were combined with festivals in honour of gods and the Emperor. Evidence of the existence of such a fair, which originated in the second century CE and perhaps even earlier, is found in the *Chronicon Paschale*, which is dated to the seventh century CE. According to this Byzantine source, after the revolt of Bar Kochba the Emperor Hadrian held a fair in Gaza, named after him, in which Jewish prisoners were sold. During the assemblies known as *Panegyris Hadriane* (πανήγυρις Ἀδριανή), which apparently took place on the day of the emperor's visit to the town, speeches in his honour were made; and, according to this source, they were made 'to this very day'.[77] It may be that the anonymous mention of 'the fable of a king who went to Hammat-Gader and took his sons with him' (*Midrach Esselesastes Rabbah* 3, 20, Buber ed., p. 131; *Tanhuma,*

---

[74] The explanation is according to Albek (1959): 325–326; On these festivals see Blaufuss (1909): 11–21; Bickerman (1929): 4–23; Krauss (1948): 68–74; Lieberman (1963): 8–9; Epstein (1964): 482; Urbach (1988): 159–162; Bickerman (1929): 4–23; Bunson (1994), s.v. 'Festival of the Roman Year'; Hayes (1997): 48–49.

[75] Urbach (1988): 135; Safrai (1984): 153, note 97) assumes that this testimony is from the Usha period.

[76] Klein (1939): 17; Fuks (1983): 88; Herman (1991): 222–223.

[77] *Chronicon Paschale*, I, 3–9; Avi-Yonah (1964a): 134; Fishman-Duker (1984): 238–239; Dan (1984): 198, 201; Safrai (1984): 152–153; According to Kindler (1975: 63) the Hadrianic counting of Gaza is connected to the panegyric assemblies, which were celebrated in the city annually.

Kedoshim 8, Buber ed., p. 76) refers to the emperor Hadrian, who visited the soldiers of the Tenth Legion, which was stationed permanently in the vicinity of Hammat-Gader, used the baths because of his medical problems, and perhaps even participated in the fair which was held there.[78] It may be that the *Mishnaic* text in *Avoda Zarah* 4, 6, refers to him:

> An idol whose devotees have abandoned it in time of peace is permitted [= to be made use by the Jews], but if in time of war it is prohibited. Baths for kings—these permitted since they were set up when the kings pass by.

However, the text might be referred also to Emperor Caracalla. This idea can be derived from a silver coin depicting an eagle with a wealth between its legs, inside which are the Three Graces, first appears in the city of Gadara in the days of Caracalla. The image of the Three Graces—the emblem of Gadara mint—appears between the eagle's legs also on the Roman provincial silver tetradrachms, which were minted in the city during the reign of Caracalla. The three Graces have a fascinating link with the medicinal baths at Hammat-Gader; it has been shown, that the original name of these baths was 'Baths of the Three Graces'. In view of the appearance of this emblem at that particular time it may be assumed that the baths of Hammat-Gader were officially inaugurated in the days of Emperor Caracalla.[79]

The Rabbinic literature shows clearly that the complex of prohibitions on participation in fairs was gradually rescinded. From a clear prohibition in the days of the *Tannaim* there developed a series of partial concessions in the second generation of Palestinian *Amoraim*. In the *Jerusalem Talmud, Avoda Zarah* 1, 4 [39d] a series of halakhic judgments lightening the prohibition on participating in a fair is quoted in the name of Rabbi Yohanan, of the third century CE.[80] These stemmed from the dictates of the economic situation in Palestine, in which the

---

[78] On the intents of the Emperors at the spas in the eastern Mediterranean, see Dvorjetski (1994d); idem, (1997b); For Hadrian's aims, see idem, forthcoming [b].

[79] Dvorjetski (1993): 404–406; idem, (1994c): 110–111, Fig. 3; idem, (1997b): 580, especially note 69; cf. Hirschfeld (1997): 478; See also Meshorer (1985): 82–83.

[80] On Rabbi Yohanan's position in the Jewish society and his attitude toward the relations between Jews and Gentiles, see Blidstein (1974): 154–161; Kimelman (1982–1983): 329–358; Herman (1991): 219–241; Urbach (1971), s.v. 'Rabbi Yohanan'; See also the reference in chapter 7.1 on his treatment by a Gentile woman physician regarding Emmaus.

fairs were an important element, and from the Rabbis' desire to help
the Palestinian Jews to become integrated in economic life, as well as
from the change in their attitude when they ceased to fear the threat
of idolatry.[81]

One of the most characteristic features of the fair was that goods
were sold there. In Hammat-Gader, in the centre of the pagan fair, a
local pagan cult was celebrated in which expensive objects and pastry
were sold:[82]

> Rabbi Hanina of Ein Te'enah went with Rabbi Ze'ira to Hammat-Gader
> and bought Rabbi Ze'ira *kluskin* [= cakes].
>
> (*Jerusalem Talmud, Terumot* 2, 1 [41b])

And spicy dishes:[83]

> Rabbi Samuel bar Nathan in the name of Rabbi Hama bar Hanina
> [= said], 'Father and I went up to Hammat-Gader, and [= on the Shabbat]
> they served us eggs as small as crab-apples, and their flavor was as good
> as that of *pankrisin* [= peaches].
>
> (*ibid., Shabbat* 3, 1 [5d])

Vegetables, fruit, tools, and, apparently, medical appliances were also
sold. In the *itliz* at Emmaus food was sold, including cattle meant for
sacrifice which had been rejected.[84]

By comparing parallel passages in Rabbinic literature it emerges that
the name of the curative bath is not specifically mentioned in the texts;
it is an interesting fact that the failure to name Hammat-Gader, a site

---

[81] Safrai (1984): 150; Bacher (1909): 148–152; Krauss (1909): 294–311; Klein
(1910a): 22–25.

[82] On wholesalers and merchants who visited the fairs for renewing their stocks, see
Kleiman (1986): 477–478; Safrai (1986): 485–486; On the *kluskin*, either cakes, scones
or white and delicate bread, see Jastrow (1950): 246; Kohut (1926): VII: 107; On
kluskin in the fair see *Jerusalem Talmud, Avoda Zarah* 1, 4 [39c]; On Rabbi Hanina from
Ein Te'enah, see Margalioth (1976): I: 350; On Ein Te'enah, east of Sepphoris, see
Avi-Yonah (1984): 134; For the permanent spelling mistake 'Hammat-Gerar' instead
of 'Hammat-Gader' here and elsewhere in the Talmudic literature, see Rabbinovicz
(1839): II: 240; Klein (1939): 47; Miller (1992): 190.

[83] Cf. *Jerusalem Talmud, Terumot* 2, 3 [41c]; *Pankrisin* is a kind of a vegetable, probably an apricot according to Jastrow (1950): 1191; More suitable is Feliks's suggestion
(1994: 230) that it is an peach based on the parallels in the Graeco-Roman literature;
Meshorer (2004: 30) indicates that these eggs were thrown into the boiling Suphur
waters and changed their coulor and taste; On the luxury food in the baths, see Sukenik
(1935a): 20, and the discussion about *The Public Baths and Spas: The Roman Leisure Culture*
in chapter 3.5; On Rabbi Hama bar Hanina, see Margalioth (1976): I: 318–319.

[84] *Mishnah, Kritut* 3, 7; *Babylonian Talmud, ibid.,* 15a; *ibid., Makkot* 14a.

which Rabbis also visited to be cured, is apparently tendentious. It is mentioned in two ways: by the use of the term 'another place' or by the general phrase 'that inn'. From these parallels it appears that the Rabbis systematically refrained from revealing the name of the place where they were accustomed to stay, since they found the atmosphere of decadence and adultery there objectionable. A certain opprobrium of Hammat-Gader healing site, when it was visited by the Sages, can be discerned when comparing four parallel Talmudic passages in one of each pair the place remains anonymous:[85]

Jerusalem Talmud, Shabbat 18, 1 [16c]: Rabbi Ze'ira in the name of Rabbi Hanina… 'Once we were going up with Rabbi to *Hammat-Gader*. He found would say to us: 'Choose for yourselves smooth pebbles, and you will then be permitted to carry them about tomorrow' [= on the Shabbat].	*Babylonian Talmud, Shabbat 125b*: Rabbi Hanina, and some say Rabbi Ze'ira n the name of Rabbi Hanina, said: 'Once Rabbi went to *a certain place* and there a block of bricks.'
Jerusalem Talmud, Shabbat 3, 1 [5d]: Rabbi Samuel bar Nathan in the name of Rabbi Hama bar Hanina: 'Father and I went up to *Hammat-Gader*, and they brought before us eggs as crab-apples, and they tasted as luscious as peaches'.	*Babylonian Talmud, Shabbat 38a*: Rabbi Hama bar Hanina said, 'My Master and I were once guests *in a certain place*, and eggs shrunk to the size of crab-apples were brought before us, and we ate many of them'.
Jerusalem Talmud, Eruvin 6, 4 [23c]: Rabbi Hiyya, and Rabbi Assi, and Rabbi Yohanan went up to *Hammat-Gader*. They said, 'We shall wait till The Elders of the South will come here'.	*Babylonian Talmud, Eruvin 65b*: Resh Lakish and the scholars of Rabbi Hanina once happened to be *in a certain inn*. He said to them, 'We shall rent, and when we come to our Rabbis at the South we shall ask them'.

---

[85] For the inn and its characteristics, see Krauss (1929): I/1: 134–139; Safrai (1985), s.v. 'Pundak'; For the innkeeping in Jewish society, see Rosenfeld (1998): 133–158; For the phenomenon of the prostitution in the inns, see Firebaugh (1928); Kleberg (1957): 57–59, 120–121; Evans (1991): 135; Dyson (1991): 175–176; Rosenfeld (1998): 136–137; On the unique stance of the Rabbinic sources towards Hammat-Gader, see Klein (1931): 23; Lieberman (1980): 10; Dvorjetski (2003); idem, forthcoming [a]; For the food in the Roman period, see André (1961); Alcock (2001); Dalby (2003); and Broshi (1987), for the food in Palestine.

Jerusalem Talmud, Eruwin 6, 4 [23c]:	*Babylonian Talmud, Eruvin 65b*:
Rabbi Hiyya, Rabbi Assi, Rabbi Ami went up to *Hammat-Gader*. They asked Rabbi Hama bar Joseph and he allowed. Rabbi Yohanan heard and said, 'You have done well'.	Hanina bar Joseph, Rabbi Hiyya bar Abba and Rabbi Assi once happened to come *to a certain inn* whither a heathen, the owner of the inn...They asked Rabbi Yohanan, and he answered, 'You have done well'.

The Sages were obviously reluctant on principle to name the site which they visited because they disapproved of certain activities which took place there. Therefore, the only hinted at its identity, which was known to all.

Another example of special goods bought from Gentiles at a fair is found in a *Baraitha* to the *Jerusalem Talmud* dealing with food that it is permitted to eat:

> Rabbi Ami went up with Rabbi Judan Nesi'ah to Hammat-Gader and allowed [= Jews] to eat *halut* [= dumplings prepared by] them to be eaten.
>
> (*Jerusalem Talmud, Avoda Zarah* 3, 9 [42a])

The dumpling, *halut* in Hebrew, was a wheat product, whose details are not given. *Halut* may be an orthographical error for χάριτ, which was known as a delicious cake made of flour and honey and was eaten in the fairs dedicated to the Three Graces.[86] The term *halut* also appears in connection with Rabbis' visits to Emmaus, the headquarters of the Roman army during the Great Revolt of 66–70 CE:

> Rabbi Aha went to Emmaus and ate *their halit*, Rabbi Jeremiah ate *hamtzin*, and Rabbi Hezekiah ate *kamtzin*.
>
> (*ibid., Avoda Zarah* 5, 4 [44d])

Some scholars maintain that the Rabbis ate the food of the Samaritans in Emmaus; the *baraitha* describes local customs, where the Jews were in a minority among Christians and Samaritans, until the Byzantine period.[87]

---

[86] Several explanations were given to the *halut*: a dumpling made of flour and water; mixture of kinds of dates or any food done by flour; See Sokoloff (1990): 202; Kohut (1926): III: 402; Jastrow (1950): 466; It seems that it might be cookies made by flour and honey, which were distributed between the celebrators in the festivals in hounor of the τρεῖς χάριτες; On these specific events, see Escher (1899): 2160–2163; Gsell (1963): 1664.

[87] See, for example, Sachs (1914): 20; Schwartz (1986): 121; idem, (1982): 188.

It is important to note that the place-names Emmaus, Hammatha, and Emmatha are frequently interchanged in Rabbinic literature; it is, therefore, impossible to know for certain whether the incident occurred in Hammat or in Emmaus.[88]

The Sages also used medical products when they visited therapeutic baths. It is not impossible that the medical aids which the bathers used were bought on the spot.[89] Thus for instance:

> Rabbi Ami went up with Rabbi Judan Nesi'ah to Hammat-Gader. He injured his finger and put a plaster on it.
>
> *(ibid., Avoda Zarah 2, 2, 40d])*

This bandage (*ispelanit* in Hebrew) was covered with viscous material, which stuck fast to the body and did not melt as a result of body heat.[90] This also applies to the pebbles, which were used for therapeutic purposes, in addition to spreading peloma on the body or on particular parts of it.[91] In the words of the *baraitha* to the *Jerusalem Talmud, Shabbat* 18, 1 [16c]:[92]

> Rabbi Ze'ira in the name of Rabbi Hanina said, 'Once we were going up with Rabbi to Hammat-Gader. He would say to us, "Choose for yourselves smooth pebbles, and you will then be permitted to carry them about tomorrow."' [= on the Shabbat].

Goods were not only purchased in the baths; they were also loaned. Once, when Rabbi Judan Nesi'ah and Rabbi Ami visited the Hammat-Gader baths, they were asked a question connected with daily life at this place of healing: whether vessels borrowed from non-Jews had to

---

[88] For a philological discussion on these names in Aramaic, Syriac and Greek, see the *Introduction* in chapter 1; See also Josephus, *Bellum Judaicum* 4.11; idem, *Antiquitates Judaicae* 18.36; Rapoport (1857): 110–113.

[89] On the medical supplies at the spas, see the survey on *The Military Presence at the Medicinal Hot Springs and Healing Spas in the Graeco-Roman World* in chapter 3.4 and the discussion on *The Healing Properties of the Spas* in chapter 5; See also Dvorjetski (1994b); idem, (1996c); idem, (2002).

[90] *Ispelanit* was a kind of emplastrum (plaster) related to the Greek σπλενίον, more or less equivalent to the Hebrew term *retiyyah* (compress). See Kohut: (1926): I: 188; Goldstein and Shechter: (1956): I: 74; Kottek (1996): 2926–2927.

[91] On the use of the *peloma*, see Buchmann (1955): 287–292; Dvorjetski (1995a); For various explanations of the pebbles, see Krauss (1909–1910): 49; Hirschberg (1920): 233–234; Sperber (1986): 64–65.

[92] See parallel version in *Jerusalem Talmud, Shabbat* 4, 6 [7a]; On Rabbi Hanina bar Hama, see Margalioth (1976): I: 327–333; Miller (1992): 175–200; Dvorjetski (2002): 43–44.

be immersed in water [in order to make them kosher]. The *Amoraims'* discussion of this question shows clearly that in this matter, too, Rabbi Yohanan's attitude was quite permissive. In Tractate *Avoda Zarah* 5, 12, of the *Mishnah* we read 'Whoever takes vessels from a Gentile—whoever is accustomed to immerse them, let him immerse; whoever is accustomed to boil them, let him boil; whoever is accustomed to whiten them in the sun, let him whiten them in the sun'. The *Mishnah* sets out rules for the purification of various vessels obtained from non-Jews, and the *Babylonian Talmud, ibid.*, 75b, adds 'It was taught: And they must all be immersed in forty *seah*'. Some Sages extended this *halakhic* injunction, and applied it to borrowed vessels. The *baraitha* in the *Jerusalem Talmud, ibid.*, 5, 15 [45b] says:

> It was taught: Rabbi Hoshaia [= said], 'One has to immerse'. [= cups or other utensils for food]. This is in line with the following: Rabbi Ami went up with Rabbi Judan Nesi'ah to Hammat-Gader. They borrowed silver from those of *Ossinus*. They asked Rabbi Jeremiah [= whether even the silver had to be immersed]. He instructed them to immerse the coins, for they had come forth from the uncleanness pertaining to a gentile and had entered the sanctification pertaining to an Israelite].

Jewish visitors, who did not bring their own vessels, were possibly compelled to use utensils borrowed from local inhabitants of the spa, most of them Gentiles. Jastrow, Kohut, Klein, and Herman conjecture that the reference is to money loaned by the money-changers of the house of *Ossinus*.[93] Hirschberg, however, explains that the reference may be to silver vessels borrowed from *Aineissi*—those suffering from nervous desease.[94] Lieberman maintains that the question of silver was connected with silver jewellery belonging to a Roman family called the Ausones (Αὔσονες), who lived in Hammat-Gader. In his view, these were not eating utensils; they were silver ornaments, which also had to be immersed, since they were passed on from unclean Gentiles to righteous Jews, and even jewels had to be immersed before use.[95] According to Hirschfeld, 'the house of *Ausinos*' was a kind of a hostel built with public funds.[96]

---

[93] Jastrow (1950): 315; Kohut (1926): III: 97–98; Klein (1939): 45; Herman (1990–1991): 234.
[94] Hirschberg (1920): 245; cf. Horowitz (1923): 25.
[95] Lieberman (1968): 106; Lieberman is followed by Kimelman (1982–1983): 349.
[96] Hirschfeld (1994): 8; It might be simply a house as remarked by Urman (1995): 598.

The large number of visitors to the thermo-mineral baths made it necessary to provide accommodation for them. During the fairs, in the course of the bathing season, and at other times, inns and hostels, whether privately owned or financed by the spa like the one at Gadara, provided accommodation in the town. These possibilities are documented in Rabbinic literature and the *Itineraria* of the pilgrims.[97] The *Ilin d'Aussinus* was apparently a private or public hostel which supplied the varied requirements of the public, such as the provision of food, the loan of various sorts of apparatus including silver jewellery, accommodation for visitors, money-changing and the sale of medical equipment.

One of the *halakhic* discussions, which centered on Hammat-Gader and served as a standard for thermo-mineral baths in general appears in Rabbinic literature in several versions, and bears witness to the Rabbis' uncertainties about daily life there. The question was whether the residents of Hammat-Gader were permitted to go to Gadara on the Shabbat, and whether the residents of Gadara were permitted to go to the spa-suburb Hammat-Gader on the Shabbat. The *Tosefta, Eruvin* 4, 16 (Lieberman ed., p. 110) states:

> An old shepherd came before Rabbi and said to him, 'I recall that the townsfolk of Migdal Gader[98] would go down to Hammtha, up to the outermost courtyard near the bridge'. And Rabbi permitted the townsfolk to go down to Hammtha up to the outermost courtyard, by the bridge. And Rabbi further permitted the townsfolk of Gader to go down to Hammtha and to go up to Gader.

Rabbi Judah the Patriarch's ruling that the residents of Hammat-Gader were not allowed to walk to Gadara, whereas travel in the opposite direction was permitted, raised controversy in the *Jerusalem Talmud* as well as the *Babylonian* Talmud. The Sages tried to explain the ruling in various ways. In the *Jerusalem Talmud, Eruvin* 5,7 [22d] is reported:

---

[97] Safrai (1995): 199–201; Alon (1971): 186–188; Dan (1984): 117; See also Antoninus Placentinus's evidence about Hammat-Gader and of Michael the Syrian about Hammei-Tiberias in chapter 4.1 on *The Historical-Archaeological Analysis of Hammei-Tiberias* and in chapter 5 on *The Healing Properties of the Spas.*

[98] The word 'Gader' is missing in Erfurt and London Codices; From this *baraitha* Klein (1925: 39) thought that Jews were living in Gadara at the end of the second century CE and in the beginning of the third century CE, while Sukenik (1935b: 43) assumed that Jews were living in Hammat-Gader; Hirschberg (1920: 232–233) is convinced that Rabbi Elazar ben Simeon had a permanent academy in Migdal Gader.

Rabbi Mana said because of the [= Roman] authorities. Rabbi Yose ben
Rabbi Bun, 'not because of this reason but because we learnt that the
people of a large town traverse the entire area of a small town [= located
within the limits of the large town]. But the people of a small town may
not traverse the entire area of the large town'.

Rabbi Mana said that the reason was 'because of the authorities', while
Rabbi Yose claimed that the problem stemmed from the difference
between 'the men of a big town and the men of a small town'; the
consequence was that the boundary of the area in which the people
of Hammat-Gader were permitted to walk on the Shabbat was in the
middle of the big town of Gader. Since they were not allowed to go
to the end of the town, they were forbidden to go there at all.[99]

In the *Babylonian Talmud, Eruvin* 61a, various other possibilities are
advanced. Some connected with the architectural structure and planning
of these towns 'a town built in the shape of a bow', some with the town
wall of Gadara, and—most relevant to the present discussion—some
with the character of the inhabitants:[100]

> Rabbi permitted the inhabitants of Gader to go down to Hammthan
> but did not allow the inhabitants of Hammthan to go up to Gader. Now
> what could have been the reason? Obviously, that the former did put up a
> barrier while the latter did not put up a barrier. When Rav Dimi came he
> explained: The people of Gader used to molest the people of Hammtha,
> and 'permitted' meant 'ordained'. Then why should Shabbat be different
> from other days? Because intoxication is not uncommon on such a day.
> Would the people of Gader not molest the Hammthan people when they
> come to Hammthan?—No; a dog in a strange town does not bark for
> seven years. Now then, might not the people of Hammthan molest those
> of Gader?—No; The people of Gader were not so submissive as all that.
> Rav Safra explained: Gader was a town that was built in the shape of a
> bow. Rav Dimi ben Hinena explained: The former were the inhabitants
> of a large town while the latter were inhabitants of a small town. Thus
> taught Rav Kahana. Rav Tabyomi, however, taught as follows: Rav Safra
> and Rav Dimi ben Hinena differ, one explaining that Gader was a town
> built in the shape of a bow, while the other explains that the latter were
> the inhabitants of a small town while the former were the inhabitants
> of a large town.

---

[99] On intensive activities of the Roman rule in the Galilee between 66 CE and
135 CE, see Oppenheimer (1977): 53–83; idem, (1992): 115–125; Isaac (1988): 9–16;
idem, (1993): 235–242.
[100] See also Elitzur (1980): 20–21; Epstein, *Babylonian Talmud, Eruvin* 61a: 427.

Rav Dimi, one of the most famous of the Babylonian *Amoraim*, put forward another reason, connected with the bad relationships between the inhabitants of Gadara and those of Hammat-Gader. When the people of the small settlement of Hammat-Gader came to the town of Gader, the people of Gader used to beat them. When the men of Gader came to Hammat-Gader, the people of Hammat-Gader took care not to attack them. Therefore, according to Rav Dimi, Rabbi Judah the Patriarch forbade the people of Hammat-Gader to visit Gader, simply in order to prevent quarrels and fights.

The objective of Rabbi Judah's ruling chimes well with other acts of his. His aims were to ensure that broad sections of the community should observe religious ordinances, to create a single obligatory legal system, and to edit the *Mishnah*. He also aimed at strengthening the Jewish communities in mixed cities and key regions in Palestine, while observing the principle of 'for the sake of peaceful relations', in theory and in practice.

The Sages visited Hammat-Gader therapeutic site for the bathing season and held semi-official meetings there. They may have been held separately from the fairs, or at times when there were no fairs; there is, therefore, no evidence in our sources that the Sages took part in the fairs.[101] One of these occasions was a fascinating encounter between Rabbi Hanina bar Hamma, the presiding judge at Sepphoris, Rabbi Yonathan, and the 'Elders of the South', whose activities were centered principally on the academy of Lydda.[102] The *halakhic* question in the *Jerusalem Talmud, Eruvin* 6, 4 [23c] discussed was whether it was permitted to hire a piece of ground, a building or a courtyard from an inn-keeper for the Shabbat. The central question arising from the *halakhic* discussion was the significance of the phrase: 'since the Gentile comes and takes me out', Which Gentile is meant here?

> 'Is it proper to rent premises from an innkeeper for the Shabbat?' Rabbi Hanina and Rabbi Yonathan went up to Hammat-Gader. They said: 'Let us wait until the elders of the South come here'. Rabbi Nathan the Southerner came. They asked him [= the above question] and he

---

[101] Safrai (1984): 146.

[102] Oppenheimer (1991): 132; idem, (1978): 90; See also Ne'eman (1991): 22, note 4; Rabbi Yonathan, who was sneering toward Rabbi Samlai and the 'Southerns', is associate to the offer waiting for Southern Elders; Schwartz (1986): 211; idem, (1983): 102–109; On the academy in Lydda, see Oppenheimer (1988): 115–136; Schwartz (1991), s.v. 'Darom', Daroma'; Rosenfeld (1997): 40–57, 141–148.

allowed it. When Rabbi Simeon ben Lakish heard it he said: 'Since the
Gentile can come and remove us, the renting is of no avail. Simeon bar
Abba reports: Rabbi Yohanan asked: Does it follow that our houses do
not belong to us either?' To this Yusti ben Simeon in the name of Rabbi
Boethus replied: [= 'There is a difference between our private homes and
an inn]; our homes are not our own [= in the sense that the Romans
may] lodge with us but do not drive us out, whereas from an inn we are
liable to be ejected'.

In the discussion of this question the arbitrary actions of the Roman
administration are described.[103] According to the *halakha*, it is forbidden to carry objects from one room to another or from a house to a
courtyard, on the Shabbat, unless they are both under the control of
one person. In the case of a gentile, the Jew can evade the prohibition
by hiring the place for the whole of the Shabbat. Judging from the
names of the Rabbis who visited the baths of Hammat-Gader, it is
clear that the event described took place in the first half of the third
century CE. The *Amoraim* dissented, as follows: Rabbi Simeon ben
Lakish claimed that, since the gentiles were liable to come and expel
them from the inn, it was pointless to hire the place. Rabbi Boethus
maintained that there was a difference between a private house and an
inn: the Romans might come and stay in the Jews' houses, but would
not turn them out, whereas those who stayed in inns could be expelled
at any time. Thus, the question centered on the fact that guests could
be expelled from an inn at any time. It should be noted that Rabbi
Simeon ben Lakish disagreed with the southern Sages, even though
he adopted their viewpoint on a parallel case in the *Babylonian Talmud,
Eruvin* 65b:[104]

> Resh Lakish and the scholars of Rabi Hanina once happened to be in a
> certain inn while its tenant was away but its landlord was present... Resh
> Lakish said to them: 'Let us rent it and when we arrive at our Masters
> in the South we might submit the question to them'. On submitting the
> question to Rabbi Afes he replied, 'You have acted well in renting it'.

---

[103] Lieberman (1946): 354–355; idem, *Eruvin*, (1935): 312–313; Urbach (1976):
125–126; On the massive presence of the Roman army in the Levant in general and
in the Galilee in particular, see Avi-Yonah (1970): 77–88, and see especially p. 83;
Goodman (1983): 471; Millar (1996); Goodman (1997); See also note 99 above.
[104] From this text it is apparent that the Galilean Sages wished to to consult with
Rabbi Afes. This tradition clarifies the status of the Sages of Southern Judaea; According to the *Babylonian Talmud, Eruvin* 65b we could deduce of affinity between Resh
Lakish and the Sages of the South, but the issue in the *Jerusalem Talmud, ibid.*, 6, 4 [23c]
undermine this conclusion; Zuri (1934): III/1: 133; On Resh Lakish, see Margalioth
(1976): II: 791–797.

Another question arising from the issue discussed in the *Mishnah* was presented in the *Jerusalem Talmud, Eruvin* 6, 4 [23c] until what time was it permitted to cancel the gentile's authority? On the Shabbat eve, only until sunset, or on the Shabbat, too?

> Rabbi Hiyya, Rabbi Yose, Rabbi Ima [= Ami] went up to Hammat-Gader. They asked Rabbi Hama bar Joseph, and he permitted doing so. Rabbi Yohanan heard about the ruling and said, 'You have done the right thing'. Rabbi Simeon ben Lakish heard and said, 'You have not done the right thing'. Do they then differ? Rabbi Ze'ira said, 'By no means. They do not differ. He who has said, 'You did the right thing' that you rented [= the right of domain from a gentile landholder in the courtyard, who was not at home prior to the advent of the Shabbat but came home on the Shabbat day itself]. He who has said, 'You did not do the right thing, that you carried objects about in the courtyard' [= without first renting the right of domain from the gentile]. Rabbi Ba said, 'They indeed differ. He who has said, 'You did the right thing', meant, 'You did the right thing in renting out the gentile's right of domain and also that you carried objects in the courtyard'. He who has said, 'You did not do the right thing', meant, You did not do the right thing in renting the gentile's right and in carrying objects about in the courtyard'.

A similar complaint from the third century CE is found in *Sifre on Deuteronomy* 320 (Finkelstein ed., p. 367):[105]

> 'And I shall provoke them with those who are not a people' (*Deuteronomy* 32, 21), read not *beloam* [= with not a people], but *bilway am* [= with associates of a people, I shall provoke them with] those who come from among the nations and kingdoms and expel them from their homes.

Lieberman and Urbach both emphasize that the Jews were frequently harassed by being evicted from their homes by the Roman auxiliaries.[106] Lieberman also claims that an inscription from the time of the question discussed in the tractate *Eruvin* 6, 4 [23c] of the *Jerusalem Talmud* casts light on the discussions of the *Amoraim*. In his reply to the inhabitants of Paneas in the Trachon, who complained of oppression by the Roman legions stationed there, Juilius Saturninus declared, 'Since you have an inn, you will not be compelled to receive your guests in your homes'. From this Lieberman concludes that where there were inns there was no

---

[105] Lieberman (1946): 355; On the relations between the Roman army and the Jews after the destruction of the Second Temple, see Safrai (1971): 124–129; Sperber (1969): 164–168; Safrai (1992): 103–114.

[106] Lieberman (1946): 355; Urbach (1976): 126; See also Avi-Yonah (1970): 83.

reason for the soldiers to be billeted in private homes. Now it is obvious
why Rabbi Boethus maintained that it was unnecessary to rent an inn,
since as soon as the Roman soldiers arrived the inn would be 'legally'
under their control, and the Jewish guests would be expelled.[107]

Another fascinating document, dating from 238 CE, the days of
Emperor Gordianus III, illustrates the sufferings of the inhabitants of
the village of Scaptopara in Thrace at the hands of the Roman soldiers,
'because of the hot springs' in the vicinity of their village.[108]

According to Hirschberg, the Sages used the spa 'also at times of
political confusion, persecution and hostile legislation'. He adds that
this was particularly the case when the bathing season was exploited for
national meetings, thus escaping the notice of the Romans.[109] Simply
from the remark 'let us wait until the Elders of the South arrive' it
can be understood that the Rabbis of Galilee and of the south met
together to discuss questions which were posed in Hammat-Gader site,
far from the centre of the country. It might be also on the contrary,
that is to say, the Sages made use of the medicinal hot springs for asking a question.

In addition to these cultic and commercial aspects, the fair served
as a place of social gathering and entertainment, and prostitution was
an accepted phenomenon there. The frequent visits of Rabbis and
patriarchs attracted the attention of the non-Jews. Since the non-Jewish
dignitaries visited the spot for the sake of debauchery and licentiousness, they assumed that the Patriarch, too, came for the same purpose.[110] Epiphanius states that the son of one of the patriarchs bathed
in Hammat-Gader during the fair together with his companion, one
of the Sages, and there met his beloved, a Christian woman.[111] Alon
maintains that the stories of the Church Fathers about the debaucheries

---

[107] Lieberman (1946): 356; Lieberman's idea is based on Dittenberger (1977): *OGIS*,
II: 305–306, no. 609.

[108] Dittenberger (1960): *SIG*, II: 605–606, no. 888; See Rostovtzeff (1957): 427, 623;
Alon (1971): 187; Dvorjetski (1992a): 165; idem, (1997a): 468. See also the discussion
in chapter 3.4 on *The Military Presence*.

[109] Hirschberg (1920): 231–232; Bedouins still thought during the 19th century that
the sites of hot springs were neutral. See Baedeker (1876): 185.

[110] Hirschberg (1920): 233.

[111] Epiphanius, *Adversus Haereses* 30.7, note 35 above; Epiphanius's descriptions are
partial, and their accuracy is questionable, however, the main point is probably not
fabricated; On the significance of the evidence, see chapter 4.2 on *The Historical-
Archaeological Analysis and Healing Cults of Hammat-Gader*; See also Rubin (1983): 105–116;
Tsafrir (1968): 81–82; For the connections between the annual celebration at Hammat-
Gader and the Maioumas festivals, see Efron (1988): 317; Dvorjetski (2001a): 99–118;
idem, (2001b): 79–93; idem, forthcoming [c].

of patriarchs and other Sages ignorant of the Torah and given over
to worldly pleasures should be viewed sceptically. However, Alon does
not deny that 'there were patriarchs who sought luxury', and adduces
as proof the practice of the patriarchs from the days of Rabbi Judah
the Patriarch onwards.[112] And, indeed, from the time of Rabbi Judah
the Patriarch Hammat-Gader was well known for its debaucheries,
and the story of the Neoplatonic philosopher Iamblichus about mixed
bathing of men and women, and more, is proof of this.[113]

It seems that mixed marriages of Jews and non-Jews were customary
in Hammat-Gader. Lieberman maintains that Roman noblemen were
accustomed to visit the spot, and that, therefore, 'many children of
non-Jews were born to Jewish women'. In his view this is not surprising,
since these thermo-mineral baths were famous throughout the world.[114]
These contentions and others appear in a *Braita* in the *Jerusalem Talmud*,
Qiddushin 3,14 [64c–d]:[115]

> Rabbi Hama bar Hanina was going up to Hammat-Gader. He came to
> his father and said to him, 'Take note that there are people there who are
> invalid. Be careful not to meet with them'. Even though Rabbi Simeon
> ben Judah said in the name of Rabbi Simeon ben Yohai, 'A gentile or
> a slave who had sexual relations with an Israelite girl—the offspring is
> valid', he concedes that if it was a daughter, she is invalid to marry a
> priest. Even though Rabbi Joshua said, 'He who has sexual relations with
> his sister—the offspring is valid', he concedes that if she was a female,
> she is invalid to marry into the priesthood.

Rabbi Hanina advised his son 'Be careful not to meet with them' that
is, that he should not go there with their daughters, lest they bear sons
prohibited from marrying.[116] This warning shows that many Jewish
women bore children there to non-Jews and slaves. The Sages' opinions
on the birth of those prohibited from marrying were divided. Some
called them bastards, others called them polluted. The *halakha* dealt with
the problems of daily life, and it may be that the following Talmudic

---

[112] Alon (1970): 19.
[113] See note 111 above; According to Schwabe's translation (1949: 236–237) Hammat-Gader was a bathing site for hermaphrodites.
[114] Lieberman (1980): 10; idem, (1974): 137.
[115] Lieberman (1959): 75–81; Klein (1939): 48; Satlow (1995): 86–88; See also Bar-Ilan (2000): 125–170; According to Sachs (1914: 21) the illegitimate infants were born from the Samaritans' inhabitants of Hammat-Gader; For the discussion if slaves could habitually use the baths as customers, see Fagan (1999b): 25–34.
[116] Hirschberg (1920): 234.

discussion of the *Jerusalem Talmud* (*Qiddushin* 3, 14 [64d]), is an example
of a solution to a real and difficult problem in the spas:[117]

> Rabbi Yonatan went up with Rabbi Judah the Patriarch to Hammat-
> Gader. He taught there that the offspring is valid. Said Rabbi Ze'ira, 'As
> to that offspring, as he goes onward, he gets promoted. 'Rabbi declared
> his offspring to be unfit, and the son of his son treats him as wholly valid'.
> Rabbi Ba bar Zabeda gave instructions in the presence of all the rabbis,
> 'The offspring is valid'. Rabbi Bibi said before Rabbi Ze'ira in the name
> of Rabbi Hanina, 'The offspring is valid'. Said Rabbi Ze'ira, 'Do they
> learn the law from this report? They do not learn the law from rumor!'
> Said Rabbi Hezekiah, 'I know the beginning and the end of it'.

Rabbi Yonathan and Rabbi Judah the Patriarch taught in Hammat-
Gader that the 'the child is legitimate'. Rabbi Ze'ira was very surprised
at this legitimization, and called out 'This child!' And as time went on
the Sages of that generation pronounced the child legitimate. Rabbi
Judah the Patriarch decided that the child prohibited from marrying
was polluted, whereas he had previously been thought a bastard. And
the grandson of Rabbi Judah—Rabbi Judah Nesi'ah—made him
legitimate.[118]

Rabbi Judah the Patriarch found in Hammat-Gader many bastard
children of Jewish women to Gentiles and slaves, and legitimized
them. Not everybody is convinced that Rabbi Judah the Patriarch was
meant. Francus claims that the reference is to his grandson, Rabbi
Judah Nesi'ah, the son of Rabban Gamaliel, the son of Rabbi Judah
the Patriarch. In his view, when Rabbi Ze'ira heard that Rabbi Judah
Nesi'ah declared that the child was legitimate, he said that this child,
born to a Jewish woman of a non-Jew or slave, was vainglorious; whereas
Rabbi Judah the Patriarch decided that the child was a bastard. His
son, Rabban Gamaliel, said that the child was polluted, that is to say
ineligible for the priesthood, whereas his grandson, Rabbi Judah Nesi'ah,
claimed that he was legitimate.[119] In short, the standpoint of the last
generation of Palestinian *Amoraim* was that the child was legitimate,
though it was not clear whether he was eligible for the priesthood.

---

[117] Cf. *Jerusalem Talmud, Yevamot* 7, 6 [8b]; On Rabbi Yonathan, see Margalioth
(1976): II: 516–517.
[118] Hirschberg (1920): 235.
[119] Francus (1988): 98–103.

It is reasonable to suppose that such crucial questions concerning matters of legitimacy were discussed seriously and publicly in the local academy or the synagogue at the thermo-mineral baths. Foerster uncovered two strata underneath the 'late' Byzantine synagogue of Hammat-Gader.[120] He dated the first stage of the synagogue at the third century CE, according to the evidence of the pottery, even though the plan of the earlier stage has not yet been exposed. This discovery may throw some light on the discussions of the *Tannaim* and *Amoraim* on the matter of the life of luxury, debauchery and immorality in the baths in the outskirts of Gadara as early as the time of Rabbi Judah the Patriarch.

There is reason to believe that some Rabbis, even apart from the Patriarch, took more liberties than the codified *halakha* allowed. An outstanding example in the region is that of the suburb of Gadara—Hammat-Gader therapeutic site—the favorite resort of some Rabbis in the third and fourth century CE. The well known site was thoroughly pagan in character. Not only did all the springs and baths have mythological names, but the annual festival that took place there, as well as the common practices of incubation and commemoration of miraculous cures, clearly indicates that the spa was not simply a place of recreation to the many visitors, but also functioned as a shrine to the Three Graces, to Aesculapius, god of medicine, to his daughter Hygieia, goddess of health, and to Sarapis. Schwartz emphasizes the fact that the *Mishnah* admittedly permits the use of baths and gardens owned by temples, but it is hard to see how a bath that was a temple could have been permitted. The willingness of some Rabbis to patronize a place like Hammat-Gader demonstrates what we might have supposed anyway—a greater diversity of Rabbinic behaviour and opinion than the Rabbinic sources indicate.[121]

Archaeological findings in the vicinity of the spas of Palestine, namely the synagogues, also bear witness to healing and relationships between Jews and Gentiles, who lived side by side throughout the Byzantine period. The donors' inscriptions in the synagogues within the baths, as well as coins and cameos, show mutual influence between the various

---

[120] Foerster (1983): 11–12; Urman (1995): 598; See below the discussion concerning the involvement of Gentiles in the dedicatory inscriptions at the synagogues in the spas and in chapter 5.4 about *The Epigraphical Material.*

[121] Schwartz (2001): 174.

sectors of the population of the country at this period. Such influence would have been impossible had there not been mutual relationships and contacts between Jews and non-Jews.

In the excavations of the synagogue of Hammat-Gader, dated to the first half of the fifth century CE, Sukenik found a number of coins. On one of them is the Greek inscription Χ^{ε} [=Χριστὲ] βοήθ(ει) Ἀνδρεᾳ: 'Christ [= Lord], help Andrea'. On the other, a seal ring, three animals—an eagle, a lion, and a snake—are engraved one above the other, as well as a Byzantine oil lamp, with a cross at the bottom.[122] Opposite the opening to the hall of the inscriptions in the Hammat-Gader baths is an inscription with the date 455 CE, which says: 'In this holy place may the memory of Marcus the scribe, and his sons Joshua, also known as Theodoros, Daniel, also known as Antoninus, born of his marriage to Nona, be preserved. Amen'. The inscription is decorated with crosses, but the names mentioned in it indicate Jewish ancestry. In the year 438 CE the Emperor Theodoros II published two anti-Jewish edicts, the first of which restricted the employment of Jews in the civil service. According to Di Segni, it may be that the father of the family, who was a state official, became Christian in order to keep his appointment.[123]

Many of the donors mentioned in the Aramaic dedicatory inscriptions at Hammat-Gader have Roman and Greek names. The names are not in themselves sufficient proof, but it is known that during the Temple period non-Jews made donations to the Temple, and also that Gentiles made substantial donations to synagogues.[124] For instance, we read in the *Babylonian Talmud, Hullin* 13b:

> As regards Israelites, you may accept sacrifices from the righteous but not from the wicked, but as regards gentiles you may not accept sacrifices from them at all?—You cannot entertain such a view, for it has been

---

[122] Sukenik (1935a): 70–71; Bagati (1984): 279; cf. Urman (1995): 604; The decorations on the ring can hint to the Legion's symbol—the eagle; the lion to the synagogue's motive on the mosaic floor; and the snake—to the attribute of Aesculapius, god of medicine; Sukenik (1935a: 59) excavated the remains of the synagogue and dated its erection between the fourth century and the first half of the fifth century CE, while Avi-Yonah (1993: 56–568) dated the synagogue to the mid-sixth century CE, at the earliest.

[123] Di Segni (1994): 41; idem, (1997): 189–190.

[124] On donations from non-Jews, see, for instance, *Lucas* 7, 4–5; Josephus, *Bellum Judaicum* (17.412–417); *Jerusalem Talmud, Megilla* 3, 2 [74a]; Lifshitz (1967): I: no. 33; Roth-Gerson (1987): 88–93; idem, (1987): 67; On the many visitors who came to the site, see Di Segni (1997): 186–266; Dvorjetski (1999b): 133–141; idem, 23–25.

taught; [= It would have suffice had Scripture stated] a man [= (*Leviticus* 22, 18)] why does it state, 'a man, 'a man'? To include gentiles, that they may bring either votive or freewill-offerings like an Israelite.

Several Aramaic inscriptions found in the synagogue at Hammat-Gader contain Greek words transliterated into Aramaic, such as κύρις = κύρος [= lord] and κύρια = κύρα [= lady]. They also contain Greek names, such as Ὅπλης [= Hoples], Πρῶτων [= Proton], Λεόντις, [= Leontis], Καλλινίκη [= Kelnik]; and on the grating of the synagogue there is a Greek inscription: 'the son of Παραγυρίος' [= Paragurios]. All this is generally thought to prove that the Greek language was quite well known in the Jewish community of Hammat-Gader, and that Greek influence reached parts of the population.[125] Moreover, it must be noted that in these inscriptions there are details which are not found in inscriptions from other synagogues, and not only in this period. The biggest financial contribution by a family of donors, the names of the donor's relatives—his wife, his sons, his in-laws, the geographical extent of the places of origin of the contributors (mainly from Galilee such as Sepphoris, Kefar Aqavia, Kefar Nahum, Arbel and Sussita), titles and appointments apparently held by those with official connections, the great number of female donors—all this creates the impression that not all the donors were Jews. It may be that some of them visited the baths for therapeutic purposes, and believed that donations to the holy place would contribute to their cure.[126] If the assumption that there were non-Jews among the donors is correct, the dedicatory inscriptions in Hammat-Gader, almost all of them written in a standard formula ('May...be remembered in this holy place')[127] (See, for instance, Figs. 15, 17, and 18), are an accurate reflection not only of the particular phenomenon of rich visitors to the spa, but also of good relationships and mutual respect between Jews and Gentiles.

It is said of most of the contributors to the Hammat-Tiberias synagogue, which is dated to the fourth century CE that they made their contributions as the result of a vow, and the inscription states that they have fulfilled the vows.[128] (See Fig. 31). Generally speaking, no clue

---

[125] Roth-Gerson (1987): 132–133.
[126] On the geographical distribution of donors, their titles, professions, and unique collection of foreign names, see Sukenik (1935a): 39–57; Naveh (1978): 11–12, 54–64; Dvorjetski (1999b): 140–141; idem, forthcoming [d].
[127] Di Segni (1997): 185.
[128] Dothan (1983): 53–62.

is given as to the reason for the vow, which includes a request and a commitment connected with the fulfillment of the request.[129] Roth-Gerson suggests that this is connected with a request for bodily health in the therapeutic baths of Tiberias. This suggestion is confirmed, to some extent, by the unusual formula of the blessing, σωζέστω or ζήσῃ ['may he be alive' or 'to survive safely'] which is found five times, and is unknown in other Jewish inscriptions. Such a blessing, praying for life for the donors, is appropriate to invalids coming to a therapeutic site. Here, too, it may be assumed that there were non-Jews among the donors, since there are many Greek and Latin names in the inscriptions, including some, such as Είορτάσις, which are extremely rare among Jews. Other names, such as Προφοτῦρος, ᾿Ιοῦλλος, Σευῆρος, Καλλίνικος and Ζωΐλος are almost unknown among Jews, and others again, such as Μάξιμος and Καλλίνικος, appear in Jewish contexts only very occasionally. The inscription says that Severus was 'a scholar of the distinguished Patriarchs; it appears, therefore, that a man with a distinctly Roman name grew up and was educated in the household of the patriarchs. Roth-Gerson is of the opinion that he may have been a non-Jewish slave, who acquired a positive attitude to Judaism when he lived in the Patriarchs' household, and after attaining his freedom and amassing wealth, played an important part in the renovation of the synagogue in Hammat-Tiberias.[130] It is well known from the Rabbinic literature that there were non-Jewish slaves in the household of the patriarchs. Male and female slaves were employed permanently in the household of Rabban Gamaliel of Jabneh. One of them, 'Tavi my slave, who is a scholar', is mentioned several times in the Rabbinic literature. Mention is also made of Gothic and German bodyguards at the time of Rabban Gamaliel son of Rabbi Judah the Patriarch and later on.[131] Even if, as has been remarked, the names are not sufficient evidence, such a list, appearing in the Jewish town of Tiberias, creates the impression that not only Jews are referred to.

Several scholars, relying on Christian traditions and archaeological evidences, discuss the relationships between Jews, Samaritans and Christians in Emmaus. One such finding is a magic amulet, beaten onto

---

[129] Roth-Gerson (1987): 67.
[130] Roth-Gerson (1987): 65–68, 185–186.
[131] *Mishnah, Sukka* 2, 1; *ibid., Pesahim* 7, 2; *ibid., Berakhot* 2, 7; See also Krauss (1948): 160, 202; On Rabbi Abbahu who was helped by two Gothic servants at the *demosin* of Tiberias, see *Jerusalem Talmud, Besa* 1, 6 [60c].

a thin silver tablet, which was found in a grave in Emmaus. This is a Jewish-Aramaic cameo in mystical style with demonological symbols, from the third century CE. (See Fig. 28). According to Vincent it was made by a Jewish artist at the request of a Christian.[132] The mythological creature in the amulet, in the form of a snake, may allude to the healing qualities of the waters of Emmaus, which are described in Church writings as good not only for human beings but also for animals. It may also allude to the well-known symbol of medicine, Aesculapius. The oath in the cameo is addressed to a god, the angels or the spirits, and asks that the symptoms of the invalid be removed from his eyes, his head, his muscles, his ears and his testicles.[133]

Spas provide a unique reflection of the relationships between Jews and Gentiles in the period of the Mishnah and the Talmud. The characteristics of medicinal baths in the classical world are similar to those of the baths of Palestine, which were famous for their healing qualities in Palestine and throughout the world. The Sages discussed fundamental *halakhic* questions concerning daily life in the spas, taking into account the dictates of reality and, in particular, points of contacts with the non-Jewish world, and suggested suitable solutions to various problems. Judging from the different questions which were discussed in Hammat-Gader, it is clear that the principle of 'or the sake of peace' was a consistently dominant theme in the approach of Rabbis and Patriarchs. On the other hand, the Sages maintained close supervision of other spas, such as those of Emmaus-Nicopolis and Hammei-Tiberias, which were close to large Jewish communities. The archaeological findings on the sites of the spas: inscriptions, cameos and coins, provide evidence of the mutual relationships and contacts between Jews and non-Jews. It is not impossible that non-Jews made contributions to synagogues in Hammei-Tiberias and Hammat-Gader, when they came to these places to be healed, and therefore made their vows 'in this holy place'. In the Roman and Byzantine periods the combination of a sacred spring, medicinal baths and religious buildings afforded the many people who visited them a special blend of comfort, medical services, and ways of worship. The mutual relationships between Jews and Gentiles in the

---

[132] *CIJ*, II: 1185; Vincent (1908): 382–394; Schwartz (1986): 121.

[133] Vincent and Abel (1932): 403–425; cf. Naveh and Shaked (1985): 60–63; See also *The Historical-Archaeological Analysis and Healing Cults of Emmaus-Nicopolis* in chapter 4.8 and *The Healing Properties of the Spas in Ancient Times* in chapter 5.

baths, against a background of leisure culture, medical facilities and buildings designed for entertainment, were natural and relaxed.[134]

In conclusion, the thermo-mineral baths in the eastern Mediterranean were places of bathing, of ritual, of therapy and of entertainment—including licentious immorality. They were social institutions, with a wide range of activities, and were frequented by many different groups and circles. Their use by the Jewish inhabitants created a fascinating conflict between the popular need, especially for healing, and the religious restrictions, which were discussed and decreed by the Talmudic Sages. The Rabbinic literature adds a significant layer to the properties of the therapeutic sites in the eastern Mediterranean, which can be classified to specific maladies. For some centuries, the spas survived as rare 'preserves' of classical culture within the declining of late Roman civilization. The aggregation of sacred springs, therapeutic baths and cultic installations offered a special combination of religious, medicinal and social conveniences to the very many Jews and non-Jews, who visited the sites during the Roman-Byzantine period.

---

[134] For the theatre facilities between the other entertainments, see Dvorjetski (1994): 51–68; idem, (1999c): 117–143; Levine (2000): 106–108; Weiss (1995): 2–19; Feldman and Reinhold (1996): 233; Weiss (2001): 427–450.

CHAPTER SEVEN

ROMAN EMPERORS AT THE SPAS IN THE EASTERN
MEDITERRANEAN BASIN

'The nature of a republican provincial governor's duties was such that
when he was not marching with an army he was traveling from city to
city in his province dispensing justice', wrote Millar in his most important study on *The Emperor in the Roman World*.[1] He added that not only
the Emperor's imperial journeys within his province, but his travels to
and from it, involved for the provincials on the one hand a burden of
organizing supplies and stopping-places, and elaborate rituals of greet-
ing, entertainment and farewell, and on the other the possibilities of
gaining favour, and for the leading men, of establishing personal links
which would be valuable for the future. Such a journey thus involved
complex and potentially important choices on both sides.[2]

Our best evidences for the impact of prospective imperial journeys
are supported by a reasonable thought and extended activeness. The
Romans erected magnificent public baths throughout the Empire. At
sites which had hot springs, medicinal baths were erected. These places
flourished and attracted many who sought healing for their ills there.[3]
Many Roman military and civil officials as well as some Emperors,
visited settlements in the East, both during military operations and in
times of peace. The Rabbinic literature expresses a gamut of different
attitudes towards the projects of the Roman Empire in Palestine as
illuminated above.[4] On the one hand, these sources express a negative
appraisal of the baths, the theatres, and the various taxes and duties
as methods for increasing the state's income. On the other hand, elsewhere in these sources, one discerns the Sages' positive opinion about
the Roman activities, which introduced the culture of the baths into

---

[1] Millar (1992): 28.
[2] Idem, (1992): 28.
[3] Jackson (1990): 5–13; idem, (1988), s.v. 'spas'; Yegül (1992): 92–127, 355, 379.
[4] See the discussion in chapter 6 on *The Daily Life at the Thermo-Mineral Baths according to Rabbinic Literature.*

the country.[5] In this chapter the aims and activities of the Emperors Vespasian, Hadrian and 'Antoninus'—Caracalla at the spas, as reflected in the Classical literature and especially in the Rabbinic sources, will be discussed.[6]

7.1 VESPASIAN

Vespasian (69–79 CE) was a new kind of Roman Emperor: middle-class rather than patrician, and a man with wide experience in the provinces and the army, rather a mere urban courtier. He gave the Empire a period of stable and efficient government after the disturbances of the year 69 CE. His tolerance and humour won him friends, and his conscientious attention to the welfare of Rome and the provinces set the Empire on a new and firmer footing.[7]

Vespasian served as a military tribune in Thrace, was a *quaestor* in Crete and Cyrene, *aedile* in 38 and *praetor* in 40 CE. He married Flavia Domitilla, by whom he had three children, Titus, Domitian and Domitilla, but his wife and daughter died before he became Emperor. His military career received a boost when he commanded the Second Legion *Augusta* in the conquest of Britain in 43–47. Vespasian was rewarded with the consulship in 51 CE, then the governorship of Africa some 12 years later. Under Nero he became an official 'companion' of the Emperor and traveled with him to Greece. Nero soon had need of him to suppress the rebellion of the Jews. In 67 CE Vespasian was appointed governor of Judaea with an expeditionary force of three legions. He was bringing the war steadily to a successful conclusion when news broke of Nero's suicide and the events of the fateful year 69 CE were set in train. The capture of Jerusalem brought the Jewish War effectively to a close, though the stronghold of Masada held out until 74 CE, and Vespasian and Titus, celebrated a joint triumph for their victory in June the following year.[8]

---

[5] Dechent (1884): 173–210; Krauss (1909–1910): 32–50; Hirschberg (1920): 215–246; Dvorjetski (1992a): 154–186; idem, (1992b): idem, (1994a): idem, (2001–2002): idem, (2004).

[6] This chapter is an expanded version of my papers: Dvorjetski (1994): 58–66; idem, (1997b): 567–581.

[7] Scarre (1995): 64.

[8] Idem, (1995): 65–67; Grant (1999): 50–53.

Vespasian strengthened the frontiers by to better lines in Britain and Germany, and he brought part of Armenia and Commagene into the Empire. Taxes were on goods and services, even public urinals. He revoked immunities on a wide scale, and with the money thus gained he restored the deficiencies caused by Nero's extravagance and the devastation of the Civil Wars. It is without doubt that he was one of Rome's greatest imperial builders. He initiated an extensive construction programme, and gave the city a new look. He reconstructed the Capitol, built a new forum and erected many new temples. His most famous building, however, is the *Amphitheatrum Flavium*, known in later as the Colosseum.[9]

Suetonius gives us a sketch of the Emperor's daily routine. He rose before dawn, every day, and spent the first part of the day meeting friends and officials, and reading official reports. Then he would have a drive and a sleep. After his siesta he would go to the baths, and then have dinner. The Roman historian also described him as a strong, square-bodied man with a curious strained expression on his face. He enjoyed excellent health and took no medical precautions for preserving it, except to have his throat and body massaged regularly in the ball alley, and to fast one whole day every month.[10] One of the most important event reported by Suetonius was during his ninth consulship while visiting Campania. He gives a health profile of the Emperor that will be illuminated below.

Vespasian was the first Emperor to visit in Palestine actually before he became Emperor. Josephus relates that:[11]

> He broke up the camp which he had pitched in front of Tiberias at Ammathus (Ἀμμαθοῦς),[12] (this name may be interpreted as 'warm bath', being derived from a spring of warm water within the city possessing curative properties) and proceeded to Gamala.

Elsewhere Josephus relates that at the beginning of the Great Uprising against the Romans, Emmaus surrendered to Vespasian—like the other Gentile cities nearby: Antipatris, Lydda and Jamnia [= Jabneh].

---

[9] Hazel (2002): 320–321; Meijer (2004): 42–43.

[10] Suetonius, *De Vita Caesarum, Vespasian* 20–21; See Graves (1986): 250; Grant (1999): 55.

[11] *Bellum Judaicum* 4.11; See also Josephus, *Antiqutates Judaicae* 18.36; On the surrender of Tiberias and the involvement of the Legion X, see *Bellum Judaicum* 3.445–461.

[12] On the Greek name Ἀμμαθοῦς and its affinity to the words *Hammat*, or *Hammtha*, or *Hammthan*, see the discussion on *Terminology* in chapter 1.4.

Locating a camp of the Legion V *Macedonia* at Emmaus (Ἀμμαθοῦς)—known as Hammtha in Judaea—was part of the encirclement of the rebellious Judaea and of the preparations for Vespasian's
campaign against Jerusalem.[13] Levick follows Smallwood, who points to
Emmaus and its settlers as a place where owners were dispossessed.[14]
Military and other, absentee landowners in full legal possession are
listed in the *Midrash de-Bei-Rav*: consuls, hegemons, *cleruches*, non-com-
missioned officers, centurions, senators, and well-born women. They
are all 'harassers', but there was no radical reorganization of Judaea
and Jews were free to buy the confiscated land.[15]

A number of inscriptions and tombstones of the Legion's soldiers,
which were found in the area of Emmaus, usually give the soldier's
name, his position, his place of origin and the unit to which he
belonged, his age and his length of service. The statue of an eagle
from the Roman period also provides evidence for the presence of
the Roman army in the area.[16] Because of its strategic location on the
main road from the coast to Jerusalem, Emmaus was incorporated into
the network of Roman roads.[17] Echoes of this military presence at the
site appear in the Rabbinic literature.[18] Emmaus lies to the south-west
of its neighbour, Gophna, where Rabban Yohanan ben Zakkai met
Vespasian and prophesied that he would become Emperor.[19] The episode of the departure of Rabban Yohanan out of besieged Jerusalem,
his move to Jabneh and his meeting with Vespasian, appears in the
Talmudic literature five times,[20] and has been discussed extensively.[21]

---

[13] Josephus, *Bellum Judaicum* 4.444–445; See also Vincent and Abel (1932): 316–335;
Schürer (1991): I: 512–513.

[14] Levick (1999): 149; Smallwood (1976): 343–344.

[15] Applebaum (1977): 385–395; See also Levick (1999): 149, note 75.

[16] Vincent and Abel (1932): 426–427; Hirschfeld (1988): 14–15; Bar-Kochva (1980):
188.

[17] Roll (1976): 41–42; Fisher (1989): 186–187; Isaac (1990): 428–429; See chapter
4.8 on *The Historical-Archaeological Analysis of and Healing Cults of Emmaus-Nicopolis*.

[18] *Midrash Lamentations Rabbah* 1, 17, 52; See also Lieberman (1932b): 454–455;
Safrai (1965): 115–116.

[19] On Gophna, which was used as an arrested place for the giving up surrenders, see
Alon (1967): 237, 242–243; On the Emperor's identification whom Rabban Yohanan
met with (Vespasian or Titus), see idem, (1967): 223–224.

[20] *Avot de Rabbi Nathan* 4, Version A: 22–24; *ibid.*, 6, Version B, 19; *Lamentations Rabbah*
1, 5, 31; *Babylonian Talmud, Gittin* 56a–56b; *Midrash Mishle* 15, 125–126.

[21] Alon (1967): 219–252; Urbach (1953): 61–72; Neusner (1962): 157–166; Baer
(1971): 127–190; Lieberman (1973): 990–992; Schalit (1975): 208–327.

An interesting detail of their meeting is documented in the *Babylonian Talmud, Gittin* 56a–56b:[22]

> At this point a messenger came to him from Rome saying, Up, for the Emperor is dead, and the notables of Rome have decided to make you head [= of the State]. He had just finished putting on one boot. When he tried to put on the other he could not. He tried to take off the first but it would not come off. He said: 'What is the meaning of this?' Rabbi Yohanan said to him: 'Do not worry: the good news has done it, as it says, "Good tidings make the bone fat" (*Proverbs* 15, 30). What is the remedy? Let someone whom you dislike come and pass before you, as it is written, "A broken spirit drieth up the bones" (*ibid.*, 17, 22). He did so, and the boot went on. He said to him: 'Seeing that you are so wise, why did you not come to me till know?' He said: 'Have I not told you?'—He retorted: 'I too have told you.'

Although this Talmudic story is probably imaginary, it has nevertheless found its place subsequently among the German legal tomes of the thirteenth century. The chapter, which deals with the Laws of the Jews, includes a curious historical explanation which indicates, that the author seeks to reconcile the tale with the tradition which was prevalent among the Christian authors—namely, that it was Josephus who healed Titus:[23]

> A Christian, who has killed a Jew or harmed him, will be brought to trial because he has broken the King's peace. This peace Josephus acquired for them [= the Jews] from Vespasian, after he cured his son Titus of gout.

Both Levy and Kisch—who published parallel studies that featured Josephus as a successful healer according to German medieval sources—mention that the story of Josephus curing Titus from gout has a parallel in the Rabbinic literature.[24] Schäfer notes that it seems rather improbable that Josephus could have been influenced by the legend featuring Rabban Yohanan, as it could hardly have been circulated so shortly after historical period involved.[25] Schäfer quotes Saldarini, who postulates that both Josephus and the *aggadah* used a story that circulated after the Great Revolt on the relationship between captured Jewish

---

[22] Epstein, *Babylonian Talmud, Gittin* 56a–56b: 255–260; Alon (1967): I: 273–219.

[23] Eckhardt (1973): 92; Aronius (1902), no. 458.

[24] Levy (1969): 266–274; Kisch (1938–1939): 105–118; This story is included in some history books without any explanation. See, for instance, Gratz (1908): VI: 229; Stobbe (1866): 13; Dubnov (1955): IV: 192; V: 89; Fischer (1931): 6.

[25] Schäfer (1979): 83–88.

leaders and the dreaded Roman generals.[26] On the other hand, Kottek adds that the Talmudic story dates back at least to the third century CE, and its historicity cannot be established with certainty, although the academy of Yavneh was definitely established after the destruction of Jerusalem and with the permission of the Roman authorities.[27] Furthermore, Kottek indicates that if Rabban Yohanan ben Zakki had some 'medical' training that enabled him to give useful advice for 'curing' the feet of the Roman general, he nevertheless requested from Vespasian, among granting the lives of some persons and the right to maintain Jewish learning in the academy of Jabneh, to send physicians to Jerusalem in order to treat Rabbi Zadoq, who had fasted so long that he had become unable to swallow anything and was nearly dying. Hence, Rabban Yohanan apparently did not consider himself as a physician, but rather as a Sage who knew how to restore to the general his disturbed spirits, which had caused him the affection in the feet.[28] It seems that Josephus cannot be considered anachronistic while mentioning Vespasian in Jotapata (*Bellum Judaicum* 4.622–629), whereas Rabban Yohanan could only have met Titus, since Vespasian had then already left for Rome—this historical detail may give preeminence to the authenticity of Josephus' narrative.

Regarding the aforementioned gout, joint disorders and pains were commonly referred to by medical writes,[29] although some of these descriptions were of a more specific joint disease: gout. This condition was apparently known to physicians at least as early as the first century CE,[30] but it was not always differentiated in the medical literature. Caelius Aurelianus, of the fifth century CE, speaks in his treatise *On Acute Diseases and on Chronic Diseases*, of 'de pedum dolore quem podagram appellant'.[31]

True gout is due to a metabolic disorder caused by an excess of uric acid in the blood. This results in the deposition of urate crystals in the joint tissues, which gradually degenerate with consequent destruction of the joint surfaces.[32]

---

[26] Idem, *ibid.*; Saldarini (1975): 189–204; Schochat (1960): 163–165.
[27] Kottek (1994): 194.
[28] Idem, *ibid.*
[29] See, for example, Celsus, *De Medicina* 4.29–31; 5.18.32–36.
[30] Aretaeus, *Chronic Diseases* 2.12.
[31] Caelius Aurelianus, *De Acutis Morbis* 5.2; See also Jackson (1988): 88.
[32] Jackson (1988): 177–178; Rogers and Waldron (1995): 78–86.

The same episode appears at even greater length and in more details in the book *Historia Miscella* of circa CE 1,000, where it is ascribed to the work *The Roman History* by Paulus Diaconus of Lombardy:[33]

> When Titus was told from Rome, that his father had become Emperor, his joy was so great that his right foot became swollen and he could not put his shoe on. His foot returned to normal on the advice of Josephus, the leader of the Jews...

An indication regarding the relationship between Josephus and healing may be found in an episode which, according to Josephus' testimony, occurred in the presence of Vespasian (*Antiquitates Judaicae* 8.45–49). It features an exorcism performed by a certain Eleazar, the Essene. Josephus considers that this performance was a sequel of King Solomon's wisdom, which included the power of healing and the knowledge of roots and incantations.[34]

Clearly the details of this story are very peculiar but the underlying fact probably cannot be denied that gout, which was one of the commonest rheumatic afflictions in antiquity, and particularly in the Roman era, afflicted both father and son, and hence the Flavian dynasty.[35] Some support to this assumption can be drawn from Suetonius' work, *Lives of the Twelve Caesars* and Cassius Dio, *Historia Romana*. Both of them imply that Vespasian used spring waters routinely to alleviate the discomfort of gout. The former relates that Vespasian 'put on his shoes himself', perhaps to hide his health problem from the public or to reduce the pain caused by this procedure.[36]

The Emperor was accustomed to spend his summers in the region of Cutiliae and Reate, the land of his birth. In 79 CE, he became ill in Campania. Rather than seek out Baiae or Aquae Sinuessanae, he returned to Rome. He than traveled to his villa and sought relief by using the cold waters of Aquae Cutiliae near Rome, a similar treatment

---

[33] Eyssenhardt (1879): 194; See also Levy (1969): 267.

[34] Kottek (1994): 195; This prophecy is related also by Suetonius, *De Vita Caesarum, Vespasian* 5, as well as Cassius Dio, *Historia Romana* 65.1.4; See also Ball (2000): 57, note 104.

[35] Dvorjetski (1992a): 140–141; Yaretzky (1982): 427–432; On the Gout, see Preuss (1993): 168; Rosner (1977b): 833; On the diagnosis of gout see also Kottek (1994): 195, and especially the discussion in chapter 5 on *The Healing Properties of the Spas.*

[36] Suetonius, *De Vita Caesarum, Vespasian* 8.21.24; Cassius Dio, *Historia Romana* 66.26.

to that which had previously proved successful Augustus.[37] Suetonius and Dio Cassius imply that Vespasian used spring waters routinely to alleviate the discomfort of gout. The former narrates that Vespasian was injured by 'creberrimo frigidae aquae usu' at Cutiliae, but leaves it unclear what method injured the Emperor. On this occasion, the springs, which were famous for their healing properties, did not afford a cure and too much cold water is said to have damaged Vespasian's intestines. He was suddenly taken by a fit of diarrhea and died standing, held up by those around him.[38] Titus died in the same place as Vespasian.[39] Plutarch says that he too was victim to a misuse of bathing.[40]

It seems, therefore, that Vespasian's interim encampment at the Tiberias therapeutic springs and his permanent base at the thermal springs of Emmaus were not dictated by purely military requirements. Possibly, he received treatment from the doctors that were attached to the supreme commander of the army.[41] At the same time there is evidence for gentile doctors, who treated various patients who visited the remedial sites of Palestine. Thus we know of a lady doctor, the daughter of Domitianus, who treated the scurvy of Rabbi Yohanan bar Nafha in Tiberias.[42]

The fame of Emmaus was based mainly on its description of 'a beautiful place' with 'good and nice waters', which refers to its public baths which served also as a site of entertainment and attracted large crowds.[43] A comparison with other public baths in the Roman Empire reveals, that the baths at Emmaus were modeled on a prototype from Antioch in northern Syria.[44] The remedial properties of the waters of

---

[37] *Suetonius, De Vita Caesarum, Augustus* 81.1; See also Jackson (1990a): 3; idem, (1999): 108; Allen (1998): 12.

[38] Suetonius, *De Vita Caesarum, Vespasian* 24; Cassius Dio, *Historia Romana* 66.17; See also Graves (1986): 251; Allen (1998): 104, 123–124; Grant (1999): 55; On Vespasian's death, see Jones (1984): 114, 154–155; Levick (1999): 196–209.

[39] Cassius Dio, *Historia Romana* 66.26; Suetonius, *De Vita Caesarum, Titus* 11.

[40] Plutarch, *De Tuenda Sanitate Praecepta* 3.

[41] See, for example, Yavetz (1974): 374; Jackson (1988): 112–137; Le Bohec (1994): 48–53.

[42] *Jerusalem Talmud, Shabbat* 14, 4 [14d], Venice ed., 1523; *ibid.*, *Avoda Zarah* 2, 2 [40d]; On Domitianus, who is not identify with the Emperor Domitianus, see Beer (1982): 280.

[43] *Avot de Rabbi Nathan* 14, version A: 59; Hirschberg (1920): 224; Gichon (1977): 101–110; idem, (1977–1978): 125–126; Hirschfeld (1989): 197–204; Gichon (1993): 387–389.

[44] Hirschfeld (1988): 22; Butler (1908): II, B: 300–303.

Emmaus are even linked to Rabban Yohanan ben Zakkai in person: they very likely helped to cure him of the illness of Bulimia.[45]

7.2   HADRIAN

Emperor Hadrian (117–138 CE) was a man of great versatility: soldier, statesman, humanist, and political innovator. His legal, administrative and military reforms made possible the most splendid and tranquil epoch of the Roman Empire. He erected buildings whose vitality, beauty and rhythm still influence architects in our own age.[46] Many Roman Emperors travelled, whether for war, inspection or mere curiosity, but none so extensively as Hadrian. His journeys took in practically the whole of the Roman world. His first itinerary began with a visit to Gaul, the Rhineland and Britain. He then travelled to Spain and Mauretania, before taking ship for Asia Minor, Greece and the Danube lands. Afterwards he visited also Tunisia, Syria, Judaea, Egypt, and Libya.[47]

Various reasons prompted Hadrian to tour his provinces: military organization and defense; administrative co-ordination; the need to recognize and guide provincial aspirations by showing himself as their common symbol; and his own desire to learn provincial conditions, especially in the Hellenized areas.[48] Only in Judaea was his policy questionable: the building of a shrine to Jupiter Capitolinus on the site of the Temple at Jerusalem. Dealing with the significance of the imperial journeys, some scholars tried to show the exact date of Hadrian visiting Judaea. Some scholars thought about 117 CE, [49] and the next visit in 129/130 CE;[50] in 131/132 CE, or during the Bar Kochba war of 132–135 CE,[51] or other options.[52]

---

[45] *Midrash Ecclesiastes Rabbah* 7, 12, 1; See also Vincent and Abel (1932): 414–416; Simon (1978a): 33; Dvorjetski (1994b): 42; idem, (1996a): 42.

[46] Perowne (1960); Speller (2002): 45–47, 54–56, 68–69, 181–182, 199–200.

[47] Scarre (1995): 99; Speller (2002): 62–63, 81–91.

[48] Den Boer (1969); Thornton (1975); Millar (1977): 28–40; Haffmann (1986); Barness (1989); Carson (1990); Syme (1991); Millar (1996): 105–108; Birley (1997): 231–234, cf. Fagan (1999a): 191–192; Boatwright (1987); idem, (2000), especially p. 209.

[49] Durr (1881); Gray (1923).

[50] Stinespring (1939).

[51] Strack (1933): 132–139; Jones (1972): 152; Haffmann (1986): 209; Syme (1988): 167; Barness (1989): 254; Boatwright (2000): 200–203, note 168.

[52] Scarre (1995): 99; Dvorjetski (1997b).

Our central task in this section will be to prove that the Emperor's aims and deeds at the thermo-mineral baths in Palestine reflect Hadrian's private life as well as his visiting his army at the spas in the eastern Mediterranean basin during his reign. It will be shown by means of the following central topics, which provide an important source for the recognition of the properties, culture and daily life of the therapeutic baths: The authenticity of the dialogue between Hadrian and a girl with skin disease at Hammat-Gader; The Talmudic legends which portray the personality of Hadrian at Hammat-Gader and at Hammei-Tiberias; Was Hadrian visiting one of his legions at Hammat-Gader, the suburb of Hellenistic-Roman city of Gadara? The archaeological evidences and the numismatic documentation of his visit to Palestine; The panegyric assemblies and rituals in honor of Hadrian in the Levant; and, finally, does the Talmudic expression 'his bones be ground to dust' relate to the medical history of Hadrian?

A *baraitha* about Emperor Hadrian, which has survived in the Rabbinic literature, in several versions, relates the following episode:[53]

1. *Midrash Tannaim, Deuteronomy* 26, 19 (Hoffman ed., p. 262):

> It was said: When Hadrian climbed the slope of Hammat-Gader he found there a little Jewish girl. He asked her: 'Who are you?' She answered: 'I am a Jewish girl'. All of a sudden he came out from his carriage and bowed down to her. All the royal nobles were angry at him and asked him: 'Why did you humiliate yourself and bowed down to this dirty and filthy?' He answered them and said: 'All of you are so silly since all nations will bow down to them'.

2. *Midrash HaGadol on the Pentateuch, Deuteronomy* 26, 19 (Fish ed., p. 603):

> It was said: When Emperor Hadrian climbed the slope of Hammat-Gader he found there a little Jewish girl covered with sore boil. He asked her: 'Who are you?' She answered: 'I am a Jewish girl'. All of a sudden he came out from his carriage and bowed down to her. All the royal nobles were angry at him and asked him: 'Why did you humiliate yourself and bowed down to this dirty and filthy?' He answered them and said: 'All of you are so silly, since all nations will bow down to them'.

---

[53] Herr (1971): 123–124; Dvorjetski (1994d): 59; idem, (1997b): 571–572; In *Seder Eliyahu Zuta* 15 [(Ish-Shalom ed.) Vienna (1904:199)—the event took place in Rome and the Jewish baby was covered in sores thrown in the garbage; See also Klein (1939): 74; Dvorjetski forthcoming [b].

3. *Seder Eliyahu Zuta* 15 (Ish-Shalom ed., p. 199):

> Rabbi Yose said: 'Once I was walking in the metropolis of Rome and I saw an Emperor riding on a horse with all the dignitaries of Rome. He saw a little Jewish baby covered in sores thrown in the garbage. Since he saw her, he got off his horse and bowed down to her. All the Roman dignitaries were angry at him and asked him: 'To such a humiliate and filthy are you bowing down?' He answered them: 'Don't be so evil, since all nations will bow down to them.'

The original sources of this text have been regarded by scholars as suspect, yet the account of this meeting, between Emperor Hadrian and a Jewish girl with skin sores at Hammat-Gader, contains a number of features which merit detailed discussion. It will be seen that it possible to link the story to the historical actuality in Palestine at the time of Hadrian.

Dialogues between Roman dignitaries and Jewish sages are frequently reported in the Talmudic literature. The best known conversations are of Rabban Yohanan ben Zakkai with Emperor Vespasian; Rabban Yohanan with a certain *prefectus, hegemon*; Rabbi Joshua with Emperor Hadrian; (or else 'the Emperor', without any closer identification); between Rabbi Akiva and Tineius Rufus; Rabbi Yose ben Halafta and a Roman matron, and between Rabbi Judah the Patriarch and Antoninus, probably Emperor Caracalla. This phenomenon is not confined to the world of the Jewish sages, but appears among other peoples, such as the dialogues between Greek philosophers and Gymnasiarchs on the one hand and Roman Emperors and notables on the other. This literary genre arises both in the Jewish and the Greek world at the beginning of the Hellenistic era and reaches it zenith in the second century CE. The topics of the dialogues were certainly not random.[54]

The Romans' curiosity about Jews and Judaism, which started prior to the Destruction of the Temple, did not cease thereafter. On the contrary, it actually increased. The period from the Destruction to Hadrian's anti-Jewish edicts was the apogee of conversion to Judaism. Curiosity about the Jewish religion in some Roman circles increased and sometimes assumed a semi-official character.[55]

Of particular importance were the conversations in which Hadrian revealed interest in the Jewish people, the Torah, the Sabbath, Moses

---

[54] Herr (1971): 124–126.
[55] Stern (1964): 156.

and God. This Emperor was known for his inclination towards philosophy, and according to the evidence he was:[56]

> curiositatum omnium explorator [= inquisitive and investigating everything].
>
> (*Scriptores Historiae Augustae, De Vita Hadriani* 20.1)

Tertullian, one of the greatest of the early Christian writers in Latin, indicates that Hadrian was fond of debating with sages and various scholars about philosophical matters.[57]

It was customary for Emperors and other persons in authority, both in the metropolis and in the provinces, to talk with any person even if they had been abusive. With regard to the first twelve Caesars, Suetonius provides a rich source of gossip in this field. For the second and third centuries CE, the Latin work *Scriptores Historiae Augustae* provides a similar, albeit less reliable, source.[58] It relates in *Scriptores Historiae Augustae, De Vita Hadriani* 17.5, that Hadrian used to bathe with the ordinary public in the public baths:[59]

> publice frequenter et cum omnibus lavit [= He often bathed in the public baths, even with the common crowd].

There is nothing particularly strange or puzzling in the episode narrated in the *baraitha* above, regarding the encounter of Hadrian with the Jewish girl on the slope from the baths at Hammat-Gader to Gadara city. It corresponds with the third century historian Cassius Dio, who mentions that while Hadrian was walking in the street and accosted by a woman loudly lamenting and trying to present a petition:[60]

> Once, when a woman made a request of him as he passed by a journey, he at first said to her, 'I haven't time,' but afterwards, when she cried out, 'Cease, then, being Emperor,' he turned about and granted her a hearing.

He refused, saying he had no time, but the woman retorting, 'If you have no time, you should not be emperor'. He immediately stopped and listened to her case.

---

[56] *Scriptores Historiae Augustae, De Vita Hadriani* 20.1; Herr (1971): 127; See Lieberman (1939a): 57; Speller (2002): 4–5, 66–67, 69–70.
[57] Bacher (1922): I/1: 126.
[58] Millar (1964): 124; Goodman (1997): 4–5, 69.
[59] *Scriptores Historiae Augustae, De Vita Hadriani* 17.5.
[60] Cassius Dio, *Historia Romana* 69.6.3; Pringsheim (1934): 143.

The text corresponds also with the fourth century CE description of Emperor Hadrian in *Scriptores Historiae Augustae, De Vita Hadriani* 20.1:[61]

> In conloquiis etiam humillimorum civilissimus fuit, detestant eos qui sibi hanc voluptatem humanitatis quasi servantes fastigium principis inviderent [= Most polite in his conversations even with the most humble, he detested those who, in the belief that they were thereby maintaining the imperial dignity, begrudged him the pleasure of such friendliness].

In a popular anecdote in *Scriptores Historiae Augustae, De Vita Hadriani* 17.5–7, Hadrian was surprised to see an army veteran acquaintance in the public baths rubbing his back against the marble wall because he could not afford to keep slaves or pay the bath attendants to massage him. The Emperor promptly donated some slaves to him, along with funds for their upkeep. When visiting the baths on a later occasion, Hadrian was confronted by a crowd of old men scraping themselves busily against the walls and columns, in the hope of exciting his generosity. The witty Emperor disappointed them by saying that they should take turns rubbing each other down.[62]

It is reported in *Historia Augusta, De Vita Hadriani* 22.7, that under Hadrian's reign 'none but invalids were allowed to bathe in the public baths before the eighth hour'. It may indicate that it was customary for the sick to use the public baths along with the healthy but Hadrian exempted them from the restrictions placed on the opening hours' or it may imply that public baths were used by the sick for treatment only during certain hours. This passage is given, according to Yegül in the context of the civic regulations Hadrian imposed upon Rome, underscoring his passion for discipline and order as well as his kindness, especially to the underprivileged and the infirm.[63]

There are other Talmudic legends that portray the personality of Hadrian. One tells of an encounter between the emperor and an old

---

[61] *Scriptores Historiae Augustae, De Vita Hadriani* 20.1; See also Herr (1971): 123; It might be translated also as 'Most democratic in his conversation, he denounced all', or 'in conversation he was civil even to the lowliest, detesting those who feigned to serve the *priceps* by trying to deny him that humane pleasure'.

[62] *De Vita Hadriani* 17, 5–7; See also: Yegül (1992): 429, note 17; cf. Fagan (1999a): 190–192.

[63] Yegül (1992): 463, note 25; Merten (1983): 63–64; Künzl (1986): 495; cf. Fagan (1999a): 191.

man. The topic is a common popular motif, but it reproduces the attitude of Hadrian's servants as quoted in *Historia Augusta*:[64]

> Hadrian, his bones be ground to dust, once passed along the paths leading to Tiberias and saw an old man standing and digging trenches to plant shoots of fig-trees...'By your life old man! How old are you this day?' 'A hundred years old'...Do you ever hope to eat of them?' He replied: 'If I am worthy I shall eat, and if not, then as my forebears have worked for me so will I work for my children'...He said to him:...'If you are privileged to eat of them, let me know'. In the course of time the trees produced figs. Said he: 'Now it is time to let the king know'...He filled a basket with figs and went and stood at the gate of the palace...Thereupon Hadrian exclaimed...'I command that you empty this basket of his and fill it with *denarii*'. His servants said to him: 'Will you show this entire honor to that old Jew?' He answered them: 'His Creator honours him, and shall not I honour him too?'
>
> (*Midrash Leviticus Rabbah* 25, 5)

Similar text also appears in *Midrash Tanhuma, Kedoshim* 8 (Buber ed., p. 76), omitting his conversation with his servants, but with a significant addition, which emphasizes the time of the episode:[65]

> It happened that King Hadrian was at war, marching with his forces to fight a state which had rebelled against him, and he encountered an old man who was planting fig saplings...He spent three years at war, and returned after three years. What did that old man do? He took a basket and filled it with the first fruits of beautiful figs, and drew near Hadrian...

This traditional tale suggests that the Bar Kochba war did last three years, perhaps corroborating the statement in the *Babylonian Talmud, Sanhedrin* 93b: 'Bar Koziba reigned two and a half years'.[66]

Emperor Hadrian is given in the story the title king, and with a possible fascinating reference to the known place Hammat-Gader—analogous to the text in *Midrash Lamentations Rabbah*:[67]

> Rabbi Hiyya taught: It may be likened to a king who went to Hammat-Gader and took his sons with him. Once they provoked him, and he vowed not to take them but he kept remembering them and wept saying: 'I wish my sons were with me even though they provoke me'.

---

[64] See Margulis ed. (1993): 576–578.

[65] On this *Aggadic* story and the moral lesson expressed by the author's homiletical interpretation, see Licht (1991): 1–23.

[66] *Babylonian Talmud, Sanhedrin* 93b, Epstein (1935): 9; Issac and Oppenheimer (1985); Ben-Shalom (1983): 20.

[67] *Midrash Lamentations Rabbah* 3, 20 (Buber ed., p. 131).

Another question that is raised by the *baraitha* above, regarding the Jewish girl 'covered in sores on the slope of Hammat-Gader', concerns the purpose of Hadrian's presence there. Was he visiting one of his legions, which was permanently stationed in the area?

After the destruction of the Second Temple, the permanent Roman occupation force in the Provincia Judaea was the Legion X *Fretensis*, which had distinguished itself in the battles generally, and particularly in Jerusalem. It was accompanied by some auxiliary units of cavalry and infantry and was stationed at Jerusalem on the south-western hill.[68] Inscriptions and seal impressions of the Tenth Legion on bricks, tiles and pottery pipes were discovered in the city, in Giv'at Ram (Sheikh Bader) and Ramat Rahel.[69] A bathhouse of the Legion dating from the end of the first century CE was discovered on the eastern slopes of the upper city.[70] Although the relationship between legion and colony is unclear at Jerusalem, it may be assumed that here too the stamps of the legion indicate a military presence. There is therefore no reason to doubt that both before and after 135 CE the legionary fortress was in Jerusalem.[71] The Legion X *Fretensis* also fought at Machaerus, Herodium and Massada. During Trajan's battle with the Parthians, the Legion sent an auxiliary force to Mesopotamia. Subsequently, this Legion bore the heavy burden of the battles against Bar Kochba, and continued on station in the country during the second and third centuries CE.[72]

At the beginning of the Bar Kochba uprising the rebels inflicted defeats on the Legion X *Fretensis*, which was stationed in Jerusalem, as mentioned.[73] The Roman tactics consisted of the encirclement of small groups of rebels and their capture, advancing step by step. Cassius Dio mentions this method:[74]

> Then, indeed, Hadrian sent against them his best generals. First of these was Julius Severus, who was dispatched from Britain, where he was governor, against the Jews. Severus did not venture to attack his opponents in

---

[68] Avigad (1983); Geva (1984); Ben Dov (1985); Issac (1992): 354.

[69] Barag (1967): 244–267; Mazar (1971): 5, 22; Isaac (1980–1981): 31–32; Avigad and Geva (1993): II: 759–760; Germer-Durand (1892): 382–384; Johns (1950): 152–153.

[70] Avi-Yonah (1950b): 19–21; Ciasca (1962): 69–72; Tsafrir (1984): 106–107.

[71] Isaac (1980–1981): 32.

[72] On the Roman dispositions after the destruction of the Second Temple, see Smallwood (1981): 331–334; Stern (1982): 7–11; Herr (1984): 316–318.

[73] Oppenheimer (1982a): 60, 64–65; On the Roman legions, who stayed in Judaea during the Bar-Kochba revolt, see Isaac and Roll (1979a): 54–66; idem, (1979b): 149–156.

[74] Cassius Dio, *Historia Romana* 69.13.3.

the open at any one point, in view of their numbers and their desperation but by intercepting small groups, thanks to the number of his soldiers and his under-officers, and by depriving them of food and shutting them up, he was able, rather slowly, to be sure, but with comparatively little danger, to crush, exhaust and exterminate them.

(*Historia Romana* 69.12–14)

And it is confirmed in the Talmudic literature, which mentions the construction of forts and other positions:[75]

Hadrian...positioned three guard forces, one at Hammatha and one at Kefar Lekitia and one at Beit el D'Yahud. He said: whoever escapes from here, will be caught from there and whoever escapes from there, will be caught from here.

(*Midrash Lamentations Rabbah* 1, 45)

In *Midrash Lamentations Rabbah* 1, 392, according to the Romi manuscript—the version differs:[76]

Hadrian...positioned three guard forces, one at Hammat-Gader, and one at Bethlehem and one at Kefar Lekitia.

Modern scholars do not agree with the opinion that the Bar Kochba rebellion spread also to the Galilee and to the Trans-Jordan.[77] Nevertheless, even if the version in *Midrash Lamentations Rabbah* does refer to the Bar Kochba rebellion in its limited geographical spread, and the place mentioned is indeed Hammat-Gader, the location of a Roman guard force there, can still be explained. It would have been vital in view of the important strategic location of Gadara, Hammat-Gader's mother-town.[78] There is undeniable evidence for the presence of the Legion X *Fretensis* in the region of Hammat-Gader. In addition to its seal impressions, there is epigraphic testimony and there are specific symbols of the X Legion on the coins of Gadara city.[79]

---

[75] *Midrash Lamentations Rabbah* 1, 16, 45; In the *Geniza* manuscript (Rabinovitz 1976: 136) is written: 'One in Hammtha, one in Kefar Lekitia and one in Bethlehem of Judea'; See Rabinovitz's remarks; It may be also the site Ἐμμαθᾶ, Hammtha in Judaea; The version 'Hammtha' appears in Defus Rishon (Pisaro 1709), and it seems that this is the correct version; See also Oppenheimer (1982a): 67.

[76] *Midrash Lamentations Rabbah* 1, 392 (Buber ed., p. 82); Oppenheimer (1982a): 67.

[77] Oppenheimer (1991): 37–44; Mor (1991): 103–116.

[78] Abel (1938): II: 458; Avi-Yonah (1984): 159–160; Schürer (1991): II: 132–134; Dvorjetski (1988): 17–42; Steuernagel (1927): 46–80; Schumacher (1890): 46–80.

[79] Clermont-Ganneau (1898): 299–300; Dvorjetski (1991); idem, (1994c).

Hadrian reached the eastern Mediterranean basin from Syria in the autumn of 129 CE, on his way to Egypt. He spent the winter in Gerasa in Trans-Jordan. A triumphal arch set up in Gerasa to celebrate the imperial visit.[80] In the spring he visited several places in Provincia Arabia and Judaea. In the summer of 130 he left the country for Egypt, where he remained to the end of the autumn. At the beginning of the winter of 131 CE, he passed through The Land of Israel again on his way back to Syria.[81] This event was commemorated by an issue of bronze *sestrii* and *dupondii* by the mint of Rome. On these coins the Emperor is depicted standing facing a woman, the personification Judaea and the surrounding legend reads: ADVENTVI AVG(ustus) IVDAEAE [= the arrival of the Emperor in Judaea]. On the local coinage his visit is shown in various ways.[82] Three cities Jerusalem-Aelia Capitolina, Gerasa and Petra began their coinage only in Hadrian reign.[83] The city of Petra names itself in appreciation of the Emperor benefactions.[84] Sepphoris was renamed Diocaesarea in the Emperor's honour.[85] A monumental building south of Nysa-Scythopolis, perhaps a triumphal arch, apparently bore Hadrian's name. At the site of the fort itself parts of a splendid bronze statue of the Emperor have been found.[86] Special era related to Hadrian's visit in 130 CE is mentioned beside the era of the city of Gaza and in some cases also beside the era of Ascalon.[87] In Gaza, festive assemblies, πανήγυρις Ἀδριανή, were held in his honour, at which orations in praise of the Emperor were given once a year.[88] The *Chronicon Paschale* states clearly that the festive assemblies were celebrated since the days of Emperor Hadrian.[89] Quite possibly, the panegyric assemblies at Hammat-Gader, which are clearly reported, had their origins for the same reason. Caesarea received an aqueduct built by legionary vexillations.[90] In Caesarea and Tiberias Temples to

[80] Welles (1938): 143–145, nos. 30, 58.
[81] Steinespring (1939): 360–363; Herr (1984): 349; See also Kraeling (1938): 390.
[82] Mattingly (1936), nos. 1655–1661; MacCormack (1972): 424; Jones (1990): 4–5.
[83] Kindler (1974–1975): 61–67.
[84] Hill (1922): 35, no. 8; Boatwright (2000): 104–105.
[85] Smallwood (1981): 432; Hecker (1961): 175–186; Mor (1985): 208; Schwartz (2001): 139.
[86] Foerster (1985); Isaac (1992): 307, 353.
[87] Hill, (1914): 146, no. 14; Kindler (1963); Millar (1983): 55; Boatwright (2000): 99, 110.
[88] Kindler (1974–1975): 62; Avi-Yonah (1964a): 134; Dan (1984): 201–202.
[89] *Chronicon Paschale* 474; See also de Ligt (1993): 255–256.
[90] Issac and Roll (1979a): 59–60; Isaac (1992): 353; Clermont-Ganneau (1898): II: 299–300; Dvorjetski (1994c).

Zeus-Jupiter were built which were named Ἀδριανεῖον in honor of
Emperor Hadrian and were depicted on the coins.[91] According to the
Rabbinic literature,[92] and to the Church Father Epiphanius,[93] in front
of the *Hadrianium* and beside the thermo-mineral baths of Tiberias
stood a statue named 'Hadorei' in honor of Hadrian.[94] Other coins of
Tiberias, issued 119/120 CE, represent Tyche holding a bust of what
is likely to be Hadrian, symbolizing the allegiance of the city to the
Emperor.[95] It is very important to point out that Hammei-Tiberias was
known of the medicinal qualities since the second century CE. On a
coin of Tiberias under Emperor Trajan (99/100 CE), is a figure of
Hygieia, the goddess of health, feeding the serpent from a bowl, and
sitting on a rock from beneath which breaks a spring.[96]

Although an historical survey of the site of Hammat-Gader estab-
lishes, that the medicinal properties of its baths were not mentioned
before the fourth century CE, the reputation of the thermae of the
Three Graces at Hammat-Gader on the bank of the Yarmuk River,
north of the city Gadara, could well have prevailed much earlier.[97] It has
become evident from the results of the excavation that the baths complex was built in the mid-second century, most probably from the time
of Emperor Hadrian. From the literary account of the fourth century
Greek biographer Eunapius it transpires that people in search of a cure
flocked from Athens to Hammat-Gader 'inferior only to those at Baiae
in Italy, with which no other baths can be compared'.[98] The therapeutic
baths of Hammat-Gader appear also in the description of Epiphanius
at the same time. He states that at the festive assembly, the ritualistic
paneguris, held there every year, women and men and hermaphrodites

[91] Hill (1914): 8, nos. 23–28; Kindler (1961): no. 7b; Jones (1971): 278; Smallwood
(1981): 432; Goodman (1983): 46; Meshorer (1985): 34–35, no. 81; Schäfer (1990):
284; Isaac (1992): 353; Schürer (1991): I: 542; Schwartz (2001): 140.
[92] *Jerusalem Talmud, Avoda Zarah* 3, 13 [43b]; *ibid., Shabbat* 14, 4 [14d]; *ibid., Berachot*
2, 1 [4b]; *ibid., Sheqalim* 2, 7 [47a].
[93] *Adversus Haereses* 30, 12, 2.
[94] Klein (1967): 99–100; Sepp (1863): 152; Dechent (1884): 181; Robinson (1841):
268–269.
[95] Hill (1914): XI: nos. 29–31; Kindler (1961): 38, no. 9; Isaac and Roll (1979): 63;
Meshorer (1985): no. 82.
[96] de Saulcy (1847): 335; Kindler (1961): 54; Meshorer (1985): 34–35; Smith (1904):
432–433; Rose (1968): 443.
[97] Dvorjetski (1988): 90–98; Jaffé, Dvorjetski, Levitte, Massarwah and Swarieh
(1999): 34–49.
[98] *Vitae Sophistarum*, 368.

bathed for medicinal purposes and for enjoyment.[99] Of great importance are the reports of Antoninus of Placentia, the pilgrim who visited
the Levant in 570 CE. He spoke about the name of the site and on
the traditions and methods of healing the lepers in the baths.[100] At his
time the inhabitants of the site adopted the Biblical tradition about
the prophet Elijah and named the baths after him 'Baths of Helias'.
The lepers bathed and were treated by the method of incubation, as
was practiced at the ancient centres of Aesculapius—in a large basin
opposite the door of the *clibanus*.[101] The details of Antoninus' description regarding the bathing procedures which the lepers underwent there
correlate closely both with the characteristics of the double-sloped pool
which has been entirely excavated and with the particular terracotta oil
lamps which were found in it.[102] The special inn built and maintained
by the local inhabitants for the leper testifies to the fame of Hammat-
Gader as a place of healing for leprosy.[103]

It may be concluded, in view of all the above considerations, that the
Talmudic text, which describes the meeting between Hadrian and the
Jewish girl, who was covered in sores at the ascent of Hammat-Gader,
could very well be historically authentic. At this stage it is important to
point out Hadrian's medical problems. He was the first Roman Emperor
to be depicted wearing a beard. This may have been another instance
of his love of all things Greek, but the *Historia Augusta, De Vita Hadriani*
26, 1, gives another explanation for the beard:[104]

> Statura fuit procerus, forma comptus, flexo ad pectinem capillo, promissa
> barba, ut vulnera, quae in facie naturalia errant, tegeret, habitudine,
> robusta [= He was tall of stature and elegant in appearance; his hair
> was curled on a comb, and he wore a full beard to cover up the natural
> blemishes on his face].

Hadrian was, by any standards, a successful ruler, in giving the Empire
firm frontiers and stable government for over 20 years. Modern writers
have tended to portray him as a confirmed homosexual. The picture

---

[99] Epiphanius, *Panarion, Adversus Haereses* 30.7, *PG* 416–417; Dvorjetski (1992a):
106–107, 160.

[100] *Itinerarium* 7, *CCSL* 132.

[101] Green and Tsafrir (1982): 32; Dechent (1884): 194.

[102] Hirschfeld and Solar (1981): 209–211; idem, (1984): 30, 33; idem, (1993): II:
570.

[103] Dvorjetski (1988): 10; idem, (1992b): 433–434; idem, (1994b); idem, (1996a).

[104] *Scriptores Historiae Augustae, De Vita Hadriani* 26.1; Henderson (1923): 265; Ramage
and Ramage (1995): 198.

presented by Roman writers is of a man of mixed sexual proclivities. Rumours of Hadrian's homosexuality surfaced quite early in his life, and several named individuals have been suggested as his sexual partners. Suggestions of sexual impropriety and excess were commonplace in accounts of Roman nobility. The Historia Augusta criticizes his passion for males and also his adultery with married women to which he is said to have been addicted:[105]

> et hoc quidem vitiosissimum putant atque huic adiungunt quae de adultorum amore ac nuptarum adulteries, quibus Hadrianus laborasse dicitur, adserunt, iungentes quod ne amicis quidem servaverit [= And, indeed, as for this habit of Hadrian's, men regard it as a most grievous fault, and add to their criticism the statements which are current regarding the passion for males and the adulteries with married women to which he is said to have been addicted, adding also the charge that he did not even keep faith with his friends].

In another place the same writer remarks:[106]

> in voluptatibus nimius. nam et de suis dilectis multa versibus composuit. amatoria carmina scripsit [= He ran to excess in the gratification of his desires, and wrote much verse about the subjects of his passion. He composed love-poems too].

Though to our disappointment—he does not give any further details.[107]

The relationship between Hadrian and beautiful young Bithynian named Antinous, beloved of the Emperor, was regarded by the Romans with considerable distaste as can be seen from the following documents:[108]

> peragrata Arabia Pelusium venit et Pompeii tumulum magnificentius exstruxit. Antinoum suum, dum per Nilum navigat, perdidit, quem muliebriter flevit. de quo varia fama est, aliis eum devotum pro Hadriano adserentibus, aliis quod et forma eius ostentat et nimia voluptas Hadriani [= He then travelled through Arabia and finally came to Pelusium, where he rebuilt Pompey's tomb on a more magnificent scale. During a journey

---

[105] *Scriptores Historiae Augustae, De Vita Hadriani* 11.7; Speller (2002): 4–5, 66, 108.
[106] *Scriptores Historiae Augustae, De Vita Hadriani* 14.9.
[107] Scarre (1995): 101.
[108] *Scriptores Historiae Augustae, De Vita Hadriani* 14.5–7; Matthews (1994): 121–123; Bell (1940); Sijpesteijn (1969): 110–113; Boatwright (1987): 236–260; Birley (1997): 253–257; Boatwright (2000): 99–100, 193–195; cf. *Historia Romana* 69.11.1–4; See also Speller (2002): 267–273, 283–296; Cassius Dio, *Historia Romana* 69.11.2–3.

on the Nile he lost Antinous, his favorite, and for this youth he wept like a woman. Concerning this incident there are varying rumours; for some claim that he had devoted himself to death for Hadrian, and others—what both his beauty and Hadrian's sensuality suggest].

(*Scriptores Historiae Augustae, De Vita Hadriani* 14.5–7)

Antinous was from Bithynium, a city of Bithynia, which we also call Claudiopolis; he had been a favourite of the emperor and had died in Egypt, as Hadrian writes, or, as the truth is, by being offered in sacrifice. For Hadrian, as I have stated, was always very curious and employed divinations and incantations of all kinds. Accordingly, he honoured Antinous either because of his love for him or because the youth had voluntarily undertaken to die.

(Cassius Dio, *Historia Romana* 69.11, 2–3)

Christian writers took offense at the relationship between the two,[109] and even certain pagan writers of the third and fourth centuries CE, illustrated above, a period of ever-increasing asceticism, raise an eyebrow at Hadrian's hedonism and Antinous' 'infamous' service to him.[110] Foucault has linked the growing intolerance of homosexual behavior with the 'invention' of homosexuality in the Roman world, itself perhaps connected with a growth of ideas about male premarital virginity and chastity.[111] Hammat-Gader was well known for sexual debaucheries.[112] This may have been an additional motive for Hadrian's visits to the well known place in the eastern Mediterranean.

Hadrian's ill health is well documented.[113] In 136 CE Hadrian, now 60 years old, found himself in failing health.[114] Cassius Dio describes his malady as a flow of blood from the nostrils:[115]

He now began to be sick; for he had been subject even before this to a flow of blood from his nostrils, and at this time it became distinctly more copious. He therefore despaired of his life.

(*Historia Romana* 69.17.1)

---

[109] Lambert (1984): 7–12, 94–95.

[110] Williams (1999): 60–61, 289–290, note 266; See his suggestion about the parallel that can be drawn between Hadrian's relationship with Antinous and Jupiter's with Ganymede; See also Kampen (1996): 269; Johns (1984): 102.

[111] Foucault (1990): 228.

[112] On Hammat-Gader as a libertine place, see in chapter 4.2 on *The Historical-Archaeological Analysis and Healing Cults of Hammat-Gader* and in chapter 6.2 on *The Sages at the Therapeutic Sites—Aims and Deeds.*

[113] Barnes (1968); Baldwin (1970); Birley (1997): 279– 300.

[114] Scarre (1995): 104.

[115] Cassius Dio, *Historia Romana* 69.17.1.

He is portrays with creases in his ear lobs, which can hint to the illness he suffered from, such as high blood pressure, Atherosclerosis, or
coronary atherosclerotic heart disease.[116] Another idea is liver disease,
which fits of the timing of the symptoms and Hadrian's movements and
reactions. Liver disease causes the fluid retention, the haemorrhages,
and the headaches and crucially the volatility of temperament that was
so marked in Hadrian's last years. Hadrian might have understood his
mood as melancholic rather than as depressed, but that too, along with
a degree of paranoia, is a notable concomitant of liver failure.[117]

Hadrian's final days were indeed far from happy. His illness grew
worse, and left him for long periods in great distress. It was described
as a form of dropsy: 'Hadrian became consumptive as a result of his
great loss of blood, and this led to dropsy'. [118]

He tried to lay his hands on poison or a sword to end his life, according to Cassius Dio, but his attendants kept these from him:[119]

> By certain charms and magic rites Hadrian would be relieved for a time
> of his dropsy, but would soon be filled with water again. Since, therefore,
> he was constantly growing worse and might be said to be dying day by
> day, he began to long for death; and often he would ask for poison or a
> sword, but no one would give them to him].
>
> (*Historia Romana* 69.22.1–3)

Such a dreadful feeling is described by *Scriptores Historiae Augustae*:[120]

> statimque testamentum scripsit nec tamen actus rei publicae praetermisit.
> Et post testamentum quidem iterum se conatus occidere subtracto pugione
> saevior factus est. petiit et venenum a medico, qui se ipse, ne daret, occidit
> [= Once more, however, after making his will, he attempted to kill him-
> self, but the dagger was taken from him. He then became more violent,
> and he even demanded poison from his physician, who thereupon killed
> himself in order that he might not have to administer].
>
> (*De Vita Hadriani* 24.11–13)

Hadrian was influenced by Stoicism in dealing with suicide, if it were
due to pain or weariness of life.[121] He died soon afterwards, on 10 July
CE 138.

---

[116] Petrakis (1980); Birley (1994): 202–203.
[117] Speller (2002): 237–238.
[118] Cassius Dio, *Historia Romana* 69.20.1.
[119] Cassius Dio, *Historia Romana* 69.22.1–3.
[120] *De Vita Hadriani* 24.11–13.
[121] Pringsheim (1934): 144.

The expression 'his bones be ground to dust' almost in every reference related to Hadrian in the Talmudic literature does not explain clearly his medical history, specially dermatological or rheumatic diseases. It may be a Talmudic curse. His cruel suppression of the Bar Kochba war and his policy of building a shrine to Jupiter Capitolinus on the site of the Temple at Jerusalem might have been a reasonable attitude towards him, but it is obvious that the lack of more information makes a final conclusion impossible.

The Emperor sought remedies for his illness, which he suffered a considerable time. At some stage it confined him to his palace. He left Rome for the medicinal springs in the Bay of Naples at Puteoli and particularly at the resort of Baiae. This means that Hadrian had clear motivation for seeking the curative powers of the baths:[122]

> Post haec Hadrianus Baias petiit Antonino Romae ad imperandum relicto [= After this Hadrian departed for Baiae, leaving Antoninus at Rome to carry on the government].
>
> (*Scriptores Historiae Augustae, De Vita Hadriani* 25.5)

As is well known, these remedial sites became very famous in the Roman era due to their healing properties. Although he may have chosen Baiae spa as his destination because the imperial villa there guaranteed a comfortable place to spend his final moments, it seems more likely that he continued to maintain some hope of recovery and believed that it might be acquired in the resort.[123]

Finally, too large a quantity of medicine was administered to him, and thereupon his illness increased, and he died in his sleep, according to *Scriptores Historiae Augustae*:[124]

> Commodus autem prae valetudine nec gratias quidem in senatu agree potuit Hadriano de adontione. Denique accepto largius antidoto ingravescente valetudine per somnum periit ipsis kalendis Ianuariis [= Moreover, because of his ill-health, Commodus could not even make a speech in the senate thanking Hadrian for his adoption. Finally, too large a quantity of medicine was administered to him, and thereupon his illness increased, and he died in his sleep on the very Kalends of January].
>
> (*De Vita Hadriani* 23.15)

---

[122] *Scriptores Historiae Augustae, De Vita Hadriani* 25.5; See also Golan (1989): 22, 70–73; Allen (1998): 119; Speller (2002): 9–10, 238–239.

[123] Jackson (1990a): 5–13; Dvorjetski (1996a); idem, (1997a); Allen (1998): 121; Boatwright (2000): 71, 207.

[124] *De Vita Hadriani* 23.5.

There is evidence for an association between Hadrian and symbols of healing on coins and reliefs. There are numerous Roman coins depicting healing deities such as Aesculapius, Hygieia, Apollo and Serapis. These may have been representations of thanks by the Emperor for recovery from a particular illness or, in some cases, a supplication to the gods for a cure from illness. An interesting depiction is that of Heracles. According to a *Dictionary of Ancient Roman Coins*,[125] Heracles was given the surname of Alexicacus (one who drives away illness), a name also given to Apollo. Heracles was also a presiding deity over hot springs, which could be used for medicinal purposes.[126]

One of the silver types of an issue struck in 126 CE to celebrate the return of Hadrian from his first journey through the provinces was of Hercules Invictus, 'the Invincible'. The god is seated to the right upon a cuirass, a round shield and a helmet behind it, holding a club on the shield with his right hand and a Victoriola in his left. Instead of a Victory he sometimes holds a distaff, an apple or two arrows, but there is no reason to suppose that these variants represent different statues. A roundel of Hadrianic date in the Arch of Constantine shows Hadrian dedicating a lion's skin to a statue of Hercules, who is seated in identical pose, holding his club and a Victoria, and it is this statue, which must have been the model for the coin-type. Five years earlier, in 121 CE an issue celebrating Hadrian's first journey upon which he was then engaged had included *aurei* with the type of Hercules in the same pose, but facing and holding a distaff or two arrows in his left hand.[127]

It may be concluded, in view of all the above considerations, that the *baraitha* which describes the meeting at the ascent of Hammat-Gader, between Hadrian and the Jewish girl who was covered in sores, could very well be historically authentic. Since there is strong circumstantial historical evidence to support the story in the Talmudic texts, that Hadrian visited the spa at Hammei-Tiberias and at Hammat-Gader and to postulate his aims. He probably passed through the places either on his way to southern Trans-Jordan in the winter of 129/130 CE, or perhaps during his return from Egypt to Syria through Judaea in 131 CE. He used the whole Mediterranean world as a stage on which his journeys were the great evolving drama not just of his own life but

---

[125] Stevenson (1889): 455.
[126] Penn (1994): 114–115; Dvorjetski (1997a): 465–468.
[127] Hill (1989): 93–94.

of the lives of the millions who inhabited his Empire.[128] His purpose may have been to visit the Tenth Legion before the Bar Kochba war, or the thermo-mineral baths in Palestine for leisure, pleasure, therapy, or both.

7.3 'Antoninus'—Caracalla

Caracalla (188–217 CE) was the elder son of Septimius Severus and Julia Domna, and reigned as Emperor from 211 CE until his death. He was born in Lugdunum (Lyons), the capital of Gaul, and was later given the official name Marcus Aurelius Antoninus after his adoptive grandfather, the Emperor of that name. He is better known by his nickname Caracalla derived from the hooded Gallic, Celtic or German military greatcoat in origin (*caracallus*), which he often wore after he became Emperor in defiance of the law that military garb could not be worn in the city. This nickname 'Caracalla' never appears on coins. In 202 CE he married Fulvia Plautilla, the daughter of the praetorian perfect, Plautianus, but he caused the death of her father in 205 CE, and killed her in 212 CE after a long exile. Caracalla was at odds with his brother Geta, and when on Septimius' death the two became joint rulers through his will, their mother, Julia Domna, prevented a partition on the Empire. Geta was to have the Asiatic provinces, while Caracalla would be left in possession of Europe and the north-west of Africa. Their joint reign had lasted little than ten months. Caracalla murdered his brother in 212 CE, and carried out a reign of terror against his brother's supporters. The same year issued an imperial edict the *Costitutio Antoninianus*, extending the franchise to all free men in the Empire. He completed the most impressive monuments of imperial Rome, the notable Thermae named after him, which his father had begun. In 213 CE he went to Germany, where he defeated the Alemanni and strengthened the wall along the frontier. In 214 CE he was on the Danube frontier on his way to the East and fought the Carpi and reorganized Pannonia. He also levied an army based on that of Alexander the Great, whom he admired and wished to emulate. The next year he attacked Armenia unsuccessfully, and in 216 CE he moved against Media, spending the following winter at Edessa, which he had

---

[128] Speller (2002): 5.

added to the province of Osroene in north-western Mesopotamia. In April 217 CE he was about to set out again for the east when he was assassinated near Carrhae in Mesopotamia by the praetorian perfect Macrinus, who succeeded and deified him.[129]

Cassius Dio, the historian of Rome (164–230 CE), reflects in his *Historia Romana* the highly critical opinions of Caracalla held by the senators. He was shrewd, we are told, and capable of expressing himself with force, having been given a very through intellectual training by his father. However, as time went on he showed a marked preference for physical activity, energetically riding and swimming and engaging in blood-thirsty sports. It was his habit to blurt out recklessly whatever came into his head, and he would not ask advice, regarding experts, and indeed people who were good at anything at all, with strong aversion.[130]

The journeys of Caracalla produce vigorous complaints from Cassius Dio, a well-placed witness who was with the Emperor at Nicomedia over the winter of 214/215 CE:[131]

> But apart from all these burdens, we were also compelled to build at our own expense all sorts of houses for him whenever he set out from Rome, and costly longings in the middle of even the very shortest journeys; yet he not only never lived in them, but in some cases was not destined even to see them. Moreover we constructed amphitheatres and racecourses wherever he spent the winter or expected to spend it, all without receiving any contribution from him.
>
> (*Historia Romana* 77.9.5–7)

His short reign was a catalogue of disasters, for he was as despotic in temper and seemingly almost as mentally distributed as Commodus. Obsessed by a desire for military glory, he considered himself an incarnation of Alexander the Great in whose footsteps he sought to tread, adopting Macedonian costume and recruiting a special of Alexander's generals. At Ilium he paid a visit to the tomb of Achilles. His ill-temper

---

[129] Green (1993): 36; Scarre (1995): 138–146; Ball (2000): 106, 404–407–411, 430–431; Hazel (2002): 52–53; Hornblower and Spawforth (2004): 139; According to Cassius Dio (*Historia Romana* 77.5.4), Caracalla planned to kill Geta, but refrained because he was very ill; After many measures directed against persons and in violation of the rights of communities he was seized with an illness and underwent great suffering. Yet even toward those who nursed him he behaved most brutally.

[130] Grant (1999): 120; Yegül (1992): 146–162; Fagan (1999a): 190; DeLaine (1997).

[131] Millar (1992): 33.

and caprice may have been made worse by the constant ill health from he suffered, the exact nature of which we do not know.[132]

Some Emperors minted the coins at time of ill health; this was especially true of Caracalla, whose temples visits suggest psychoneurosis rather than physical ill health. His life and the coins he issued have much of medical interest.[133] He does seem to have been suffering both mentally deranged and physically sick after the death of his father and his brother. His ill-temper and caprice may have been made worse by the constant ill health from he suffered, the exact nature of which we do not know. Cassius Dio gives an interesting description of the illnesses of Caracalla and his responses:[134]

> For he was sick not only in body, partly from visible and partly from secret ailments, but in mind as well, suffering from certain distressing visions, and often he thought he was being pursued by his father and by his brother, armed with swords...But to Antoninus no one even of the gods gave any response that conduced to healing either his body or his mind, although he paid homage to all the more prominent ones. This showed most clearly that they regarded, not his votive offerings or his sacrifices, but only his purposes and his deeds. He received no help from Apollo Grannus, nor yet from Aesculapius or Serapis, in spite of his many supplications and his unwearyingly persistence. For even while abroad he sent to them prayers, sacrifices and votive offerings, and many couriers ran hither and thither every day carrying something of this kind; and he also went to them himself, hoping to prevail by appearing in person, and did all that devotees are wont to do; but he obtained nothing that contributed to health.
>
> (*Historia Romana* 77.15.6)

Caracalla, as mentioned above, went in person to seek help in search of a cure and visited the shrines of Celtic deities, Apollo Grannus at Baden-Baden, then called Aurelia Aquensis, from Asculapius at Pergamum in Asia Minor, and from Serapis at Alexandria. His personal attendance and his lavish gifts were no more successful than the prayers, sacrifices and benefactions his servants had previously made on his behalf. Caracalla's pilgrimage also indicates that some gods were indeed viewed more widely than others as effective protectors and sources of healing.[135]

---

[132] Green (1993): 36.
[133] Penn (1994): 109–115; Hart (2000): 176–177.
[134] Cassius Dio, *Historia Romana* 77.15.6; See also Penn (1994): 109–110.
[135] Halfmann (1986): 226–229; Green (1993): 37; Scarre (1995): 144; Nutton (2004): 275.

Why Caracalla visited the East is not totally clear, but he left Rome in the spring of 214 CE to set up his base in Nicomedia, fixed firmly Penn.[136] Probably in the autumn of 214 CE he visited Pergamum, a visit which is commemorated by the issue of a magnificent set of coins. The ceremony of the *adventus*, the official welcome that a provincial city paid to a visiting Emperor had evolved by the third century CE into a complicated procedure during which the Emperor met the gods of the city, its officials and the people. He visited shrines, repaired temples and bestowed gifts and privileges and attended sacred festivities. After the visit of Caracalla, the citizens of Pergamum issued the coins which recorded the main events of his stay. The obverse has, in general, the bust of Caracalla wearing a cuirass ornamented with a Gorgoneion. The reverses of the coins record the Emperor's visit in pictorial sequence. They start with the arrival of the Emperor and the welcome at the city's gates. Further coins record the meetings with the city's gods and the sacrifices made to them. Yet other coins record the generosity of the Emperor in restoring temples. Varied scenes represent the cult statue of god of medicine, Aesculapius. His depiction on coins also symbolized health for the Emperor and the Roman state. On some coins the cult statue is presented to the Emperor by a magistrate, and on others Tyche or city goddess of Pergamum, wearing the mural headdress of a protective goddess, holding a statue of Aesculapius, symbolized the city and the cult of Aesculapius. Caracalla is shown also in military dress holding a *patera* over an alter, while the Aesculapius is holding his snake encircled staff is standing on the other side of the alter facing the Emperor. Other coins offer a complex and dramatic picture of the sacrifices. One shows Caracalla, holding a *patera*, facing Aesculapius with a humped bull between them. Another shows Caracalla, this time in a toga, holding a *patera* in his right hand and a scroll in his left. He is standing in front of a temple seen in perspective which has Aesculapius inside. Between them a figure is striking at a sacrificial humped bull. The function of the scroll may be as a petition to Aesculapius.[137]

A park next to the *Asclepion* at Pergamum housed the oracular serpents and a cult figure of Telesphorus, one of Aesculapius's sons and the guardian of convalescence, who was also a local divinity reputed to have been the founder of Pergamum. It may have formed part of an

[136] Penn (1994): 109.
[137] idem, (1994): 111–112; See also Hart (2000): 42, 134; Schmitt and Prieur (2004): 356–357.

issue celebrating the undertaking of vows for the Emperor's health.[138] Another coin shows Caracalla in military dress, carrying a spear in his left hand, saluting with upraised right hand the snake of god of medicine, Aesculapius, coiled around a tree. Between the snake and the Emperor is the figure of Telesphorus.[139]

Three temples are depicted on a coin of this series of the city. The obverse has the bust of Caracalla wearing a cuirass ornamented with a Gorgoneion. Two temples are shown in perspective, and the third is *tetrastyle* and shows a seated Aesculapius holding a serpent. The construction and restoration of temples was a major part of the Emperor's visit and this coin perhaps celebrates Caracalla's repair of the Asclepion and the temples deified Augustus and Trajan.[140]

Caracalla also issued other coins illustrating his interest in Aesculapius and various healing deities. For instance, in 215 CE, the year after his visit to Pergamum, an *aureus* was issued at Rome. The Emperor is in military dress attended by a figure in a toga and sacrificing out of a *patera* over a flaming altar. He is looking at a temple showing four columns in front of which a statue of Aesculapius probably copied from the cult statue in the temple on the Isola Tiburina.[141]

Even coins of Apollo Medicus were struck by Caracalla. According to Hill, the Emperor issued a denarius in 214 CE, to celebrate vows undertaken for his health. On the reverse of this coin Apollo is depicted sitting almost naked, except for drapery around his thighs, holding a laurel branch in his right hand and with his left elbow resting on a lyre set on a tripod. Another version of Apollo Medicus was issued by Caracalla in 215 CE. The Emperor, accompanied by attendants, is sacrificing before a temple of, apparently, the Ionic order. The figure of Aesculapius, undoubtedly copied from the cult statue, is shown as presiding over the ceremony, which must have been the understanding of vows for Caracalla's failing health.[142]

Another interesting depiction is that of Heracles. A denarius of Caracalla shows Heracles on the reverse with an olive branch in his right hand and in his left a club and the skin of the Nemean lion. As

---

[138] On the Pergamon Asclepieion, see Jackson (1988): 152–157; Yegül (1992), s.v. 'Pergamon'; Hart (2000): 64–69.

[139] Penn (1994): 112; Hill (1989): 78; Hart (2000): 42.

[140] Penn (1994): 112.

[141] Penn (1994): 113–114.

[142] Hill (1989): 38, 91; Penn (1994): 39, 47–48.

was explained above regarding Emperor Hadrian, Heracles was given the surname of Alexicacus—one who drives away illness. Heracles was also a presiding deity over hot springs, which could be used for medicinal purposes.[143] The hot springs at Himera in northern Sicily, which presumably were thought to have curative and restorative properties, were said to have been opened by the Nymphs to refresh Heracles after he was wearied in his journey around Sicily. They are symbolised on a tetradrachm dating to the fifth century BCE (465–415 BCE).[144] Heracles was also given the general epithet of Prophylax. The modern term 'prophylaxis' meaning preventive treatment against disease is similarly derived.[145]

The Rabbinic literature probably adds a layer to Caracalla's aims and deeds to seek a cure for his illness. In the light of recent research, there is a tendency to identify Emperor 'Antoninus', the close friend of Rabbi Judah the Patriarch, with Emperor Caracalla.[146] One of the numerous meetings between Rabbi Judah and the Roman Emperor Antoninus took place in Tiberias in which Rabbi Judah had arrived in order to bathe in its thermo-mineral baths because of his chronic health problems.[147]

The Roman Emperors owned territory in eastern Mediterranean, parts of which almost certainly remained imperial property even during the Byzantine era.[148] It is well known, that the wealth of Rabbi Judah the Patriarch included tracts of land that he received from the Emperor either on lease or as an award.[149] Traditions report about the lands of Rabbi Judah in the Tiberias region (*Jerusalem Talmud, Ma'aser Sheni* 4, 1 [54d]), and Beth Shearim is also included among his tracts.[150]

---

[143] Penn (1994): 114–115; Dvorjetski (1997a): 465–468.

[144] Dvorjetski (1992a): 38–39; Krug (1993): 181–182; Dvorjetski (1997a): 466; Penn (1994): 29; See also Ziegler (1919): 2385.

[145] Jones (1986): 108; Penn (1994): 115.

[146] On this possibility and others, see Urbach (1968): 208; Guttmann (1959): 422–424; Herr (1971): 291–192; Avi-Yonah (1970): 51–56; Safrai (1975): 52; Marmorstein (1977): 1116.

[147] *Babylonian Talmud, Avoda Zarah* 10a; *ibid., Shabbat* 40b; Dvorjetski (1995a): 43–52; idem, (2000a): 232–236.

[148] Applebaum (1967): 284–287; See Vespasian's explicit order about the leasing or selling of all the lands of the Jews: Josephus, *Bellum Judaicum* 7.216–217; Hadrian's estate in Judaea is mentioned clearly in the Talmudic literature, see *Jerusalem Talmud, Ta'anit* 4, 8 [69a]; *Midrash Lamentations Rabbah* 2, 4 (Buber ed., p. 104).

[149] Krauss (1910): 17–26; Alon (1971): II: 114, 132–133; Avi-Yonah (1970): 33.

[150] Oppenheimer (1991): 66, 68, 70; Applebaum (1989): 149; Safrai (1958): 211.

In some cases his possessions are mentioned without indicating their location. There are details about cattle belonging to Rabbi and to the Emperor, which 'came within each other', and this tells us about the Emperor's pastures and collaboration in the raising of cattle (*ibid., Shevi'it* 6, 1 [36d]).[151] The information in the *Jerusalem Talmud*, tractate *Ma'aser Sheni* 4, 1 [54d], that 'Rabbi was taking the first-ripe marrows to the authorities' is more likely to indicate tenancy payments or leasing fees than ordinary land taxes. Elsewhere, there is mention of two thousand portions of land, probably in the Bashan and the Golan areas,[152] about which it is stated that: 'Antoninus gave Rabbi two thousand units of land as tenancy' (*ibid., Shevi'it* 6, 1 [36d]). This land was clearly awarded to Rabbi Judah by Antoninus. Levin claims that this comment applies to most of Rabbis properties, if not to all of them.[153] Press is convinced that Rabbi Judah had his own fields in the vicinity of Gadara city—but he does not amplify his supposition.[154]

The good relationship between the Jewish Presidency and the Emperors are illustrated in a fascinate manner on the coins of the cities of Sepphoris and Gadara, particularly in the days of Emperor Caracalla. The coins of Sepphoris emphasize the bond of brotherhood and friendship between the 'Holy Council' of Diocaesarea—i.e., Sepphoris—'the autonomous, the faithful and the Senate of the Roman People'.[155] The governing institutions during the presidency of Rabbi Judah the Patriarch were located in Sepphoris, and these coins bear evidence of the recognition and status which were bestowed upon them by the authorities.

A silver coin depicting an eagle with a wreath between its legs, inside which are the three Graces, first appears in the city of Gadara in the days of Caracalla. The image of the Three Graces—the emblem of the Gadara mint—appears between the eagle's legs also on the Roman provincial silver tetradrachms, which were minted in the city during the reign of Caracalla.[156] The Three Graces have a fascinating link with the medicinal baths at Hammat-Gader, and the original name of these

[151] *Midrash Genesis Rabbah* 20, 6 (Theodor and Albeck ed., p. 190).
[152] Klein (1911–1912): 545–550; Krauss (1910): 17, 21, 26; Safrai (1958): 211; Levine (1982): 100.
[153] Levine (1982): 102.
[154] Press (1948): I: 148.
[155] Meshorer (1978b): 185–200.
[156] idem, (1985): 83; Dvorjetski (1992a): 190–192.

baths was 'The Baths of the τρεῖς χάριτες', [= The Three Graces].[157]
In view of the appearance of this emblem at that particular time it
may be assumed, that Hammat-Gader spa was officially inaugurated
in the days of Caracalla, and it is possible that the following *Mishnah,
Avoda Zarah* 4, 6 refers to him: [158]

> An idol whose devotees have abandoned it in time of peace is permitted
> [= to be made use of by Jews], but if in time of war it is prohibited.
> Baths for kings—these are permitted since they were set up when the
> kings pass by.

It is reasonable to assume, that as a result of the encampment of the
Legion X *Fretensis* in the area of Hammat-Gader, the lands of the city
passed to the ownership of the Army as *territorium legionis*, namely tracts
which became judicially the Emperors' property. Possibly the baths of
Hammat-Gader became the imperial estate of Caracalla, and they were
given to Rabbi Judah on lease or as an award—not only because of
Caracalla's policy of awarding territory to Rabbi Judah the Patriarch,
but also as a result of their deep friendship. Caracalla was also in the
habit of inaugurating baths throughout the Roman Empire wherever he
went.[159] According to Cassius Dio's evidence, when the ailing Emperor
Caracalla undertook his 'Temple Tour' around the Empire, he was in
the habit of sacrificing to the healing deities in the medicinal baths in
order to obtain relief for his maladies.[160] It is not inconceivable, that
Caracalla also tried the healing powers of Hammat-Gader, which were
known throughout the Roman world: 'And in Syria there are hot baths,
which are second only to those at Baiae, with which no other baths
can be compared throughout the Roman world'.[161]

---

[157] Dvorjetski (1990): 134–137; idem, (1993): 390–406.
[158] *Mishnah, Avoda Zarah* 4, 6, Blackman (1967): 471; See also Albek (1959): 327.
[159] Yegül (1992), s.v. 'Caracalla'.
[160] Cassius Dio, *Historia Romana* 78.15.3–7; Engelmann, Knibbe and Merkelbach
(1980): 148–149, no. 802.
[161] Eunapius, *Vitae Sophistarum* 459; Dechent (1884): 174; Sukenik (1935a): 21;
Hirschfeld (1987): 104; idem, (1997): 5; Dvorjetski (1994a): 16–17; idem, (2004): 19.

CHAPTER EIGHT

THE NUMISMATIC EXPRESSION
OF THE MEDICINAL HOT SPRINGS

The Romans minted their coins mainly in Rome itself or in auxiliary mints, while keeping to a clear separation of powers between the Emperor and the senate. However, the expansion of the empire and especially the annexation of the East with its Hellenistic traditions, brought about a new fiscal policy, and the Romans now began to strike silver and probably also gold coins in central eastern mints. Most of the city coins minted in the eastern mints were issued between the late first century and middle third century CE. They were inscribed in Greek, rather than Latin inscriptions, since Greek was the language spoken by the people in the Roman East. The Romans embarked on a policy of granting minting rights to cities, some of which they had founded or re-founded. A number of these cities were even raised to the rank of a colony, a status which conferred important privileges on the local inhabitants, including Roman citizenship and exemption from the taxes paid by other people living in the provinces. One of the important rights granted liberally to a growing number of Roman provincial cities was the right to mint bronze coins, while silver were continued to be minted only in the few above mentioned important cities. Generally speaking, the circulation of the city coins did not extend beyond the limited geographical area of the city where they were minted and of its surroundings.[1]

Together with this monetary development, the Romans came to realize that coins which are passed from hand to hand and from region to region are a highly efficient means of spreading information rapidly over extensive areas. In a world lacking mass means of communication this was an important advantage and the Romans, more than any other nation before them, knew how to exploit it. They began to use symbols, inscriptions and designs on the coins in order to publicize political ideas, social events and religious, military or economic messages. Thus within

---

[1] Meshorer (1985): 6–7; Hendin (2001): 347–349.

a short period of time, in the first and second centuries CE, the coins
became a most important source of information. The city-coins are an
incomparable mine of information, providing material for reconstructing the history of the city which minted the coins, as well as affording
insight into the character of the inhabitants, their religion, their local
economy, political, and cultural expression.

One particular group of cities is known as the Decapolis, a league
of Syrian-Hellenistic cities in Trans-Jordan and the northern Jordan
Valley during the Roman and Byzantine periods. Most of the Decapolis
cities date their eras from the time of Pompey's conquest of the area in
63 CE, some believe that the Decapolis was founded by Pompey himself
when he freed the cities which had been conquered earlier by King
Alexander Jannaeus. Cities of the Decapolis were self governing, and
maintained the right to mint their own coins. The Decapolis was of
special importance because they were located along the key trade routes
between Syria and northern Arabia. Frequently, the city coins bear the
portraits of the Emperors under whom they were issued. However, the
coins are not dated by regnal years, but mainly according to eras of
each individual city.[2]

The Numismatic finds, with the ritual characteristics of the curative sites, likewise shed light and uncover a veritable treasure about
the spas. The ritual worship characteristics of the spas in the eastern
Mediterranean basin are expressed in most interesting types of coins
from Tiberias, Gadara, and Pella.[3]

8.1   TIBERIAS (HAMMEI-TIBERIAS)

On one of the most famous coins of Palestine and especially outstanding among the coins of Tiberias, Hygieia, daughter of Aesculapius,

---

[2] On the Decapolis see, for example, Bietenhard (1963): 24–58; Jones (1971): 459;
Parker (1975: 437–441) rejects the long-held view that the Decapolis ever formed a
league or confederation; Bietenhard (1977): 220–261; Spijkerman (1978); Isaac (1981):
67–74; Barghouti (1982): 209–229; Bowsher (1987): 62–69; Lenzen and Knauf (1987):
21–46; Dvorjetski (1988): 26–35; Weber (1991): 223–235; Sartre (1992): 139–156;
Bowsher (1992): 265–281; Graf (1992): 1–48; Zeyadeh (1992): 101–115; Freeman
(2001): 440–452; Walmsley (2002): 137–145.
[3] This chapter is based on my following researches: Dvorjetski (1988): 126–139;
idem, (1990): 134–137; idem, (1992a): 187–199; idem, (1993): 387–406; idem, (1994a):
11–15; idem, (1994c): 100–115; idem, (2001–2002): 500–503; idem, (2004): 20–21, 26;
idem, (2005): 439–467; idem, forthcoming [e].

the god of healing, appears seated upon a rock from which water is flowing. She is wearing a long *chition* and holds a serpent in her right hand and feeds him from a *patera* [= bowl] she is holding in her left. This should undoubtedly be seen as a reference to the hot springs of Tiberias, whose waters steam from between the rocks and whose healing quality is emphasized by the image of the goddess of health, Hygieia. This type of important coin was minted in Tiberias in great quantities during the reign of Emperor Trajan (99/100 and 108/109 CE), and also in a limited quantity and in a cruder form during the reign of Emperor Commodus (188/189 CE). In the latter coin Hygieia is wearing long *chition* and *peplos*, seated to right on rock, below which water flows.[4] (See Fig. 8).

The equivalent of the Greek goddess Hygieia is the Roman Salus, which means 'Health, welfare'. Sometimes the concept is extended to include not only physical health but also the general welfare of the Roman people, the army and the state. During the Roman Empire a figure representing the personification of Salus appears on a number of coins. Her attributes are a scepter, a *patera*, a feeding snake (which connects her with the Greek Hygieia and the cult of Aesculapius), and occasionally a rudder or ears of grain, which may link her with Ceres or, more probably, with *Annona*. Sometimes Salus herself is not shown and the idea is conveyed by a figure of Aesculapius. In addition to *Salus Augusta* or *Augusti*, legends expand the idea of Salus with additions such as *Italiae, Romanorum, Exerciti* or *Militum*. The Emperor Galba claimed to be responsible for the *Salus Generis Humani*, 'The welfare of the Human Race', and Trajan copied this claim.[5]

These coins doubtless served as publicity vehicle to spread the fame of the Tiberias thermo-mineral healing waters, so that people would come to be healed by them. On the third century CE coins in the days of Emperor Caracalla (211–217 CE) and Emperor Elagabal as well (218–222 CE), Hygieia and her father Aesculapius appear standing opposite one another, holding serpents in their hands. Traces of an

---

[4] Kindler (1961): 55, 99, no. 15; Meshorer (1985): 34–35; idem, (2000): 50; Wallack-Samuels, Rynearson and Meshorer (2000): 119; Hendin (2001): 410; On Hygieia cult see, for instance, Wroth (1885): 82–101; Sobel (1990); Compton (2002): 312–329.

[5] Thrämer (1951): 554–555; Hammond and Scullard (1970): 948; Scullard (1981): 55, 170; Grimal (1986): 411; Marwood (1988); Jones, (1990): 276–277; Adkins and Adkins (2000): 102, 198; Compton (2002): 320.

inscription indicate that at that time Tiberias was a colony.[6] It may well
be that statues of Hygieia, both seated and standing beside Aesculapius,
as they appear on the coins, were most probably erected for worship
in sanctuary in the vicinity of the thermal springs. A passage in the
Jerusalem Talmud, Sanhedrin 7, 13 [25d] refers to a *kipa* [= cupola], which
has already been explained as a niche in the baths where the statue of
Hygieia, the goddess of health, was erected.[7]

Aesculapius was identified with oriental deities such as Sarapis or
Serapis in Egypt and Ashmon in Phoenicia. Serapis is a syncretistic
god originating in Hellenistic Egypt by Ptolomy I in order to provide
a cult in which both Greeks and Egyptians could take part. The name
derived from a combination of the Egyptian god Osiris and the sacred
bull Apis. He was represented as a bearded figure with the attributes of
various deities additional to Aesculapius, such as Osiris, Zeus-Jupiter,
Hades-Pluto, and also occasionally those of Helios-Sol, Poseidon-
Neptune and the Nile. Although Serapis was the chief god in the cult
of Egyptian deities, in the Roman Empire he was usually eclipsed by
the associated cult of Isis. His portrayed with a benign and bearded face
and figurehead surmounted by ornamented *modius* [= corn-measure],
a symbol of fertility, and his hair confined with *taenia*, is represented
only once on an undated coin from the era of Emperor Commodus.[8]
This type is very common in the repertoire of the second century CE
Palestinian city coin-types in Aelia Capitolina, Caesarea Maritima and
Shechem-Neapolis.[9] It is therefore natural, that we should find Serapis in
his capacity as god of medicine represented on the coins of Tiberias, the
city of the thermo-mineral waters. The administrators of the city were

---

[6] de Saulcy (1874): 335; Kindler (1961): 54; Rosenberger (1977): 67; Meshorer (1985):
35; Dvorjetski (1990): 134–135; idem, (1992a): 187–189; idem, (1994a): 11–15; idem,
(2001–2002): 500–501; idem, (2004): 26; For the many ancient Graeco-Roman coins
depicting medical themes also reveal the close connection of Hygieia and Aesculapius,
see Penn (1994): 30–31; McCasland (1939): 221–227.

[7] Kindler (1961): 54; Meshorer (1985): 34–35; Avi-Yonah (1984): 140; On the
importance of the *kipa*, see the discussion in chapter 6.2 on *The Sages at the Therapeutic
Sites—Aims and Deeds*.

[8] Thrämer (1951): 549; Kindler (1961): 40; Ferguson (1970): 36–37; Hammond and
Scullard (1970): 951; Witt (1971); Helck (1972): 1549; Jones (1990): 286; Witt (1997);
Adkins and Adkins (2000): 202; Compton (2002): 323–324.

[9] For Aelia Capitolina, see Kadman (1956): I: nos. 18, 19, 47, 48, 60, 79, 80, 91,
101, 105, 130–133, 183; For Caesarea Maritima, see nos. 28, 36, 39–41, 52, 53, 59,
64, 68–70, 76, 82–84, 89, 194, 205; and for Shechem-Neapolis, see Hill (1914): 62,
nos. 106–108.

well aware of the value of the curative springs and coins were issued bearing the effigy and Serapis in his quality as god of health.[10]

Moreover, the city-goddess, Tyche, is represented on coins from the days of Trajan and Commodus standing on a galley holding rudder and cornucopia in her hands. The latter is a symbol of prosperity, while the galley indicating the maritime character of the city. It is a pure maritime symbolism refers to the nautical activities of the Tiberians citizens on the Sea of Galilee. Two crossed *cornucopiae* were struck twice under Trajan in the years 99/100 CE and 108/109 CE with palm-branch between. It might be that it is a reflection of the most flourishing condition of Hammei-Tiberias at that days.[11]

The figures of Hygieia and Aesculapius also appear on the coins of other cities in the Levant that have no connection with natural hot springs such as Hammei-Tiberias and Hammat Gader. On the coins of Shechem-Neapolis from the days of Antoninus Pius (138–161 CE), it seems that they are linked to the therapeutic qualities still to this very day ascribed to the spring of Joseph at the foot of the mountain Gerizim. Aesculapius is holding a staff upon which a serpent is entwined; He and Hygieia standing opposite one another. A coin from the time of Philip the Arab (244–245 CE) has figures of Aesculapius and Hygieia standing opposite one another. He holds a staff with the entwined serpent, and she is feeding the serpent from a bowl. Between them, on top, is Mt. Gerizim. A coin from the time of Trebonianus Gallus (251–253 CE) on the right, Aesculapius offering a libation upon the alter while holding a staff with the serpent entwined upon it, and, opposite him, Hygieia is feeding the serpent from a bowl. Above them is Mt. Gerizim.[12] On a coin from Jerusalem at the time of Etruscus and Hostilianus (250–251 CE) there is the figure of Hygieia, goddess of healing, seated upon a rock and feeding a coiled serpent at her bosom. This perhaps is symbolic of the therapeutic qualities of the waters of

---

[10] Kindler (1961): 30, 40; Belayche (2001): 157–160; On the intensive worship of Aesculapius in the Decapolis, see Weber (1997): 334–338; See also the survey in chapter 5.4 on *The Medicinal Properties in the Light of the Archaeological Finds.*

[11] Kindler (1961): 42, 56, 61; Meshorer (1985): 34, no. 79; 35: no. 84; Hendin (2001): 410–411, nos. 912, 913.

[12] Meshorer (1978): 63; idem, (1985): 49–51, nos. 127, 128, 142, 143; Meyshan (1973: 9) thinks that there might be seen a building, which served as an *Asclepion* and a cave within was a therapeutic spring on the coin depicting Mt. Grizim. Generally it is a nice idea, but these descriptions cannot be seen at all.

the Siloah to which such healing powers have been constantly attributed from highest antiquity even though they are non-mineral. Their
clarity and cleanliness, as compared to the waters of the wells within
the city itself, gained them their therapeutic reputation. The well of
Siloah, in whose history Jesus played a role, originates at the foot of
the Temple Mount and follows into a pool. A man blind from birth
came to Jesus who spat on the ground, made dough from the spittle,
stroked it over the blind eyes and ordered him to wash in the Siloah
pool (*John* 9, 1–7). Tradition maintains another efficacy of this pool.
When the priests eaten much meat from sacrifices at the time of the
Temple, they drank of the waters of the Siloah and digested thereby the
meat like normal food (*Avot de Rabbi Nathan*, Version A, 35, Schechter
ed., p. 105). This is to the best of my knowledge, the only account in
Talmudic literature concerning the internal use of mineral water with
medical intent. From a religious viewpoint, to the Jews, the waters of
the well of the well of Siloah were endowed with an extraordinary
cleansing power (*Jerusalem Talmud, Ta'anit* 2, 1 [65a]; *Lamentations Rabbah*
19, Buber ed. p. 15).[13] The appearance of Aesculapius on the coinage
of Aelia Capitolina is presumably connected with the few remains that
have been uncovered at the excavations in the area of the Santa Anna
Monastery near the Lions' Gate in Jerusalem. These remains might be
indicative of the Aesculapius worship connected with the large poll of
water and already known from the end of the Second Temple period.[14]
Hygieia is also known from a coin struck in Caesarea Maritima from
the days of Trebonianus Gallus. Hygieia's sculptures and relief are
common in Caesarea. The explanation for her appearance there might
be connected to Ein Tsur spring, which has been excavated so far and
famed by its fertility healing qualities.[15]

The coins from Tiberias represent symbolically the hot springs of its
suburb, Hammei-Tiberias, whose curative properties were famous in
the ancient world. They served as a means of advertising the spa and
attracting people to come and bathe in their healthful waters.

---

[13] Funk (1912): 191, 222; Preuss (1993): 531; Kottek (1994): 54; Dvorjetski (1999d):
13.
[14] van der Vliet (1950); Meshorer (1982): 17–18; idem, (1989): 56–57; Dvorjetski
(1990): 134–135.
[15] Kadman (1957): 160, no. 31; Meshorer (1967): 107–109; Levine (1972): 134–140;
Finkliesztejn (1986): 419–428; Hirschfeld (1995): 43–44; Gerest (1999), s.v. 'Hygieia';
Barkay (2000): 377–419.

8.2   Pella (Hammat-Pella)

There are two clues on the coins of ancient Pella, in the foothills of the north Jordan Valley that indicate how great was the fame of its healing site Hammat-Pella. One is a symbol of Athena from the reign of Emperor Commodus (177 CE). She is helmeted and holding spear and shield.[16] This completes the hypothesis that thermo-mineral waters in the classical world were dedicated to Athena as well. The other clue is the description of a *nymphaeum*, which was built alongside the therapeutic baths, in great details. This highly complex building had three stories and a splendid facade richly decorated with columns and statues. It is identified on the coins as a NYMΨ[EΩN] *Nymphaeum*, and the full inscription is translated from the days of Elagabal as: 'of the people of Pella Philippi at the Nymphaeum' (220 CE). This is the only instance of a building specifically named on a coin of the eastern Mediterranean basin.[17] The coins depicting the *nymphaeum* are larger than usual, so that the wealth of architectural details can be shown. An interesting medallion struck under Commodus (183 CE) provides a view of the city. Pella is seen as a high hill surrounded by a wall or a colonnaded street with arched gates. An unidentified statue stands within the temple. The inscription around reads: 'of the people of Philippopolis which is also Pella, near the *Nymphaeum*, and free city'.[18] (See Fig. 23).

The notion of the *nymphaeum* was not uniformly employed in antiquity. Water, with its different optical, acoustical and haptic qualities, gained in importance already in Hellenistic fountain architecture. Reflecting surfaces, the rippling, splashing and even evaporation of water, and the coolness and the pleasing, moist scent which was produced were all incorporated into the design of fountain structures as symbols of

---

[16] Smith (1973): 58–59; Spijkerman (1978): 215; Meshorer (1985): 92; See also the discussion in chapter 3 on *The Medicinal Hot Springs and Healing Spas in the Graeco-Roman World*.

[17] Seyring (1959): 69; Spijekerman (1978): 211, 215; Price and Trell (1977): 44, Fig. 72; Nicolet (1981): 51; Meshorer (1985): 92, no. 251; Schürer (1991): II: 147, note 329; Dvorjetski (1992a): 197–199; idem, (1994a): 14–15; idem, (1996a): 40*, 44*; On another *nymphaea* impressed on coins such as Rome, Hadrianopolis in Thrace, Nicopolis in Moesia and Neocaesarea in Pontus, see Hill (1989): 98–99; Tameanko (1999): 89, 93.

[18] Smith (1973): 53–54; Meshorer (1985): 121; Bowsher (1987): 63; Dvorjetski (1992a): 197–199; idem, (1994a): 14; Wallack-Samuels, Rynearson and Meshorer (2000): 116.

the life-giving element. Water sanctuaries are frequently classed among *nymphaea*. The difference between them can be seen in the fact that in the water sanctuaries the building concept is firmly rooted in temple architecture. The traditional temple placement was in front of large basins, which however were not integrated into it, as on the contrary is the case for the exedra and façade *nymphaea*.[19]

The *nymphaeum* from the Roman period is monumental architectural expression of the 'site of the Nymphs', divinities of junior rank in Greek mythology, built in a variety of architectural forms and incorporating fountains. The *nymphaea* of the classical period were sacred sites around springs, streams or caves from which fountains flows. Very often the Nymphs serve as patronesses of the medicinal springs and as such are connected with Aesculapius. The *nymphaeum* is a decorated structure with a decorative pool in the front. The water served as the main component in the decorative complex of the *nymphaeum* structure.[20] *Nymphaea* are common in the Roman period as building which combine architectural extravagance with the provision of water, and they were often donated to the cities by Emperors or wealthy individuals.[21]

The *nymphaeum* depicted on Pella's coins is joining a remarkable list of *nymphaea*, which thus far been revealed in the eastern Mediterranean basin, such as Philippolis, Kanata, Bosra, Suweida, Philadelphia, Gadara, Beth Shean-Nysa-Scythopolis, Sussita-Hippos, Petra and Kallirrhoe.[22] Two of the most elaborate fountain structures built during the Roman period were in the Decapolis in Philadelphia and Gerasa. The *nymphaeum* of Philadelphia was located near Wadi Amman and near the main streets of the city. The two-story limestone *nymphaeum* had an imposing central wall with a large apse. This 'baroque' building with its arches, columns, niches, and gables must have made quite

[19] On the *nymphaeum* in the Greek, Hellenistic and Roman architecture, see Neuerburg (1967): 19–21; Settis (1974): 661–745; Aupert (1974); Walker (1987): 60–71; Glaser (2000): 437–449.
[20] Liddel-Scott (1985): 580; Harvey (1937): 289; Kerényi (1951): 177–180; Graves (1959): 149–150, 162–163; Hangmann (1968): 615; Danbabin (1989): 13–16; See also Weller (1903): 263–288.
[21] Segal (1995b): 161–162; Jones (1990): 223.
[22] Brünnow and Domaszewski (1909): 90, 142–143, 216–220; Klengel (1971): 100; Schumacher (1888a): 194–206; Butler (1915): I: 54–59, 355; Fisher (1938): 21–22; Hadidi (1978): 210–222; Segal (1988): 9–11, 59–63; Weber (1988): 349–352; idem, (1989): 606–607; On *Kallirrhoe*, see chapter 4.4 on *The Historical-Archaeological Analysis and Healing Cults of Kallirrhoe*.

an impressive sight in Philadelphia. The individual fountains were on the second floor, which one reached after going up a wide set of stairs. The *nymphaeum* of Gerasa, built in 190 CE, was located almost in the centre of the city and is considered the most magnificent of all the urban structures in that city. The three-story building is a 24 meters long façade built in the form of a large central apse with smaller ones and niches along the sides.[23] The *nymphaeum* at Beth Shean is located between the temple and the central monument and basilica. This *nymphaeum*, like the one in Gerasa, was in the forms of an apse-shaped façade and was a number of stories high. A Greek inscription identifies the building as a *nymphaeum* built by Flavius Artemidoros, apparently in the fourth century CE. The inscription undoubtedly refers to the reconstruction or renewal of the building, which was originally built at the end of the second century CE.[24]

8.3   GADARA (HAMMAT-GADER)

The Gadara coins provide most instructive information about the city's political history, about its cultural character in general and its therapeutic hot springs in particular. One of the major deities in the pantheon of the city Gadara was Heracles, to whom it was customary to dedicate spas. The annual fair at Hammat-Gader baths revolved around a ritual festival in honor of the mythical hero Hercules, who was, in the opinion of Safrai, the patron and protector of traders.[25] Heracles is standing in front of column on which rests a basket with snakes; a lion jumps up against the column and another animal stands on the left from the reign of Elagabal.[26] He is also described in a collection of engraved gems from Gadara city, attributed to the period between the first century BCE and the second century CE.[27]

A mintage unique among the coins of Roman Palestine is that of the Three Graces appearing on the Gadara coins starting with the

[23] Butler (1907): IIA: 54–59; Ward-Perkins (1981): 338–339; Tsafrir (1984): 77; Hirschfeld (1989): 22; Segal (1993): IV: 371, 1448; Sperber (1998): 178.

[24] Foerster (1993): II: 227–228; Sperber (1998): 178.

[25] Safrai (1984): 158; See also the discussion in chapter 3.3 on *The Ritual Worship of the Medicinal Hot Springs and Healing Spas in the Graeco-Roman World*.

[26] Spijkerman (1978): 137–151; Meshorer (1985): 80, 83; Dvorjetski (1993): 388–389, Figs. 1a–b.

[27] Henig and Whiting (1987): 18–19, 27–28.

days of Caracalla (211–217 CE), Elagabal (218–222 CE), and Gordian III (238–244 CE), showing a silver *sela* with a bird of prey with wings spread and between the bird's legs a wreath in which there are three nude female figures, the Three Graces. On the provincial Roman silver tetradrachms minted in the city during the reign of Caracalla and Macrinus the statue of the three Graces appears between the claws of an eagle as the mintmark of Gadara. This testimony reflects clearly that a cult of the Three Graces was apparently practiced in Gadara, likely associated with that of Hearacles.[28] (See Fig. 22).

Graces is the Latin term for the 'graceful and beautiful' goddesses of Greek mythology called the Χάριτες. The Three Graces or *Gratiae* (the number sometimes varies in ancient literature) were personifications of charm and beauty. They were a sort of three-fold Aphrodite-Venus, Goddess of Love, and they are represented as naked maidens holding each other's shoulder and symbolizing the forces of growth. Being the Underworld goddesses, their image served as an amulet. As we have seen before, to the Romans the spring was not merely a source of hot water but a sacred place where mortals could communicate with the deities of the Underworld. Especially evident is the Graces' many-sided relationship with water.[29] They are called θαλάσσιαι, that is 'daughters of the sea', and their mother is the daughter of Oceanus. The Graces dwelt on the Olympus with the Muses with whom they occasionally formed a choir. Incidentally, one of the Gadara residents designates his city by the distinctive Greek word χρηστομουσία, which means a distinguished sanctuary of wisdom.[30] Often they accompany Apollo, Artemis, Athena, Dionysus, and especially Eros and Aphrodite. Eros, the god of love, almost always escorted the Graces, and it should be mentioned that two of the springs of Hammat-Gader were called Eros and Anteros. The springs might be identified with the hot spring *'Ain el-Maqle*, around which the bath complex was erected. Another spring with cool, moderating waters—a candidate is *'Ain Būlus*—located about

[28] Spijkerman (1978): 82–83, 91–92, 97–98, 151–155; Meshorer (1985): 82–83; idem, (2000): 52; Dvorjetski (1992a): 190–193; idem, (1993): 390–397; idem, (1994c): 100–115; Wallack-Samuels, Rynearson and Meshorer (2000): 111; Hendin (2001): 372.

[29] Escher (1899): 2150; Zielinski (1924): 158–163; Krappe (1932): 155–162; Gsell (1963): 1658–1659; Jones (1990): 129; Dvorjetski (1993): 392–393; idem, (1999a): 127–128; idem, (2004): 26.

[30] Schürer (1991): II: 132.

200 meters to the northwest.[31] (See Map 4). The Graces bathe and oil Aphrodite, and she dances and sings with them. Celebrations known as χάρισα or χαριτησία were sort of festivals in their honor taken especially at nights and accompanied by songs and dances. Various epigrams in the Greek Anthology link them with the baths. In the Greek mythology baths and springs are very closely connected with both the Nymphs and the Graces, for the Nymphs are the goddesses of the natural springs and waters, and the Graces dwell alone in the bath buildings. Later on, the Graces were seen as the symbol of health, and it is in this sense that they are associated with Aesculapius and Hygieia, who was also the patroness of the therapeutic springs.[32] A small relief of the Roman period, preserved in the Vatican Museum, shows Aesculapius with the Graces, naked, by his side. Here they symbolize both gratitude to the healer of the sick and the joy of returning to health.[33]

Gadara seems to be the outstanding place in the region of the worship of the Graces, and their likeness served as the symbol of the Gadara mintmark. In the ruins of Gadara, which is Umm Qais Jordan, four kilometers from Hammat-Gader, a silver ring from the first half of the third century CE was discovered. On one side, Zeus is seated in a temple and on the other, the Three Graces appear exactly as they do on the city coins, but they are standing in a temple.[34] In light of this find, one may assume that a temple was erected in their honor, which may have existed near the thermo-mineral springs, in the area of the baths. (See Fig. 33).

In the Hellenistic period Gadara was an important cultural centre, and Philodemus the Epicurean, the poet Meleager, Menippus the Cynic and satirist as well as Oenomaus the cynic, and the orator Apsines were the renowned sons of Gadara. Meleager and Menippus named their treatises *The Graces.* It can be assumed that the reasons for these names were as a result of an inspiration of the Graces' model in the academy of those two intellectuals, or that they were influenced from

---

[31] Eunapius, *Vitae Sophistarum*, 459; Geiger (1986): 375–376; Hirschfeld (1987): 104.

[32] Stevenson (1889): 438; Escher (1899): 2157–2166; Oesterley (1923): 88–106; Hangmann (1949): 227; Kerényi (1951): 99–101; Rose (1989): 124; Gsell (1963): 1662–1665; Schmitz (1967): 686–687; Avi-Yonah and Shatzman (1981): 118; Green and Tsafrir (1982): 88–89; Dunbabin (1989): 12–17; Dvorjetski (1993): 392–393; On the various epigrams, see Robert (1948): 84; Paton (1969): III: 607, 609, 616, 623.

[33] Escher (1899): 2163; Gsell (1963): 1663.

[34] Meshorer (1979): 221–222, Pl. XXV.

their sanctuary adjacent to the springs or within the baths or it could have been or both.[35]

The Three Graces are also described among the collection of intaglios and cameos from Gadara, attributed to the first-second century CE.[36] They are shown nude in their typical stance, except for one detail: they wear helmets, imparting a distinctly military atmosphere to the scene. These evidences, as well as other historical proofs, indicate that the soldiers belonged to the Legion X *Fretensis*, whose members were also engaged in building baths,[37] built the *thermae* of the *Three Graces* in the suburb of Gadara, Hammat-Gader, for their own use and for the enjoyment of the inhabitants of the region.[38]

In the *Jerusalem Talmud*, Tractate *Shabbat* 3, 4 [6a], we read of two contemporaries of Rabbi Judah Nesi'ah, Rabbi Aha bar Isaac and Rabbi Abba bar Memel, who went to bathe in the bathhouse named after the Three Graces. Had the Gadara coins not been found, this text would have remained historically unauthenticated to this very day. Here we have an instructive picture of the therapeutic hot springs acting as a sort of nature preserve of Classical culture, a preserve of the Three Graces at the Hammat-Gader therapeutic site, where the Sages did not hesitate to come and bathe. From analysis of the text in the *Jerusalem Talmud*, it appears that the πανήγυρις, the pagan festival was held, first and foremost, in honor of the *Three Graces*, which was also the original name of the Hammat-Gader spa.[39]

The Three Graces were known in the region not only by means of as a mintmark on coins. The Mosaic of the Four Seasons discovered at Shahba, ancient Philippopolis, combines an acanthus scroll border with an *emblema* which depicts Gê [= the Earth], offering the gifts of the Seasons to Dionysus and Ariadne under the supervision of Ploûtos [= Wealth]. Next to the Roman villa which yielded this mosaic, a set

---

[35] Hengel (1974): I: 85; Geiger (1985): 3–16; Luz (1988): 222–231; Schürer (1991): II: 49–50; Luz (1992): 42–80; Geiger (1994): 221–230; Dilts and Kennedy (1997); Luz (2003): 97–107.

[36] Henig and Whiting (1987): 28.

[37] Tsafrir (1984): 106–107; Arubas and Goldfus (1995); Mazar (1999): 59; Stiebel (1999): 74–75.

[38] Dvorjetski (1988): 61, 133–139; idem, (1993): 397–406; idem, (1994c): 100–115.

[39] See the discussions in chapter 4.2 on *The Historical-Archaeological Analysis and Healing Cults of Hammat-Gader* and in chapter 6.2 on *The Sages at the Therapeutic Sites—Aims and Deeds.*

of four rooms of another villa with mosaic floors In three rooms, geometric motifs interrupted by panels enclosing a series of heads, surrounded *emblemata* which depicted Orpheus and the beasts, the wedding of Aphrodite, and Ares, God of War and the Three Graces.[40] The excavation of a mid-sixth century hall under the atrium and narthex of the Church of the Virgin at Madaba, disclosed three remarkable panels framed by an inhabited acanthus scroll. The upper panel showed Aphrodite and Adonis, the Three Graces—each named as Χάρις, four *Erotes* and a peasant-woman (*Agroikis*).[41] Another mosaic pavement is that of Sheikh Zouède in northern Sinai, exhibited nowadays in the Ismailiya Museum, Egypt. This mosaic floor together with other coloured mosaics paved several rooms of a large building, whose function is unknown, but it seems to have been a villa. Three Greek inscriptions inserted in the mosaic are interrelated by their content. All three praise the beauty of art in general and the splendid mosaic pavement in particular, and invite the guest or visitor to 'enter gladly into this grand hall' and enjoy the beauty of the work of art. The lower panel includes a Greek inscription within a *tabula ansata*, surrounded by various birds, plants motifs, a snake, and a basket. The middle and the upper panels include mythological scenes: Phaedra and Hippolytus, Dionysus's triumphal procession (*triumphus*), satyrs and maenads.[42] These poetic inscriptions have a classical character, as others of the early Byzantine period, such as those from Hammat-Gader and Apollonia.[43]

At this stage one can sum up, that coins of the cities Tiberias, Gadara and Pella, which contained therapeutic springs, served as a means of spreading their reputation far and wide so that people would come to be cured there, thus boosting the city economy. Furthermore, we can certainly see in the spas a 'nature reservations' of the classical culture.

---

[40] Dentzer and Dentzer-Feydy (1991): 143, nos. 8, 59, Pls. C–F; See also Dauphin (1997): 16.

[41] Piccirillo (1989): 51–60; See also Dauphin (1997): 24.

[42] Ovadiah, Gomez-de Silva and Mucznik (1991a): 181–191; Ovadiah, Mucznik and Gomez-de Silva (1991b): 122–126; Ovadiah (1997): 441–443; idem, (1998): 15–18.

[43] Green and Tsafrir (1982): 77–96; Di Segni and Hirschfeld (1986): 250–268 (Hammat-Gader); Birnbaum and Ovadiah (1990): 182–190; idem, (1989): 279–288 (Apollonia); See Ovadiah, Gomez-de Silva and Mucznik (1991a): 190; See also the discussion in chapter 4.2 on *The Historical-Archaeological Analysis and Healing Cults of Hammat-Gader.*

8.4   Nautical Symbols and the Tenth Legion
Fretensis—A Reassessment

The Gadara mint was one of the larger municipal mints in the region of the Levant, and its coins reveal fascinating data concerning the political history and character of the city, and the medicinal hot springs in the suburb, Hammat-Gader and a unique affinity to one of the Roman Legions—*Legio Decima* [= Tenth] *Fretensis*.[44]

This Legion was one of the 45 backbones of the Roman army, supported by auxiliary troops. It was founded in 41/40 BCE by Augustus for arresting Sextus Pompey's occupation of Sicily, which put the grain supply of Rome into peril. After Augustus's victory at Actium in 31 BCE, many Roman soldiers were pensioned off. Several subunits of *Decima Fretensis* were stationed at Cyrrhus, where they guarded the route from the Euphrates to Antioch. It is likely that the legion was sent to suppress the rebellions of the Jewish messianic claimants Judas, Simon, and Athronges after the death of King Herod the Great in 4 BCE. The unit, together with Legion III *Gallica*, Legion VI *Ferrata*, and Legion XII *Fulminata*, must have taken part in the campaign led by the famous governor of Syria Quirinius to Judaea in 6 CE, which had become restless after the Augustus had exiled Herod Archelaus. For almost half a century we have no evidence for the whereabouts and actions of *Decima Fretensis*, except for the fact that veterans were deduced to a new colonia at Acre-Ptolemais. From 67 CE onward, the Legion fought in the war against the Jews. The supreme commander of the Roman forces in Judaea was Vespasian, who was to become Emperor during the civil war that broke out after the suicide of Nero in 68 CE. After the first year of war, Legion X *Fretensis* and Legion V *Macedonia* had their winter camp at Caesarea (67/68 CE), and after the capture of Gamala, Legion X moved to Beth Shean-Nysa-Scythopolis. In 70 CE, X *Fretensis* took part in the siege of Jerusalem and was to stay in Judaea for more than a century and a half. Jerusalem became its new base and several archaeological finds in the vicinity of Jerusalem and the city itself—bricks, tiles, coins and countermarks with the name of emblem of the Legion—prove its presence. Like the other Legions in the Levant, *Decima Fretensis* served during Trajan's campaign against

---

[44] This survey is based on the following researches: Dvorjetski (1988): 128–133; idem, (1992a): 193–196; idem, (1993): 387–406; idem, (1994c): 100–115.

the Parthian Empire (115–117 CE). During the reign of Hadrian, it was involved in the war against the leader Simeon Bar Kochba, one of the greatest disasters that ever befell the Roman Empire. The Tenth Legion had to evacuate its fortress at Jerusalem, where the Jews restored the proper cult in the Temple. This was duly commemorated: many Jewish coins show the restored sanctuary and imply the Roman loss of their base. To prevent future Jewish wars, the VI Legion *Ferrata* was transferred to Palestine. In the course of the third century CE, *Decima Fretensis* was transferred to Aila, modern Eilat. From now on, the Legion begins to disappear from the historical documentations. A subunit of horsemen was active in the west during the age of the independent Gallic Empire (260–274 CE). *Decima Fretensis* was at some stage awarded the title *Pia Fidelis*. The unit is not mentioned as part of the Roman army of the fourth century. Many sources referring to this legion prove that its soldiers took part in many kinds of military building operations.[45] The emblems of the *Legio Decima Fretensis* were the bull—the common symbol of any Legion created by Julius Caesar—a boar, an eagle (aquila), a dolphin, and several maritime symbols.[46]

8.4.1   *Coins of Gadara City and Their Link to Nautical Symbols*

The coins of Gadara are distinguished by numerous images, including dolphins, ship' ramming prows, *aphlaston* [= decoration on the war-galley's stern], long oars, and a helmsman holding a long steering oar, with a tall banner behind him. Thus, for example, a medallion from the days of the Emperor Marcus Aurelius bears a Greek inscription ΓΑΔΑΡΕΩΝ/ΝΑΥΜΑ/ΔΚΣ [= 'of the people of Gadara / *Naumachia*/ (year 224)' = 161 CE]. There are galley sailing with ramming prow, a rudder and eight oarsmen; the same symbols appear on a medallion from the reign of the Commodus. The Greek inscription reads as follows: ΠΟΜΠ/ΗΙΕΩΝ/ΓΑΔΑΡΕΩΝ/ ΕΤ. ΓΜΣ [= 'of the people of Pompeian Gadara, year 243' = 180 CE]; another coin is dated to the

---

[45] For the history of the *Legio Decima Fretensis*, see Keppie (1986): 419–424; Mor (1986): 581–582; Bohec (1994), s.v. 'Jerusalem', 'Judaea'; Goldsworthy (2003), s.v. 'Judaea'; Mazar (1971); Tsafrir (1984): 106–107; Geva (1984): 239–254; Isaac (1986): 635–640; Dąbrowa (1993): 11–21, with extensive bibliography; Magness (2002): 189–212) demonstrates a study of the pottery associated with the Legion at Jerusalem and Masada, which provides valuable insights on the manner in which the Roman army operated while in the field and when stationed in permanent camps; Jona Lendering at: http://www.livius.org/lelh/legio/x_fretensis.html.
[46] See, for example, Barag (1967): 244–267.

days of Emperor Elagabal 'ΑΠC' [= 281 = 218 CE], with the same
Greek inscription. The galley with details is clearly visible, and below
the galley two dolphins. On a coin dated to the reign of Gordian III
is a war-galley with *aphlaston* and oars and oarsmen sit within as well
as the latter Greek inscriptions, except the year 'ΓΤ' [= 240 = 303
CE].[47] (See Fig. 34).

This fact is somewhat surprising, as far less emphasis is given to
nautical themes on the coins of Roman cities which are located on
the Mediterranean coast, such as Acre-Ptolemais, Dor-Dora, Caesarea,
and Ascalon.

Various explanations have been offered for the appearance of ships on
the coins of Gadara, the mother city of Hammat-Gader. Some maintain
that the first inhabitants during the Roman conquest were seafarers
by origin, while others presume that the reason lay in the proximity
of the city to the Sea of Galilee, which is navigable.[48] It is obviously
impossible to prove the former assumption, whereas the latter seems
plausible, especially in view of the various opinions noted below.

Firstly, we should mention the view held by Clermont-Ganneau who
was of the opinion that the image of a rowing boat symbolized the victory of the X Legion in the naval battle on the Sea of Galilee during
the First Jewish War, after the Legion had captured the city of Taricheae
on its western shore as accounted in *Bellum Judaicum* 3.532–542.[49]

This opinion was repudiated by Meshorer, who claims that no real
naval battle took place during that war and that such an unimportant
engagement would have had no impact on citizens of Gadara, who
would have been unable to see it in any case. He has suggested that
the ships symbolize the conquest of the country by Pompey, following
his naval victories over the pirates controlling the eastern coast of the
Mediterranean basin.[50] According to Meshorer, it is understandable
that the only city which was rebuilt by Pompey and named after him

[47] de Saulcy (1874): 294, Pl. XV; Head: (1963): 787; Rosenberger (1978): 36–50;
Spijkerman (1978): 288–289, Pls. 26, 30–32; Meshorer (1985): 80–83; Dvorjetski
(1993): 398–401, Fig. 6; idem, (1994c): 101–102, Figs. 2A, 2B, 2C; Hendin (2001):
374, no. 860.
[48] Stahl (1986): 15–16.
[49] Clermont-Ganneau (1898): 299–301.
[50] Meshorer (1966): 28; idem, (1985): 82; Wallack-Samuels, Rynearson and Meshorer
(2000): 111; See also Hendin (2001): 372.

would portray a ship on its coins. It is also noteworthy that in 161 CE, during the reign of Emperor Marcus Aurelius, a *naumachia*, a staged naval battle, was held at Gadara in honour both of its foundation and of Pompey and his naval victories. Yet, our knowledge of this nautical performance stems solely from the medallions minted to commemorate the event.[51] Meshorer claims that the site of this *naumachia* at Gadara can be identified at a place on the Yarmuk River, known by the Latin name Hieromices, at the point where it widens before reaching the area of Hammat-Gader. At that point, according to Meshorer, the river formed a wide basin, capable of accommodating all the ships which were required to reenact Pompey's battle with the pirates. However, Meshorer's assumption is surprising in view of his statement in an earlier article,[52] that during the reign of Marcus Aurelius *naumachiae* were no longer held. He emphasizes, moreover, that the tradition of *naumachiae* ceased at the end of the first century CE, and that there is no description of a *naumachia* in the second and third centuries.

Taking a different line, Nun explains the portrayal of ships on coins by the fact that Gadara was the largest and most magnificent of the Hellenistic towns around the shores of the Sea of Galilee, and that its limits extended to the sea shore. He points out that there are clues indicating that the south-eastern corner of the sea was within the city's territory. He cites the New Testament story, which gives the land of the Gadarenes as the location for the Miracle of the Swine that plunged into the sea (*Mark* 5, 1–20; *Luke* 8, 26–39).[53] Nun suggests that Tel Samara—now the Kibbutz Ha'on camping ground—was the naval suburb of Gadara, while the adjacent large harbour was built by the Greek city for its fleet and naval communications. According to his view, the harbour also served the thousands of visitors who steamed to the Hammat-Gader spa for healing and recreation. Nun also opposes Meshorer's opinion, quoted above, that the naval games were held in a pool on the River Yarmuk, as no remains of a catchment facility of this kind have been discovered there. He sees a much more suitable location for the *naumachia* in the large harbour basin and the surrounding piers, whose total length, 500 meters, could have accommodated the spectators.

---

[51] Meshorer (1985): 83; See also Avi-Yonah (1976): 54; Dan (1984): 203) explains that it was due to Pompey's victory over the pirates; Kadman and Kindler (1963): 105.

[52] Meshorer (1985): 82; idem, (1966): 28.

[53] Nun (1987b): 1–18.

Avi-Yonah, on the other hand, did not believe that the city's borders extended as far as the Sea of Galilee.[54] This was firstly because, in the parallel version of the Miracle in *Matthew* (5, 21) and in some manuscripts of *Mark* and *Luke*, the name appears as 'Gerasenes' and not Gadarenes; secondly, because *naumachiae* were held at the hippodromes of land-locked cities, far from the sea; and thirdly, whereas the swine in the story of the Miracle ran down a steep mountainside, the land by the south-east shore of the Sea of Galilee is quite flat.

Dalman was the first to record the acquisition of a medallion of this type.[55] Although he did not publish a photograph or a drawing of it, he read the legend as follows: ΓΑΔΑΡΕΩΝ ΤΗΣ ΚΑΤΑ Π(Ο)Τ(ΑΜΟΝ) ΝΑΥΜΑ(ΧΗΣ). In his view, the *naumachia* took place in the city baths, or on the Yarmuk, or in a pool specially constructed for the purpose. Hirschfeld also considers that the performances took place in the Yarmuk River itself; but in his view it is more likely that an artificial lake was created in the natural depression in Hammat-Gader through which the waters of *Ἀin eǧ-Ǧarab* flow. Today this depression is the site of a large bathing-pool.[56] Ten huge basalt seats were discovered in 1938 by Makhouly while clearing the area northwest of the thermal baths.[57] There is no evidence that the seats at Hammat-Gader were part of any sanctuary. It is more likely, according to Hirschfeld that they were designated for the elders and notables of the city, as part of either a waiting area annexed to the thermae or the city council (*bouleuterion*). Another possibility of Hirschfeld is that they were connected to the water festivals celebrated at Hammat-Gader. According to him if the basalt seats did over-look an artificial lake created for the events of the *naumachia*, they might have been reserved for the nobles of the city of Gadara.[58] In light of three coins, Lichtenberger suggested another interpretation of the abbreviated legend as ΓΑΔΑΡΕΩΝ ΤΗΣ ΚΑΤΑ Ι(ΕΡΟΜΥΚΟΥ) ΓΥ(ΑΛΟΝ) ΝΑΥΜΑ(ΧΗΣ) [= 'of the Gadarenes which have a *naumachia* in the valley of the Hieromices'].[59] In view of this

---

[54] Avi-Yonah (1944): 6; See also Klausner (1977): 222; On the idea that the miracle of the swine occurred in Koursi, see Avi-Yonah (1984): 159; Abel (1927): 113; Dalman (1967): 190.
[55] Dalman (1912): 54–55; idem, (1914): 143.
[56] Hirschfeld (1987): 116; idem, (1992): 366.
[57] Makhouly (1938): 59–62, Figs. 1–4.
[58] Hirschfeld (1987): 115–116; See also Belayche (2001): 273.
[59] Lichtenberger (2000–2002): 192–193.

reading, the location for a *naumachia* of Gadara is the Yarmuk River. Another concept for an appropriate place of the mock naval battle performed on the occasion of municipal games and festivals in the domain of Gadara—will be illuminated below.

We can conclude that the common denominator of the views cited above is the obvious link between the image of the ship and maritime activity. It remains to ascertain whether ships or other nautical images appear on the coins of the other cities not directly on seashore, and to elucidate whether the depiction of a boat has any additional significance.

8.4.2   *Nautical Images on Coins of Inland Cities*

Nautical images are indeed common on the coins of cities situated far inland. Such motifs appear on the coins of Samaria-Sebaste, Shechem-Neapolis, Moab-Rabath-Mōba, and Jerusalem-Aelia Capitolina.

At Samaria-Sebaste, coins from the reign of Domitian (81–96 CE) have been found, which bear countermarks of the *Legio Decima* in the shape of a galley, a boar, and a dolphin, as well as the Legion's initials: LXF. Meshorer remarks that many of the coins of Samaria from the time of Domitian present an interesting features. They bear countermarks which had been added after the coins had been in circulation. These coins had already been taken out of circulation and the countermarks were meant to convert them into tokens for special purposes, such as use in legionary camps.[60]

At Jerusalem-Aelia Capitolina, coins from the reign of Hadrian (117–138 CE) also bear emblems associated with the X Legion, which had captured Jerusalem and was stationed there. The eagle and boar, which symbolize the military character of the Legion, predominate; but the war-galley in sail and the dolphin are also represented, symbolizing the Legion's naval activities in the field of transportation and in battle. A set of three coins from the reign of Antoninus Pius (138–161 CE) has been found, depicting three of the emblems of the X Legion, an eagle at the top of a standard, a boar, and a galley with a ramming prow and oars. As noted above, the Legion's veterans settled in the city and were among the first inhabitants of Aelia Capitolina.[61]

---

[60] Meshorer (1985): 44, no. 113.
[61] Meshorer (1985): 60, 62, 164–165.

At Rabath-Mōba a coin from the reign of Emperor Caracalla (211–217 CE) was found; it bears the classical image of Poseidon. Standing on deck, holding a dolphin and leaning on a trident, his name even appears in the inscription: 'of the people of Rabath-Mōba, Poseidon. A coin from Neapolis, dating to the reign of Trebonianus Gallus (251–253 CE) indicates that the Tenth Legion was stationed there at the time. It depicts Poseidon standing on the bow of a ship, leaning on a trident and with a dolphin in his right hand. Behind him to the right is Mount Gerizim, and opposite him is a wild boar beneath an eagle-topped standard—all emblems of the Tenth Legion.[62]

It is evident, therefore, that the Tenth Legion *Fretensis* is characterized by two types of symbols: animals such as a boar, an eagle, and a bull, and maritime symbols. The predominant nautical emblems are the galley, Neptune, and the dolphin.[63] Mommsen surmised that the Legion was named *Fretensis* ('of the sea straits'), only after it had excelled in the naval battle against Sextus Pompey in 36 BCE, which took place near Fretum Siculum—the straits between Italy and Sicily and was active during the battles at Mylae and Naulochus.[64] Barag supported this assumption when he stressed the great importance which the Legion attributed to naval emblem.[65] A combination of these maritime symbols is also present on the coins of Gadara: a galley with a ramming prow, a steering oar, and oarsmen. These signify the presence of the Legion X *Fretensis* in the area of Hammat-Gader, probably stationed on a regular basis. These symbols have been found on coins from the reign of Commodus, as evidenced by the Greek inscription and date 'of the people of Pompeian Gadara, year 243' [= 180 CE], and from the reign of Elagabal.[66] The details of the ships on the coins of the latter are remarkably clear: the ship is sailing to the left, it has a ram on the prow, and carries a flag; eight rowers are visible and a helmsman sits in the stern. Below the ship a pair of dolphins can be seen. One of the coins has a Greek inscription and is dated: 'of the people of Pompeian Gadara, year 283' [= 220 CE), and this is also true of coin of 281 [= 218 CE]—as shown above.

---

[62] For Rabbath-Moba, see Meshorer (1985): 102, no. 273; For Neapolis see idem, (1985): 50, no. 139; See also Dvorjetski, forthcoming [e].

[63] Ritterling (1899): 1071–1077; Cagnat (1963): 1084–1085; Parker (1958): 261–263; Barag (1967): 245–247.

[64] Mommsen (1883): 69.

[65] Barag (1964): 250.

[66] Meshorer (1985): 82, no. 223–224.

8.4.3   Evidences for the Presence of the Tenth Legion
Fretensis in the Area of Hammat-Gader

Further indications of the presence of the Tenth Legion *Fretensis* in the area of Hammat-Gader are listed below:

A. Seal impressions, countermarks, of the Legion X *Fretensis* appear not only on the coins of Gadara, but also on coins from Caesarea, Sebaste, and Ascalon. These seals testify to the presence of units from the Tenth Legion in these cities.[67] *Decima Fretensis* was stationed permanently in Jerusalem from the suppression of the First Jewish Revolt until the end of the third century CE—a period of more than 200 years. During this long period, the Legion's installations were built, repaired, and modified many times.[68]

B. When Emperor Hadrian visited Judaea in 130 CE, various cities in Palestine minted coins in his honour, among them Aelia Capitolina, Gaza, Ascalon, Caesarea, Gerasa, Petra, and Philadelphia, as well as Gadara. There is concrete evidence of the presence of the Legion in all of these cities during the reign of Hadrian and thereafter, and a connection can be presumed between the minting of the coins and the presence of the Tenth Legion.[69]

C. The Talmudic literature also associates Hadrian with a military presence in the Hammat-Gader area. *Midrash Tannaim to Deuteronomy* 26, 19 (Hoffman ed., p. 262), relates: that when Hadrian climbed the ascent to Hammat-Gader he found a Jewish girl at the upward slope of Hammat-Gader, and in *Midrash HaGadol to Deuteronomy* 26, 19 (Fish ed., p. 603): 'It was said, when Emperor Hadrian climbed

---

[67] Hill (1914): 113; Kindler (1958): 75–76; Heyman (1963): 49–50, Pl. 2–3; Barag (1967): 118–119; Rosenberger (1978): 81, 84; Mor (1986): 582, especially note 30; Applebaum (1983): 235, 392, note 55) comments that Gadara might have been within the area of control of the Legion VI *Ferata* from 127 CE, but provides no reasons or proof for this premise. Clues to the stationing of the Roman army at various locations in Palestine can be found in Josephus, *Bellum Judaicum* 7.216–218, 252; idem, *Vita* 76, 96, 420–422, and elsewhere.

[68] On the Roman military dispositions after the destruction of the Second Temple, see Stern (1982): 7–11; Herr (1982): 316–318; See also Vincent (1902): 428–433; Mazar (1972): 83–84; Sarfatti (1975): 151; Isaac (1980): 341.

[69] Lifshitz (1963): 784, no. 3; Barag (1964): 250; Negev (1972): 523; Olami and Ringel (1974): 44–46; Kindler (1974–1975): 61–67; Stahl (1986): 92; On Gerasa see Kraeling (1938): 390, no. 30; The topic here deals with an inscription dedicated to Hadrian from the soldiers of the X Legion in Gerasa; See also Steinspring (1939): 360–363.

the ascent to Hammat-Gader', he found a sick Jewish girl at the approach to Hammat-Gader. In *Midrash Lamentations Rabbah* (Buber ed., p. 82), according to the Romi manuscript, 'Hadrian placed three guards: one in Hammat-Gader, and one in Bethlehem and one in Kefar Lekitia'.[70]

D. An inscription found at Gadara includes a dedication to Hadrian from the Tenth Legion *Fretensis*. It can be dated, like the inscriptions at Caesarea, to Hadrian's visit to Palestine in 130 CE, or to the era of the Second Jewish Revolt. In the margin of the inscription there is a carving of Neptune with his trident, a dolphin in his hand, and his foot on a ship's prow. At the edge of the X Legion's inscription on the aqueduct at Caesarea there is also a dolphin.[71]

E. Poseidon-Neptune appears on a carved gem from Gadara, which is dated to the second century CE. He is standing on a dolphin and holds a ball in his right and trident in his left hand. The sea beneath the dolphin is indicated by diagonal lines.[72]

F. A tombstone inscription discovered at Byblos further corroborates our hypothesis on the connection between Gadara and the soldiers of the Legion X *Fretensis*.[73]

Among the engraved gems from the mother city Gadara mentioned above, there is one which possibly combines the two motifs that appear on the city's coins—the Three Graces, and the insignia of the Tenth Legion. On this gem the Three Graces are shown nude in their typical stance, except for one detail: they wear helmets, imparting a distinctly military atmosphere to the scene.[74]

---

[70] See the discussion in chapter 7.2 on *Hadrian at the Spas in the Eastern Mediterranean*; See also Rabinovitz (1976): 136; Oppenheimer (1982): 67.

[71] *CIL* III, no. 13589; For the year 130 CE see Clermont-Ganneau (1895): I: 171; For the opinion that it dates to the era of the Second Jewish Revolt, see Gera (1977): 42; On a similar monumental inscription, see Meshorer (1984): 41–45; See also Mor's description (1991): 111; Oppenheimer (1991: 41) claims that a Roman soldier's epitaph from Legion XIV *Gemina* which was found in Gadara (*CIL* III, no. 12091) gives no definite evidence about that soldier's death in the battles in the Galilee or in the Trans-Jordan during the Bar Kochba revolt.

[72] Henig and Whiting (1987): 10, no. 39.

[73] *CIL* III/2, no. 181; *ibid.*, III/1, Supp. no. 6697; See Renan (1864): 191; Clermont-Ganneau (1898): II: 299–301; cf. Jeremaias (1932): 78–79; Schürer (1991): II: 135; For the new interpretation of the Byblos inscription, see Dvorjetski and Last (1991): 157–162.

[74] Henig and Whiting (1987): 28, no. 272.

The τρεῖς χάριτες, the Three Graces—the emblem of the Gadara mint—also appear on the Roman provincial silver tetradrachms minted in the city during the reigns of Caracalla and Macrinus. They are shown within a garland, between the claws of an eagle. Many tetradrachms of Caracalla and a few of Macerinus, have been discovered in Palestine, mostly as hoards in buried jars.[75] According to Kadman and Kindler, the tetradrachms of Caracalla and Macerinus were minted for a specific and single purpose—namely the payment of soldiers' wages. These coins were not issued for general circulation in the country, and only in the course of time did they find their way to the hands of merchants and other civilians. They claim that at the time of the severe inflation, in the mid-third century CE, when all silver coins were removed from circulation, those who possessed coins preferred to conceal them in the ground and await more opportune times, rather than suffer the loss.[76] Therefore, the minting of such coins at Gadara indicates that the headquarters of these forces was located in the city. As we have shown, these soldiers belonged to the *Legio Decima*, whose members also engaged in building baths.[77] They built the baths of the τρεῖς χάριτες, the Three Graces in the suburb of Gadara, Hammat-Gader, for their own use and for the enjoyment of the inhabitants of the region.

Hirschfeld and Solar hold that a Semitic, non-Jewish population built the baths from local basalt. In their opinion, this population was influenced by the Roman culture, due to the fact that Gadara was one of the Decapolis.[78] In my opinion, this imposing architectural complex, the magnificent creation of a Roman town, must have been built by experts, namely soldiers of the Tenth Legion, although possibly the inhabitants of Gadara and Hammat-Gader might have assisted them.

---

[75] Bellinger (1940): 90–91; Gilmore (1984): 40–41; Meshorer (1979b): 222: idem, (1985): 83; Dvorjetski (1992a): 189–193; On other baths in the Roman period named after their gods, see, for example, Elmslie (1911): 48–49; See also Kadman and Kindler (1963): 46–47.

[76] Kadman and Kindler (1963): 46–47.

[77] On the widespread role of the Legion X *Fretensis* in building projects, including the erection of baths at Ramat Rahel, Motza, and Emmaus, see for example, Germer-Durand (1892): 382–384; Johns (1950): 152–153; Avi-Yonah (1950b): 19–21; Ciasca (1962): 69–72; Press (1954): III: 558–559; Tsafrir (1984): 106–107; On the road network which was constructed in Judaea in the days of Hadrian, see Isaac (1978): 47–60; Geva (1993): 759–760.

[78] Hirschfeld and Solar (1984): 39.

8.5   Kefar Agon, the Domain of Gadara and Its Affinity to
       Leisure and Amusement Culture

Kefar [= village] of Agon was situated on the southern shore of Lake
Kinneret, within the boundaries of the Hellenistic-Roman city Gadara
(Γαδάρα) in eastern Trans-Jordan, which was one of the cities of the
Decapolis. (See Map 3). Today Kefar Agon, Kefar Agin or Kefar
Gon, is identified with the Arab village of Umm Juni, on whose land
Kibbutz Degania *Aleph* was built. It is about a half km south-west of
Degania *Beit*, close to the spot where the Jordan emerges from Lake
Kinneret, on the east bank of the Jordan. The name Degania is a styl-
ized version of the ancient name, Umm Juniya.[79] The Arabic names
Umm Juniya and Umm Juni are derived from Guni, the name of one
of the sons of Gad: 'Ahi the son of Abdiel, the son of Guni, chief of
the house of their fathers. And they dwelt in Gilead, in Bashan, and
in her towns' (*I Chronicles* 5, 15). From verses 16–17 it appears that
the family of Guni was one of the families of the tribe of Gad which
settled in Bashan and Gilead in the time of Jeroboam II, and it may be
that its name is preserved in the place-name. It may also be surmised
that their territory extended to the southern tip of the Kinneret. One
of the families of the tribe of Naphtali was called Guni, or HaGuni
(*Genesis* 46, 24; *Numbers* 26, 48; *I Chronicles* 7, 13). Some scholars maintain, therefore, that the site was given to the children of Naphtali at
the time of Joshua. The meaning of the name Guni is obscure.[80] Noth
has suggested that it should be interpreted, as in Arabic, as the name
of a bird.[81] The earliest archaeological finds on the site—for instance,
remains of walls, basalt tools, and hundreds of potsherds—date from
the Early Bronze age, at the beginning of the third millennium BCE;
others are from the Byzantine and early Muslim periods. Kefar Agon
was of strategic importance, since in ancient times it was an important
crossing-point for traffic between the Hauran in the north and western
Trans-Jordan.[82]

---

[79] Avi-Yonah (1944–1945): 6; idem, (1976): 71; idem, (1984): 150–160; Klein (1932):
1124; Press (1946): I: 25; III: 475; Ne'eman (1971): II: 22–23; Vilnaey (1977): 1600–
1604, 3696; Dvorjetski (1988): 20–22; idem, (2002c): 65–75; idem, (2005): 439–467.
[80] Levinstam (1965): 458; Press (1946): I: 25; Klein (1967): 118, 146; Ne'eman (1971):
II: 22–23; Abel (1938): II: 64.
[81] Noth (1928): 230; See also Rothstein and Haenel (1927): 98.
[82] Saarisalo (1927): 22–26; Zimbalist-Zori (1943–1944): 122; Oded (1971): 192–195;
Dvorjetski and Segal (2001): 17–52.

8.5.1   *The Domain of Gadara and the New Testament Traditions*

According to Josephus, the territory of Gadara or Gader, extended as
far as the Jordan, since it bordered on Galilee: 'In the south Galilee
borders on Samaria and Scythopolis, as far as the River Jordan. In the
east it borders on the territory of Hippos ("Ιππος) [= Sussita], Gadara
(Γαδάρα) and the Golan (Γαυλανῖτις), and the boundaries of the
kingdom of Agrippa are also there' (*Bellum Judaicum* 3.3). In the south
Wadi at-Taiyibe separated the territories of Gadara and Pella (Πέλλα)
[= Paḥel], and the boundary ran north of Arbel (Ἄρβηλα) [= Irbid],
which was within the bounds of Paḥel. In the east the territory of
Gadara extended as far as el Khureibe, whence an aqueduct brought
water to the city. The territory of the city of Beit Rêsha was appar-
ently originally included in that of Gadara. In 96 CE the Emperor
Nerva founded a city called Capitolias (Καπιτωλιάς). It is unlikely that
he intended to cause any disturbance to the border with his allies, the
Nabataeans, whose kingdom had not yet been annexed to the Empire.
The road from Edrei (Αδράα) to Amman (Φιλαδέλφια) was not in the
territory of Gadara, for it was built only in the time of the Emperor
Trajan, after the annexation of the province of Arabia. In the north,
the border of Gadara ran along the Yarmuk (Hieromices). The whole
of the valley of Hammat-Gader, known by the Greek name Ἐμμαθᾶ
(el-Ḥamma), was within the city boundaries. The thermo-mineral
springs there were famous throughout the eastern Mediterranean and
the Roman Empire. In Hammat-Gader there have been found a theatre,
residential districts, a Roman tomb, basalt pews, a synagogue, ritual
buildings, a Byzantine church, and parts of an urban street system, as
well as what may have been the site of mock naval battles *Naumachiae*
(ναυμάχιαι).[83]

Gadara functioned as the capital city of a broad area, known to
its inhabitants as 'the land of the Gadarens' (ΓΑΔΑΡΕΩΝ). The city
mint was one of the biggest in the region, and its coins provide useful
information about the character of the city. It originally had the prestigious status of an autonomous city. Coins struck in the first century
BCE, until the time of Augustus, bear the head of Tyche, the goddess
of the city, and on the reverse side a cornucopia or caduceus, with

---

[83] This survey is based on Avi-Yonah (1936): 168; idem, (1984): 159–160; Smith
(1920): 597–606; Schürer (1991): II: 136; See also Sukenik (1935a); Hirschfeld (1987):
101–116; Dvorjetski (1988); idem, (1992a): 104–115; Hirschfeld (1997).

the inscription (ΓΑΔΑΡΕΩΝ)—'of the people of Gadara'. At a certain point in its history, after its reconstruction by Pompey in 63 BCE, it was called Gadara Pompeiana or 'of the people of Gadara Pompeiana' (ΠΟΜΠΗΙΕΩΝ ΓΑΔΑΡΕΩΝ). Of all the cities in the Levant reconstructed by Pompey, only Gadara was named after him.[84] (Fig. 34).

In the New Testament there is an account of Jesus' travels in the Decapolis. He performed a number of miracles in the biggest of its cities—Gadara, with curative springs in its outskirts (*Mark* 5, 20–21; *Luke* 8, 26–39; *Matthew* 8, 28–34). Here, as opposed to other places, he deemed it necessary to say to a man who had been healed: 'Go home to thy friends, and tell them how great things the Lord hath done for thee' (*Mark* 5, 19). *Mark* (5, 1) refers to 'the land of the Gerasenes' (εἰς τὴν χώραν τῶν Γερασηνῶν), and the manuscripts read 'the land of the Gadarenes' (Γαδαρηνῶν) and 'the Gergesenes' (Γεργεσηνῶν); in *Luke* 8, 26 and 37, we find 'the land of the Gerasenes' (εἰς τὴν χώραν τῶν Γερασηνῶν), and 'the land of the Gerasenes' (περί χωροῦ τῶν Γερασηνῶν), and in the manuscripts 'the land of the Gerasenes' (Γερασηνῶν), and 'the land of the Gergesenes' (Γεργεσηνῶν) and 'the Gerasenes' (Γερασηνῶν), while *Matthew* (8, 28) speaks of 'the land of the Gadarenes' (τὴν χωράν τῶν Γαδαρηνῶν), and the manuscripts have 'Gerasenes' (Γερασηνῶν) and 'Gergesenes' (Γεργεσηνῶν).[85] According to the story, Jesus wanted to get away from the crowd around him, and set out by sea from Kefar Nahum (Capernaum). When the boat was caught in a storm, his disciples panicked, and asked their master to help. Jesus rebuked them, calling them 'men of little faith'. He rebuked the storm, which calmed down, and the boat reached shore safely. At this point there began the 'miracle of the swine', which took place in the land of the 'Gergesenes' or the 'Gadarenes' (*Matthew* 8, 28–33). Jesus performed a miracle there, by casting out devils from human bodies. The devils entered into a herd of swine belonging to the local inhabitants, and the swine jumped from a steep place into Lake Kinneret, and 'perished in the waters'.

Gergesa (Γέργεσα) was in the territory of Sussita (Ἵππος), and is identified as Chorsia (Χορσία—Kursi). In the opinion of Origenes, the third century CE Church Father, Gergesa was 'an ancient city', and

---

[84] Meshorer (1985): 82–83; Dvorjetski (1993): 398–402; Avi-Yonah (1944–1945): 6; Klausner (1983): 143; idem, (1999): 98–99; Schlatter (1918): 90–110.
[85] Berry (1989); According to Lindsey (1969: 16–63), *Luke* is the ancient of all four Gospels; Freyne (1992): 83–84.

derived its name from the fact that the men who drove out Jesus after the miracle lived there, as stated in *Matthew* (8, 34).[86] It seems, therefore, that Origines had difficulty with the nomenclature. He claimed that the phrase 'the land of the Gadarenes' was not logical, since 'Gadara is a city in Judaea, with famous baths nearby, and there is no sea or lake in the vicinity'. He also rejected the name 'Gerasa', for similar reasons. Thus, the version which he possessed read 'the Gadarenes' and, in parallel, 'the Gergesenes'; since this version seemed illogical to him, he emended it according to his own judgment. Clear confirmation of this is found in the writings of scholars who assumed that the text was emended in the third century CE.[87] Eusebius, fourth century CE and author of the *Onomastikon*, also had difficulties with this matter. It is clear from his account that he had different variants before him. He puts forward Origenes' account, that the miracle of the swine took place close to the city of Gergesa, but adds that in his time the place was known as Gerasa.[88] From Hieronymus' Latin translation, dating from the fourth century CE, it is clear that he, too, had the same difficulty in identifying the location of the miracle.[89] Thus, as a result of Christian influence Kursi is called Gergesa or Gerasa in the pilgrims' literature and maps. Its inhabitants, however, called it Kursi, and this is mentioned in Christian and Arabic sources.[90]

It appears that the reason for the different versions is connected with the administrative status of the territories of Gadara and Sussita, which changed over the years. In the first half of the first century CE Kursi was transferred from the jurisdiction of Gadara to that of Sussita. Neither Origenes nor Hieronymus, following him, was familiar with 'Gerasa (Gargesa), in the land of the Gadarenes'. Nor were Cyril of Scythopolis, Saint Willibald, Autychius of Alexandria, al-Yāqūt and others; for in their day Kursi was not in the land of the Gadarenes. This was, perhaps, the reason why they amended the text, which seemed to them to be incorrect in light of the situation in their time. The monastery and church in Kursi, dated at the fifth century CE, match the topographical conditions described in the account of the miracle.

---

[86] Origens, *Commentary on John* 6, 41; Gergashtha was a village in the eastern Sea of Galilee, see *Midrash Song of Songs Zutta* 1, 4 (Buber ed., p. 11).
[87] Buttrick (1952): 156.
[88] Eusebius, *Onomastikon* (Klosterman ed., p. 74).
[89] Hieronymus, *Onomastikon* (Klosterman ed., p. 75); Riches de Levante (1874).
[90] Abel (1927): 113; Nun (1987a): 183–187.

When they were excavated, the site was recognized as the place where Jesus performed the miracle.[91]

In the light of the references to 'the land of the Gadarenes' in the gospels, commentators have tried to 'extend' the territory of Gadara as far as Lake Kinneret, in the vicinity of Tzemach, using as evidence the coins of Gadara which depict a mock sea battle (ναυμαχία). Avi-Yonah has expounded the reasons for rejecting this thesis. First of all, the parallel version of the gospel (*Matthew* 5, 21) and several manuscripts of *Mark* and *Luke* read 'Gergesa', and not 'Gadara'. Secondly, Origen's interpretation of *John* 1, 28, rests on the fact that Gadara has no coastline; he would not have written as he did had the town's limits reached Lake Kinneret; thirdly, *naumachiae* were conducted in the hippodromes of inland towns; and, fourthly, even if we suppose that Gadara possessed part of the coast of the Kinneret between Tzemach and the Jordan, there are there no steep places like those so prominent in the gospel stories.[92]

Gadara was the capital of Gilead in the time of the Seleucids. There have been found on the site two theatres, a fortified acropolis, cultic sites, statues, a basilica, paved streets, baths, remains of residential buildings, graves and coffins, mosaic floors, and remains of the Jewish inhabitants—reliefs of candelabra on marble slabs and three basalt lintels. Gadara's ancient name is preserved in Wadi Jadar, close by. Today it is the Arab village of Umm Qais in Jordan, 364 metres above sea level and looking down on a beautiful view of Lake Kinneret, the Jordan Valley, Galilee and Mount Hermon.[93]

In Avi-Yonah's view, the territory of Gadara did not reach Lake Kinneret, but it did include Kefar Agon, situated on the Jordan. In Talmudic times there was a clear administrative division between the Valley—the territory of Tiberias—and Upper Galilee. Thus, the borders of the territory of Naphtali were the borders of the administrative area of Tiberias, while the territory of Asher was the administrative area of Upper Galilee. Safrai emphasizes this fact, and adds that a narrow

---

[91] Tzaferis (1993): 893–896; idem, (1983): 1–51; Nun (1987a): 183–187; Dalman (1967): 190.

[92] Avi-Yonah (1944–1945): 6.

[93] Schumacher (1890): 46–80; Steuernagel (1927): 497–498; On the main recent publications of the last decade on the archaeological remains of Gadara, see Weber (1989); idem, (1991): 223–235; Wagner-Lux, Vriezen et al.: (1993): 64–72; Nielsen, Andersen and Holm-Nielsen (1993); Weber (1995); idem, (2002).

strip of the coast south of Kinneret was attached to the territory of Tiberias, even though the area south of the Kinneret belonged to the Hellenistic city of Gadara. Hence, he believes that the administration's planners were faithful to the principle that an administrative district had to be congruent with an economic unit, and there should never come about a situation in which a worker from one district makes use of land in another.[94]

8.5.2   *Kefar Agon in Rabbinic Literature*

The name of the settlement of Kefar Agon is mentioned in Rabbinic literature in a variety of linguistic forms, as a result of corruption of the name. Sometimes it appears as Kefar Agin, instead of Kefar Agon, apparently as the result of a copyist's error:

> Rabbi Hanina bar Pappa went to visit [= on the Shabbat] Rabbi Tanhum bar Hiyya of Kefar Agin, who was in mourning, and the latter came out to meet him wearing his *santerin* [= best clothes].
>
> (*Genesis Rabbah* 100, 7, Theodor-Albek ed., p. 1292)

The name of the place appears in connection with Rabbi Tanhum's son, Rabbi Yose:

> Rabbi Yose ben Rabbi Tanhum of Kefar Agin was in Asia,[95] and a certain man wanted to go sailing between Feast of Tabernacles and Hanukkah. A matron saw him, and said to him, 'Is this the time for sailing?' His father appeared to him in a dream, and said 'And he also did not even have a funeral'. Nonetheless he did not listen either to this one or to that one, but he went to sea, and died there.
>
> (*Jerusalem Talmud, Shabbat* 2, 3 [5b])

Kefar Agin is also the version which appears in *Sefer Yafeh Mar'eh*—a collection of legends from the *Jerusalem Talmud*.[96] In *Midrash Ecclesiastes*

---

[94] Safrai (1980): 191–192.

[95] On Asia, see Ne'eman (1971): I: 112; Rapoport (1857): 154–155; Hirschberg (1920): 225; Klein (1924): 116–127; Tokatzinski (1970): 28–39; Reland (1714): 776; Neubauer (1868): 38; Dvorjetski (1992a): 78–81; See also the discussion in chapter 4.7 on *The Waters of Asia*.

[96] Askenasi (1590): 97a; On Kefar Agin, see Levy (1963): 388; Romanoff (1937): 20; Neubauer (1868): 260; Kohut (1926): I: 24; Klein (1939): 90; On the Talmudic reality in the sailing period between the *Sukkot* [= Tabernacles Feast] taking place in September and *Hanukkah* [= Festival of Lights] (occurs in December) compared to the Roman Vegetius of the fourth-fifth century CE, see Sperber (1986): 100.

Rabbah (3, 2) this story is repeated, but the name is given there as Kefar
Agon, and the name of the Sage as Rabbi Joshua. In *Midrash Genesis
Rabbah* 6, 5, (Theodor-Albeck ed., p. 45), the content of the story is
identical, the name of the Sage is Joshua, and the name of the place
is Kefar Hagin. Apparently the corruption in the place-name was the
result of the substitution of the letter *ḥet* for *aleph*.[97] The story is also
told in a fragment of the *Jerusalem Talmud* in the Geniza, *Shabbat* 2, 3
[5b], but the name of the place does not appear in the text.[98] Kefar
Egoz, another version of the name, appears in connection with Rabbi
Joshua, but this time without mentioning that Rabbi Tanhum bar Hiyya
was his father; the story is told in the name of Rabbi Tanhum bar
Hiyya alone. To sum up the above: Rabbi Yose or Rabbi Joshua, the
son of Rabbi Tanhum bar Hiyya, did not take the advice either of a
certain matron or of his own father, who appeared to him in a dream
and warned him not to go to sea, since if he were to go to the sea he
would drown and not be buried. He went to sea in the wintertime,
and was drowned.

The place name Kefar Agon sometimes appears in the Rabbinic
sources with the *aleph* syncopated, as Kefar Gon. In the *Jerusalem Talmud*,
Baba Bathra 5, 1 [16a]), the chapter 'He who sold the boat' says:

> Rabbi Tanhum of Kefar Gon in the name of Rabbi Eleazar ben Rabbi
> Yose: 'They are four gather grasses anywhere, on condition that one does
> not pull up the grass by the roots. And people may relieve themselves on
> the other side of a wall [= anywhere]'. Rabbi Eleazar ben Rabbi Yose
> in the name of Rabbi Tanhum: 'That applies to a place in which one
> may sneeze without being heard. And they may pasture a flock in forest,
> even a flock belonging to the tribe of Judah in the territory of the tribe
> of Naphtali. And they assign to Naphtali a complete strip of land south
> of the lake, as it is said, *"O Naphtali, satisfied with favor and full of the blessing
> of the Lord, possess the lake and the South"* (*Deuteronomy* 33, 23), the words of
> Rabbi Yose the Galilean'. Rabbi Akiva says, 'The reference to the sea
> here is to the sea of Samkho, and the reference to the south refers to
> the sea of Tiberias'.

In a fragment of the *Jerusalem Talmud* from the Genizah (MS Antonin
of Petersburg, Tractate *Avoda Zarah* 5, 4 [45a]) the name Kefar Gon

---

[97] On the substitution of the letter *ḥet* for *aleph*, see Klein (1924): 42–43; Alternatives
formulas for Kefar Hagin in *Genessis Rabbah* 6, 5 (Theodor-Albek ed., p. 45) are as follows: 'Agin' in Romi and London manuscripts; 'Anon—Paris manuscript; and 'Egoz'
according to Oxford manuscript.

[98] Ginzberg (1909): 74.

is preserved.[99] Despite the corruptions and the many versions of the name Kefar Agon, in most of the texts it is connected with sources of water, and it is quite possible that the context is Lake Kinneret.

In the *Babylonian Talmud*, Rabbi Tanhum, son of Rabbi Hiyya, a Palestinian *Amora* of the third century CE, is usually called 'a man of Acre' (*Berakhot* 63b; *Ta'anit* 7b; *Mo'ed Qatan* 16b; *Yevamot* 45a; *Bekhorot* 57b). Romanoff, author of *The Onomastikon of Palestine*, maintained that the names Kefar Acre, Kefar Achus, Kefar Ichus and Kefar Achis were interchangeable in Rabbinic literature, and that they could be corrupted to Kefar Agon or Kefar Agin.[100] Margulis adds that the place names Kefar Agin and Kefar Agon were unknown in Babylonia, and were therefore altered to the more familiar Kefar Acre.[101]

8.5.3 *The Origin, Meaning and Development of the Term Agon*

The literal meaning of the word *agon* (ἀγών) in Greek is 'contest, competition, war, battle', and it has a similar significance in Syriac. The *agonos* (ὁ ἀγῶνος) became a standard term, parallel to *arena*, or *stadium*, for the place in which competitions and games—in particular, the Greek festivals at which the Olympic games (ἀγὼν Ολυμπικὸς, ἀγὼν Ολυμπίας), took place—were held.[102]

The sporting spirit and the aspiration to compete for excellence and superiority are expressed in classical Greek literature, beginning with the Iliad and the Odyssey. Expressions such as νεῶν ἐν ἀγῶνι; λῦτο δὲ ἀγών; ἵζανεν εὐπὺν ἀγών and in the plural κατ' ἀγῶνας, frequently appear in these works, signifying both a gathering or competition between men to play and strive for excellence and a place where competitive sports took place.[103] After the end of the heroic period, the *agon* became the concern of the masses. At first it was confined to one region, only the inhabitants of that region participated in it, and it took place close to the temple of the god in whose honour it was conducted. The number

---

[99] Epstein (1932): 246; Liberman (1931): 88, note 24; Romanoff (1937), s.v. 'Kefar Gon'; 'Kefar Agon'; 'Kefar Agin'; For some more variants of the name Kefar Agon, see Dvorjetski (2005): 445–448.

[100] For the variants of the place Kefar Acus, see Romanoff (1937): 192–197, 203; Hildesheimer (1886): 12; On Rabbi Tanhum of Kefar Agon, see Hyman (1964): II: 737; Palmoni (1969): 46–50.

[101] Margalioth (1976): II: 833–834.

[102] Liddell, Scott and Jones (1940): 18–19; Payne-Smith (1957): 3; Brockelman (1893): 18; See also Gardiner (1967), s.v. 'Agon', especially pp. 222–229.

[103] Homer, *Iliad* 23.258; 24.1; 15.428; Homer, *Odyssey* 8.259.

of participants in the *agon* gradually increased, and it encompassed people outside the vicinity of the temple. The Amphiktyons, associations of a number of tribes which settled round a particular shrine, led to the broadening of the bounds of the *agon*, and an increase in the number of participants. For various reasons certain shrines became famous throughout Hellas, and the *agones* which were celebrated in honour of their gods—the pan-Hellenic games—became important to the whole of Greece. Examples of such Pan-Hellenic *agones* are the Olympic Games, in honour of Zeus, at Olympia in Elis; the Pythian Games, in honour of the Delphic Apollo; the Isthmian Games, in honour of Poseidon, in Isthmus near Corinth; and the Nemean Games, in honour of Zeus, at Cleonae near Argos. The Greeks generally distinguished between three types of *agon*: gymnic, hippic and musical. The Gymnic Games were so called because the competitors appeared naked (in Greek, *gymnos* = naked), and were based on various athletic exercises. The hippic games consisted primarily of horses or chariot-races. The musical games were based on poetry, dance, and theatrical performances. Only males of Greek nationality participated in the games, apart from barbarian women and slaves. The victors in the Pan-Hellenic *agones*, particularly the Olympic Games, achieved fame throughout Greece. In their home cities statues of them were erected, and their names engraved on monumental inscriptions. The prize for victory in the Pan-Hellenic games was modest in worth, but most honorific: a garland of olive or laurel leaves. In the less prestigious games which took place from time to time valuable prizes were also given.[104]

In the fifth century BCE the historian Herodotus mentioned the competitions in Olympia, ὁ ἐν Ὀλυμπίῃ ἀγών, competions for prizes in athletic games (ἀγών γυμνικός), horse-races (ἀγών Ἱππικός), and musical contests (ἀγών μουσικός). In Herodotus, as in other writers, poets and historians, *agones* (ἀγῶνες) is a metaphorical expression for struggles between various nations and their enemies; for instance, πολλοὺς ἀγὼν δπαμένται οἱ Ἕλληνες—'the Greeks waged many battles for their existence'.[105]

The custom of conducting *agones* spread all over the Hellenistic world. In the Hellenistic and the Roman periods *agones* were organized

---

[104] Krause (1841); Neutsch (1949); Olivová (1984): 77–153.
[105] Herodotus, *Historiae* 2.91; 6.127; 7.11; 8.102; 9.60.

by professional artists, and slaves or freedmen participated in them. In
the New Testament, the Apocrypha, the works of Josephus and Philo
and early Christian writings the term *agon* appears in the sense both
of an athletic contest and of a battle, or, in general, of a struggle.[106]
Here are a few examples of this expression and the contexts in which
it appeared: 'Let us run with patience the race that is set before us'
(*Hebrews* 12, 1); 'We were bold in our God to speak unto you the gospel
of God with much contention' (I *Thessalonians* 2, 2); 'Throughout all
time it marches, crowned in triumph, victor in the contest for prizes
that are undefiled' (*Wisdom of Solomon* 4, 2); 'He [= Herod the Great]
instituted games which were held every five years, and called them, too,
by the name of the emperor, and gave valuable prizes' (*Bellum Judaicum*
1.415); 'Herod gave a donation in common not only to all Greece, but
to all the habitable earth, as far as the glory of the Olympic Games
reached. For when he perceived that they were come to nothing, for
want of money, and that the only remains of ancient Greece were in
a manner gone, he not only accepted the presidency of a session of
the four-year games at which he happened to be present in the course
of his journey to Rome, but settled funds upon them in perpetuity to
ensure that the games should continue' (*ibid.*, 1.426–427); 'The battle
continues for seven days' (*ibid.*, 2.424); 'In the light of future battles'
(*ibid.*, 4.88); 'Therefore he trained his soldiers for the battle like athletes'
(*ibid.*, 4.91); 'One may properly be amazed at the generosity of Vespasian
and Titus who acted with moderation after the wars and great struggles
which they had with us' (*Antiquitates Judaicae*, 12.128); 'To honour him
with a garland of gold, the usual reward according to the law, and to
erect his statue in brass in the temple of Demos and of the Graces;
and that this present of a garland shall be proclaimed publicly in the
theater, in the Dionysian shows and in the gymnaic shows also' (*ibid.*,
14.153); 'Immediately after the dedication [= of Caesarea] there was a
great festival, with most lavish arrangements. For he had announced a
contest in music and athletic exercises, and had prepared a great number
of gladiators and wild beasts and also horse races and the very lavish
shows that are to be seen at Rome and in various other places. And
this contest too he dedicated to Caesar' (*ibid.*, 16.137–138); 'He gave

---

[106] Arndt and Gingrich (1967): 14; Rami (1973): II: 398; Berry (1989), s.v. 'αγων';
Schalit (1968): 16; Harris (1972): 31–125; On the Hellenistic entertainment culture
and its influence upon Jews, See Smith (1956): 67–81; Bergman (1937): 146–151; Herr
(1977–1978): 22–23; idem, (1989): 89–92; Levine (2000): 108–110.

the festival greater dignity in respect of sacrifices and other ceremonies. For his munificence in this matter he had his name recorded by the people of Elis as perpetual president of the games' (*ibid.*, 16.149); 'My friend, never enter any competition for evil, and do not strive for first prize' (Philo, *On Agriculture*, 111); 'Like runners in a competition who leap forward from the starting gate' (idem, *Life of Moses* 2.71); 'This is what runners imitate in their biennial festivals, which take place in every nation in public stadiums, and they present it as a brilliant and most honorable achievement' (idem, *On the Unchangeingness of God* 36); 'They are victorious not thanks to the strength of the victors but because their opponents are weak in this sort of competition' (idem, *That the Worse is Wont to Attack the Better* 35); 'After he had trained his people, Moses called on them to show the results of his training. They presented themselves like competitors in the sacred games, and demonstrated their absolute readiness for the struggle as clear proof of their true character. Then it was proven that true moral athletes did not disappoint the hopes which their trainers—the *mitzvot*—had placed in them' (idem, *On Reward and Punishment*, 4); 'For they become famous by throwing punches in the air in the absence of any opponent; but when they take part in a real contest they will fail miserably' (idem, *That the Worse is Wont to Attack the Better* 41); 'The athlete who participates in a boxing match or a *pankratium* and strives to win the crown of victory fends off with one hand or the other the blows that are meant for him' (idem, *On the Cherubim* 81); 'Let the man who enjoys vigour of body be the prop of those who are weaker, and let him not, like the men at the *pankratium* in the gymnastic contests, use violence to overthrow those who are inferior in strength. (idem, *On the Special Laws* 4.74); 'Which man who takes part in the games of life has never been thrown? Which man has never failed? (idem, *On Dreams* 2.145).

In Latin, too, the word *agon* means competitions in public games. In ancient Rome, as in Greece, these were in the fields of athletics, music, poetry and drama.[107] The most famous *agones* in the period of the Roman Empire was the Agon Neronianus, founded by the Emperor Nero in 60 CE as part of the Olympic Games, and intended to be held every five years. It included chariot racing, athletic contests, and musical contests for voice and instrument. Another *agon*, founded in 86

---

[107] Lewis and Short (1879): 77; Harvey (1986): 13.

CE, in the reign of the Emperor Domitian, was also an imitation of the Olympic Games. It was held every four years, and included athletic and musical competitions. Another great *agon* took place in 248 CE, in honour of the millennium of the foundation of the city of Rome.[108]

Both Greeks and Romans attributed great importance to competitive games, and viewed the *agones as* preparation and training for war. They also served as an unfailing source of entertainment and dissipation for the masses throughout the empire. The Graeco-Roman concepts of sport reached Palestine, and the Sages approved of them, as long as there was no suspicion that one of the three major prohibitions—idolatry, bloodshed and incest—might be infringed. Because of the customs of the non-Jews and the immoral nature of the games the rabbis forbade participation in them on religious or moral grounds; but the way in which the *Amoraim* related to Roman leisure culture and amusements differed from that of their predecessors, the *Tannaim*. The *Tannaim* set their faces unambiguously against Roman recreational institutions and strictly forbade any contact with them, using the words 'forbidden', 'no', 'never'; the *Amoraim*, however, did not condemn or explicitly forbid them, but argued their case, emphasizing the differences between the people of Israel and the society around them in order to persuade them not to take part in such entertainments. The more moderate attitude of the *Amoraim* is an expression of the social and cultural situation in their time. They understood that they had to speak in a more moderate tone than that of their predecessors; otherwise they would simply be ignored, since Jews visited places of entertainment both as spectators and as participants.[109] Nonetheless, the Sages' prohibitions did not only stem from the dissolute nature of the games. They also feared that a Jew who visited these centres of entertainment would forget his religion as a result of seeing the varied performances.[110] Moreover, it appears that the Sages permitted sports which were somewhat different from those of the non-Jews, among them running, swimming, wrestling, the hunting of animals and birds and more. This is pointed up in the use

---

[108] Guhl and Koner (1994): 547, 554: Seyffert (1891): 18; Ringwood-Arnold (1960): 245–251; On the survey of games in the Graeco-Roman world, see Toner (1995); Swaddling (1999); Beacham (1999): 214–219; Wiedermann (2001).

[109] Krauss (1948): 119–120; idem, (1911): I: 209–210; III: 113–114; Lieberman (1963): 70–73; On the principal viewpoint of the Sages toward leisure culture and its historical development, see Weiss (2001): 427–450; idem, (1995): 2–19; Dvorjetski and Segal (1998): 83–94; Herr (1994): 105–119; Dvorjetski (1994): 51–68.

[110] Jacobs (1998b): 327–347.

of certain intriguing expressions, such as 'who changed the custom', or 'because he is different'. It can be illustrated by considering the way in which Jews engaged in running. The *Tosefta* (*Shabbat* 16, 22) says: 'One should not run on the Shabbat for exercise'. Abba Saul, writing after Bar Kochba revolt, concluded that Jews ran for exercise on the Shabbat, and this had to be forbidden. At the very least, it can be said that they ran regularly on week-days 'for exercise'. The *Mishnah* (*Baba Qamma* 3, 6) says: 'Two people went in public, one walking, and the other running. If both were running, and harmed each other, both are exempt'. It follows that both were permitted to run in public. The *Jerusalem Talmud* (*ibid.*, 3, 3 [4d]) expands the *Mishnaic* saying: 'Yose HaBavli says that a man who ran in public and did harm was liable, since he violated the custom'. The meaning of this may be that a man is entitled to run freely in private. The *Babylonian Talmud* (*ibid.*, 52a) relates to the *Mishnaic* saying quoted above: 'A runner is liable because he is exceptional'. 'Runner' here is emphatically a noun: not 'a running man', but a man who devotes some of his time to running as part of his leisure culture. This 'runner' is 'exceptional' because he has changed the accepted custom: apparently this was to run and take exercise in special agonistic facilities, as in many other branches of sport.[111]

Various branches of sport existed in Palestine because of the intense activity of Herod the Great (*Antiquitates Judaicae* 15.267–276).[112] The festivals he instituted included, among other activities, musical competitions, gymnastic exercises, gladiatorial contests, hunting, and horse-races. In addition to the historical sources and the evidences from Rabbinic literature, over the past few decades various sites dedicated to entertainment and sport dating from the periods of the Second Temple, the Mishnah and the Talmud have been uncovered: in Jerusalem (*ibid.*, 15.268–271; *ibid.*, 339–341; *Bellum Judaicum* 1.415);[113] in Caesarea (*Antiquitates Judaicae* 16. 341; *Bellum Judaicum* 1.415; *ibid.*, 2.172); in Maioumas-Shuni; Tiberias (*Bellum Judaicum* 2.618; *ibid.*, 3.539–540; *Vita* 17.64; *Jerusalem Talmud, Eruvin* 5, 1 [22b]); Taricheiai (*Bellum Judaicum*

---

[111] On the Jews occupation in running, see Shorek (1977): 42–43; On aquatics and swimming installations, see idem, (1977): 61–70; Pintsover (1945): 279–281; Muntner (1983): 11–16.

[112] Lichtenberger (1999): 74–79; Roller (1998): 91–94, 116–118; Lämmer (1971): 10–14.

[113] Lämmer (1972): 51–70; Ballou (1970): 70–81; Shorek (1981): 8–10; On the findings from Jerusalem and the various possibilities of their location within the city, see Schick (1898): 224–229; Vincent and Abel (1914): II: 14, 34; Kloner (2001): 75–86; Reich and Biling (2000): 37–42; Patrich (2002): 173–188.

2.598); in Jericho (*ibid.*, 1.659; *Antiquitates Judaicae* 17.193); in Sepphoris; in Beth Shean-Nysa-Scythopolis; in Samaria-Sebastia; in Shechem-Neaopolis; in Ascalon; in Gaza; in Beth Guverin-Eleutheropolis; and in other places.[114] To these sites must be added places of popular entertainment, baths and therapeutic baths where, in addition to bathing or receiving medical treatment at the allotted times, people spent many hours watching various performances and enjoying other types of diversion. It is known that these places were often centres of crime and prostitution.[115]

8.5.4   *Competitions, Games and Competitors in Talmudic Sources*

Greek and Latin names of competitions, games and competitors are preserved in Talmudic sources. Here are some examples among many: *agon* (ἀγών)—a contest; *athlet* (ἀθλητής)—an expert at wrestling; *luder* (ludarius)—a gladiator, who performs in the theatre, takes part in a chariot race or wrestles in the arena; *monomachos* (μονομάχος), a hero, a fighter; *dromeos* (δρομεύς)—a swift runner; *dromos* (δρόμος)—the running track; *eniochos* (ἡνιοχός)—charioteers; arena or *ris*—the place where

---

[114] For the entertainment and sport facilities that have been uncovered, see the following. On Caesarea: Frova (1965): 167–174; Porat (1995): 15–17; Segal (1995): 64–69; Humphry (1996): 121–129; Patrich (2001): 269–283; On Maioumas-Shuni, see Conder and Kitchener (1881–1883): II: 66–67; Shenhav (1997): 56–70; Segal (1995): 65–66; Dvorjetski, forthcoming [c]; For the stadium of Tiberias, see Schwabe (1949): 238–241; Harris (1973): 52; Lämmer (1976): 37–76; Smallwood (1981): 183–184; On the theatre there, see Hirschfeld (1991c): 19–20; For amusement and sport installations in Jericho, see Netzer (1980): 104–107; idem, (1995): 135–141; idem, (2001): I: 56–59; Segal (1995): 87–89; On Sepphoris, see Waterman (1931): 29; Weiss and Netzer (1997): 3–8; Segal (1995): 41–43; On Beth Shean-Nysa-Scythopolis, see Fuks (1983):123–141; Bar-Nathan and Mazor (1994): 117–137; Foerster and Tsafrir (1992): 117–139; Segal (1995): 41–43; On Samaria-Sebaste, see Crowfoot, Kenyon and Sukenik (1942): 57–62; Zayadine (1966): 576–580; Segal (1995): 77–78; For Shechem-Neaopolis-Nablus, see Magen (1987): 269–277; Segal (1995): 78–80; On Ascalon, see the evidence of Theophanes [τέατρον καὶ ᾠδεῖον] in Schwabe (1957): 181–185; For the baths in Ascalon, see Josephus, *Bellum Judaicum* 1.423; These entertainment installations have not been uncovered; As a very popular place for recreation and pleasure in Ascalon, see Dvorjetski (2001a): 99–118; Gaza's leisure buildings have not been found yet, but in the Madaba Map—dated to the second half of the sixth century CE—it is seen obviously. See for this: Avi-Yonah (1953): 74; Piccirillo and Alliata (1999): 92; On Beth Guverin-Eleutheropolis, see Kloner (1989): 279–295; Kloner and Hubsch (1996): 85–106; For general survey of baths and spas, see Harris (1967), map no. 4; Lifshitz (1977): 509–510; Gichon (1978): 35–39; Tsafrir (1984): 115–127; Schürer (1991): II: 44–48; Dvorjetski (1992a); Dan (1984): 200–221.

[115] On these central places for sin and prostitution, see Kiefer (1994): 155–177; Dunbabin (1989): 6–46; Toner (1995): 101–116; Dvorjetski (1999a): 117–129; Dalby (2000), s.v. 'prostitutes'.

the contest or performance took place; *astadion* or *itztadion* (στάδιον, stadium)—the place where the games were conducted.[116]

The word *agon* (ἀγὼν), in its meaning in classical Greek and Latin literature, was absorbed into Talmudic literature.[117] The *Haggadat Yelamdenu*, chapter *Emor*, discussing the Bible portion *ulekachtem b'yom rishon* says 'there was a struggle (*agon*) in the state', but does not say what the state was like, or what its geographical position was.[118] *Agonia* (ἀγωνία), which means in Greek a battle, struggle, or contest, appears in the *Tanhuma* (*Mishpatim* 5) in a conversation between Aqiles the proselyte and the Emperor Hadrian: 'You gave the general an *aguna*,[119] unless he took up his weapon himself'. *Genesis Rabbah* (56, 11) says: 'Like one who jumped with [*shiver*] his *agin* into a stormy river, and made his son jump in with him'. An emended Romi manuscript (*ibid.*, Theodor-Albeck ed., pp. 608–609) reads 'after he had jumped into the pond (*agum*) and made his son jump with him'. Similarly, a fragment from the Geniza, overlooked by Theodor and Albeck, reads 'after he had jumped into the pond and made his son jump with him'.[120] Commentators have been hard put to explain the word *agino* in the text, and have suggested that is derived from *gina* (garden), or the Syriac word *agan* (basin), or from *ogen* (rim).[121] Lieberman has suggested that this may be an example of an ancient game: one person leapt, or jumped in contest (*agon*) at the place where competitive games (*agon*) took place, and showed his bravery by making his son jump also. He conjectures that they may have called a barrier through which one had to jump *agum* or *agun* (*nun* and *mem* interchanged, as often happens): *totum pro parte*, the whole for the part.[122] The conclusion is that these texts deal with aquatic sports—a dive into the *agon*, the place where the games and competitions took place.

In *Midrash Tanhuma* (*Emor* 18), the *agin* is mentioned in connection with a victory in court: 'The king judged them, but the people did not

---

[116] Krauss (1911): I: 219; *Ris* means stadium or hippodrome (*Midrash Song of Songs Rabbah* 1, 3), or an ancient unit of length, parallel to Greek 'stadium', 266 *Amot*, which are around 150 metres (*Mishnah, Baba Kamma* 7, 7).

[117] Arndt and Gingrich (1967): 14; Levy (1963): 28; Krauss (1911): II: 8.

[118] Krauss (1911): I: 209 Jastrow (1950): 11; Kohut (1926): I: 23.

[119] Ἀγωνια means a combat, a competition; See Levy (1963): 20; Kohut (1926): I: 24.

[120] Lieberman (1939a): 54.

[121] See various explanations in *Genesis Rabbah* 56, 11 (Theodor-Albeck ed., p. 609); Kohut (1926): I: 24 notes that the word Agin derives from the Syriac *agan*, which means garden.

[122] Lieberman (1939a): 54; See also idem, (1939b): 28.

know who prevailed over his friend. The king said that it should be known that whoever went out with an *agin* in his hand was the winner. Similarly, Israel and the nations of the world are judged on *Yom Kippur*, and the nations do not know who prevailed. The Lord said "take palm fronds in your hands, so that all shall know that you prevailed in judgment"'. *Psikta Rabbati, Ulekachtem lachem* 27, reads *denesev b'agin* (who dealt with an *agin*), and the *Psikta de Rav Kahana* 27 (Mandelbaum ed., p. 406) *denesev b'yayin* (who dealt with wine). The Oxford and Safed manuscripts, however, keep the word *agin*. In *Midrash Leviticus Rabbah* 30, 2 (Margulis ed., p. 694) it is said that 'this is a palm frond, likened to one who is victorious and disqualified'. *Midrash Psalms* 17, 5 (Buber ed., p. 128) corrects the corruptions of the other versions: 'Like somebody who is victorious and becomes as naught. In the way of the world two charioteers run in a horse-race. Who takes the *b'ayin*? The winner'. *Yalkut Shim'oni, Psalms* 670, explains: 'What is the meaning of "conquer by thy right hand"? Rabbi Abbahu said: 'This is the palm-frond, which is like somebody who is victorious and takes it in his right hand. [*b'ayin*] In the way of the world, two charioteers take part in a horse-race. Who takes the palm-frond in his right hand? The winner'.[123] It may be pointed out that the Greek word *baion* (βάϊον) means a date-branch, or a rod woven from palm-branches, which was a symbol of victory for heroes in battle or victors in a competition.[124]

8.5.5   *Kefar Agon: 'Village of Competitions and Games'*

In the Graeco-Roman world the word *agon*, which as has been pointed out, means competition or confrontation, came to mean 'competitive games'. From the place-name Kefar Agon, 'the village of competition', or 'the village of competitive games', we can learn much about everyday life in this village in general, and in the domain of the city of Gadara in particular.[125] Agon's proximity to the theatre and the

---

[123] Krauss (1948): 220; Wiedermann (2001): 101, Fig. 17; Köhne and Ewigleben (2000): 93.

[124] See the explanation in *Midrash Leviticus Rabbah* 30, 2 (Margilies ed., p. 694, note 5), and *Midrash Psalms* 17, 5 (Buber ed., p. 128)—referring to the charioteers; See also Sperber (1982): 22–26.

[125] Here we have a Semitic-Hebrew and Greek tradition to the same place; Other sites with such toponimic traditions are, for instance, Acre [= Ἀκή], which means healing; and Raphia [= Ῥαφή] is a seam; The implication of their names is shown on their coins. See Kasher (1988a): 35; Meshorer (1985): 14, 32; Dvorjetski, forthcoming [e].

therapeutic baths of Hammat-Gader, and its position on the southern shore of Lake Kinneret, may give some indication of the particular sports which took place there. In 1967 Harris, the great scholar of Greek sport, pointed out in his book *Greek Athletes and Athletics* that this is one of the sites in Palestine where sporting facilities have been found;[126] and in 1977 Shorek repeated this claim.[127] Neither of them, however, proved or illustrated this contention with the aid of historical sources, or with the archaeological evidence which has been published since their works appeared.

A collection of precious stones and cameos from Gadara, published in 1987, gives an indication of the sporting activity which character-ized the city. Together with the many gods depicted in them there are horses, riders, chariots, athletes, an arena, and a warship with its rowers. These are dated between the first and third century CE.[128] As we have presented above, in the coins of Gadara the great number of nautical symbols stands out. On many of them there appear, among other such figures, Roman ships, a battering-ram, rowers holding long oars, and a helmsman holding a tiller, with a flag behind him.

In Dalman's view in 1914, that at the time of the celebration there took place both ναυμαχία and fair (πανήγυρις) in honour of the therapeutic baths of Hammat-Gader, mentioned by the fourth-cen-tury CE Church Father Epiphanius.[129] Epiphanius' remarks about the annual fair at this spot, and its various elements, are reminiscent of the sermon attributed to Rabbi Meir in *Ecclesiastes Rabbah* (5, 10): 'the masses bring things to sell and to buy'. From the days of Rabbi Meir, in the middle of the second century CE, onwards, Hammat-Gader is pictured as an animated place, with inns, shops and dwelling-places. It served as a model for inter-religious meetings in the Levant in the Roman and Byzantine periods.[130] It is important to note that, in addi-tion to its commercial and ritual functions, the fair was also an occa-sion of entertainment. Sozomenus, the Christian historian of the fifth century CE, states in his *Historia Ecclesiastica* that until the time of the

---

[126] Harris (1967).

[127] Shorek (1977).

[128] Henig and Whiting (1987): 29–31, 33.

[129] Dalman (1914): 143–144; Dalman rely upon Epiphanius, *Haversus Haereses* 30, 7; See also Lifshitz (1977): 511.

[130] On Epiphanius's documentation, see Rubin (1983): 111–112; Dvorjetski (1994a): 7–27; idem, (2003): 9–39; On the town-plan of Hammat-Gader, see Hirschfeld (1987): 101–116.

Emperor Constantine there used to take place in Bothna (Beit Ilanim, near Hebron) an important festive fair in which Jews, Christians and pagans participated.[131] There is also evidence of the existence of fairs in other places in Palestine, among them Gaza, Ascalon, Beth Guverin-Eleutheropolis, Beth Shean-Nysa-Scythopolis, and Emmaus-Nicopolis, and other places.[132] In Hammat-Gader there was a unique combination of a fair and a centre of entertainment, and prostitution was rife there. This suburb of Gadara was an important spa, well-known in the East, and during the relatively short bathing period, from Passover until Pentecost, there took place every year a cultic festivity for the region. Crowds of people came to the spa, and the annual festival was like the celebrations of the *Maioumas* (μαιούμας)—the licentious aquatic festival.[133]

As shown above, there have been various conjectures as to the symbolism of the ships on the coins of Gadara as well as the assorted locations of the *naumachia* (ναυμαχία) of Gadara, such as in the city baths; in an artificial lake was created in the natural hollow where the present bathing-pool of the Hammat-Gader site is situated; in the dammed-up Yarmuk-Hieromices, or in the river itself; or in the Kinneret, the Sea of Galilee. We would like to offer a new idea based on the proximity of Kefar Agon to the therapeutic baths and theatre of Hammat-Gader, and its position on the south bank of Lake Kinneret. It may give some indication of the quality of everyday life in this place, which encompassed the variegated elements of Roman leisure culture, including water sports and athletic competitions. These could well have taken place on the River Jordan, too, at its ancient outlet from Lake Kinneret.

8.5.6   *'The Delights of Sons of Men are Pools and Baths'* (*Babylonian Talmud, Gittin 68a*)

Today, the outlet of the Jordan from Lake Kinneret is not the original one: the ancient outlet was north of Tel Beit Yerah, and not to its south, as it is today. This ancient outlet can be plainly seen in the present topography of the area in aerial photographs, and even in general

[131] Sozomenus, *Historia Ecclesiastica* 2, 4, *PG* 67, 944.
[132] Safrai (1984): 150–153.
[133] Efron (1988): 317; See also Lieberman (1980): 10; Goodman (1983): 48; Safrai (1984): 146, 153; Dvorjetski (1992a): 104–108; idem, (2001a): 99–118.

388   CHAPTER EIGHT

topographical maps.[134] Ancient Beit Yerah was situated on the bank
of the Jordan, at the point where it left the Kinneret and began to
flow south. The rabbis believed that the main part of the Jordan was
south of Beit Yerah: 'What is the Jordan? From Beit Yerah downward'
(*Tosefta, Bekhorot* 7, 4), or 'The real Jordanic is only from Beit Yerah
and below' (*Babylonian Talmud, ibid.*, 55a). The opening of the Jordan
from the sea is known as Bab a-Tom, 'The Gate of the Mouth', since
it is like a mouth, and the waters of the Jordan flow through it to the
south: 'It meanders and flows downwards until it reaches the mouth of
Leviathan, as is written: "He trusteth that he can draw up Jordan into
his mouth" (*Job* 40, 23)' (*Babylonian Talmud, Baba Bathra* 74b).

An examination of the seabed of the lake east of the former outlet
of the river shows that it is quite possible that immediately after the
formation of the existing Kinneret, the Jordan emerged from it half a
kilometre east of this outlet. Ben-Arieh maintains that as the southern
coast of the lake retreated, this opening moved more and more to the
west, in line with the coast at this point. Further, he claims, the ancient
outlet of the Jordan was west of the lake because of the gradient of
the delta of the plain south of the lake. It may be that the direction
of the current in the lake was a contributory factor, for in this sector it
flows westwards. Similarly, there may be a weak interface at this point,
since it is a meeting-place between the sediment of the tongue series
and calcareous and basaltic rocks; moreover, it is possible that there
is a fault-line or fissure in this area. The original outlet of the Jordan
was some distance away, inside the lake, and this explains its winding
course after its present exit from the Kinneret.[135]

It is still not certain why the outlet of the Jordan moved from its
ancient channel to its present one. In 1932 Picard suggested three factors which could have contributed to this change: first, a drop of two
metres in the level of the lake, which prevented the river from emerging in its old channel; secondly, an advance of the southern shore of
the Kinneret, which allowed the river to emerge in its new channel;
and, thirdly, human intervention.[136] Schattner suggested two reasons
for the change: that when the Jordan flowed south of Tel Beit Yerah

[134] Ben-Arieh (1965): 47; Velnaey (1977): 'Bab a-Tom', 448; 'Beit Yerah', 737;
'Jordan', 3031.
[135] Ben-Arieh (1965): 47.
[136] Picard (1932): 169–337.

it turned eastward at such an acute angle that when the coast of the lake withdrew southwards it reached the turn, and thereby created a new point of emergence from the lake; or that the Jordan arrived at its new position because of the existence of a fault line or some other weakness in an east-west direction at this point.[137]

Ben-Arieh maintains that Picard's third conjecture, that the change was the result of human intervention, seems the most probable. It is very likely that a channel or moat, even one filled with water, was dug between the Kinneret and the Jordan south of Beit Yerah for purposes of defence. This is the factor most likely to have created the present outlet from the lake. It is obvious why the old channel was abandoned and the new one became the main outlet: the old channel was influenced by streams which bring down alluvium from the hills in the west; the new channel, on the other hand, is further east, in a level stretch which is unaffected by such factors. From the Arabic name for Beit Yerah, Hirbet Krach—a fortified place—it may be deduced that at some historical period the inhabitants fortified the town by surrounding it with water on all sides. Later, when the settlement was abandoned, the waters of the lake broke into the channel and turned it into the main outlet of the river.[138]

The first time the new outlet of the Jordan River is mentioned is in 1106, at the beginning of the Crusader period, in an account written by the Russian Christian Cardinal Daniel, who saw two streams issuing forth from the Kinneret, and joining together:[139]

> The Jordan flows from the Sea of Tiberias in two streams, which foam along in a marvelous way; one of these is called Jor and the other Dan. Thus the Jordan flows from the Sea of Tiberias in two streams, which are three bow-shots apart, and which, after a separation of about half a verst [= 600 metres], reunite as one river, which is called Jordan, from the name of the two arms. The course of the Jordan is very rapid and sinuous. The water is very pure; and it very much resembles the river Snov in its width, depth, and sheets of stagnant water. At the source fish abound; and there two stone bridges, very solidly built upon arches through which the Jordan flows, span the two streams.

Ibn Fadl Allah al-ʿUmari, a scholar and writer of the first half of the fourteenth century, whose works on the administration of the Mamluk

---

[137] Schattner (1962): 9–66, Fig. 18; Ben-Arieh (1965): 48–49 disfavors the two possibilities.

[138] Ben-Arieh (1965): 48–49.

[139] de Khitrowo (1889): 59–60; See also Wilson (1888): 60–61; Raba (1986): 80.

dominions of Egypt and Syria became standard sources for Mamluk history—gives a similar account.[140]

In the nineteenth century travellers still saw water flowing in the original channel of the Jordan. In the winter of 1837–1838 the American traveller Edward Robinson, the pioneer of research of the historical geography of Palestine, saw Tel Beit Yerah surrounded on three sides by branches of the Jordan. He mentions that Richard Pocock, an Englishman who visited the region between 1783 and 1785, as well as Charles Irby and his colleague James Mangels, who visited the area in 1818, maintained that Hirbet Krach gave the impression of having been enclosed by water for purposes of defence.[141] Wilson and Anderson, who were among the founders of the Anglo-Palestine Exploration Fund and made maps of the whole of the Kinneret and Lower Galilee in the winter of 1865–1866, saw a similar sight.[142]

The Scottish Christian John MacGregor, one of the boldest of nineteenth century Palestine tourists, who conducted pioneering research on the sources of the Jordan and the Huleh swamps, visited the area of Beit Yerah between January 29th and 31st 1869. He related that Beit Yerah was separated from the mainland by an artificial lagoon, and that there were signs indicating how to get to there when it was cut off. He claimed to possess a map given to him by Wilson and Anderson which showed Beit Yerah as an island surrounded on both sides by branches of the Jordan. He surmised that the map was drawn when the lake was high, and that this was not the normal state of the site. He ventured to correct their map, therefore, and made an exact drawing of the situation as he saw it at the time of his visit.[143] The authors of the original map accepted his amendment.[144]

In the light of the archaeological researches of Bar-Adon, it may definitely be assumed that throughout ancient times, from the Chalcolithic era until after the Byzantine period, Tel Beit Yerah was connected on its southern and south-eastern sides with the level part of the Jordan Valley and not separated from it by the Jordan. At that time, the

[140] Ibn Fadl Allah al-ʿUmari, *al-Taʿrif bi-al-mustalah al-sharif* 3; See also Hartmann (1916–1917): 1–4.

[141] Robinson and Smith (1841): 100–102.

[142] In the PEF map of 1877 one can see very clearly that nearby Kibbutz Menahemia Hirbet Anin is marked, identified with Kefar Agon, Kefar Agin = Umm Juni.

[143] MacGregor (1904), Map no. 7.

[144] Ben-Arieh (1965): 50.

Jordan flowed not from the south of Tel Beit Yerah, as it does today, but from the north and north-west, immediately below it. The remains of the Roman bridge, immediately below the mound and close to the cemetery of Kinneret, are further evidence that when the bridge was built water still flowed in the old channel of the river. It appears that during the Roman period it was feared that the Jordan would break into a new channel in the south, particularly during the winter flood-time. A strong dam was built, therefore, and its remains are still to be found on the seashore, south of the mound, close to the present-day channel of the Jordan.[145]

Only in 1932, when the Rutenberg electricity project in Naharaim deepened the present channel of the Jordan by three metres, was it cut off from its former channel. Today, anybody going from Degania to Kinneret can see clearly the difference between the two outlets. The previous outlet, in the hollow of Rachel Garden, is 200 metres wide, while the present one is only 40 metres wide. There are fishponds in the previous outlet.[146] It seems, then, that the area north-west of Kefar Agon on the southern coast of Lake Kinneret—a kind of lagoon, lake or pond—served in the past as the site of contests, and particularly aquatic games. The Sages were not mistaken when they said ' "The delights of the sons of men" (*Ecclesiastes* 2, 8) are pools and baths' (*Babylonian Talmud, Gittin* 68a). Thus, in ancient times Kefar Agon— literally 'a village of competitions and games'—constituted in its essential characteristics a genuine expression of the culture of leisure and entertainment in the region.

---

[145] Bar-Adon (1936): 50–55.
[146] See, for example, Nun (1996): 270–271.

CHAPTER NINE

PILGRIMAGE TO THE SPAS IN THE EASTERN MEDITERRANEAN DURING THE LATER ROMAN AND BYZANTINE PERIODS

From the time Christianity became the predominant religion, from the fourth century CE on, the Holy Land was a desired destination of travelers and pilgrims from countries around the globe. Indeed, from the early existence of the Christian religion, pilgrimage occupied a central place in the religious conception of the Christian. It should be seen as a spontaneous phenomenon of popular faith that fulfilled an emotional need for the pilgrim rather than as part of the established religion. Christian pilgrimage is a kind of active fulfillment of the Christian recognition of the temporariness of man's existence in this world. The Latin term for pilgrim is *peregrinus*, which implies a stranger, a wayfarer. In the Byzantine period, Jerusalem became the most important centre for pilgrimage for Christians and the archetype of pilgrimage to the holy places in general as it had been for the Jews in the past.[1]

The earliest pilgrims, like Bishop Melito of Sardis in Asia Minor, or Origenes, went to the holy places from motivations related to the study of the Bible, and their journey had a didactic and intellectual value. Origenes was a scholar and important Christian theologian in his time, with significant influence on future generations. The presence of a teacher of Origenes's stature could not pass without influencing Christian spiritual life in Israel and the propagation of the religion. Eusebius' compositions, too, emphasized the value of the holy places for knowing the Bible, and his *Onomastikon* is indeed a clear attempt to bring together geographical and historical knowledge of the holy places for the purposes of teaching the Bible. Most pilgrims arrived out of a religious sentiment. A minority did so out of an adventurous inclination or for commercial reasons. Although Origenes (230 CE) and

---

[1] Newton (1926): 39–66; Wilkinson (1977); Turner and Turner (1978); Hunt (1982): 50–82; Frend (1985): 567–571; Turner (1987); Ousterhout (1990); Walker (1990); Leyerle (1996): 345–357; Limor (1998); idem, (1999).

Eusebius (340 CE) were not pilgrims in the common sense, and both were Church Fathers who resided in Caesarea, their writings are among the most cited sources on Palestine, as we will face later on.

Testimonies about Christian pilgrimage are found in varied sources—historical, literary, geographical, theological, and even archeological—from the Byzantine period. Nevertheless, the principal, concentrated information about the phenomenon exists in the *itineraria*, the literature of the pilgrims themselves. This genre was composed mainly in Latin by travelers from the West.[2]

The various descriptions in the pilgrims' writings evidence the accelerated process of building churches and ritual places on a large and magnificent scale, most of them in places related to stories in the Bible and the New Testament. Pagan temples were torn down or turned to churches, and many Christians streamed to the Holy Land in order to visit the places mentioned in the Scriptures, places that were directly connected to Jesus and to his Disciples; sites that were sanctified at the initiative of the authorities or on behalf of church institutions; and sites that were sanctified by various Christians sects. The holy sites were concentrated in Jerusalem, in Nazareth, and in the area of the Sea of Galilee because most of the stories bought forth in the Gospels took place there. Hostels were built in the vicinity of the churches, and services for pilgrims installed in them. They were managed by monks who resided there and who became in the course of the fourth century CE responsible for the holy places and were entrusted with the spiritual welfare of the pilgrims—instruction and guidance—as well as with the physical arrangements of their stay.

Especially instructive among the main compositions of this literature in its early days were descriptions of the journey, such as that written by Antoninus of Placentia in northern Italy in 570 CE. Appended to the information is also first-hand, authentic testimony of the personal experience and behavior at the holy places. Moreover, one can even learn about a description of paths not only from Jerusalem to the various sites in the Holy Land, but also of his walking from Acre to the Galilee and afterwards southward to Jericho via the Jordan, and from there ascending to Jerusalem.

Although pilgrimage was a popular phenomenon at base and had very large dimensions, the sources necessarily highlight the pilgrim elite,

---

[2] See the discussion on *The Source Material* in chapter 1.1.

which in part chose in the final analysis to settle in the Holy Land. This refers to a class and intellectual nobility for whom pilgrimage was a stage in a complete change in their way of life. The Emperor Constantine and his mother Helen in the fourth century CE; Eudocia, the wife of the Emperor Theodosius II in the fifth century CE; and Justinian in the sixth century CE—not only did they influence the economic development of Jerusalem from their wealth, but they also served as exemplars for a full line of generous nobles at the top of Roman society. Alongside them, mention should be made of the learned monks who went to Jerusalem and chose to live there for longer or shorter periods of time. The most famous was Jerome [= Hieronymus], who resided in Bethlehem, where he worked on a translation of the Bible and a commentary. Even Empress Eudocia's visit in the fifth century CE manifests the interest of the empress' court in Jerusalem and in the holy places. The period of her residence in Jerusalem was one of the most glorious in the history of building in the city and an attraction for the distinguished regime figures. Thus, Petrus from Iberia was a Georgian prince who had become a monk and supported the monophist faith as Eudocia herself did. He came to Jerusalem in 437 CE, built a monastery in the area of the citadel and hosted pilgrims there. Afterwards, he became the monophist bishop of Maioumas-Gaza.

As one of the most sacred regions in Christian tradition, the area of the Sea of Galilee has attracted many visitors and pilgrims, as well as scholars and writers. In this framework, the place of thermo-mineral baths is not absent, and extensive attention has been paid mainly to two central healing sites in the eastern Mediterranean: Hammei-Tiberias and Hammat-Gader—both of which flourished in the Roman-Byzantine period.[3]

Baths in general remained an important element of urban culture during the Late Roman period, functioning as centres of leisure and social intercourse. Separate facilities were provided for men and women, and the interiors were sumptuously decorated with marbles and statuary. Even clergy and monks used public baths, which were occasionally decorated with objects from Christian iconography.[4]

---

[3] Dvorjetski (1994a): 7–27; idem, (1999a): 117–129; idem, (1999b): 133–141; idem, (2001–2002): 485–512; idem, (2004): 16–27; Reuling (2004): 243–260.

[4] Kazhdan (1991): 271; See also Croutier (1992): 87–89; For the Christian attitude to the Roman baths, see Yegül (1992): 314–349; Nielsen (1993): 81–96; Dvorjetski (2006–2007): 19–22.

396   CHAPTER NINE

The chapter will, at first stage, illuminate the objectives and activities
of the central personages in the Christian tradition, and the contribution
of their compositions to the study of the curative baths in the region of
the Sea of Galilee and along the Syro-African Rift. Were the healing
baths in the Levant holy places in the eyes of the pilgrims? What made
them sanctified? How were they referred to in Christian sources, and
what did the many Christian visitors, who came from all corners of the
Later Roman Empire, seek to see in them? Was their pilgrimage mainly
for therapy or for amusement motivation? In the second stage, we will
examine the position of the Church toward baths, bathing, and mixed
bathing, and bathing as a medical measure; The third stage of the study
will demonstrate the contribution of Christian epigraphic finds to the
special nature of the therapeutic baths in Christian public consciousness
in everyday life in the Late Roman Empire and Byzantine periods.

9.1   THE PERSPECTIVE OF THE CHURCH FATHERS AND PILGRIMS
                TO THE THERAPEUTIC SITES

9.1.1   *Thermal Baths of Tiberias*

The flowering and publicity of the Hammei-Tiberias were described
in favorable terms throughout the generations. The baths brought not
only economic blessing, but also a new bathing culture, which had great
impact on the lives of the residents. (See Map 1 and Fig. 9).

The Christian pilgrim Antoninus of Placentia from north Italy visited the region in 570 CE. He extols the salty and sweet water of the
thermal springs of Tiberias for its therapeutic properties:[5]

> Deinde venimus in civitate Tiberiade, in qua sunt termas ex se lavantes
> salsas, nam aqua maris ipsius dulcis est [= From here we went to the city
> of Tiberias, where there are baths <pools> of salt water, though there
> is also sweet water].

Similar details are known from Arculfus, a Frankish Bishop of the
latter part of the seventh century CE. On his return from a pilgrimage to the Holy Land about the year 670 CE or 690 CE, he was cast
by a tempest on the shore of Scotland. He was hospitably received by

---

[5] Antoninus, *Itinerarium* 7; Stewart (1896): 6; Dvorjetski (2006–2007): 14.

Adamnan, the abbot of the island monastery of Iona, to whom he gave a detailed narrative of his travels in the Holy Land.[6]

Saint and historian Bede Venerabilis, a monk at the Benedictine community at Jarrow, known as the 'Father of English History', documented the holy places in 729 CE: 'Tiberias thermal and salubrious springs'.[7]

The head of the Christian community in Antioch, the twelve century historian Michael the Syrian, who visited the Holy Land, tells of the uniqueness of Hammei-Tiberias, the hotels and inns close-by the baths:[8]

> The baths were built by [= King] Solomon son of David...For the use of those who want healing, there were also pottery jars in it that were artistically arranged, with writing on every one of them: the frequency with which it activated the stomach of a person who drinks from it.

The thermal waters of Tiberias were known as being a medicine for various illnesses when this water is drunk; its special natural attributes were known for urinary and digestive tracts according to the Literature of the Sages and to Maimonides, a contemporary of Michael the Syrian.[9] Today only some poor remnants are left of the magnificent baths of Hammei-Tiberias from the Roman-Byzantine era. (See Tab. 2 and Fig. 9).

9.1.2   *Hammat-Gader*

The site earned many titles from the Church Fathers and pilgrims, who serve as reliable witnesses to the effervescent life and colorful atmosphere that prevailed there in the Roman-Byzantine period, as well as to the names of the site, and its daily functioning.[10] (See Map 1 and Fig. 10).

---

[6] Arculf, *De Locis Sanctis* 26–27; Macpherson (1896): 40–41; Dvorjetski (2006–2007): 14.

[7] Bede Venerabilis, *De Locis Sanctis* 316; Dvorjetski (2006–2007): 14.

[8] Michael the Syrian, *Chronique* 466; See also Assaf and Meir (1954): 10; Buchmann (1956): 24; Dvorjetski (2006–2007): 14.

[9] Kindler (1961): 12–27; Buchmann (1967): 195–202; Meiri (1971): 32–33; Dvorjetski (1992a): 93–103; See also chapter 4.1 about *The Historical-Archaeological Analysis and Healing Cults of Hammei-Tiberias*.

[10] Sukenik (1935a); Hirschfeld and Solar (1984): 22–40; Hirschfeld (1987): 101–116; Dvorjetski (1988); idem, (1992a): 53–61, 104–115; Schürer (1991): II: 132–136; Dvorjetski (1994c): 100–105; Hirschfeld (1997); Dvorjetski (2004): 16–27; idem, forthcoming [a].

The first to mention the most impressive monumental baths in the Levant was the well known theologian Origenes (185–254 CE). He interprets the verse in *John* 6, 41:[11]

> Gadara is a city in Judaea, next to which are famous thermae (θερμά).

It is clear from this testimony that the thermo-mineral baths were in use in the mid-third century CE. Thus, they were constructed at the beginning of that century or even earlier, in the second century CE, and their fame spread. The explicit testimony of the Church Father Origenes for the first time comprises a decisive contribution to the history of Hammat-Gader.

In 363 CE a famous earthquake devastated Palestine. In a Syriac manuscript, a late copy of a letter attributed to Cyril bishop of Jerusalem, Cyril names the towns destroyed by the earthquake, including *Aina de Gader* [= the spring of Gader].[12] According to the many rebuildings of the baths, which were excavated in 1979–1982, it is able to attribute much of this work to the repair of damage caused by this earthquake. Several alterations and building repairs can be distinguished; and the testimony of Cyril can be related to this.[13] The residents of the mother city Gadara and its suburb Hammat-Gader, under the guidance of the Legion X *Fretensis*, exploited the renovation work that was undertaken following the earthquake in order to improve and beautify the spa.[14]

Emerging from the descriptions of the Church Father Epiphanius— bishop of Salamis, who founded his monastery at Beth Guverin-Eleutheropolis in the fourth Century CE—is a colorful atmosphere that prevailed at the site, which attracted people seeking healing from throughout the Empire. A kind of annual fair πανήγυρις was conducted there during which men and women bathed together. Epiphanius objects loudly to the corruption and the low morality during the annual festive assembly. He also related that the Patriarch's son accompanied by Joseph the *Comes*, spent time at the baths with youths, who tried to drag women into the nearby caves and tempt them into carnal acts. A

---

[11] *Commentaria in Evangelium Joannis* 6, 41.
[12] Brock (1979): 276.
[13] Hirschfeld and Solar (1981): 68.
[14] Dvorjetski (1993): 387–406; idem, (1994c): 100–105; idem, (2006–2007): 15–17; This idea is based on the original survey of surgeries in Roman baths done by Künzl (1986): 491–509.

Christian virgin who during bathing there was molested by that young man, drove him away with the sign of the cross.[15]

The central event of the Πανήγυρις was the regional ritual honoring Heracles, patron and defender of merchants,[16] while the *Jerusalem Talmud* (*Shabbat* 3, 4 [6a]) discusses the fair as being intended first and foremost to honor the τρεῖς χάριτες [= The Three Graces]. The atmosphere of corruption and adultery is also manifested in the literature of the Sages, particularly in discussions by the Sages of the many illegitimate children found there and the various proposals for solving this complicated *halakhic* problem.[17] (See Fig. 22).

The most interesting literary reference appears in the *Itinerarium* of Antoninus from Placentia in northern Italy:[18]

> Three miles from the city [= Gadara] there are hot springs, called the baths of Elijah. There lepers cleanse themselves; they receive meals from a hospice...In the evening hours the baths fill up...there is a large bath-tub. When it is full, all the openings are closed, and they [= the lepers] are sent inside with candles and incense...They sit in this bathtub the whole night. When they fall asleep, a person who is to be cured has a certain vision, and when he relates it, the baths themselves are not used for 7 days, and within seven days, he is healed.

According to Antoninus's testimony, a public hospice was built in order to provide therapeutic services and entertainment for the visitors. In the Byzantine period, the residents of Hammat-Gader and Gadara adopted the Biblical traditions about Elijah, and called the medicinal baths or part of it after him *Thermae Heliae*. The lepers were sent inside with candles and incense, sitting there the whole night. They were cured by way of incubation, as was customary in the ancient medical centres of Aesculapius, in a large bathtub. This bathtub was separate from the overall complex that served all the bathers. The details regarding the bathing procedures which the lepers underwent there correlate closely both with the characteristics of the double-sloped pool, which has been entirely excavated and with the particular terracotta oil lamps

---

[15] *Panarion* 30.7; Williams (1987): 125; Hirschfeld (1987): 104–105; Dvorjetski (1988): 93–94; idem, (1992a): 106–107; idem (1994c): 24–25; Hirschfeld (1997): 5; Dvorjetski (2001–2002): 492–493; For women and mixed bathing, see Ward (1992): 125–147; Dupont (1992): 264; Merten (1983): 79–100.

[16] Safrai (1984): 158.

[17] Dvorjetski (1994a): 18; idem, (1994c); idem, (1999a): 127–128; idem, (2000b): 91–93.

[18] Antoninus, *Itinerarium* 7.

which were found in it. They are all very similar in style, and all lack
the soot, which characterizes a lamp after use. The lepers used these
lamps as an element of some ritual ceremony conducted at the pool.
On the basis of archaeological appraisals, the pool and its hall have
been dated to the third-fourth centuries CE.[19]

The place certainly served as a centre for curing leprosy in particular
and skin diseases in general already at the time of Hadrian according
to the Talmudic literature. During his reign, and perhaps even with
his aid, the foundations were laid for the edifice of the thermal baths
in Hammat-Gader, whose publicity as a place of healing assisted its
reputation and its profits.[20]

Furthermore, a Byzantine church stood once in the eastern sector
of Hammat-Gader, north of 'Ain er-Rih spring. It seems that the many
visitors prayed in this church donated generously to the place. Among
the architectural fragments discovered and reported by Makhouly in
1938, were four Corinthian capitals; one capital was decorated on each
side with a cross, and a basalt pillar base.[21] Hirschfeld assumes that on
or adjacent to the spot where the Byzantine church stood, there may
have originally been a pagan sanctuary. The purification of pagan
ritual sites and their conversion into Christian places of worship was
very common during the Byzantine period. An archaeological clue
to the existence of a previous Roman sanctuary at this locale temple
is the marble Corinthian capital of secondary use that was found in
the church, which was built in the typical style toward the end of the
Roman period, second–third century CE.[22]

The existence of a Byzantine church near the *Thermae* and the theatre is not surprising. Therapeutic springs were considered sacred and
bathing in their waters was accompanied by various rituals. Many of
the dedicatory inscriptions, which were found during the excavation
of the Thermae and will be shown later on—open with the formula:
'In this holy place'.[23]

---

[19] Hirschfeld and Solar (1984): 22–40; Hirschfeld (1997): 79–83; See also Dvorjetski (1992b): 425–449; idem, (2004): 20.

[20] Dvorjetski (1997b): 567–581; idem, forthcoming [b]; See also chapter 4.2 about *The Historical-Archaeological Analysis and Healing Cults of Hammat-Gader.*

[21] Makhouly (1938): 59–62.

[22] Hirschfeld (1987): 113.

[23] Di Segni (1997): 185–186; Dvorjetski, forthcoming [b].

9.1.3   *Thermal Baths of Livias*

Julias was rebuilt and fortified by Herod Antipas and named Julias in honor of the wife of Augustus. Eusebius, Jerome and Syncellus give the name as Livias instead of Julias. Josephus alone uses the official designation Julias. The town is also frequently referred to elsewhere as Livias by Pliny, Ptolemy, Eusebius, Hierocles, Gregory of Tours and Petrus the Iberian.[24] Another example of bestowing holy names on therapeutic baths is found in the biography of Petrus the Iberian (409–488 CE) about Hammei-Livias. It was written originally in Greek by his disciple, Johannes Rufus and remained in its Syriac translation. Rufus relates that when his master was ill suffering from dermatological disease and weakness, he left his monastery in Maioumas-Gaza and went to take a cure by bathing in the thermal waters of Livias, which were called the Baths of Moses.[25]

The most accurate description of the site is given by the Christian pilgrim Theodosius, who visited the region in 530 CE and emphasizes the 'aquae calidae' [= the hot springs] as follows:[26]

> In this Livias Moses struck the rock with his rod, and the waters flowed out. Thence emerges a rather large stream which irrigates the whole of Livias...There Moses departed his life, and there are the warm waters where Moses bathed. In these warm waters lepers are cleansed.

Antoninus of Placentia reports mainly about the baths of Moses and their properties:[27]

> Nearby is a city called Livias...in that place are natural hot springs, which are called the Baths of Moses. In these also lepers are cleansed. A spring there has very sweet water, which they drink as a cathartic, and it heals many diseases...In the evening they wash in these Baths of Moses. From time to time by the will of God one of them is cleansed, but for most of them it brings some relief.

9.1.4   *Thermal Bath of Ba'arah*

This bathing place has very hot mineral springs, which are also potable; it is located near Wadi Zarqa Ma'in, east of the Dead Sea, and its

---

[24] Schürer (1991): II: 176–178.
[25] Petrus the Iberian, 81–82; See also Kofsky (1997): 209–222; Dvorjetski (2006–2007): 17–18.
[26] Theodosius, *De Situ Terrae Sanctae* 145.
[27] Antoninus, *Itinerarium* 134; Stewart (1896): 40–41.

waters pour out to the sea along with those of the stream. Josephus
describes Βααρας very picturesquely in *Bellum Judaicum* as having both
bitter water and sweet water springs. It 'cures every sickness and especially sickness of the nerves.'[28]

The description of the springs of Ba'arah appears in the biography
of Petrus of Iberia. Petrus went to the thermal waters of Ba'ar in order
to heal his body, which had become weakened from self-mortification.
The site is mentioned as 'a desolate place with very hot and curative
springs'.[29] This account is the most precise description of the place,
and it corresponds to the one given by Josephus.[30]

The Semitic name Ba'arah is derived from the root bar which
means 'burning', and traces of an underground fire are noticeable at
the location. The very mention and description of Hammei-Ba'arah
in the Madaba map dated to the second-half of the sixth century CE,
testifies to the importance of the springs as it has been discussed.[31]
(See Fig. 25).

9.1.5   *Thermal Baths of Emmaus-Nicopolis*

Many Christian sources mentioned traditions about Jesus and his resurrection in connection with Emmaus-Nicopolis. The place had become
a focus of pilgrimage in the Christian world.[32]

The Christian historian Sozomenus of the fifth century CE brings
testimony of great value to clarify why Emmaus-Nicopolis became a
famous city in Palestine in his *Historia Ecclesiastica*:[33]

> In front of this city…there was the place where Jesus walked in the
> company of Cleopas and his retinue after his resurrection. There is the
> spring of Jesus, whose waters give a cure not only to the illnesses of
> people who bathe in it, but also to various animal diseases. They say
> that when the Messiah stayed with his disciples, he deviated from the
> path one day to wash his feet in this spring, and from then on its waters
> had a special quality of removing all types of illnesses and suffering from
> humans and animals.

---

[28] Josephus, *Bellum Judaicum* 7.186–189.
[29] Petrus the Iberian, 81–82, 87.
[30] Donner (1982): 175–180; Dvorjetski (1992a): 64–70; Clamer (1993): 222–224;
Dvorjetski (2006–2007): 18.
[31] See the discussion on *Terminology* in chapter 1.4.
[32] On the sources related to Jesus, see below; See also Dvorjetski (2006–2007):
18–19.
[33] Sozomenus, *Historia Ecclesiastica* 5.21; Walford (1855): 239; Dvorjetski (1992a):
121–122.

Theophanes, a ninth century CE monk and chronicler, also notes the well-known spring in Emmaus and adds that Emperor Julian the Apostate ordered the spring to be blocked because of the wonders of healing that were generated in it. Despite the damming of the spring, its location was well documented in the years that followed due to the monk Saint Willibald in the eight century CE, the chronographer George Cedrenus from the eleven century CE, Michael the Syrian, twelve century CE Patriarch of Antioch, and more.[34]

The special qualities of the waters of Emmaus, as presented above, are clearly legendary in every way. Apparently this assumption is somewhat invalidated because of the epigraphic find of an Aramaic magic amulet, dating to the third century CE found in a grave in Emmaus in 1896.[35] The actual remains of the Roman bath at Emmaus were excavated in 1977 and covered an area of about 14×7.5 metres. These excavations did furnish tangible proof of seismic activities in Emmaus.[36]

To date, the hot springs have not been discovered in or around ancient Emmaus, which was over built by the Arab village ʿImwās. Gichon suggests that the hot springs might have been blocked during an earthquake, possibly as late as 1546.[37] Gichon's opinion finds no support either by mineralogical analysis or by the evidences of the many Church Fathers. (See Figs. 29 and 30).

At this stage one can sum up, that the evidence of the Church Fathers, chronographers and pilgrims shows several common denominators. Firstly, the spas were considered as centres of culture and therapy; secondly, people of all kinds bathed there; thirdly, certain places gained great fame because of their healing qualities and their effectiveness in curing health ailments, especially dermatological conditions, general debilitation, rheumatism, and nervous diseases; and most importantly, without the Christian evidences the historical reconstruction of the thermo-mineral baths in Roman-Byzantine Palestine could not have been accomplished.

---

[34] Theophanes, *Chronographia* 5854; Saint Willibald, *Itinerarium* 293; Cedrenus, *Historiarum Compendium* 582; Michael the Syrian, *Chronique* 187; See also Vincent and Abel (1932): 414–420; Dechent (1884): 209–210; Abel (1938): I: 315.

[35] Vincent (1908): 382–394; See also Goodenough (1958): 71–80; idem, (1964): XI: Fig. 290.

[36] Gichon (1979): 101–110; idem, (1980): 228–234; idem, (1986–1987): 54–57; idem, (1993): 385–389.

[37] Gichon (1979): 102.

9.2   CHRISTIAN ETHICS TOWARDS MIXED BATHING
AND BATHING AS A MEDICAL MEASURE

Baths remained one of the popular institutions of late antiquity and early Byzantine cities. The public baths or thermae were one of the adornments of the city, and were extremely popular.[38] Bathing at the baths were so important to the Roman Citizen that it is inconceivable to think that the Christians would have ignored this deep rooted social and cultural habit, as Yegül points out:[39]

> Bathing in the ancient world, especially in the world of the Romans, went far beyond the functional and hygienic necessities of washing. It was a personal regeneration and a deeply rooted social and cultural habit—in the full sense of the word, an *institution*. For the average Roman a visit to the public baths in the afternoon was an irreplaceable part of the day's routine...It would have been unrealistic to expect the Church to take a consistent stance against an institution [= that is, bathing in the Roman baths] that had become a deeply ingrained part of daily life.

The position of the Church toward baths and bathing was, at best, ambivalent. It is clearly evident that Christians in the first two centuries did in fact visit the baths regularly, and this is fairly well documented. Some of the Apostles' deeds are related to bathe and bathing. John frequented the baths at Ephesus, the capital of the Roman Province of Asia Minor.[40] Reading the testimony of Eusebius bishop of Caesarea in Palestine (263–339 CE), for instance, who was the first great Church historian, it is clear that John the Apostle had gone to the baths with the intension of bathing. Seeing someone, whom he regarded as a heretic inside, John left the baths in haste.[41] This episode and others are mentioned in such a matter of fact that it clearly show that it was not unusual for a disciple that had known Jesus to bathe at the baths. Furthermore, in the apocryphal acts of John and elsewhere there are number of texts show a similar belief in demons that haunt the baths.

---

[38] Cameron (1973): 149–150; Heinz (1983); Brödner (1983); DeLaine (1988): 11–32; Nielsen (1990); Kazhdan (1991): 271; Toner (1995): 53–64; Weber (1996); Fagan (1999a); Gatier (1999): 227; Dalby (2000): 237–240; Ball (2000): 219–220; Goldsworthy (2003): 106–107; Cruse (2004): 91–93, 131–134; McGinn (2004): 23–26, 121–122, 206–214; DeLaine (2004): 113–115.
[39] Yegül (1992): 1–5.
[40] Dunbabin (1989): 35.
[41] Eusebius of Caesera, *Historia Ecclesiastica* 3.28.

The demon was sometimes in the habit of strangling a youth or maiden. This makes clear the possible danger of exposure to the Evil Eye.[42]

The Church Fathers did not normally prohibit Christians from bathing or urge them to curb the habit; in fact they bathed themselves like everyone else. Among the earliest references to Roman baths by Christians, no ethical reservations about going to bathe are suggested. Tertullian of Carthage (155–225 CE), who is regarded as one of the greatest Western theologians and writers of Christian antiquity, in his *Apologeticum*, an impassioned defense of Christians against pagan charges of immorality, economic worthlessness and political subversion—addressing the Roman governors and states that 'the Christians are no different from other people: they go to the forum, to the marcellum [= market], and to the baths (*balneia*)'.[43] As for Tertullian himself, he notes:[44]

> How it is we seem useless in your ordinary business, living with you and by you as we do, I am not able to understand. But if I do not frequent your religious ceremonies, I am still on the sacred day a man. I do not bathe in the early dawn on the *Saturnalia*, lest I should waste both night and day; still I do bathe at the hour I should, one which is conductive to health and which protects both my temperature and my life's blood. To become stiff and ashen—I can enjoy that when I am dead!

Tertullian also states that the baths are full of idols, though he includes them in a list of places which Christians living in the world have to frequent:[45]

> Why, even the streets and the market-place, and the baths, and the taverns, and our very dwelling-places, are not altogether free from idols. Satan and his angels have filled the whole world. It is not by merely being in the world, however, that we lapse from God, but by touching and tainting ourselves with the world's sins.

Elsewhere he speaks of worship offered at the doorways of baths: 'For we see too that other entrances are adored in the baths'.[46] Dunbabin remarks: 'Christian apologists do not normally include the presence

---

[42] See, for example, Bonner (1932): 204–208; Dunbabin (1989): 35–36.
[43] Tertullian, *Apologeticum* 42.2; Tertullian indicated that he bathed for hygienic purposes: *ibid.*, 42.4; On Tertullian's motivation in medicine, see Amundsen (1982): 343–345.
[44] Tertullian, *Apologeticum* 42.2.
[45] Tertullian, *De Spectaculis* 8.
[46] Tertullian, *De Idolatria* 15.6.

of the pagan gods as one of the items which the good Christian has to fear in the baths, and it is noteworthy that the Christianization of the Empire has only limited effects on the choice of subjects. "Pagan" themes, such as Venus, the Nymphs etc., disappear from some of the inscriptions'.[47] The continuing cult of the Nymphs can be attested, at least in connexion with thermal springs. There may have been many who paid their respects to the Nymphs or Asclepius when they bathed.[48]

Bathing could be a dangerous exercise. There was an undoubted possibility of real accidents. Tertullian mentions the possibility of drowning in the pool as if it were a standard and recognized danger in his treatise *De Anima*. He speaks of evil and unclean spirits inhabiting in *balneis piscinae*, which seize on men and points out:[49]

> In certain sacred rites they are initiated by means of a bath [= so as to belong to] Isis perhaps or Mithras. Also they carry their gods out [= in procession] for washings. Moreover they ritually purify their country and town houses, their temples, and whole cities, by carrying water about and sprinkling it. If they suppose water receives healing power from religious usage, what more effective religious usage is there than the acknowledgement of the living God? Here too we observe the devil's zeal in hostility to the things of God...If so, he will be pulling down his own work, and washing away the sins he himself inspire...apart from this, without any sacred significance, unclean spirits do settle upon waters, pretending to reproduce that primordial resting of the divine Spirit upon them: I as witness shady springs and all sorts of unfrequented streams, pools in bathing-places, and channels or storage-tanks in houses, and those wells called snatching-wells-obviously they snatch by the violent action of a malignant spirit: for people also use words like 'esetic' and 'lymphatic' and 'hydrophobic' of those whom water has drowned, or has vexed with madness or fear.

A contemporary of Tertullian, namely Clement of Alexandria, who fled the persecution of Septimius Severus in 202 CE, was the head of the Christian catechetical school in Alexandria. The Exhortation to Conversion was designed to win pagans to the Christian faith. In *The Educator*, Clement warns against bathing too long and several times a day, which was unhealthy. He writes:[50]

---

[47] Dunbabin (1989): 32.
[48] Dunbabin (1989): 12–13, 22–23.
[49] Tertullian, *De Baptismo* 5.4.
[50] Clement, *The Educator* 3.10.

There are four reasons prompting us to frequent the baths (it was at this point that I digressed a while back in my discussion): either for cleanliness, for warmth, for health, or for the satisfaction of pleasure. We must not think of bathing for pleasure, because we must ruthlessly expel all unworthy pleasure. Women may take use of the bath for the sake of cleanliness and health; men, only for the sake of their health...The motive of seeking warmth is scarcely urgent, since we can find relief from cold in other ways. The continued use of baths undermines a man's strength, weakening the muscles of his body and often inducing lassitude and even fainting spells...We ought not bathe on every occasion...

Clement recommended frugal living, because a voluptuous life is alien to refined pleasures, and love of wealth induces one to stop being ashamed of what is shameful. Baths are used for cleanliness, heat, health, or pleasure; but Clement suggested women use them for cleanliness and health, and men only for cleanliness, since they can use gymnastic exercise for health. With respects to the evidence of Clement and others, Ward comments in his article entitled 'Women in Roman Baths' that 'Clement did not forbid his Christian readers from going to the baths; he allowed men to use the baths for the sake of health (ὑγίεια) and women for cleanliness (καθαριότης) and health (ὑγίεια). He counseled that Christians should not bathe often. It is clear from Clement that in Alexandria at the end of the second century—contemporaneous with Irenaeus, bishop of Lugdunum, and Tertullian—mixed bathing by all classes was not only customary but also a popular activity in which Christian men and women engaged'.[51] Certainly, women who were concerned about their respectability, did not frequent the baths when the men were there, but of course the baths were an excellent place for prostitutes to ply their trade. Prostitutes of both sexes often frequented the baths, and the bath attendants could either perform that function or serve as pimps. There could even be rooms set aside as a brothel. Finally, the body's other needs could be satisfied, in that most baths had personnel for anointing, massage and depilation.[52]

Christian women continued to engage in mixed bathing according to *Didascaliae Apostolorum*, written in Syria about 250 CE. The books deal with Christian ethics, the duties of the clergy, the Eucharistic liturgy, and various church problems and rituals. Women who were

---

[51] Ward (1992): 143.
[52] See, for example, Jones (1964): II: 976–977; Dunbabin (1989): 6–46; Toner (1995): 53–64; Dauphin (1996): 47–72; McGinn (2004), s.v. 'baths'; See also the intensive discussion in chapter 1.5 on *Leisure-Time Activities and Places of Entertainment.*

obliged to bathe in men's baths are advised not to do so naked and to avoid the busy period. The instructions that are given to women are as follows:[53]

> Avoid also that disorderly practice of bathing in the same place with men; for many are the nets of the evil one. And let not a Christian woman bathe with an hermaphrodite; for if she is to veil her face, and conceal it with modesty from strange men, how can she bear to enter naked into the bath together with men? But if the bath be appropriated to women, let her bathe orderly, modestly, and moderately. But let her not bathe without occasion, nor much, nor often, nor in the middle of the day, nor, if possible, every day; and let the tenth hour of the day be the set time for such seasonable bathing. For it is convenient that thou, who art a Christian woman, shouldst ever constantly avoid a curiosity which has many eyes.

The church viewed the baths with displeasure. Mixed bathing it naturally condemned as an incitement to sin, but it also disapproved of bathing in general. 'He who has once bathed in Christ has no need of a second bath', wrote Saint Jerome.[54] After leaving Rome for the East, Jerome writes a letter to Asella in 385 CE to refute the calumnies by which he had been assailed, especially as regards his intimacy with Paula and Eustochium. He contrasted the ascetic lifestyle of Melania with that of other women in Rome:[55]

> Of all the ladies in Rome, the only ones that caused scandal were Paula and Melania, who, despising their wealth and deserting their children, uplifted the cross of the Lord as a standard of religion. Had they frequented the baths, or chosen to use perfumes, or taken advantage of their wealth and position as widows to enjoy life and to be independent, they would have been saluted as ladies of high rank and saintliness.

Jerome's own position was even more extreme, and he opposed virginal women bathing with women. In a letter to Laeta, the daughter-in-law of Paula, written in 403 CE—how she ought to bring up her infant daughter—Jerome opposed Christian virgins bathing with eunuchs or with married women but also of any virgin bathing naked at all:[56]

> As regards the use of the bath, I know that some are content with saying that a Christian virgin should not bathe along with eunuchs or with

---

[53] *Didascalia Apostolorum* 87–89; For the *Didascalia*, see Ferguson (1990): 263.

[54] Jerome, *Epistulae* 14.10; See also Jones (1964): II: 976–977; For Jerome's background and education see, for example, Amundsen (1982): 331.

[55] Jerome, *Epistulae* 45.4; See also Ward (1992): 145–146.

[56] Jerome, *Epistulae* 107.11.

married women, with the former because they are still men…and with the latter because women with child offer a revolting spectacle. For myself, however, I wholly disapprove of baths for a virgin of full age. Such a one should blush and feel overcome at the idea of seeing her undressed. By vigils and fasts she mortifies her body and brings it into subjection. By a cold chastity she seeks to put out the flame of lust and to quench the hot desires of youth. And by a deliberate squalor she makes haste to spoil her natural good looks. Why, then, should she add fuel to a sleeping fire by taking baths?

Saint Augustine of Hippo (354–430 CE) allowed nuns to go to the baths only once a month unless by doctor's order. Pious Christians had doubts even about this. A letter was sent to Augustine by Publicola in 398 CE and the later listed a number of questions in which he seeks answers. One of these, question 15 he asks:[57]

May a Christian use baths in places in which sacrifice is offered to images? May he use baths which are used by pagans on a feast day, either while they are there or after they have left?

The first thing that someone might notice is that the question was not 'May Christians visit the baths', but rather if they did, what should they do if sacrifices to images were being made, or if 'pagans' were celebrating a feast day at the time. Clearly, at this time Christians did visit the baths.

In another letter to the consecrated virgins written in 423, Saint Augustine claims:[58]

The washing of the body, also and the use of baths is not to be too frequent, but may be allowed at the usual interval of time, that is, once a month. In the case of illness, however where there is urgent need of bathing the body, let it not be postponed too long, but let it be done without objection for medical reasons. If the patient herself objects, she must do what health requires to be done at the bidding of the Superior… if a handmaid of God has a hidden pain in her body and tells what ails her, she should be believed without reserve, but when it is not certain whether pleasant would be good for her, a doctor should be consulted. If they go to the baths or wherever they have to go, let there be not less than three.

---

[57] Augustine, *Epistulae* 46; See also Jones (1964): II: 977; On the significantly thoughts that Augustine had been deeply influenced, see Amundsen (1982): 330–331, 334, 337, 349.

[58] Augustine, *Contra Academicos* 2.2.6.

The Church Father, great preacher and Patriarch of Constantinople, John Chrysostom (347–407 CE) mentions the infernal racket of the baths. The noise there was like that in the theatre or the market-place. He also says: 'Let food and baths and dinners and the other things of this life have their appointed time', but he goes on in the next sentence:[59]

> For the things of this life, baths, I mean, and dinners, even if they are necessary, yet being continually repeated, render the body feeble.

In general John Chrysostom refused invitations to banquets, gave no dinner parties, and ate the simplest fare in his solitary chamber. He denounced unsparingly luxurious habits in eating and dressing, and enjoined upon the rich the duty of almsgiving to an extent that tended to increase rather than diminish the number of beggars who swarmed in the streets and around the churches and public baths. In his days those who were of his party celebrated Easter in the public baths, which are called Constantinae, and thenceforth left the church.[60] He deplored the vanity of mothers, who spoiled their daughters with worldly luxuries and refinements such as baths, but he did not object to visiting the baths himself nor did he stop his followers from performing baptisms in a major bath in Constantinople. He also criticizes the bad habit of exhibiting golden jewelry in the bath and the talkativeness of women there. However he recognizes the necessity of bathing for women.[61]

It is seen from several sources that it gradually became common for the baths to stay open at night, especially in the fourth century. Special clientele frequented the baths at night, and the Church Father Ambrosius, Bishop of Milan (died 397 CE) states that while it was acceptable for Christians to bathe in the daytime, it was sinful to visit the baths at night.[62]

In this sphere the church's censure was utterly ignored save by a puritanical minority. The baths remained a great social institution

---

[59] Chrysostom, *Homilae in Ioannem* 18.4; See also idem, *De Sanctis Martyribus Sermo* 2; Hanoune (1980): 260–261; On Chrysostom's education, faith and medicine, see for example, Amundsen (1982): 330, 334, 340.

[60] Mentioned while describing Empress Eudoxia's silver statue by Socrates Scolasticus, *Historia Ecclesiastica* 6.18.

[61] Chrysostom, *Matthaeu Homilae* 51.239, 56.536, 60.218; See also Hanoune (1980); Berger (1982): 24, 37, 39–40, 53–54; Nielsen (1990): I: 137, 145–146; Yegül (1992): 314.

[62] See Hunter (1987): 48; Ward (1992): 145.

among rich and poor alike. Even the clergy did not always conform to the church's teachings. The continued popularity of the baths, even among Christians, is attested by Socrates Scholasticus's account of Bishop Sisinnius, Patriarch of Constantinople (died in 427 CE). Sisinnius shocked his Novatian congregation by bathing twice a day in the public baths. He proudly announced 'when someone asked him "why he, a bishop, bathed himself twice a day?" He replied, 'Because it is inconvenient to bathe thrice'.[63]

That mixed bathing continued to be a problem for some Christians men can be seen from Canon 30 of the Synod of Laodicea in Phrygia in the middle of the fourth century CE. This regulation declared that 'no priests or clerics or ascetics are permitted to bathe in the baths with women, nor any Christian or laic, for this is the greatest reproach among the gentiles'. At the Council of Chalchedon in 451 CE, a bishop was criticized for bathing with females.[64]

Furthermore, the Syrian bishop Theodoret, who in the mid-fifth century CE complains about pagan sculpture still being produced and displayed in public, was himself a bath builder. When Theodoret speaks of pagan sculpture displayed in public, he is probably referring to the baths. His own building was hardly furnished with this type of sculpture, despite the fact that Dionysus and his attendants, by tradition, were particularly favored for the baths; rather he installed some decent philosophers, who could also be met in such surroundings. Apollonios from Tyana, who is frequently reproduced in sculpture in Late Antiquity, could have been present. As Bishop Theodoret tells us, the production of pagan sculpture continued beyond the period of the decisive victory of Christianity. Pagan motifs appeared in other art forms as well, and it is evidenced from private context that sculpture in the classical tradition was still produced for the decor of stately homes throughout the fifth century CE. In some cases it is evidenced that traditional sculpture was also created for the baths.[65]

Although many monks refrained from washing, the majority of saints were not adverse to the use of baths. The Palestinian hermit Barsanuphius from Gaza, who lived at the days of Emperor Justinian

---

[63] Socrates Scholasticus, *Historia Ecclesiastica* 6.22; See also Jones (1964): II: 977; Chestnut (1986): 184; Nielsen (1990): I: 137; Yegül (1992): 314.

[64] See for example Ward (1992): 145.

[65] http://www.archaeologie-sachbuch.de/Fleischer/index1.htm?/Fleischer/Texte/Hannestad1.htm

(died in 540 CE), took an intermediate view. In his opinion bathing
was not forbidden to people if necessity forced them there. Therefore,
if they were sick and needed to use a bath, it would not be wrong. But
for healthy people taking a bath meant that they were pampering their
bodies, which led to relaxation, which led to weakness. He was asked
if it was a sin to bathe if someone is ill and the doctor ordered him
to take baths. He replied:[66]

> Bathing is not absolutely forbidden to a man in the world, when need
> demands. So if you are ill and need it, it is not a sin. But if a man is
> healthy, it cossets and relaxes his body and conduces to lust.

This query is typical of many and illustrates the permissive position
taken by the Church with respect to medicinal and curative bathing.
Visits to mineral springs for purely health reasons were permitted. Some
leading Church figures, such as Saints, Bishops and Theologians: Basil
the Great, Gregory of Nazianzus, Gregory of Nyssa, Petrus the Iberian
and Theodore of Sykeon—reported to have taken thermal baths.[67]

In a letter to Antipater, the Governor of Cappadocia, to whom Saint
Basil from Caesarea in Cappadocia, east-central Anatolia, (330–379
CE), is recommending the protection of his old friend and relative,
Palladius, written in 373 CE, he describes his health:[68]

> At present, I seem to be especially sensible of the loss which I suffer by
> my illness, when during the administration of our country by such a great
> man. I myself am compelled to be absent because of the care I must give
> my body. For the whole month already I have been taking the treatments
> of the natural hot springs in the hope of receiving some benefit from
> them. But, I seem to labor in vain in the solitude, or even to appear to
> most people to be deserving of ridicule, as one who does not understand
> the proverb which says: 'Hot springs are of no use to the dead'.

At least three passages in the writings of Saint Gregory of Nazianzus
from Cappadocia as well (330–389 CE), a life-long friend of Saint Basil
refer to the therapeutic use of natural springs. Cold and hot springs were
both considered healing in their effect. Gregory himself was obliged
by his physician to frequent those thermal springs at Xanxaris, the

---

[66] Barsanuphius, *Quaestiones* 336; See Jones (1964): II: 977; Yegül (1992): 317; Gatier
(1999): 227.
[67] Yegül (1992): 314; On the Cappadocian Fathers' background, see Amundsen
(1982): 329–330; See also the discussion below.
[68] Saint Basil, *Epistulae* 137; On the Cappadocian Fathers see, for example, Frend
(1985): 630–634.

usual resort of the people in Cappadocia, in 382 CE. Even the strictest ascetics in all monasterial orders, who otherwise forbade bathing completely, approved of therapy for disease:[69]

> Since my illness has brought me too far, and it has become necessary for me to try the hot baths of Xanxaris at the advice of my medical men, I send a letter to represent me.

A good friend of Gregory of Nazianzus and a younger brother of Basil of Caesarea was Gregory of Nyssa (335–394 CE). He testifies also that baths were still a part of the health regimen of their day. Gregory was appointed Bishop of Nyssa by his brother Basil about the same time that the latter attempted to make Gregory of Nazianzus bishop of Sasima. Another story on demons is given by him in his life of Saint Gregory Thaumaturgus, Bishop of Neocaesarea. It tells of a demon, which haunted a bath, and made it impossible to use after sunset; those who had dared to enter the water after dark, instead of the relief they had hoped for, had found only mourning and lamentations. The doorman does not wish to allow the deacon sent by Gregory to enter; when he does so, the deacon is assailed by all sorts of terrors and phantasms of fire and smoke in the form of men and beasts, by noises and smells, which grow worse, with earthquake and flames, as he goes further into the building. All vanish when he makes the sign of the cross.[70]

Despite the anecdotal character of some of the hagiographic materials pertaining to miraculous healing, certain texts are worth citing in detail because of their importance in delineating the physicians' methods and their status in the Byzantine community, as well as in showing what were the capabilities and limitations of medical science in those days. Churchmen and saints acquired great skill and knowledge in the practice of medicine. In the Eastern Church some were regarded as Doctors of the Church, a term that was bestowed on certain ecclesiastical writers who had received this title on account of the great advantage the whole Church had derived from their doctrine. There are three Doctors that were prominent: Saint John Chrysostom, Saint Basil, and Saint Gregory of Nazianzus. Saint Theodore of Sykeon was the remarkable in that he was an excellent practitioner of medicine. Like a trained physician he would send those patients, for whom surgery was the required treatment, to the most capable surgeons; others he would dissuade from

---

[69] See, for example, Berger (1982): 35, 77, 146.
[70] Gregory of Nyssa, *Opera* 952 a–d.

surgery, sending them to specific hot springs, and still others he would
send to specifically designated physicians for medicines. Besides all this,
he was also capable of recommending certain plasters for wounds and
abscesses. Saint Theodore, however, was exceptional in that he was not
hostile to the medical profession of his day.[71]

After a pilgrimage to the Holy Land, Saint Theodore of Sykeon,
who was an excellent practitioner of medicine, became a monk in
his native Galatia in Asia Minor. About 584 CE he was ordained
Bishop of Anastasiopolis in Galatia for ten years. Unique information
is documented in his *Vita* on medical instructions in the therapeutic
springs:[72]

> In the case of sick persons who were lying in their own homes their rela-
> tions would bring back oil or water that had been blessed by him and
> received them back restored to health. Those who were afflicted with
> wounds or maladies of any kind obtained healing through his prayers.
> Again if any required medical treatment for certain illnesses or surgery or
> a purging draught or hot springs, this God-inspired man would prescribe
> the best thing for each for even in technical matters he had become an
> experienced doctor. He might recommend one to have recourse to surgery
> and he would always state clearly which doctor they should employ. In
> other cases he would persuade those who wished to undergo an opera-
> tion or take some other medical treatment and would recommend them
> rather to go to hot springs, and would name the springs to which they
> should go. Or he would prevent those who wished to go to the hot springs
> at Dablioi or to take the waters, say, at Apsoda, and would advise them
> rather to drink a purging draught instead under a doctor whom he would
> name. Others again he would not allow doing that but sent them away
> to drink hot waters or to some other hot springs. Others who had been
> wounded or had abscesses and might perhaps wish for an operation he
> would send to hot springs or would advise them to use plasters of which
> he himself gave them the name. In a word, as the very best of physi-
> cians and as a disciple of the true master physician, Christ our God, to
> each one of those who came for treatment he gave exactly the suitable
> advise that each man's case demanded, and of those who carried out
> his instructions not one failed to regain his health; and thus in him was
> fulfilled the thanks-giving sung by David to God, 'Oh, Lord, Thou shalt
> preserve men and beasts' (*Psalms* 36, 6). However, if perchance one of
> those who had been advised by him neglected, or made a change in, his

---

[71] Ioannou (1884): 145–146, 491–492; Dawes and Baynes (1948): 182–183; Festugière
(1970): 114; Magoulias (1964): 128; For the Byzantine holy person, see Kofsky (2004):
261–285.
[72] Theodore of Sykeon, *Vita* 145–146; See also Dawes and Baynes (1948): 182–
183.

orders, either by consulting another doctor, not the one the Saint had named, or by using other plasters, or different treatment, or other hot springs that person's illness became incurable until he reverted to the treatment the Saint had prescribed and to the hot springs he had named and to the doctor chosen by him.

Many diseases in the Byzantine era were widespread and had a high morbidity, such as respiratory diseases, various kinds of anaemia, pestilential diseases, like quartan fever, plague, dysentery and cholera, parasitic diseases, orthopedic, rheumatic and psychiatric disorders, trachoma, and alcoholism. Other very serious and relatively frequent conditions included leprosy, mania, gout, cancerous tumours and ulcers. To protect the public's health, the Byzantine state and Church controlled the circulation and composition of remedies, their price, the function of pharmacies, and the prohibition of narcotics and poisonous essences. For the treatment of the different kinds of obesity, Byzantine physicians recommended diet, purgation, bloodletting, physicotherapy, bathing, proper climate, substances causing anorexia and diuretics.[73]

In the Byzantine world, there was, according to Aetius from Amida, today Dijarbekir, court physician of Emperor Justian I of the six century CE, a special 'doctor of the old people', who tried to give them treatment and ensure a happy old age.[74] The geriatric disorders are gouty arthritis, kidney stones, bronchitis, catarrh, cerebral vascular episodes, loss of memory, psychological problems, tremor and ileus. The medical care of old people included sanitary and dietary regimens, bathing, physiotherapy and the treatment of the age-related diseases.[75]

Byzantine scientists distinguished the different rheumatic diseases as acute rheumatisms, rheumatic arthritis, chronic deforming arthritis, retrogressive arthritis of the aged and gout. They are the first to mention the existence of rheumatic factor and the influence of rheumatism on the function of the heart, as Pantazides remarked.[76] Gout was described

---

[73] Eftychiadis (1997): 217; For the care of the sick, rational medicine and Christianity, see for instance, Leven (1996): 75–84; Ferngren and Amundsen (1996): 2971–2975; On the origin of hospital, see for example Gask and Todd (1953): 122–130; Miller (1997): 30–49, 85–88; Horden (2004): 77–99; idem, (2005): 361–389; Many institutions were staffed by monks and nuns, some of whom were physicians or medical attendants. See Ferngren and Amundsen (1996): 2974–2975.

[74] Aetius Amidenus, *Libri medicinales* I: 52, 56, 82, 85, 97; II: 163–168, (197, 237, 240; III: 278, 282, 342, 352; IV: 372–376; See also Poulakou-Rebelakou and Marketos (1999): 172–176.

[75] Eftychiadis (1997): 218.

[76] Pantazides (1879): 72.

broadly by Demetrius Pepagomenus,[77] and the proper diet by Joannes Chumnus.[78] The first use of colchicine in the treatment of an acute attack of gout is also noted.[79]

As for chronic renal failure, Oribasius Pergamenus, chief physician to Emperor Julian the Apostate in the fourth century CE,[80] generally names the patients nephritics.[81] The pharmacist Nicolaus Myrepsus describes the relationship between severe systemic diseases and chronic renal failure. Simeon Seth, a Jewish physician at the Byzantine court in Constantinople in the eleventh century CE, recognizes chronic renal temperaments due to phlegm.[82] Curative baths, bathing in natural waters and mineral springs, purgative remedies and special diets, such as asparagus, were suggested.[83]

In the Byzantine Empire, the baths continued to exist, primarily in the form of monastery baths and adjoined to churches. These are very small and simple, and give no particular priority to cold chambers. Christian churches became the model for the generally octagonal baptistery. It could be that the early Christians used the *piscinae* for baptism. An institution closely related to the baths and an integral part of them was the ancient *gymnasium*. The Church Fathers were generally suspicious of the *gymnasium* as well as the training in the *palaestra*.[84]

Church authorities who felt the need to be specific on the 'medical intent' of bathing lost no time denouncing the atmosphere of pleasure and sin that might surround a spa. The libertine world of Baiae was censured by both Saint Jerome and Saint Augustine.[85] Hammat-Gader was described by the pagan philosopher and historian Eunapius in the late fourth century CE as a place for relaxation and intellectual pleasures, 'inferior only to those at Baiae in Italy, with which no other baths can be compared'.[86] On the other hand, the Church Father

[77] Demetrius Pepagomenus (1558): 33, 41.
[78] Joannes Chumnus (1844): 220–222.
[79] Eftychiadis (1997): 219.
[80] Oribasius, *Oeuvres* III: 329–337, 362–363, 506, 509, 519, 534; IV:18–19, 355, 571; See also Eftychiadis (2002): 136–138.
[81] Nicolaus Myrepsus (1478): 13, 16, 33, 54, 68, 70, 78, 93, 95, 128–137, 168.
[82] Simeon Seth (1868): 23–28, 54, 100.
[83] Eftychiadis (1997): 220.
[84] Nielsen (1990): I: 38, 104, 138; See also Kazhdan (1991): 271.
[85] Saint Jerome, *Epistulae* 45.4.1; Saint Augustine, *Contra Academicos* 2.2.6; See also Yegül (1992): 317; Comfort (1976).
[86] Eunapius, *Vitae Sophistarum* 459; Ward-Perkins (1981): 166–168; Sukenik (1935a): 21; Lieberman (1946): 354; Hirschfeld and Solar (1981): 202; Jackson (1990a): 5; Dvorjetski (1992a): 105–106; Yegül (1992): 121.

Epiphanius, bishop of Salamis and a contemporary of Eunapius, described disparagingly the colorful atmosphere at Hammat-Gader and its baths. The devil set his snares, since men and women bathed there together. The spa from his point of view is as an abode of wantonness and black magic, where the fashion of bathing to ward off illness or to cure it was abused by unscrupulous people for their own ends, to the detriment of morals.[87]

To sum up, the Church regarded public baths as centres of immorality, issued regulations prohibiting mixed bathing, and condemned frequent visits to the baths by clergy. Monastic baths, which constitute a distinctive and important category, continued to be built throughout the Byzantine era. Under the influence of Christian ethics, the Church viewed with suspicion the habit of mixed bathing, not only for the sake of modesty, but also because of the dictates of ascetic behavior. Although there are innumerable examples for taking a bath, the Church admitted bathing only as a medial measure. Thus, this approach placed the thermal springs in the class of hallowed waters endowed with supernatural healing powers. This frame of mind is reflected in the tradition of bestowing holy names on the therapeutic baths such as the *Baths of Moses* to Hammei-Livias and *Thermae Heliae* to Hammat-Gader and in the very many inscriptions from Hammat-Gader too. These inscriptions bear expressions that the place was viewed not as a pleasure resort or a sporting site consecrated to hygiene and body cure, but as a healing place endowed with a God-given power of restoring health.

9.3   The Contribution of Archaeology to the Christians' Deeds at the Spas in the Levant

The most distinguished and significant contribution of the excavations conducted in the baths of Hammat-Gader, Hammei-Tiberias, Emmaus-Nicopolis, and remains of the Madaba mosaic map from a Byzantine church in Jordan—is the epigraphical material. Most of them were from private persons on the occasion of their visit at the sites—a visit that inspired wonder and gratitude in the presence of the healing powers of the baths.[88] (See Fig. 1).

---

[87] Epiphanius, *Panarion, Adversus Haereses* 30.7; Yegül (1992): 317; Di Segni (1997): 185–186.
[88] Dvorjetski (2003): 9–39; idem, (2004): 16–27, 60; idem, forthcoming [b].

9.3.1   *Thermal Baths of Emmaus-Nicopolis*

A magic amulet was discovered in a tomb at Emmaus-Nicopolis and
dated to the third century CE, inscribed with an incantation in Aramaic
to clear up the afflictions of the patient from his head, muscles, phallus
and ears. The description of the snake, the attribute of Aesculapius,
on the amulet seems to hint at the therapeutic qualities of Emmaus,
which are documented in Church Fathers' texts, as good not only for
humans but also for animals.[89] Vincent suggested that it was done by
a Jewish artisan at the request of a Christian.[90] (See Fig. 28).

9.3.2   *Thermal Baths of Ba'arah and Kallirrhoe*

The sixth century CE Madaba mosaic map, which laid in a Byzantine
church at Madaba in Jordan allots considerable space to the thermo-
mineral baths of Kallirrhoe and Hammei-Ba'arah, including the
inscriptions [BA]APOY *and* ΘΕΡΜΑΚΑΛΛΙΡΟΗC, (See Fig. 25) and
to two boats carrying cargo, testifying to the transport of goods on
the Dead Sea in that period. The mosaicists of the map represented
along the eastern shore of the Dead Sea three constructions.[91] Various
possibilities have been offered about the cargoes on these boats, such
as goods, sails, Bitumen, salt or import of wheat. Another option is a
maritime marketing of the healing sites characterizing thermo-mineral
baths in the Graeco-Roman world, which can be any kind of glass vessels, pottery assemblages, and medical instruments.[92] We know of boats
in the Roman world that carried various cargoes from the therapeutic
sites. Among them were glass vessels that contained liquids for healing purposes. For instance, the healing site in northern Spain, Otanẽs,
known as Salus Omeritana, gained fame from its waters, which were
exported to distant locations. Glass bottles from the thermal waters in
the Bay of Naples, Baiae and neighboring Poteoli, arrived in North
Africa; engraved on them were schematic scenes of the spas, where
the bottles were manufactured and marketed.[93]

---

[89] Vincent and Abel (1932): 416–418; Dvorjetski (1996a); idem, (2004): 20.
[90] Vincent (1908): 382–394; cf. Naveh and Shaked (1985): 60–63.
[91] Avi-Yonah (1954): 39–40; Donner (1963); Clamer (1996); idem, (1999); Dvorjetski
(1996c).
[92] Dvorjetski (1996c).
[93] Rostovtzeff (1957): 478–479; de Franciscis (1967); Painter (1975); Krug (1993):
181; Jackson (1999): 115–116; Dvorjetski (1997a).

9.3.3   *The Epigraphical Material from Hammat-Gader Thermal Baths*

The Greek dedication inscriptions from Hammat-Gader dated to the fifth-seventh centuries CE contributed greatly to the reconstruction of the history and daily life of the spa, especially the Christian ones.

Hammat-Gader reached its apex of publicity in the fifth century CE and gained momentum. Testifying to this, are the imperial building inscriptions from governors of Palestina *Secunda*, which were found in the Fountain Hall. This shows the great reputation that the thermo-mineral baths had acquired and also the healing of the sicks, who streamed to the site from throughout the Empire.[94]

The most important inscription bears the name and title of Empress Eudocia, the wife of Emperor Theodosius II (408–450 CE). (See Fig. 13). It was discovered in *situ* in the pavement of the Hall of the Fountains, and was probably composed on the occasion of Eudocia's visit to Hammat-Gader.[95] (See Fig. 12). Meïmaris suggests that Eudocia's visit to the famous baths could be associated with a medical reason.[96] The *Vita Melaniae* written by Gerontius, abbot on Mount of Olives, recounts that during the inauguration of Saint Stephen Protomartyr church in Jerusalem on May 15, 439 CE, an accident caused her severe pain in her left leg and Empress came to Hammat-Gader to cure it.[97]

At the beginning of the inscription there are crosses and a long list of private names, pagan and Christian titles, mythological figures, such as Hygieia, Galatea, Paean and parts of the baths, pools and fountains, names and titles of various people as 'Elijah the Holy', whose honor the thermae was later said to have been named *Thermae Heliae*. Eudocia's poetic inscription in Homeric style glorifies the hot springs 'for those in pain', and extols the marvels of the architectural complex.[98]

Toward the end of the Byzantine period, the location was hit by an earthquake. The destruction caused the baths is documented in a Greek-Byzantine inscription from the seventh century. The dedicatory inscription, discovered in the Fountain Hall, cites the reopening and renovation

---

[94] Di Segni and Hirschfeld (1986): 265–267.
[95] Hirschfeld and Solar (1981): 203; Green and Tsafrir (1982): 77–91; Dvorjetski (1988): 101–107; idem, (1992a): 111–112; Di Segni (1997): 228–233.
[96] Meïmaris (1983): 394.
[97] Gerontius, *Vita Melaniae* 59.244; Hunt (1982): 230–231; Clark (1984): 139–140; Habas-Rubin (1996): 112–113; Di Segni (1997): 232.
[98] Hirschfeld and Solar (1981): 203; Green and Tsafrir (1982); 77–91; Di Segni (1997): 228–223.

of the baths in the early days of the Caliph Mu'āwiya, founder of the
Umayyad dynasty, on 5 December 662 CE. The Greek language of
the inscription, the cross at its head, and the use of Byzantine dating
testify to the fact that the Arab ruler did not at first alter the existing
administrative and cultural arrangements.[99] (See Fig. 21).

Except for the small group of building inscriptions, most texts open
with the words Ἐν τῷ ἀγὶῳ or (ἱερῷ) τόπῳ μνησθῇ, which means 'in this
holy place may someone be remembered', or in plural Ἐν τοῖς ἁγίοις
τόποις μνησθῇ, 'in these holy places may someone be remembered',
or simply Ἐν τῷ τόπῳ τούτῳ μνήσθωσιν, which means 'in this place
may be remembered', and Ἐν τῷ χαριεστάτῳ τοπῳ τούτῳ μνησθῇ, 'in
this graceful place may someone be remembered'. Appeals to God,
κύριε [= Lord] and to Christ for help [= Χριστὲ] βοτήθ(ε)ι] or Lord
Christ, remember [= Κ(ύριε) Χρ(ιστ)ὴ μνήσθη] are frequency used.
(See, for instance, Figs. 16, 17, 18, and 20). There are many inscriptions surmounted by deeply carved crosses, which were later obliterated
neatly, by careful chiseling. The deletion might be carried out by the
Muslims as an anti-Christian gesture. A very obvious proof might be
learnt from the word φιλοχριστὸς, which was deleted too and would
point to iconoclasm at the hands of Muslims. It could be also in the
Byzantine period, since in 427 Theodosius II Code forbade the depiction of crosses in places where they could be trodden upon. Another
possibility was the days of Emperor Justinian, a confirmed meddler in
religious issues, who might have insisted on the fulfillment of his order
in this matter.[100]

At Hammat-Gader no less than 24 inscriptions are decorated with
one or more crosses. Most of them are deeply and carefully carved
on slabs or engraved under the script, and some are graffiti on plaster,
scratched or painted. Some of the visitors mentioned their homeland;
among them an *agens in rebus* from Gaza, a *tribunus* [= commanding
officer] from Damascus and governors from Caesarea. An acclamation in honor of Perge, the capital of Pamphylia, shows that some of
its citizens came here came from a distance as well. Several visitors
indicated their title, rank or profession among them were a notary, a
scriber, public weigher, marble worker, engraver, peddler, senior army
officers, ranks which reflected highest aristocracy such as countess,

---

[99] Hirschfeld and Solar (1981): 203–204; Green and Tsafrir (1982): 94–96; Di Segni
and Hirschfeld (1986): 265–266; Dvorjetski (1988): 109–110; idem, (1992a): 113; Di
Segni (1992): 315–317; idem, (1997): 237–240.
[100] Di Segni (1997):185, 254.

illustris specially for wives of nobility, singulais (clerk in the military or in the civil administration), and more. The stage professions, which represent the largest group—a dancer, a piper, an actress, a juggler, and perhaps a strolling actor—were not Christians. These performers were permanent or visiting members of its staff in the Roman theatre of Hammat-Gader, which was still active in the Byzantine period.[101] (See Map 3).

An onomastic examination of the inscriptions decorated with crosses revealed an impressive variety of names of men and women. It may be assumed that the many visitors mentioned prayed in the church that was east of the baths, north of ʿAin er-Rih spring, and had given a substantial donation to have their names immortalized there.

The donors' inscriptions in the synagogues at Hammat-Tiberias, dated to the fourth century CE,[102] and Hammat-Gader from the fifth-sixth century CE,[103] in addition to some little finds shed light on Jewish-Christian relations in the Late Roman and Byzantine periods. The mosaic inscriptions from both sites were dedicated in the names of donors who contributed to the synagogues' buildings. These donors might have been cured at Hammat-Gader and Hammei-Tiberias and commemorated their recovery by contributing to the development of the sites. The formula of the blessing in the inscription from Hammei-Tiberias 'May he be alive' or 'to survive safely' (ζήσῃ; σωζέστω) repeated five times, is unusual, and such a blessing, wishing the donors life, is apt for sick people, who have come to the place for a cure.[104] It may be assumed that Christians were among the donors in light of the multiplicity of Greek and Latin names, among them Μάξιμος, Ζωΐλος, Καλλίνικος, Ἰοῦλλος and Προφοτῦρος. The name Εἰορτάσις was very rare among Jews. The dedicatory inscription to Σευῆρος has these words: θρεπτὸς τῶν λαμπροτάτων πατριαρχῶν [= disciple of the most illustrious Patriarchs]. The prominent place allotted to his dedication, the special blessing accorded him, and his appearance in a second inscription—all indicate that Severus was a donor or the chief founder, who fulfilled an important task in renovating the synagogue at Hammei-Tiberias. (See Fig. 31).

[101] Di Segni (1992): 309–310; idem, (1997): 189–190, 198–200, 204–216, 218–222, 224– 225, 235–237, 241–244, 246, 251–252.
[102] Dothan (1983).
[103] Sukenik (1935a); Avi-Yonah and Hirschfeld (1993).
[104] Roth-Gerson (1987): 65–69.

Likewise, among the donors in the Aramaic dedicatory inscriptions in the Hammat-Gader synagogue are many Greek and Latin names, such as Hoplis, Proton, Leontis, Kalnikos, and Paregurius, titles like κύρος and κύρα [= Lord and Lady], holders of government posts, and wealthy visitors.[105] Gentile donors are known to have contributed to the temple and to synagogues in the Second Temple period. Therefore, it seems that not all the donors were Jewish. Some of them, who came to be healed, sought to donate to the holy place in order to express their thanks to the place or in order for its special qualities to assist in their cure. Most of the donors to the synagogues gave after having made a pledge and the inscription cites those who fulfilled their obligation.

In the excavation of the synagogue area at Hammat-Gader, rings were found. One of them bore a Greek inscription: Χ^ε [= Χριστὲ] βοτή(ει) Ἀνδρεᾳ [= Lord (Christ), help Andrea]. There was a Byzantine oil lamp and a cross at the bottom.[106] In front of the entrance to the Hall of Inscriptions at Hammat-Gader, there is an inscription dating to 455 CE: 'In this holy place may Marcus the scribe be remembered together with his sons, Joshua, also (called) Theodorus and Daniel also (called) Antoninus, (born) from his marriage with Nonna. Amen. The inscription is decorated with crosses, but the names are Jewish or Samaritan. In 438 CE, Emperor Theodosius II published decrees against the Jews, the first of which limited their occupation in the civil service. Conceivably the father of the family, Marcus, was a state official who converted his religion in order to preserve his position and to continue his career. Such a location of his dedication directly in front of the entrance indicates that he contributed a substantial sum for the paving of the sports area.[107]

In conclusion it is important to point out that the early Christians normally accepted a visit to the baths as a natural part of life. The Church Fathers testify that baths were still a part of the health regimen of their day. They did not normally prohibit Christians from bathing or urge them to curb the habit; in fact they bathed themselves, like everyone else. They were an integral part of urban life. As Tertullian

---

[105] Naveh (1978): 11, 58.
[106] Sukenik (1935a): 70–71.
[107] Di Segni (1997): 189–190.

said, 'The Christians are no different than other people: they go to the forum, to the marcellum, and to the baths'.[108]

Mixed bathing it naturally condemned as an incitement to sin. It was gradually given up, eventually to be strictly forbidden. Church fathers repeatedly condemned the temptations of the luxurious baths. The Church's interest in baths was primarily in public morality. The church was strict in proscribing this custom, allowing the use of the baths only for healing, especially the spas.

Certain places in the eastern Mediterranean gained great fame because of their healing qualities and their effectiveness in curing health ailments and disturbances. The descriptions by the Church Fathers, chronographers, and pilgrims produce an instructive picture of the medicinal baths. They add the most important layer in understanding the properties of the spas, which can be classified to specific maladies. The spas were used not only for medical proposes but also for leisure and recreation. There emerges a fascinating picture of a luxurious and immoral life. During the Later Roman and Byzantine periods, these unique sites served also as a preservation of the classical culture. Hammat-Gader was indeed a special combination of a festival, an entertainment centre and a place of social gathering for the life of debauchery.

Further evidence of the medicinal properties is provided by archaeological finds. The Greek inscriptions from Hammat-Gader faithfully tell the history and daily life of the thermo-mineral baths. Most of them were from private persons on the occasion of their visit at the sites—a visit that inspired wonder and gratitude in the presence of the healing powers of the water. The inscriptions viewed the baths of Hammat-Gader not as a pleasure resort site consecrated to hygiene and body care, but as a healing place endowed with a God-given power of restoring health. Mutual relations between Jews and Christians were natural and affable in the baths in the framework of leisure culture, healing installations, and places of entertainment. The integration of sacred springs, healing baths, and cultic installations offered a special combination of religious, medicinal and social conveniences to the many pilgrims who visited the spas in the eastern Mediterranean basin in the Later Roman and Byzantine periods.

---

[108] Tertullian, *Apologeticum* 42.2.

CHAPTER TEN

EPILOGUE

Thermo-mineral waters are found on the earth's surface where there are geological rifts. The Jordan Valley is a result of a geological rift, which extends from east Africa in the south to Asia Minor in the North. The most famous spas in the eastern Mediterranean basin are located along the Syro-African Rift in the Jordan: Hammei-Tiberias, Hammat-Gader, Hammei-Ba'arah, Kallirrhoe, Hammat-Pella, and Hammei-Livias. Another one is Emmaus-Nicopolis situated at the Ayalon Valley on the road that ascends from the west to Jerusalem.

Geologists, hydrologists and geochemists have for many years been trying to answer questions about the formation of the thermo-mineral waters and the source of their waters in the Eastern Mediterranean Basin, and have suggested various models for their creation: a magmatic source, e.g., vapors and gases rising from the boiling lava inside the earth; an ancient salt lake whose waters, trapped and preserved in reservoirs deep beneath the ground, are now surfacing as hot brine; remnants of ocean water that percolated down to the depths of the rift in the periods when the ocean penetrated the Jordan Valley; rainwater that dissolves salt deposits or grains of salt scattered in the rocks forming the Jordan depression. It is most plausible that the thermo-mineral waters—the *Hammoth*, the hot springs or warm baths—are phenomena that accompany volcanic activities that have subsided.

In antiquity there were more places with medical hot springs, but in the course of time their sources either dried up or became plugged. It is natural enough that over the generations there should be changes in the abundance of the springs and the quality of their waters. Geological researchers have also shown that springs are sometimes blocked after earthquakes. There is considerable doubt whether there was any use of hot springs as health resorts before the Roman period since there are allusions already in the Bible.

Today we know most of the components that determine the medicinal characteristics of the curative springs. Their waters are hyperthermal and contain salts, gases and basic radioactive material. The springs have been classified by their effectiveness against specific illnesses and complaints such as: rheumatic illnesses, pulmonary diseases, digestive and urinary ailments, dermatological and sexual problems, gynecological and nervous diseases. Various analyses of the water have shown that it has therapeutic qualities and that it may be drunk as mineral water. Their early use and development was related to the growing interest in bathing and medicine in the first centuries of the Roman Empire. Spas provided a new method for improving health, which combined the comforts of the bath with innovative treatments based on rational and logical medicine.

An etymological investigation indicates that the common name *Hammat, Hammtha Hammei, Hammoth* in Hebrew, Syriac or Aramaic, *Emmaous*, or *Emmatha* in Greek, and *Hamma*, or *Hammamat* in Arabic, is an adjectival noun shared by places that have hot springs. All the sites have almost identical terms since they are the dominant, inseparable component of each of the mother cities. In some Talmudic literature, the site Emmaus is called *Demosin* or *Demosit*, short for the Greek 'public bath'. Emmaus itself is a Hellenized version of the Hebrew *Hammat*, or Aramaic *Hammatha*, meaning 'hot springs', 'hot baths', or 'spa'. The common Latin words used to indicate a thermo-mineral spring are *fons* and *aquae*. In many of the Greek phases, an adjective is also attached to the noun to give a more specific meaning. In spite of that, there is no clear distinction between the words used to describe the springs and those used to describe the spas. The word *aquae* can refer not only to the springs at a spa, but to the actual spa itself, so that it is sometimes obscure which is meant. There is less confusion in the Greek texts because the writers tended to refer to a spa by name and to identify specific of springs available at a spa.

The combined literary and epigraphic sources, the archaeological findings, and the numismatic evidence since the Biblical era throughout the Hellenistic, Roman, Byzantine and early Muslim periods enabled us to examine the history, the medicinal properties and the cultural aspects of the therapeutic baths.

The evidences of Greek and Roman writers, Church Fathers, pilgrims and the Rabbinic literature show several common denominators of these sites. Firstly, the medicinal springs served the two-fold purpose of bathing and drinking; Secondly, the effectiveness of the springs was for specific ailments and disturbances, such as: dermatological conditions, urinary and digestive tracts, general debilitation, rheumatism, nervous and venereal diseases; Thirdly, the properties of the therapeutic baths can be classified to specific maladies; Fourthly, the places were used not only for bathing and medical proposes but also for leisure and recreation; Fifthly, there emerges a fascinating picture of a luxurious, reckless and immoral life. Including varied activity with pagan elements, the Sages were forced to limit and restrict the activity.

Bath-buildings were habitually combined with structures and spaces devoted to other leisure activities: libraries, lecture-halls, lounges, sports grounds, gardens and paths for walks, all put together in a clever homo-geneity and symmetry of design. Of all the leisure activities, bathing was surely the most important for the greatest number of Romans, since it was part of the daily regimen for men of all classes, and many women as well. Next to buildings used for shows, the most characteristic structures of Roman cities were undoubtedly the *thermae* or public baths. The Roman baths, above all in their public, imperially funded form, were pleasure palaces dedicated to the principle of enjoyment. They were centres of social gathering and worship where intellectual and recreational activities as well as health and hygiene were pursued.

The Romans believed that the divinities gave springs healing pow-ers that led to the successful curing of patients who worshiped them. The Romans and later the Byzantines, who ruled the eastern Mediter-ranean lands, paid particular attention to thermal water sources and developed them for curative and recreational purposes. Evidence of their engineering ingenuity can be recognized among the remnants of ancient waterworks around thermo-mineral springs: Hammei-Tiberias, Hammat-Gader, Kallirrhoe, and Emmaus-Nicopolis.

The spa institution has been a unique subject worthy of study. It has served a different purpose, and has a different architectural and technical fixtures involved with heating. Sometimes there were single-person pools, which allowed people to bathe individually and treat-ment chambers. These baths were dependent on the presence of hot and/or mineral springs, which means that they were independent of the cities and arose where nature allowed them to. Since thermal baths were usually outside cities, accommodations for housing and feeding patients must have been furnished. The temperature of the water was high, so cooling equipment was needed by means of two options either by an installation of cooling basins or mixing of hot thermal water with fresh water. Moreover, the treatments found in spas were aimed at specific needs and focused on the thermo-mineral springs. They pri-marily served medical purposes, as a kind of *valetudinarium* with medical facilities and instruments, although they were also social resorts with a wide range of activities, and many different circles frequented them.

Findings of medical instruments indicate that physicians were present at the healing sites.

Like the public baths, the use of therapeutic hot springs has its origin in ancient Roman tradition. While the public baths were an important institution in Roman society and also served as cultural centres and meeting places, the Romans also constructed magnificent bathhouses wherever there were hot springs. Ordinary bathing certainly was an important factor in the improvement of health and hygiene, but the Romans believed that the spas offered a distinct medical treatment for health problems. A military presence was the key to the development of these places. Normally it was the army and not the civilians who constructed the first elaborate bath complexes employing thermal water in newly conquered territories that did not yet have adequate installations. Only the army could provide a sufficient number of specialists for the realization of such projects in areas which had no tradition in stone building and hydraulic engineering. Since most army members were recruited from areas where bathing culture was well established, they were also the ones who felt the need for such installations. Soldiers requiring long-term care might be granted sick leave during which time they could return home, if this was feasible, or be sent somewhere suitable to recuperate, such as a spa. Thus, considerable military resources were often allotted to the building of the facilities at therapeutic sites; the military sick and wounded were sent to these places, which also served as rest and recreation centres for healthy soldiers and likewise centre of culture, education, sport, and therapy. Some of the dedicatory Greek inscriptions found at Hammat-Gader and Hammei-Ba'arah suggest that the military personnel did travel in search of cures and convalescence. The presence of soldiers spurred the economic growth of the sites, but not a few clashes developed between the soldiers and the local population.

Certain places gained great fame because of their healing qualities and their effectiveness in curing various ailments. Temples were erected at therapeutic sites. Each site had a spring that served as the dominant part of the bathhouse complex and was dedicated to a god of healing. Within the boundaries of the Roman Empire local deities were integrated with their parallel Graeco-Roman deities. The ritual worship in the eastern Mediterranean basin is expressed in most interesting types of Hygieia, Aesculapius, the Three Graces and the Nymphs. Besides the Graeco-Roman gods, Egyptian Serapis and the local Zeus Beelbaaros, the local Baal of Hammei-Ba'arah, played an important role in the nature of the spas as healing and fertility local gods. The numismatic and the epigraphic evidences and little finds with the ritual characteristics of the curative sites likewise shed light and add unique information about variegated use of medicine in antiquity, the maladies, and the relationship between Jews and gentiles at the curative baths in the eastern Mediterranean. The inscriptions faithfully tell the history and daily life of the thermo-mineral waters of Hammat-Gader. Most of them were from private persons on the occasion of their visit at the sites—a visit that inspired wonder and gratitude in the presence of the healing powers of the water. Other poetically-styled lapidary inscriptions bear witness to the high reputation of the place, their beauty, dimensions and the therapeutic properties of their hot waters. Archaeological finds from the Roman, Byzantine and Muslim periods support this reputation with evidence of the great numbers of bathers, who flocked to the site seeking cures and medical treatment. The baths would thus appear to have become the focus of interest of the rich and powerful, who, in an effort to perpetuate their names, commissioned various inscriptions in the magnificent structures of the bathhouse. The governors' concern with the healing of the sick was also reasons for the restoration of the baths during the fifth-seventh centuries CE. These inscriptions indirectly indicate also the cultural atmosphere, which prevailed at Hammat-Gader and other sites in Late Antiquity.

The theoretical basis for the use of the therapeutic springs lies in the teaching of Hippocrates. His ideas were developed systematically by Roman and Byzantine physicians. People of all kinds bathed at the sites. Many military and civil officials, Roman and Byzantine Emperors visited the curative baths in the Levant both during military operations and in times of peace, either for their maladies or for visiting the army. The spas attracted very large numbers of visitors, among whom the wealthiest made generous benefactions which sometimes brought an architectural splendor. Healed people customarily expressed their gratitude to the gods and divinities of the hot springs in the Classical world by leaving a variety of offerings: artifacts, coins, pillars and terracotta votives. Anyhow, beside the possibility for intensive body care, all thermal springs were a centre of the mental and cultural life, were able to alleviate many illnesses, and that their effectiveness in soothing and pains and afflictions were well known. A belief in the effectiveness of the water lay at the centre of the use of thermo-mineral springs for healing.

Bathing was linked to nakedness and sinfulness. For the early Christians, it was associated with evil and promiscuity. The Church regarded

public baths as centres of immorality, issued regulations prohibiting
mixed bathing and condemned frequent visits to the baths by clergy.
Monastic baths, which constitute a distinctive and important category,
continued to be built throughout the Byzantine era. Under the influence of Christian ethics, the Church viewed with suspicion the habit
of mixed bathing, not only for the sake of modesty, but also because of
the dictates of ascetic behavior. Although there are innumerable examples for taking a bath, the Church admitted bathing only as a medial
measure. Thus, this approach placed the thermal springs in the class
of hallowed waters endowed with supernatural healing powers. This
frame of mind is reflected in the tradition of bestowing holy names
on the therapeutic baths such as *Baths of Moses* to Hammei-Livias and
Thermae Heliae to Hammat-Gader and in the very many inscriptions
from Hammat-Gader too. These inscriptions bear expressions that the
place was viewed not as a pleasure resort or a sporting site consecrated
to hygiene and body cure, but as a healing place endowed with a God-
given power of restoring health.

   Church authorities who felt the need to be specific on the 'medical
intent' of bathing lost no time denouncing the atmosphere of pleasure
and sin that might surround a spa. The libertine world of Hammat-
Gader was censured by Church Fathers. Thus, for instance, Hammat-
Gader was described by the pagan philosopher and historian Eunapius
in the late fourth century CE as a place for relaxation and intellectual
pleasures, 'inferior only to those at Baiae in Italy, with which no other
baths can be compared'. On the other hand, Epiphanius, Bishop of
Salamis and a contemporary of Eunapius, described disparagingly the
colorful atmosphere at Hammat-Gader and its baths. The devil set his
snares, since men and women bathed there together. The spa from his
point of view is as an abode of wantonness and black magic, where
the fashion of bathing to ward off illness or to cure it was abused by
unscrupulous people for their own ends, to the detriment of morals.
Hammat-Gader was indeed a special combination of a festival, an
entertainment centre and a place of social gathering for the life of
debauchery. However, the sixth century CE Madaba mosaic map, which
laid in a Byzantine church at Madaba in Jordan, allots considerable
space to the thermo-mineral waters of Kallirrhoe and Ba'arah. This
map served, among other things, as a guide for those wishing specifically
to visit particular spas, presumably with the intent of taking advantage
of the healing benefits of the spring waters.

   The descriptions by Church Fathers, chronographers and pilgrims produce an instructive picture of the medicinal baths. They add the most important layer in understanding the properties of the spas, which can be classified to specific maladies. The spas were used not only for medical proposes but also for leisure and recreation. During the Later Roman and Byzantine periods, these unique sites served also as a preservation of the classical culture.

Baths were, apart from the issue of prostitution, highly sexualized places and they might easily acquire a reputation as centres of prostitution, especially if both sexes were present. It is plausible that the Church Fathers and the Rabbis were aware of this and not only the fear of temptation was their main reason for equating baths with lust.

The Sages for the life of frivolity and licence deprecated the cities with thermo-mineral waters. The therapeutic activity of the springs itself was interpreted negatively by them. The nature of the thermal springs has implications in law for daily life: cooking, drinking and danger of scalding; immersion; the ritual washing of the hands, and bathing. Over the generations the Sages wrestled with the various aspects of *halakhah* concerning the spas. Jewish religious laws that deal with these thermo-mineral waters, and whose concern are the Sabbath prohibitions, were adapted to take account of the benefits of the therapeutic sites. The Sages knew the healing qualities of the thermo-mineral waters. There are knowledge and recommendations on these waters in the Talmudic literature. From the behavioral patterns at the baths and the laws connected with them, it is evident that the Sages did not prohibit the use of the baths per se, but rather attempted to prevent the spread of the gentile practices in them. This approach stems from the Sages' understanding that they would not be able to eliminate the phenomenon entirely; it sufficed to adapt it to their world-view. But use of the baths raised grave reservations because idolatrous statues were customarily displayed in them. In spite of that, interesting permissions were authorized by the Sages, and a vivid picture of daily life is reflected in some stories in the *Jerusalem Talmud*. In other words, their use by the Jewish inhabitants created a conflict between the popular need, especially for healing, and the religious restrictions, which were discussed and decreed by the Talmudic Sages.

There is reason to believe that some Rabbis, even apart from the Patriarch, took more liberties than the codified *halakha* allowed. An outstanding example in the region is that of the suburb of Gadara—Hammat-Gader curative site—the favorite resort of some Rabbis in the third and fourth century CE. The well known site was thoroughly pagan in character. Not only did all the springs and baths have mythological names, but the annual festival that took place there, as well as the common practices of incubation and commemoration of miraculous cures, clearly indicates that the spa was not simply a place of recreation to the many visitors, but also functioned as a shrine especially to Aesculapius, to Hygieia, to the Three Graces, and to Serapis. The willingness of some Rabbis to patronize a place like Hammat-Gader demonstrates what we might have supposed anyway—a greater diversity of Rabbinic behaviour and opinion than the Rabbinic sources indicate.

The numerous dedicatory inscriptions, frequent recommendations by medical writers and non-specialists, and the existence of many thermomineral establishments throughout the eastern Mediterranean basin and the rest of the Roman-Byzantine world, provide an unequivocal demonstration of the important role spas had in medicine in antiquity. The aggregation of sacred springs, therapeutic baths and cultic installations offered a combination of religious, medicinal and social institutions to the many who visited the curative sites through the ages, especially the Roman, Byzantine, and Early Muslim periods.

The spas were regarded highly for their ability to restore health, and at the same time the waters were treated as a source of enjoyment and delectation. The regimens and general ambience of some of these spas cannot have been so very different to those of the watering places, modern spas or health clubs, of 20th century Europe and Levant. Further study, mainly of the archaeological evidence from therapeutic sites in Israel and Jordan, will provide new results that can as yet only be suggested hypothetically.

BIBLIOGRAPHY

Primary Sources

ad-Dimašqī, Shams al-Dîn Muhammad b. Ibrâhîm, *Nuhbat ad-dahr fi aga'ib al-bar wa-l-bahr* (ed. A.F.M. Mehren). Saint-Pétersbourg, 1866. [A]

Aetius Amidenus, *Libri medicinale* (ed. and tr. A. Olivieri). I–III, Lipsiae, 1935.

al-Baladhuri, Ahmad ibn Jābir, *Kitāb futūh al-buldān* (ed. M.J. de Goeje), *BGA*. Leiden, 1866 [= (tr. P. Hitti). *The Origins of the Islamic State*. Beirut, 1966]. [A]

al-Idrīsī, Muhammad b. Muhammad, *Kitāb nuzhat al-mushtāq fi ikhtirāq al-'afāq* (eds. E. Cerulli et al.). Neapoli, 1970–1984 [= (ed. J. Gildemeister), 'Beiträge zur Palästinakunde aus arabischen Quellen', *ZDPV* 8: 117–145]. [A]

al-Istahrī, Abū Ishāq al-Fārisī, *Suwar al-aklim* (ed. M.J. de Goeje). *BGA* I, Leiden, 1888. [A]

al-Muqaddasi, *Ahsan al-taqasim fi ma'rifat al-aqalim* (ed. M.J. de Goeje). *BGA* III, Leid 1906. [A]

al-Ya'qubi, Ibn Wadiah, *Kitab al-buldān* (ed. M.J. de Goeje). *BGA* VII, Leiden, 1892. [A]

al-Yāqūt ibn 'Abd Allāh, *Mu'jam al-buldān* (ed. F. Wüstenfeld). III, Leipzig, 1868. [A]

Ammianus Marcellinus, *Res Gestae* (ed. and tr. J.C. Rolfe). *LCL*, 1963.

Antoninus Placantinus, *Itinerarium*. *CCSL*, 175, Turnhout, 1967.

Arculfus, *De Locis Sanctis* (ed. P. Mickley), *Arculf—De locis sanctis*. Leipzig, 1971: 26–27.

Aretaeus, *Chronic Diseases* (ed. and tr. F. Adams). London 1856.

Aristides, Aelius, *On Rome* (ed. and tr. C.A. Behr). *LCL*, 1973.

Aristophanes, *The Clouds* (ed. and tr. B.B. Rogers). *LCL*, 1963.

Augustine, *Contra Academicos*. *CSEL*, LXIII: 3–4.

Augustine, *Epistulae*. *CSEL*, XXXIV, XLIV, LVII.

Barsenuphius, *Quaestiones* (ed. S.N. Schoinas). Volos, 1960.

Basil, *Epistulae* (ed. P. Geyer), *PG*, XXXII: 219–220.

Bede Venerabilis, *De Locis Sanctis* (ed. P. Geyer) *Itinera Hierosolymitana*. Lipsiae, 1898: 316.

Caelius Aurelianus, *De Acutis Morbis* (ed. and tr. I.E. Drabkin). *On Acute Diseases and on Chronic Diseases*. Chicago, 1950.

Cassiodorus Aurelius, *Chronicon* (ed. J.P. Migne). *PL*, LXIX.

Cassius Dio, *Historia Romana* (ed. and tr. E. Cary). *LCL*, 1961.

Cedrenus, *Historiarum Compendium* (ed. J.P. Migne). *PG*, CXXI: 582.

Celsus, *De Medicina* (ed. and tr. W.G. Spencer). *LCL*, 1938.

Chrysostom Johannes, *De Sanctis Martyribus Sermo* (ed. J.P. Migne). *PG*, L: 2, cols. 647–648.

——, *Homilae in Joannem* (ed. J.P. Migne). *PG*, LIX: 118.

——, *Matthaeu Homilae* (ed. J.P. Migne). *PG*, LI: 239.

Chronicon Paschale (ed. L. Dindorf). *CSHB*, I: 474; *PG*, XCII: 657.

Claudian, *Carmina Minora* (ed. and tr. M. Platnauer), *LCL*, 1922.

Clement of Alexandria, *Paedagogus* (tr. S.P. Wood). *The Fathers of the Church, Clement of Alexandria*. Washington, 1954.

Demetrius Pepagomenus, Σύνταγμα περὶ ποδάγρας. Parisiis: Morelius, 1558.

Didascalia Apostolorum (ed. and tr. R.H. Connolly). Oxford: Clarendon Press: 1929.

Diodorus Siculus, *Bibliotheca Historica* (C.H. Oldfather). *LCL*, 1970.

Enoch, *The Apocrypha and Pseudepigrapha of the Old Testament* (ed. R.H. Charles). Oxford, 1913 [repr. 1977].

Epiphanius, *Panarion, Adversus Haereses* (ed. J.P. Migne) *PG*, XLI: 416–417.

Eunapius, *Vitae Sophistarum* (ed. and tr. W.C. Wright). *LCL*, 1968.

Eusebius of Caesarea, *Onomastikon* (ed. E. Klosterman) *Eusebius Das Onomastikon der biblischen Ortsnamen.* Hildesheim, 1966.

——, *Historia Ecclesiastica* (ed. E. Schwartz). *GCS* IX, Leipzig 1903–1908 [= *PG*, XX]; (ed. and tr. J.E.L. Oulton). I–II, *LCL*, 1932.

——, *Chronicorum Libri Duo* (ed. A. Schone). II, Berlin 1875.

Galen, *In Hippocrates, De Natura Hominis, CMG*, V 9.1, 106.15–21.

——, *De Method Medendi* (ed. C.G. Kühn). VIII, Leipzig, 1821–1833.

George Cedrenus, *Historiarum Compendium* (ed. J.P. Migne), *PG*, CXXI: 582.

Gerontius, *Vita Melaniae Junioris* (ed. D. Gorce), *Vie de sainte Mélanie, Sources Chrétiennes*, No. 90. Paris, 1962.

Gregory of Nyssa, *Opera* (ed. J.P. Migne). *PG*, XXXV–XXXVIII. [= ed. W. Jaeger, *Opera.* Leiden, 1966].

Gregory of Tours, *De Gloria Martyrum* (tr. R. Van Dam). Liverpool, 1988.

Herodotus, *Historiae* (ed. and tr. A.D. Godley). *LCL*, 1961.

Hierocles, *Synecdemus* (ed. G. Parthey). Amsterdam, 1967.

Hieronymus [= Jerome], *De viris illustribus* (ed. J.P. Migne), *PL*, XIII.

——, *Epistulae* (ed. J.P. Migne), *PL*, XXII. [= *CSEL*, LIV–LVI].

——, *Liber Hebraicarum Quaestionum in Genesim* (ed. J.P. Migne), *PL*, XXIII.

——, *Onomastikon* (ed. E. Klosterman), *Eusebius Das Onomastikon der biblischen Ortsnamen.* Hildesheim, 1966.

——, *Paulae et Eustochii ad Marcellam, Epistola* XLVI (A), (ed. J.P. Migne), *PL*, XXIII.

Hippocrates, *Aphorisms* (tr. T. Coar). Birmingham, 1982.

——, *Places in man* (ed. and tr. E.M. Craik). Oxford, 1998.

——, *Regimen in Acute Diseases* (ed. and tr. W.H.S. Jones). *LCL*, 1959.

Homer, *Iliad* (ed. and tr. A.T. Murray). *LCL*, 1963.

——, *Odyssey* (ed. and tr. A.T. Murray). *LCL*, 1966.

Ibn al-Kalbī, Hisham, *Kitāb al-Asnam* (ed. R. Klinke-Rosenberger). Leipzig, 1941.

Ibn Fadl Allah al-ʿUmari, Ahmad ibn Yahyá, *al-Taʿrif bi-al-mustalah al-sharif* (ed. S. al-Droubi). al-Karak, Jordan, 1992.

Ibn Hisham, Abu Muhammad ʿAbd al-Malik, *Kitāb Sirat Rasul Allah* (ed. F. Wüstenfeld). Göttingen, 1859–1860.

Josephus, *Antiquitates Judaicae* (ed. and tr. L.H. Feldman). *LCL*, 1965.

——, *Bellum Judaicum* (ed. and tr. H. Thackeray). *LCL*, 1927.

——, *Vita* (ed. and tr. H. Thackeray). *LCL*, 1965.

Livy, *Historia Romana* (ed. and tr. B.O. Foster). *LCL*, 1962–1969.

Lucianus of Samosata, *Dialogi Deorum* (ed. and tr. M.D. Macleod). *LCL*, 1961.

——, *The True History, Nigrinus* (ed. and tr. A.M. Harmon), *LCL*, 1961.

Malalas John, *Chronographia* (ed. L. Dindorf). Bonn 1831 [= (trs. E. Jeffreys, M. Jeffreys and R. Scot). Melbourne, 1996].

Martial, *Epigrammata* (ed. and tr. W.C.A. Ker). *LCL*, 1968.

Michael the Syrian, *Chronicle* (ed. J.B. Chabot). I–IV. Bruxelles, 1963. [S]

Moschus Joannes, *Pratum Spirituale* (ed. J.P. Migne), *PG*, LXXXVII/3: 3032.

Nâsir-i-Khusrau, *Tahlil-i Safarnāmah* (ed. and tr. W.M. Thackston). Tehran, 1992.

Nicephorus Klistos, *Ecclesiastica Historia* (ed. J.P. Migne), *PG*, CXLVI: 536.

Nicolaus Myrepsus, Περί συνθέσεως φαρμάκων. National Library of Athens, codex 1478.

Oribasius, *Oeuvres d'Oribase*: texte Grec, en grande partie inédit, collationnée sur les manuscrits. (eds. U.C. Bussemaker and C. Daremberg). Paris, 1851–1876.

Origenes, *Commentaria in Evangelium Joannis. GCS, Origines.* Leipzig, 1903.

Ovid, *Ars Amatoria*, R.K. Gibson (ed.), *Ovid—Book 3.* Cambridge, 2003.

Petrus of Iberia, *Petrus der Iberer. Ein Charakterbild zur Kirchen und Sittengeschichte des fünften Jahrhunderts: syrische Übersetzung einer um das Jahr 500 verfassten griechischen Biographie* (ed. R. Raabe). Leipzig, 1895.

Philo of Alexandria, Works (eds. and trs. F.H. Colson and G.H. Whitaker). *LCL*, 1958–1962.

Pindaros, *Odes* (ed. and tr. J. Sandys), *LCL*, 1961.
Pliny the Elder, *Naturalis Historia* (ed. and tr. W.H.S. Jones). *LCL*, 1958.
Plutarch, *Vitae Demetrius et Antonius Pyrrhus et Caius Marius* (ed. and tr. B. Perrin). *LCL*, 1968.
———, *De Tuenda Sanitate Praecepta. Precetti Igienici, Plutarco: introduzione, testo critico, traduzione e commento a cura di Luigi Senzasono*. Napoli, 1992.
Polybius, *Historiae* (ed. and tr. W.R. Paton). *LCL*, 1960.
Ptolemy [= Ptolemaeus Claudius], *Geographia* (ed. C.F.A. Nobbe). Hildesheim, 1966.
Scriptores Historiae Augustae, De Vita Hadriani (ed. and tr. D. Magie). *LCL*, 1967.
Simeon Seth, *Simeonis Sethi Syntagma De Alimentorum Facultatibus* (ed. B.A. Langkavel). Lipsiae, 1868.
Seneca, *Epistulae Morales* (ed. and tr. R.M. Gummere). *LCL*, 1967.
———, *Quaestiones Naturales* (ed. and tr. T.H. Corcoran). *LCL*, 1971.
Socrates Scholasticus, *Historia Ecclesiastica* (ed. P.J. Migne), *PG*, VI: 18, LXVII: 728B.
Solinus, *Collectanea Rerum Memorabilium*, in *Greek and Latin Authors on Jews and Judaism* (ed. M. Stern), II, Jerusalem, 1980.
Soranus, *Gynaecia* (ed. I. Jlberg), Lipsiae, 1927.
Sozomenus, *Historia Ecclesiastica* (ed. P.J. Migne), *PG*, LXVII: 944, 1280.
Stephanus Byzantinus, *Ethnika* (ed. A. Meineke). Berolini, 1849.
Strabo, *Geographica* (ed. and tr. H.L. Jones). *LCL*, 1959–1961.
Suetonius, *De Vita Caesarum* (ed. and tr. J.C. Rolfe). *LCL*, 1914.
Suidae Lexicon (ed. A. Adler), Lipsiae, 1931.
Syncellus, *Chronographia* (ed. M. Dindorf), *CSHB*, 1829.
Tacitus, *Annales* (ed. and tr. J. Jackson). *LCL*, 1925–1937.
Tertullian, *Apologeticum*. (ed. and tr. T.R. Glover). *LCL*, 1931.
———, *De Baptismo* (eds. A. Reifferscheid and G. Wissowa). *CSEL*, XX.
———, *De Idolatria*. (ed. J.P. Migne), *PL*, I: 663–696.
———, *De Spectaculis* (tr. G.H. Rendall). *LCL*, 1931 [repr. 1984].
Theodore of Sykeon, *Vita* (ed. A.J. Festugière), *Vie de Théodore de Sykéon*. I, Texte grec. Bruxelles, 1970.
Theodosius, *De Situ Terrae Sanctae* (ed. P. Geyer), *Itinera Hierosolymitana*. Vienna, 1898.
Theophanes, *Chronographia* (ed. J.P. Migne), *PG*, CVIII: 160.
Thucydides, *Historiae* (ed. and tr. C.E. Smith). *LCL*, 1958.
Vitruvius, *De Architectura* (ed. and tr. F. Granger). *LCL*, 1931.
Willibald, *Itinera Hierosolymitana, Itinerarium Saint Willibald ab Anonymo Confectum*. (eds. T. Tobler and A. Moliner). I, 293, Geneva, 1879.

RABBINIC LITERATURE

Avot de Rabbi Nathan, Version I–II (ed. S. Schechter). Vienna, 1887. [H]
Babylonian Talmud (ed. I. Epstein). I–XVIII, London, 1935–1961.
Batei-Midrashot, Midrash Hesed Leumim (ed. S.E. Wertheimer). Jerusalem, 1952. [H]
Jerusalem Talmud [= *Talmud Yerushalmi*]. Venice, 1523. [H]
Jerusalem Talmud (tr. J. Neusner), *The Talmud of the Land of Israel*. I–XXXIV. Atlanta, 1982–1991.
Maimonidis Commentarius in Mishna (ed. D. Sassoon). Copenhagen, 1956–1966.
Mekhilta de Rabbi Ishmael (eds. H.S. Horovitz and I.A. Rabin). Jerusalem, 1970. [H]
Midrash Genesis Rabbah (eds. Y. Theodor and Ch. Albeck). Jerusalem, 1965. [H]
Midrash Exodos Rabbah (ed. A. Shinan). Jerusalem, 1984. [H]
Midrash Deuteronomy Rabbah (tr. L. Rabbinowitz). VII, London, 1961.
Midrash HaGadol, Deuteronomy (ed. S. Fisch). Jerusalem, 1975. [H]
Midrash Lamentations Rabbah, 1619, Pesaro (edn.). [H]
Midrash Lamentations Rabbah (ed. S. Buber), *Lamentations Rabbah*. Vilna, 1899. [H]

Midrash Mishle (ed. B.L. Visotzky). New York, 1990. [H]
Midrash Proverbs Rabbah (ed. S. Buber). Jerusalem, 1965. [H]
Midrash Rabbah (tr. H. Freedman and M. Simon). I–X, London, 1939–1961.
Midrash Song of Songs Zutta (ed. S. Buber). Berlin, 1894. [H]
Midrash Tannaim, Deuteronomy (ed. D.Z. Hoffmann). Berlin, 1909. [H]
Midrash Tanhuma (ed. S. Buber). Vilna, 1885. [H]
Midrash Wayyikra Rabbah (ed. M. Margulies). *Midrash Wayyikra Rabbah*. I–V, Jerusalem, 1953–1960 [repr. 1993]. [H]
Mishnah (tr. P. Blackman) *Mishnayoth* (2nd rev. edn.). I–VIII, New York, 1967.
Psikta de Rav Kahana (2nd edn.). (ed. D. Mandelbaum). *Psiqta de Rav Kahana*. I–II, New York, 1987. [H]
Pesikta Rabbati (ed. M. Ish-Shalom). Vienna, 1880.
Pesikta Rabbati (trans. W.G. Braude). New Haven-London, 1968.
Seder Eliahu Zuta (ed. M. Ish-Shalom). Vienna, 1904.
Sifre on Deuteronomy (ed. L. Finkelstein). New York, 1969. [H]
Tanhuma (ed. S. Buber), *Tanhuma*, I–IV. Wilna, 1831. [H]
Tosefta (ed. S. Lieberman), based on Wein, Erfurt, and Venice and the Geniza Manuscripts. I–IV. New York, 1955–1988.
Tosefta (eds. and trs. J. Neusner and R.S. Sarason), I–VI. New Jersey, 1977–1986.
Tosefta (ed. M.S. Tsukermandel), based on Wein and Erfurt Manuscripts. Pozevalk, 1880. [H]

SECONDARY SOURCES

Aaland, M. (1978): *Sweat: The Illustrated History and Description of the Finnish Sauna, Russian Bania, Islamic Hammam, Japanese Mushi-buro, Mexican Temescal, and American Indian and Eskimo Sweat Lodge*. Santa Barbara, California: Capra Press.
Abdul-Hak, S. (1951): *Catalogue illustré du département des antiquités gréco-romaines au musée de Damas*. Damas: [s.n.].
Abel, F.-M. (1909): 'Une Croisière a la Mer Morte', *ZDPV* 6: 213–242.
—— (1911): *Une croisière autour de la Mer Morte*. Paris: J. Gabalda.
—— (1927): 'Koursi', *JPOS* 7: 112–121.
—— (1931): 'Exploration du Sud-Est de la vallée du Jourdain', *RB* 40: 213–226, 380–388.
—— (1933–1938): *Géographie de la Palestine*. I–II, Paris: J. Gabalda.
Abramski, S. and Parness, A. (1965): 'Bitumen', in *EB*, III. Jerusalem: Mosad Bialik: 187–190. [H]
Abramson, S. and Ginsberg, H.L. (1954): 'On the Aramaic Deed of Sale of the Third Year of the Second Jewish Revolt', *BASOR* 136: 17–19.
Abu-Ajamieh, M. (1980): *The Geothermal Resources of Zerka Ma'in and Zara*. Amman: Natural Resources Authority.
Abu-Ajamieh, M., Bender, F. and Eicher, R. (1989): *Mineral Resources of Jordan*. Amman: Natural Resources Authority.
Adams, J.N. (1992): 'British Latin: The Text, Interpretation and Language of the Bath Curse Tablets', *Britannia* 23: 1–26.
Adkins, L. and Adkins, R. (1996) [repr. 2000]: *Dictionary of Roman Religion*. Oxford: Oxford University Press.
Agishi, Y. and Ohtsuka, Y. (eds.) (1995): *Recent Progress in Medical Balneology and Climatology*. Sapporo, Japan: Hokkaido University School of Medicine.
Aharoni, Y. (1957): *The Settlement of the Twelve Tribes of Israel in Northern Galilee* Jerusalem: Magness Press, The Hebrew University. [H]
—— (1962) [repr. 1987]: *Eretz-Israel in the Biblical Period. Geographical History* (2nd edn.), Jerusalem: Yad Izhak Ben Zvi. [H]

—— (1968): 'Misrephoth Mayim', in *EB*, V. Jerusalem: Mosad Bialik: 641. [H]

—— (1979): *The Land of the Bible: An Historical Geography* (2nd rev. ed. by A. Rainey). London: Burns & Oates.

Ahituv, S. (1968a): 'Na'aman', in *EB*, V. Jerusalem: Mosad Bialik: 893. [H]

—— (1968b): 'Sodom and Gomorrah', in *EB*, V. Jerusalem: Mosad Bialik: 998–1002. [H]

—— (1984): *Canaanite Toponyms in Ancient Egyptian Documents*. Jerusalem-Leiden: The Magness Press & Brill.

Akurgal, E. (2002): *Ancient Civilizations and Ruins of Turkey: From Prehistoric Times until the End of the Roman Empire* (5th edn.). London: Kegan Paul.

Albek, H. (1953–1959): *Six Sidrei Mishna*. I–VI, Jerusalem: Mosad Bialik.

Albright, W.F. (1925): 'Bronze Age Mounds of Northern Palestine and the Hauran: The Spring Trip of the School in Jerusalem', *BASOR* 19: 5–19.

—— (1926): 'The Jordan Valley in the Bronze Age: Pehel-Fahil', *AASOR* 6: 39–42.

—— (1965): 'Hamat', in *EB*, III. Jerusalem: Mosad Bialik: 193–200. [H]

Albu, M., Banks, D. and Nash, H. (eds.) (1997): *Mineral and Thermal Groundwater Resources*. London-New York-Tokyo-Melbourne-Madras: Chapman & Hall.

Alcock, J.P. (2001): *Food in Roman Britain*. Stroud: Tempus.

Allason-Jones, L. (1989): *Women in Roman Britain*. London: British Museum Press.

—— (1999): 'Health Care in Roman North', *Britannia* 30: 133–146.

—— (2000): *Roman Woman: Everyday Life in Hadrian's Britain*. London: Michael O'Mara.

Allen, D. (1988): *Preliminary Evaluation of the Geothermal Potential of Jordan and Recommendations for Further Studies*. British Geological Survey, UK.

Allen, T.J. (1998): *Roman Healing Spas in Italy: A Study in Design and Function*. PhD thesis, University of Alberta.

Almog, Y. and Eshel, B.Z. (1956): *The Dead Sea District*. Tel-Aviv: Am Oved. [H]

Alon, G. (1967–1971): *Studies in Jewish History during the Second Temple, The Mishna and the Talmud* (3rd edn.). I–II, Tel-Aviv: HaKibbutz HaMeuhad. [H]

—— (1984) [repr. 1996]: *The Jews in Their Land in the Talmudic Age (70–640 CE)* (tr. and ed. G. Levi), Cambridge, Mass.: Harvard University Press.

Amalfitano, P., Camodeca, G. and Medri, M. (1990): *I Campi Flegrei. Un itinerario archeologico*. Venezia: Marsilio.

Amir, D. (1976): 'Raqat', in *EB*, VII. Jerusalem: Mosad Bialik: 437. [H]

Amiran, D. (1996): 'Earthquakes in Eretz-Israel', *Qadmoniot* 112: 53–61. [H]

Amiran-Kallner, D.H. (1950–1951): 'A Revised Earthquake: Catalogue of Palestine', *IEJ* 1: 223–246.

Amiran, D.H.K., Arieh, E. and Turcotte, T. (1994): 'Earthquakes in Israel and Adjacent Areas: Macroscismic Observations Since 100 BCE', *IEJ* 44: 261–305.

Amitai-Preiss, N. (1997): 'Arabic Inscriptions, Graffiti and Games', in Y. Hirschfeld (ed.), *The Roman Baths of Hammat Gader, Final Report*. Jerusalem: The Israel Exploration Society: 267–278.

'Amr, K. and Hamdan, K. (1996): 'Archaeological Survey of the East Coast of the Dead Sea. Phase q: Suwayma, az-Zara and Umm Sidra', *ADAJ* 40: 434–445.

Amundsen, D.W. (1982): 'Medicine and Faith in Early Christianity', *BHM* 56: 326–350.

André, J. (1961): *L'Alimentation et la cuisine à Rome*. Paris: C. Klincksieck.

Andreae, B. (1973) [repr. 1978]: *The Art of Rome* (tr. R.E. Wolf). London: Macmillan.

Anonymous (1964): 'Analysis Lengthwise the Channel of the Salted Waters Springs', *HA* 9: 1–6. [H]

Applebaum, S. (1967): 'The Agrarian Question and the Revolt of Bar Kokhba', *EI* 8: 284–287. [H]

—— (1976): *Prolegomena to the study of the Second Jewish Revolt (AD 132–135)*. *BAR Supp. Series* 7. Oxford: British Archaeological Reports.

—— (1977): 'Judaea as a Roman Province: The Countryside as a Political and Economic Factor', in *ANRW* II.8: 355–396.

—— (1983): 'The Results of Bar-Kokhba War', in U. Rappaport (ed.), *The World History of the Jewish People: Judea and Rome, The Jewish Revolts.* Jerusalem: Am Oved: 230–260. [H]

—— (1989): *Judaea in Hellenistic and Roman Times: Historical and Archaeological Essays.* Leiden: Brill.

Arad, A. and Bein, A. (1986): 'Saline Versus Freshwater: Contribution to the Thermal Waters of the Northern Jordan Rift Valley, Israel', *JH* 83 (1–2): 49–66.

Arad, V., Bartov, Y. and Hambright, K.D. (1998): *Lake Kinneret Research. Bibliography.* Tiberias-Jerusalem: Israel Oceanographic and Limnological Laboratory & The Ministry of National Infrastructures, Geological Survey of Israel.

Ardet, A. (1996): 'The Ancient Spa *Ad Mediam* (Baile Herculane)', *Balnearia* 4.2: 3.

Arndt, W.F. and Gingrich, F.W. (1958) [repr. 1967]: *A Greek-English Lexicon of the New Testament and Other Early Christian Literature* (2nd edn.). Chicago: University of Chicago Press.

Aronius, J. (ed.) (1902): *Regesten zur Geschichte der Juden im fränkischen und deutschen. Reiche bis zum Jahre 1273.* Berlin: Berl.

Arthur, P. (1991): *Romans in Northern Campania: Settlement and Land-Use around the Massico and the Garigliano Basin.* London: British School at Rome.

Arubas, B. and Goldfus, H. (1995): 'The Kiln-Works of the Tenth Legion Fretensis', *JRA* 14: 95–107.

Askenasi, S.J. (1590): *Sefer Yafeh Mar'eh: Explanatios and Innovations on the Aggadoth of the Yerushalmi.* Venice.

Assaf, S. (1956): *Sources and Researches in the History of Israel.* Jerusalem: Mosad HaRav Kook. [H]

—— (1958): 'The History of the Jews in Tiberias', *Sinai: The Jubilee Book.* Jerusalem: Mosad HaRav Kok. [H]

Assaf, S. and Meir, L.A. (1954): *Sefer HaIsuv*, 'Tiberias'. II, Jerusalem: The Israel Society for History and Ethnography: 10–12. [H]

Atlas, M. (1951): 'The Waters of Springs as Curative Drink, Especially of Tiberias Hot Springs', *HaRefuah* 40: 157–159. [H]

—— (1970): 'Therapeutic Springs in the Dead Sea Shore', *Mada* 15 (3): 166. [H]

—— (1971): 'Hammei-Tiberias and Their Role in Therapeutic Baths in Israel'', in A. Ya'akov (ed.), *Tiberias Hot Springs. Compilation of Essays in Medicine.* Hammat-Tiberias: Hammei-Tiberias Co.: 77–83. [H]

Aupert, P. (1974): *Le nymphée de Tipasa et les nymphées et septizonia nord-africains.* Rome: École française de Rome: L'Erma di Bretschneider.

Authier, A. and Duvernois, P. (1997): *Patrimoine et Traditions du Thermalisme.* Toulouse: Éditions Privat.

Avigad, N. (1972): *Beth Shearim.* III, Jerusalem: The Israel Exploration Society. [H]

—— (1983): *Discovering Jerusalem.* Jerusalem: Shiqmona. [H]

Avigad, N. and Geva, H. (1993): 'Jerusalem: The Second Temple Period', in E. Stern (ed.), *NEAEHL* III, Jerusalem: Israel Exploration Society & Carta: 717–757.

Avissar, O. (ed.) (1973): *The Book of Tiberias: The City of Kinnrot and Its Settlement throughout the Ages.* Jerusalem: Keter. [H]

Avi-Yonah, M. (1936): 'Map of Roman Palestine', *QDAP* 5:139–193.

—— (1944–1945): 'The City Boundaries of Roman Trans-Jordan', *BJPES* 11: 1–8. [H]

—— (1946): 'Newly Discovered Latin and Greek Inscriptions', *QDAP* 12: 84–102.

—— (1950a): 'The Foundation of Tiberias', *IEJ* 1: 160–169.

—— (1950b): 'Excavations at Sheikh Bader (1949)', *BJPES* 5: 19–24. [H]

—— (1950–1951): 'The Development of the Roman Road System in Palestine', *IEJ* 1: 54–60.

—— (1954): *The Madaba Mosaic Map.* Jerusalem: Israel Exploration Society.

—— (1962): 'Emmaus', in *EH*, III. Jerusalem-Tel-Aviv: Dvir: 847. [H]

—— (1963): 'The Bath of the Lepers at Scythopolis', *IEJ* 13: 325–326.

—— (1964a): *Essays and Studies*. Tel-Aviv: M. Neuman. [H]

—— (1964b): 'The Caesarea Inscription of the 24 Priestly Courses', *EI* 7: 24–28. [H]

—— (1965): 'Hammat', in *EB*, III. Jerusalem: Mosad Bialik: 192–193. [H]

—— (1967a): 'The Foundation of Tiberias', in H.Z. Hirschberg (ed.), *All the Land of Naphtali. The 24th Archaeological Convention, 1966.* Jerusalem: Israel Exploration Society: 163–169. [H]

—— (1967b): 'Tiberias during the Roman Period', in H.Z. Hirschberg (ed.), *All the Land of Naphtali. The 24th Archaeological Convention, 1966.* Jerusalem: Israel Exploration Society: 158–162. [H]

—— (1970): *In the Days of Rome and Byzantium* (4th edn.). Jerusalem: Mosad Bialik. [H]

—— (1976): *Gazetteer of Roman Palestine*. Qedem, 5. Jerusalem: Institute of Archaeology, The Hebrew University of Jerusalem.

—— (1984): *Historical Geography of Palestine from the End of the Babylonian Exile up to the Arab Conquest* (4th edn.). Jerusalem: Mosad Bialik. [H]

—— (1993): 'Emmaus', in E. Stern (ed.), *NEAEHL* I, Jerusalem: Israel Exploration Society & Carta: 385–387.

Avi-Yonah, M. and Hirschfeld, Y. (1993): 'Hammat-Gader', in E. Stern (ed.), *NEAEHL* II, Jerusalem: Israel Exploration Society & Carta: 565–573.

Avi-Yonah, M. and Shatzman, I. (eds.) (1981): *Illustrated Encyclopaedia of the Classical World.* Maidenhead: Sampson Low.

Avnimelech, M. (1935): 'Discovery of Volcanic Formations between Jerusalem and Jaffa', *BJPES* 2: 59–63. [H]

Ayli, M. (1987): *Workers and Craftsmen: Their Labour and Status in the Rabbinic Literature.* Givatiim: Yad La-Talmud. [H]

Bacher, B.Z. (1920–1923): *The Legends of the Tannaim* (tr. A.Z. Rabbinovitz). I–II, Berlin: Eitan Press. [H]

—— (1925–1938): *The Legends of Amoraei Eretz-Israel* (tr. A.Z. Rabbinovitz). I–III, Tel-Aviv: Dvir. [H]

Bacher, W. (1896): 'Rome dans le Talmud et le Midrasch', *RÉJ* 33: 187–196.

—— (1899): *Die Agada der Palästinensischen Amoräer.* I–III, Strassburg: K.J. Trubner.

—— (1909): 'Der Jahrmarkt am der Terebinthe bei Hebron', *ZAW* 29: 148–152.

Baedeker, K. (1880): *Southern Italy* (7th ed.), Leipzig: Baedeker.

—— (1876): *Palestina and Syria: Handbook for Travellers* (3rd rev. edn.). Leipzig: Baedeker.

Baer, Y.F. (1961): 'Israel, the Christian Church and the Roman Empire', *SH* 7: 79–145.

—— (1971): 'Jerusalem during the Great Revolt', *Zion* 36: 127–190. [H]

Bagati, B. (1947): *I Monumenti di Emmaus el-Qubeibeh e dei Dintorni.* Jerusalem: Tip. Dei Pp. Franciscani.

—— (1969): *Excavations in Nazareth* (tr. E. Hoade). I, Jerusalem: Studium Biblicum Franciscanum.

—— (1984): 'Notes on the Byzantine Period in the Holy Land', in E. Schiller (ed.), *Zeev Vilnay's Jubilee Volume. Essays on the History, Archaeology and Lore of the Holy Land.* I, Jerusalem: Ariel Publishing House: 278–279. [H]

Bainart, H. (1963): 'Salt', in *EB*, IV. Jerusalem: Mosad Bialik: 1053–1057. [H]

Baldwin, B. (1970): 'Hadrian Farewell to Life: Some Arguments for Authenticity', *CQ* 64: 372–374.

Ball, W. (2000): *Rome in the East: The Transformation of an Empire.* London-New York: Routledge.

Ballou, R. (1970): 'The Role of the Jewish Priesthood in the Expansion of Greek Games in Jerusalem', *CJHSP* 1 (2): 70–81.

Balog, P. (1976): *Ummayad, 'Abbasid, and Tulunid Glass Weights and Vessel Stamps.* New York: American Numismatic Society.

Balsdon, J.P.V.D. (1969): *Life and Leisure in Ancient Rome*. London-Toronto: Bodley Head.
—— (1974): *Roman Women: Their History and Habits* (rev. ed.). London: Bodley Head.
Balty, J.C. (1981): *Guide d'Apamée*. Bruxelles: Centre belge de recherches archéologiques à Apamée de Syrie & Paris: Diffusion de Boccard.
Bar-Adon, P. (1936): 'Sinnabra and Beit Yerah in the Light of the Sources and Archaeological Finds', *EI* 4: 50–55. [H]
Bar-Droma, H. (1958): *And This is the Boundary of the Land: The Real Boundares of Eretz-Israel according to the Sources*. Jerusalem: Beer. [H]
Bar-Ilan, M. (1999): 'The Medicine in the Land of Israel in the First Centuries', *Cathedra* 91: 31–78. [H]
—— (2000): 'The Attitude toward *Mamzerim* in Jewish Society in Late Antiquity', *Jewish History* 14: 125–170.
Bar-Kochva, B. (1980): *The Battles of the Hasmonaean: The Times of Judas Maccabaeus*. Jerusalem: Yad Izhak Ben Zvi & Ministry of Defence Publishing House. [H]
Bar-Nathan R. and Mazor, G. (1992): 'The Centre of the City (Beit Shean) and the Region of Tel Itstaba', *HA* 98: 38–43. [H]
—— (1993): 'City Center (south) and Tel Iztabba Area. Excavations of the Antiquities Authority Expedition, the Beit Shean Excavation Project (1989–1991)', *ESI* 11: 33–52.
—— (1994): 'Scythopolis: The Capital of Provincia Palastina Secunda', *Qadmoniot* 107–108: 117–137. [H]
Barag, D. (1964): 'An Inscription from the High Level Aqueduct of Caesarea, Reconsidered', *IEJ* 14: 250–252.
—— (1967): 'Brick Stamp-Impressions of the Legio X Fretensis', *BJb* 167: 244–267.
Baratte, F. (1992): 'La coupe en argent de Castro Urdiales', in R. Chevallier (ed.), *Les eaux Thermales et les cultes des eaux en Gaul et dans les provinces voisines. Actes du Colloque, Aix-les-Bains 1990*. Turin: Antropologia alpine: 43–54.
Barghouti, A.N. (1982): 'Urbanization of Palesitne and Jordan in Hellenistic and Roman Times', in A. Hadidi (ed.), *SHAJ*, I, Amman: Department of Antiquities: 209–229.
Barkay, R. (2000): 'The Coins of Horvat 'Eleq', in Y. Hirschfeld (ed.), *Ramat Hanadiv Excavations, Final Report of the 1984–1998 Seasons*. Jerusalem: Israel Exploration Society: 377–419.
Barness, T.D. (1989): 'Emperors on the Move', *JRA* 2: 247–261.
Barnett, R. (1986–1987): 'Six Fingers in Art and Archaeology', *BAIAS* 6: 5–11.
—— (1990): 'Polydactylism in the Ancient World', *BAR* 16 (3): 46–51.
Barth, J. (1909): 'Zur altaramäischen Inschrift des Königs Zkr', *OLZ* 12: 10–12.
Barton, C.A. (1992) [repr. 1995]: *The Sorrows of the Ancient Romans: The Gladiator and the Monster*. Princeton: Princeton University Press.
Bartov, V. Arad, V. and Arad, A. (1992): *The Geology of Jordan: Bibliography*. Jerusalem: Geological Survey of Israel.
Baruch, S. (1899): *The Principles and Practice of Hydrotherapy: A Guide to the Application of Water in Disease for Students and Practitioners of Medicine*. New York: William Wood and Company.
Baudisch, O. (1939): 'Magic and Science of Natural Healing Waters', *JCE* 16: 440–448.
Baumgarten, A.I. (1981): 'Rabbi Judah I and His Opponents', *JSJ* 12: 135–172.
Bazzocchini, P.B. (1905): *L'Emmaus di S. Luca*. Roma: Libreria Pontificia di Federico Pustet.
Beacham, R.C. (1991): *The Roman Theatre and Its Audience*. London-New York: Routledge.
—— (1999): *Spectacle Entertainments of Imperial Rome*. New Haven-London: Yale University Press.
Beare, W. (1963): *The Roman Stages* (3rd edn.). London-Totowa, N.J.: Methuen & Rowman & Littlefield.

Beer, M. (1982): *The Babylonian Amoraim: Aspects of Economic Life* (2nd edn.). Ramat-Gan: Bar-Ilan University Press. [H]

Beeson, P.B. and McDermott, W. (1975): *Textbook of Medicine* (4th edn.). Philadelphia: Penn.

Behr, C.A. (1968) *Aelius Aristides and the Sacred Tales.* Amsterdam: Hakkert.

Bein, A. (1976): *A Critical Review on Salinity Studies of Lake Kinneret.* Israel Geological Survey. [H]

Belayche, N. (2001): *Iudaea-Palaestina: The Pagan Cults in Roman Palestine (Second to Fourth Century).* Tübingen: Mohr Siebeck.

Bell, H.I. (1940): 'Antinoopolis: A Hadrianic Foundation in Egypt', *JRS* 30: 133–147.

Bellinger, A.R. (1940): 'The Syrian Tetradrachms of Caracalla and Macrinus', *ANS* 3: 11–92.

Belvedere, O. and Alliata, V. (1988–2002): *Himera. III, Prospezione archeologica nel territorio.* Roma: Erma di Bretschneider.

Ben-Ami, D. (1984): 'A Legend and Moral about the Marvelous of Hammat-Gader Springs', *Eretz-HaGolan* 96: 18–19. [H]

Ben-Arieh, R. (1997): 'The Roman, Byzantine and Umayyad Pottery', in Y. Hirschfeld (ed.), *The Roman Baths of Hammat-Gader, Final Report.* Jerusalem: The Israel Exploration Society: 347–381.

Ben-Arieh, Y. (1968): *The Changing Landscape of the Central Jordan Valley.* Jerusalem: Magness Press, The Hebrew University [= idem, (1965) *The Central Jordan Valley.* Tel-Aviv: HaKibbutz HaMeuhad. (H)].

—— (1973): 'Valley of Kinnarot: A Geographical Frame and Geomorphological Background', in O. Avissar (ed.), *The Book of Tiberias: The City of Kinnrot and Its Settlement throughout the Ages.* Jerusalem: Keter: 17–28. [H]

Ben-Avraham, Z. (1997): 'Geophysical Framework of the Dead Sea: Structure and Tectonics', in M. Niemi et al. (eds.), *The Dead Sea: The Lake and Its Setting.* New York-Oxford: Oxford University Press: 22–35.

Bender, F. (1968): *Geologie von Jordanien.* Berlin: Gebr. Borntraeger.

—— (1974): *Geology of Jordan. Contribution of the Regional Geology of the Earth.* Berlin: Gebrüder Bornträger.

—— (1975): *Geology of the Arabian Peninsula, Jordan.* Washington: U.S. Government Printing Office.

Ben-Dov, M. (1985): *In the Shadow of the Temple: The Discovery of Ancient Jerusalem.* Jerusalem: Keter. [H]

Ben-Horim, N. (1929–1930): 'The Eye in the Talmud', *HP* 1 (2): 121–127. [H]

—— (1933): 'Daily Routine according to the Talmud', *HP* 2 (1): 94–104. [H]

—— (1937): 'The Dietetics in the Talmud', *HP* 10: 93–99. [H]

Bennahum, D.A. (1985): 'Psoriasis, Leprosy and the Dead Sea Valley', *Koroth* 9 (1–2): 86–89.

Ben-Shalom, I. (1983): 'The Support of the Sages for Bar Kokhba Revolt', *Cathedra* 29: 13–28. [H]

—— (1984): 'Rabbi Judah bar Ila'i and His Attitude towards Rome', *Zion* 49: 9–24. [H]

Ben Shamai, M.H. (1960): 'Sulphur', in *EH*, XI. Jerusalem-Tel-Aviv: Dvir: 149–155. [H]

Ben-Yehuda, E. (1948): *A Complete Dictionary of Ancient and Modern Hebrew.* I–XVII, Jerusalem: Ben-Yehuda. [H]

Ben-Zvi, Y. (1976): *The Book of the Samaritans* (3rd edn.). Jerusalem: Yad Izhak Ben Zvi. [H]

Berger, A. (1982): *Das Bad in der byzantinischen Zeit. Miscellanea Byzantina Monacensia.* 27, München: Institut für Byzantinistik und neugriechische Philologie der Universität.

Bergman, Y. (1937): 'The Sages of Eretz-Israel and the Graeco-Roman Culture', in N.H. Torthiner et al. (eds.) *Klausner Book.* Tel-Aviv: Vad HaYovel: 146–153. [H]

Berlin, A.M. (2005): 'Jewish Life before the Revolt: The Archaeological Evidence', *JSJ* 36 (4): 417–170.

Berry, G.R. (1897) [repr. 1989]: *Interlinear Greek-English New Testament, King James Version.* Michigan: Lond. &c.

Beyer, G. (1933): 'Die Stadtgebiete von Diospolis und Nikopolis im 4. Jahrh. n. Chr. und ihre Grenznachbarn', *ZDPV* 56: 218–246.
Beyer, K. (1984): *Die aramäischen Texte vom Toten Meer*. Göttingen: Vandenhoeck & Ruprecht.
Bickerman, E. (1929): 'Die römische Kaiserapotheose', *AR* 27: 4–23.
Bidez, J. and Hanson, G.C. (eds.) (1960): *Kirchengeschichte—Sozomenus. Die griechischen christlichen Schriftsteller der ersten drei Jahrhunderte*. 50, Berlin: Akademie Verlag.
Bieber, M. (1961): *The History of the Greek and Roman Theater* (2nd ed.). Princeton, New Jersey: Princeton University Press.
Bietenhard, H. (1963): 'Die Dekapolis von Pompeius bis Trajan', *ZDPV* 79: 24–58.
——— (1977): 'Die syrische Dekapolis von Pompeius bis Trajan', in *ANRW* II.8: 220–261.
Birley, A.R. (1994): 'Hadrian's Farewell to Life', *Laverna* 5: 176–205.
——— (1997): *Hadrian: The Restless Emperor*. London-New York: Routledge.
Birnbaum, R. and Ovadiah, A. (1990): 'A Greek Inscription from the Early Byzantine Church at Apollonia', *IEJ* 40: 182–190 [= idem, (1989), *ibid.*, in I. Roll and E. Ayalon (eds.), *Apollonia and Southern Sharon: Model of a Coastal City and Its Hinterland*, Tel-Aviv: HaKibbutz HaMeuhad: 279–288]. [H]
Birnbaum, S.A. (1957): 'The Kepher Bebhayu Conveyance', *PEFQSt* 89: 108–132.
——— (1958): 'The Kepher Bebhayu Marriage Deed', *JAOS* 78: 12–18.
Blake, G.S. (1930): *The Mineral Resources of Palestine and Transjordan*. Jerusalem: Government of Palestine.
Blake, I.M. (1967): 'Jericho (Ain Es-Sultan): Joshua's Curse and Elish's Miracle, One Possible Explanation', *PEQ* 99: 86–97.
Blanckenhorn, M. (1896): 'Entstehung und Geschichichte des Todten Meeres', *ZDPV* 19: 5–59.
——— (1912): *Naturwissenchaftliche studien am Toten Meer und Jordantal*. Berlin: Friedländer & Sohn.
Blau, Y. (1982): 'Transcription of Arabic Words and Names in the Inscription of Mu'āwiya from Hammat-Gader', *IEJ* 32: 102.
Blaufuss, H. (1909): *Römsiche Feste und Feiertage nach den Traktaten über Fremden Dienst. Aboda Zara, in Mischna, Tosefta, Jerusalemer und babylonischem Talmud*. Nürnberg: [s.n.].
Blázquez, J.M. (1999): 'The Presence of Nature in the Madaba Mosaic Map', in M. Piccirillo and E. Alliata (eds.), *The Madaba Map Centenary 1897–1997*. Jerusalem: Studium Biblicum Franciscanum: 250–252.
Blidstein, J.G. (1971): 'Judah Ha-Nasi', in *EJ* X. Jerusalem: Keter Books: 366–372. [H]
——— (1974): 'Rabbi Yohanan, Idolatry and Public Privilege', *JSJ* 5: 154–161.
Boardman, J. (1988): 'Herakles', in *LIMC* IV/1, Zürich: Artemis: 797.
Boatwright, M.T. (1987): *Hadrian and the City of Rome*. Princeton-Oxford: Princeton University Press.
——— (2000): *Hadrian and the Cities of the Roman Empire*. Princeton, New Jersey: Princeton University Press.
Bonner, C. (1932): 'Demons of the Bath', in *Studies Presented to F.L. Griffith*. London: Egypt Exploration Society & H. Milford, Oxford University Press: 204–208.
Bonneville, de, F. (1998): *The Book of the Bath*. London: Thames and Hudson.
Boon, G.C. (1983): 'Potters, Oculists, and Eye-Troubles', *Britannia* 14: 1–12.
Borée, W. (1930) [repr. 1968]: *Die alten Ortsnamen Palästinas* (2nd edn.). Hildesheim: Olms.
Boren-Borenstein, R. (1971): 'The Tiberias Baths and the Vascular System', in A. Ya'akov (ed.), *Tiberias Hot Springs. Compilation of Essays in Medicine*. Hammat-Tiberias: Hammei-Tiberias Co.: 57–59. [H]
Borriello, M. and d'Ambrosio, A. (1979): *Baiae-Misenum*. Firenze: L.S. Olschki.
Boulanger, R. (1966): *The Middle East: Lebanon, Syria, Jordan, Iraq, Iran* (tr. J.S. Hardman). Paris: Hachette.

Bourke, S.J. (1993): 'Pella in the Bronze and Iron Ages: A Report on the 1992 Field Season', *Med. Arch.* 5–6: 61–163.

—— (1997): 'Pre-Classical Pella in Jordan: A Conspectus of Ten Years' Work (1985–1995)', *PEQ* 129: 94–115.

Bowersock, G.W. (1994): *Roman Arabia*. Cambridge-Mass.-London: Harvard University Press.

Bowman, D. (1997): 'Geomorphology of the Dead Sea Western Margin', in M. Niemi et al. (eds.), *The Dead Sea: The Lake and Its Setting*. New York-Oxford: Oxford University Press: 217–225.

Bowsher, J.M.C. (1987): 'Architecture and Religion in the Decapolis: A Numismatic Survey', *PEQ* 119: 62–69.

—— (1992): 'Civic Organisation within the Decapolis', *ARAM Periodical* 4 (1–2): 265–281.

Branda, F., Luciani, G., Costantini, A. and Piccioli, C. (2001): 'Indagine tecnico-scientifica sull'emblema del settore della Sosandra delle Terme di Baia', in A. Paribeni (ed.), *Atti del VII Colloquio dell'Associazione Italiana per lo Studio e la Conservazione del mosaico, Pompei 2000*. Ravenna: Edizioni del Girasole: 609–614.

Brandon, S.G.F. (1951): *The Fall of Jerusalem and the Christian Church: A Study of the Effects of the Jewish Overthrow of A.D. 70 on Christianity* (2nd edn.). London: SPCK.

Braslavsky, J. (1954): *Studies in Our Country Its Past and Remains*. Tel-Aviv: HaKibbutz HaMeuhad. [H]

—— (1956–1965): *Do You Know the Land?* (2nd edn.). I–VI, Tel-Aviv: HaKibbutz HaMeuhad. [H]

Braver, A.Y. (1928): 'The Jordan Area as a Health and Resort Place', in J. Stein et al. (eds.), *Health Resorts in Eretz-Israel (Palestine). Lectures Called on at the Special Medical Conference at Tel-Aviv on 26–27.12.1927*. Tel-Aviv: The Palestine Jewish Medical Association: 10–12. [H]

—— (1954): *Eretz-Israel* (2nd edn.). Tel-Aviv: Mosad Bialik. [H]

Brim, B.C.J. (1936): *Medicine in the Bible: The Pentateuch*. New York: Froben Press.

Brock, S.P. (1977): 'A Letter Attributed to Cyril of Jerusalem on the Rebuilding of the Temple', *BSOAS* 40: 267–286 [= (1984) *Syriac Perspectives on Late Antiquity*. X, London: Variorum Reprints: 267–286].

Brockelmann, K. (1893): 'Die griechischen Fremdwörter im Armenischen', *ZDMG* 47: 1–42.

—— (1924) [repr. 1995]: *Lexicon Syriacum* (2nd edn.). Vaduz: A.R. Gantner.

Brödner, E. (1983): *Die römischen Thermen und das antike Badewesen: eine kulturhistorische Betrachtung*. Darmstadt: Wissenschaftliche Buchgesellschaft.

Brodribb, G. (1987): *Roman Brick and Tile*. Gloucester: Alan Sutton.

Broshi, M. (1965): 'Jordan', in *EB* III. Jerusalem: Mosad Bialik: 778–787. [H]

—— (1987): 'The Diet of Palestine in the Roman Period', *Cathedra* 43: 15–32. [H]

Broshi, M. and Qimron, E. (1986): 'A House Sale Deed from the Time of Bar Kokhba', *IEJ* 36: 201–214.

Brothers, A.J. (1989): 'Buildings for Entertainment', in J.M. Barton (ed.), *Roman Public Buildings*. Exeter: University of Exeter: 97–112.

Brown, F., Driver, S.R. and Briggs, C. (1906): *A Hebrew and English Lexicon of the Old Testament*. Oxford: Clarendon Press.

Brown, F.E. (1961) [repr. 1963]: *Roman Architecture*. London: Studio Vista.

Brown, P. (1967): *Augustine of Hippo: A Biography*. London: Faber.

Browne, S.G. (1970): *Leprosy in the Bible* (3rd edn.). London: Christian Medical Fellowship.

—— (1975): 'Some Aspects on the History of Lepra', *PRSM* 68: 485–493.

Browning, I. (1979): *Palmyra*. London: Chatto & Windus.

—— (1982) [repr. 1994]: *Jerash and the Decapolis*. London: Chatto & Windus.

Brünnow, R.E. and Domaszewski, A.V. (1904–1909): *Die Provincia Arabia: auf Grund zweier in den Jahren 1897 und 1898 unternommenen Reisen und der Berichte früherer Reisender.* I–III, Strassburg: Trübner.

Brzezinski, A. (1934): *Les sources thermals de la Palestine et en particular celles de Hamei-Tiberia.* Paris: L. Rodstein.

Büchler, A. (1956): 'The Patriarch Rabbi Judah and the Graeco-Roman Cities of Palestine', in I. Brodie and J. Rabbinowitz (eds.), *Studies in Jewish History.* London: Oxford University Press: 179–244.

—— (1967): *Studies in the Period of the Mishnah and the Talmud* (tr. B.Z. Segal), Jerusalem: Mosad HaRav Kook. [H]

—— (1980): 'On the Participation of the Samaritans in the Bar-Kokhva Revolt', in A. Oppenheimer (ed.), *The Bar-Kokhva Revolt.* Jerusalem: The Zalman Shazar Center for Jewish History & The Historical Society of Israel: 115–121. [H]

Buchman, D. (1994): *The Complete Book of Water Therapy.* New Canaan: Keats.

Buchmann, M. (1928a): 'Hammei-Tiberias and Tiberias as a Healing Site', in J. Stein et al. (eds.), *Health Resorts in Eretz-Israel (Palestine). Lectures Called on at the Special Medical Conference at Tel-Aviv on 26–27.12.1927.* Tel-Aviv: The Palestine Jewish Medical Association: Tel-Aviv: 28–34. [H]

—— (1928b): 'Die Thermen von Tiberias und Tiberias als Winterkurort', *Palästina* 8–10: 364–371.

—— (1933): 'Therapeutic Springs in Israel', *HaRefuah* 6: 299–306. [H]

—— (1942): 'The Achievements of Balneology and Its Goals', *HaRefuah* 23: 139–140. [H]

—— (1947): 'Hammei-Tiberias in the Past', *HH* 20: 90–106. [H]

—— (1948): 'Hammei-Tiberias at Present', *HH* 21: 128–135. [H]

—— (1955): 'The Nature of Piloma', *AMO* 14 (11–12): 287–291.

—— (1956): *Tiberias and Its Hot Springs.* Tiberias: Hammei-Tiberias Co. [H]

—— (1957): 'Balneotherapy and Orthopaedic Diseases', *HaRefuah* 52: 35–36. [H]

—— (1962): 'The History of the Baths of Tiberias', *HH* 1:100–101. [H]

—— (1967): 'The History of Hammei-Tiberias', in A.Z. Hirschberg (ed.), *All the Land of Naftali. The 24th Annual Meeting on the Geography of the Land.* Jerusalem: Israel Exploration Society: 195–202. [H]

—— (1971a): 'Modus Operandi of the Thermo-Mineral Springs and the Treatment Results in Hammei-Tiberias', in A.Ya'akov (ed.), *Tiberias Hot Springs. Compilation of Essays in Medicine.* Hammat-Tiberias: Hammei-Tiberias Co.: 29–43. [H]

—— (1971b): 'Researches, Purposes and Limitations in Balneology', in A. Ya'akov (ed.), *Tiberias Hot Springs. Compilation of Essays in Medicine.* Hammat-Tiberias: Hammei-Tiberias Co.: 84–92. [H]

Buckingham, J.S. (1821): *Travels in Palestine through the Countries of Bashan and Gilead, East of the River Jordan.* London: Longman, Hurst, Rees, Orme & Brown.

Buhl, F. (1896): *Geographie des alten Palästina.* Freiburg-Leipzig: I.B. & Mohr.

Bunson, M. (1994): *Encyclopedia of the Roman Empire.* New York: Facts on File.

Burckhardt, J.L. (1822): *Travels in Syria and the Holy Land.* London: John Murray.

Burdon, D.J. (1959): *Handbook of the Geology of Jordan.* Amman: Government of the Hashemite Kingdom of Jordan.

Burkett, W. (1985): *Greek Religion* (tr. J. Raffan). Cambridge-Mass.: Harvard University Press.

Butcher, K. (2003): *Syria and the Near East.* London: British Museum.

Butler, H.C. (1903): *Publications of the American Archaeological Expedition to Syria, 1899–1900.* Part II: *Architecture and Other Arts.* New York: Century Company.

—— (1907–1920): *Publications of the Princeton University Archaeological Expeditions to Syria in 1904–1905 and 190.* Division II, Section A—*Southern Syria.* Division II, Section B—*Northern Syria.* Leiden: Brill.

Buttrick, G.A. et al. (eds.) (1952): *The Interpeter's Dictionary of the Bible.* I–XII, New York: Abingdon-Cokesbury Press.

Caffarelli, E.V., Bandinelli, R.B. and Caputo, G. (1967): *The Buried City: Excavations at Leptis Magna.* London: Weidenfeld and Nicolson.

Cagnat, R. (1963): 'Legio X Fretensis', in C. Daremberg and E. Saglio (eds.), *Dictionnaire des antiquités grecques et romaines.* III/2, Graz: Akademische Druck-u. Verlagsanstalt: 1084–1085.

Caillois, R. (1961): *Man, Play, and Games* (tr. M. Barash). New York: Free Press of Glencoe.

Cameron, A. (1973): 'Sex in the Swimming Pool', *ICST* 20: 149–150.

—— (1976): *Circus Factions: Blues and Greens at Rome and Byzantium.* Oxford: Clarendon Press.

Campion, M. (ed.) (1996): *Hydrotherapy: Principles and Practice.* Oxford-Boston: Butterworth-Heinemann.

Cante, A.M. (1984): 'Les plaques votives avec plantae pedum d'Italica: un essai d'interpretation', *ZPE* 54: 183–194.

Carcopino, J. (1991) [repr. 1941]: *Daily Life in Ancient Rome: The People and the City at the Height of the Empire* (tr. E.O. Lorimer). London-New York: Routledge.

Carson, R.A.G. (1989): *Coins of the Roman Empire.* London-New York: Routledge.

Case, S.J. (1923): 'The Art of Healing in Early Christian Times', *JR* 3: 238–255.

Casson, L. (1974 [repr. 1994]): *Travel in the Ancient World.* Baltimore-London: Johns Hopkins University Press.

Cassuto, M.D. (1962): 'Kemosh', in *EB* IV. Jerusalem: Mosad Bialik: 186–188. [H]

Cataldi, R. and Burgassi, P.D. (1999): 'Flowering and Decline of Thermal Bathing and Other Uses of Natural Heat in the Mediterranean Area from the Birth of Rome to the End of the First Millenium', in R. Cataldi et al. (eds.), *Stories from A Heated Earth: Our Geothermal Heritage.* California: GRC & IGA: 147–163.

Cataldi, R. and Chiellini, P. (1999): 'Geothermal Energy in the Mediterranean Before the Middle Ages: A Review', in R. Cataldi et al. (eds.), *Stories from A Heated Earth: Our Geothermal Heritage.* California: GRC & IGA: 165–181.

Chaitow, L. (1999): *Hydrotherapy: Water Therapy for Health and Beauty.* Shaftesbury: Element.

Chandler, R. (1776): *Travels in Asia Minor, 1764–1765* (2nd edn.). London: Lond.

Charpentier, G. (1994): 'Les bains de Serjilla', *Syria* 71: 113–142.

Chesnut, G.F. (1986): *The First Christian Histories: Eusebius, Socrates, Sozomen, Theodoret, and Evagrius* (2nd edn.). Macon, GA: Mercer University Press.

Chevallier, R. (1988): *Voyages et déplacements dans l'empire romain.* Paris: Armand Colin.

—— (ed.) (1992): *Les eaux thermales et les cultes des eaux en Gaul et dans les provinces voisines. Actes du Colloque, Aix-les-Bains 1990.* Turin: Antropologia alpine.

Ciasca, A. (1962): 'A Hypocaust at Ramat Rahel', in Y. Aharoni et al. (eds.), *Excavations at Ramat Rahel: Seasons 1959 and 1960.* Rome: Israel Exploration Society: 69–72.

Clamer, C. (1989): 'Ain Ez-Zara Excavations 1986', *ADAJ* 33: 217–225.

—— (1997a): *Fouilles archéologiques de 'Aïn ez-Zâra-Callirrhoé, villégiature hérodienne.* Beyrouth: Institut français d'archéologie du Proche-Orient,

—— (1997b): ''Ain Ez-Zara—Kallirrhoe: The Thermal Bath of Herod the Great', *OOr* 2 (1): 10–12.

—— (1999): 'The Hot Springs of Kallirrhoe and Baarou', in M. Piccirillo and E. Alliata (eds.), *The Madaba Map Centenary 1897–1997.* Jerusalem: Studium Biblicum Franciscanum: 221–225.

Clark, E.A. (1984): *The Life of Melania The Younger: Introduction, Translation and Commentary.* New York-Toronto: Edwin Mellen Press.

Clark, V.A., Bowsher, J.M. and Stewart, J.D. (1986): 'The Jerash North Theatre', in F. Zayadine, (ed.), *Jerash Archaeological Project 1981–1983.* I, Amman: Department of Antiquities: 205–270.

Clarke, J. (1996): 'Hypersexual Black Men in Augustan Baths', in N. Kampen (ed.), *Sexuality in Ancient Art: Near East, Egypt, Greece and Italy.* Cambridge: Cambridge University Press: 184–198.

Clermont-Ganneau, C. (1895–1898): *Recueil d'archéologie orientale*. I–II, Paris: Ernest Leroux.

Cochrane, R.G. (1961): *Biblical Leprosy: A Suggested Interpretation*. London: The Tyndale Press.

Cohen, E. (1933): 'Roman, Byzantine and Umayyad Glass', in Y. Hirschfeld (ed.), *The Roman Baths of Hammat-Gader, Final Report*. Jerusalem: The Israel Exploration Society: 396–431.

Cohen, M. (2002): 'Bathhouse from the Roman Period at Beth Guvrin', in Y. Eshel (ed.), *Judea and Samaria Research Studies*. XI, Ariel: Research institute: The College of Judea and Samaria & The Center for Judea and Samaria Studies: 187–194. [H]

Cohen, M.R. and Drabkin, I.E. (1966) [repr. 1948]: *A Source Book in Greek Medicine, Therapeutics and Hygiene*. Cambridge-Mass.: Harvard University Press.

Cohen, S.J.D. (1998): 'The Conversion of Antoninus', in P. Schäfer (ed.), *The Talmud Yerusalmi and Graeco-Roman Culture*. Tübingen: Mohr-Siebeck: 141–171.

Cohen, Y. (1975): *The Attitude toward the Gentile in the Halakha and Reality*. PhD thesis, The Hebrew University of Jerusalem. [H]

—— (1978): *Chapters in the History of the Period of the Tannaim*. Jerusalem: Education and Culture Authority. [H]

Cohen-Uzzielli, T. (1997): 'The Oil Lamps', in Y. Hirschfeld (ed.), *The Roman Baths of Hammat-Gader, Final Report*. Jerusalem: The Israel Exploration Society: 319–346.

Cohn, J. (1929): 'Die Marktbezeichnungen אטלס und ירד und ihr Verhältnis zueinander. Eine philologische Studie', in M. Gaster (ed.) *Festschrift zum 75 jährigen Bestehen des Jüdisch-Theologischen Seminars Fraenckelscher Stiftung*. II, Breslau: [s.n.]: 11–44.

Cohut, I. and Árpási, M. (1999): 'Ancient Uses of Geothermal Waters in the Precarpathian Area of Romaina and the Pannonian basin of Hungary', in R. Cataldi et al. (eds.), *Stories from A Heated Earth: Our Geothermal Heritage*. California: Geothermal Resources Council & IGA: 239–249.

Coleman, K.M. (1993): 'Launching into History: Aquatic Displays in the Early Empire', *JRS* 83: 48–73.

Coley, N.G. (1982): 'Physicians and the Chemcal Analysis of Mineral Waters', *Med. Hist.* 26: 123–144.

—— (1990): 'Physicians, Chemists and the Analysis of Mineral Waters: "The Most Difficult Part of Chemistry"', *Med. Hist.* 10: 56–66.

Colini, A.M. (1968): 'La stipe delle acque salutari di Vicarello. Notizie sul complesso della Scoperta', *RPAR* 60: 35–56.

Collingwood, R.G. and Wright, R.P. (1965): *Roman Inscriptions in Britain*. Oxford: Stroud.

Comfort, H. (1976): 'Baiae', in R. Stillwell et al. (eds.), *The Princeton Encyclopedia of Classical Sites*. Princeton, New Jersey: Princeton University Press: 137–138.

Compton, M.T. (2002): 'The Association of Hygieia with Asklepios in Graeco-Roman Asklepieion Medicine', *JHM* 57 (3): 312–329.

Conder, C.R. (1889): *The Survey of Eastern Palestine*. London: Lond.

Conder, C.R. and Kitchener, H.H. (1998) [repr.]: *Survey of Western Palestine 1881–1888: Memoirs of the Topography, Ortography, Hydrography, and Archaeology*: [London]: Archive Editions in association with the Palestine Exploration Fund.

Connolly, P. and Dodge, H. (1998): *The Ancient City: Life in Classical Athens and Rome*. Oxford: Oxford University Press.

Constable, O.R. (2003): *Housing the Stranger in the Mediterranean World: Lodging, Trade and Travel in Late Antiquity and the Middle Ages*. Cambridge: Cambridge University Press.

Copeman, W.S.C. (1964): *A Short History of the Gout and the Rheumatic Diseases*. Berkeley: University of California Press.

Cotton, H.M. and Yardeni, A. (1997): *Aramaic, Hebrew and Greek Documentary Texts from Nahal Hever and Other Sites with an Appendix Containing Alleged Qumran Texts. The Seiyâl Collection II*. Oxford: Clarendon Press.

Coulston, J. and Dodge, H. (2003): 'An Imperial Metropolis', in G. Woolf (ed.), *Cambridge Illustrated History of the Roman World*. Cambridge: Cambridge University Press: 138–169.

Cowell, F.R. (1973): *Everyday Life in Ancient Rome*. London-New York: B.T. Batdford & G.P. Putnam's Sons.

Cozzo, G. (1971): *The Colosseum: The Flavian Amphitheatre, Architecture, Building Techniques. History of the Construction, Plan of Works*. Rome: Fratelli Palombi.

Crabtree, R.D. (1983): *Leisure in Ancient Israel (Before 70 A.D.)*. PhD thesis, Ann Arbor, Michigan.

Croke, B. (1981): 'Two Early Byzantine Earthquakes and Their Liturgical Commemoration', *Byzantion* 51: 122–147.

Croon, J.H. (1967): 'Hot Springs and Healing Gods', *Mnemosyne* 20: 225–246.

Croutier, A.L. (1992): *Taking The Waters: Spirit, Art, Sensuality*. New York: Abbeville Press.

Crowfoot, J.W. (1941): *Early Churches in Palestine*. London: Publishing for the British Academy by H. Milford, Oxford University Press.

Crowfoot, J.W., Kenyon, K. and Sukenik, E. (1942): *The Buildings at Samaria*. London: Palestine Exploration Fund.

Cruse, A. (2004): *Roman Medicine*. Stroud, Gloucestershire: Tempus.

Cunliffe, B. (1984): *Roman Bath Discovered* (rev. ed.). London-New York: Routledge & Kegan Paul.

—— (1988): *The Temple of Sulis Minerva at Bath. The Finds from the Sacred Spring*. II, Monograph No. 16. Oxford: Oxford University Committee for Archaeology.

—— (1995): *Roman Bath*. London: B.T. Batsford.

Cunliffe, B. and Davenport, P. (1985): *The Temple of Sulis Minerva at Bath. The Site*. I, Monograph No. 7. Oxford: Oxford University Committee for Archaeology.

Cüppers, H. (1982): *Aquae Granni: Briträge zur Archäologie von Aachen*. Köln: Rheinland-Verlag.

Czysz, W. (1994): *Wiesbaden in der Römierzeit*. Stuttgart: Theiss.

Dąbrowa, E. (1993): *Legio X Fretensis. A Prosopographical Study of Its Officers (I–III c. AD)*. Stuttgart: Franz Steiner.

da Costa, K., O'Hea, M., Mairs, L., Sparks, R. and Boland, P. (2002): 'New Light on Late Antique Pella: Sydney University Excavations in Area 35, 1997', *ADAJ* 46: 503–533.

Dalby, A. (2000): *Empire of Pleasures: Luxury and Indulgence in the Roman World*. London-New York: Routledge.

—— (2003): *Food in The Ancient World from A to Z*. London-New York: Routledge.

Dalman, G. (1912): 'Jahresbericht des Institus für das Arbeisjahr 1911/12', *Palästina-jahrbuch* 8: 1–63.

—— (1914): 'Inschriften aus Palästina', *ZDPV* 37: 135–145.

—— (1922): *Aramäisch-neuhebräisches handwörterbuch zu Targum, Talmud und Midrasch*. Frankfurt a. Main: J. Kauffmann.

—— (1924) [repr. 1967]: *Orte und Wege Jesu* (4th edn.). Darmstadt: Wissenschaftliche Buchgesellschaft.

—— (1935): *Sacred Sites and Ways: Studies in the Topography of the Gospels*. London: S.P.C.K.

Damati, E. (1986): 'Caphareccho-Huqoq: The Unknown Fortress of Joseph Flavius', *Cathedra* 39: 37–44. [H]

D'Amato, C. (1989): 'Terme e cure termali nell'antica Roma', *Terme romane e vita quotidiana: supplemento all'edizione romana della mostra "Terme romane e vita quotidiana"*. Roma: Edizioni Quasar: 10–16.

Dan, Y. (1984): *The City in Eretz-Israel during the Late Roman and Byzantine Periods*. Jerusalem: Yad Izhak Ben Zvi. [H]

Daniel, R.W. (1988): 'A Note of the Philinna Papyrus (PGM XX 1–2)', *ZPE* 73: 306.

D'Arms, J.H. (1970): *Romans on the Bay of Naples: A Social and Cultural Study of the Villas and Their Owners from 150 BC to AD 400*. Cambridge, Mass.: Harvard University Press.

Dauphin, C.D. (1996): 'Brothels, Baths and Babes: Prostitution in the Byzantine Holy Land', *CI* 3: 47–72.

—— (1996–1997): 'Leprosy, Lust and Lice: Health and Hygiene in Byzantine Palestine', *BAIAS* 15: 55–80.

—— (1997): 'Carpets of Stone: The Graeco-Roman Legacy in the Levant', *CI* 4: 1–32.

—— (1998): 'Bordels et filles de joie: La prostitution en Palestine byzantine', in M. Balard et al. (eds.), *Eupsychia: Mélanges offerts à Hélène Ahrweiler*. I, Paris: Publications de la Sorbonne: 177–194.

Davenport, P. (1999): *Archaeology in Bath Excavations 1984–1989. BAR International Series* 284. Oxford: Archaeopress.

Davies, R.W. (1970): 'The Roman Military Medical Service', *SJ* 27: 84–104.

Davis, E.J. (1874): *Anatolica: or, the Journal of a Visit to Some of the Ancient Ruined Cities of Caria, Phrygia, Lycia, and Pisidia*. London: Grant.

Dawes, E. and Baynes, N.H. (1996) [repr. 1948]: *Three Byzantine Saints: Contemporary Biographies Translated from Greek*. Crestwood, N.Y.: St.Vladimir's Seminary Press.

Dechent, H. (1884): 'Heilbäder und Badeleben in Palästina', *ZDPV* 7: 173–210.

de Franciscis, A. (1967): 'Underwater Discoveries around the Bay of Naples', *Archaeology* 20: 209–216.

Dehn, W. (1941): 'Ein Quellheiligtum des Apollo und der Sirona bei Hochscheid Kr. Bernkastel', *Germania* 25, 104–111.

Deines, R. (1993): *Jüdische Steingefässe und pharisäische Frömmigkeit: ein archäologisch-historischer Beitrag zum Verständnis von Joh 2,6 und der jüdischen Reinheitshalacha zur Zeit Jesu*. Tübingen: Mohr-Siebeck.

de Khitrowo, B. (1899): *Itinéraires Russes en Orient: Vie et Pelerinage de Daniel, Hégoumène Russe 1106–1107*. Genève: Imprimerie Jules-Guillaume Fick.

DeLaine, J. (1988): 'Recent Research on Roman Baths', *JRA* 1: 11–32.

—— (1989): 'Greek to Roman Baths in Hellenistic Italy', *Med. Arch.* 2: 111–125.

—— (1993): 'Roman Baths and Bathing', *JRA* 6: 348–358.

—— (1997): *The Baths of Caracalla: A Study in the Design, Construction, and Economics of Large-Scale Building Projects in Imperial Rome*. Portsmouth: JRA.

—— (1999): 'Introduction: Bathing and Society', in J. DeLaine and D.E. Johnston (eds.), *Roman Baths and Bathing, Proceeding of the First International Conference on Roman Baths held at Bath, 1992. JRA, Supp. Series* 37: 7–16.

—— (2004): 'Baths', in S. Hornblower and A. Spawforth (eds.), *The Oxford Companion to Classical Civilization*. Oxford: Oxford University Press: 113–115.

de Levante, E.R. (ed.) (1874): *Hexaglot Bible*. London: Lond.

DeLigt, L. (1993): *Fairs and Markets in the Roman Empire: Economic and Social Aspects of Periodic Trade in a Pre-Industrial Society*. Amsterdam: J.C. Gieben.

Den Boer, W. (1969): 'Religion and Literature in Hadrian's Policy', *Mnemosyne* 8: 123–144.

Dentzer, J.-M. and Dentzer-Feydy, J. (1991): *Le djebel al-ʿArab. Histoire et Patrimoine au Musée de Suweida*. Paris: Éditions Recherche sur les civilisations.

Dermage J. and Tournage D. (1990): *Study of the Potential and Uses of the Geothermal Resources in Jordan*. CFG, France.

de Sandoli, S. (1980): *Emmaus-Qubeibe: The Sanctuary and Nearby Biblical Sites*. Jerusalem: Studium Biblicum Franciscanum.

de Saulcy, F. (1874): *Numismatique de la Terre Sainte: Description des monnaies autonomes et impériales de la Palestine et de l'Arabie Pétrée*. Paris: J. Rothschild.

Dessau, H. (ed.) (1892–1916): *Inscriptiones Latinae Selectae*. I–III. Berolini: Weidmannos.

de Vaux, R. (1938): 'Une Mosaïque Byzantine a Ma'in (Transjordanie)', *RB* 47: 227–258.

—— (1956): 'Fouilles de Khirbet Qumran', *RB* 63: 533–577.

—— (1959): 'Fouilles de Feshkha', *RB* 66: 225–255.

de Vaux, R. and Steve, A.M. (1950): *Fouilles à Qaryet el-'Enab et Abū Gôsh*. Paris: J. Gabalda.

de Zanche, P. (1988): *Thermal Therapy in the Euganean Basin*. Regione Veneto: Terme Euganee.

Di Capua, F. (1940): *L'idroterapia ai tempi dell'impero romano*. Roma: Istituto di studi romani.

Dickie, M.W. (1994): 'The Identity of Philinna in the Philinna Papyrus', *ZPE* 100: 119–122.

Dieppe, P.A. Doherty, M. Mcfarlane, D.G. and Maddison, P. (eds.) (1985): *Rheumatological Medicine*, 'Seronegative Spondarthritidies', Edinburgh: Churchill Livingstone: 65–92.

Di Segni, L. (1988): 'The Inscriptions of Tiberias', in Y. Hirschfeld (ed.), *Tiberias: From Beginnings until the Muslim Conquest*. Jerusalem: Yad Izhak Ben Zvi: 70–95. [H]

—— (1992): 'Greek Inscriptions of the Bathhouse in Hammat-Gader', *ARAM Periodical* 4: (1–2): 307–328.

—— (1994): 'The Inscriptions of Hammat-Gader', in Y. Hirschfeld, *Hammat-Gader and Its Thermae*. Jerusalem: Israel Exploration Society: 37–42. [H]

—— (1997): 'The Greek Inscriptions of Hammat Gader', in Y. Hirschfeld (ed.), *The Roman Baths of Hammat-Gader, Final Report*. Jerusalem: The Israel Exploration Society: 185–266.

Di Segni, L. and Hirschfeld, Y. (1986): 'Four Greek Inscriptions from Hammat-Gader from The Reign of Anastasius', *IEJ* 36: 250–268.

Dilke, O.A.W. (1975): *The Ancient Romans: How They Lived and Worked*. Newton Abbot: David & Charles.

Dilts, M.R. and Kennedy, G.A. (eds.) (1997): *Two Greek Rhetorical Treatises from the Roman Empire*. Leiden-New York-Köln: Brill.

Dittenberger, W. (1960): *Sylloge Inscriptionum Graecarum* (4th edn.), I–II. Hildesheim: Georg Olms.

—— (ed.) (1977): *Orientis Graeci Inscriptiones Selectae*. I–IV. Hildesheim: Georg Olms.

Dodge, H. (1990): 'Impact of Rome in the East', in M. Hening (ed.), *Architecture and Architectural Sculpture in the Roman Empire.* Oxford: Oxford University Committee for Archaeology. Monograph No. 29: 108–120.

—— (1999): 'Amusing the Masses: Buildings for Entertainment and Leisure in the Roman World', in D.S. Potter and D.J. Mattingly (eds.), *Life, Death, and Entertainment in the Roman Empire*. Ann Arbor: University of Michigan Press: 205–255.

Donner, H. (1963): 'Kallirrhoë. Das sanatorium Herods des großen', *ZDPV* 79: 59–89.

—— (1979): *Pilgerfahrt ins Heilige Land: die aeltesten Berichte christliche Palaestinapilger (4.–7. Jahrhundert)*. Stuttgart: Katholisches Bibelwerk.

—— (1982): 'Mitteilungen zur topographie des Ost-jordanlandes anhand der mosaikkarte von Mādebā. I: Die Thermen von Baaras', *ZDPV* 98: 175–180.

—— (1992): *The Mosaic Map of Madaba—An Introductory Guide*. Kampen: Kok Pharos.

—— (1995): *Isis in Petra*. Leipzig: Ägyptologisches Institut & Ägyptisches Museum der Universität.

Donner, H. and Cüppers, H. (1967): 'Die Restauration und Konservierung der Mosaikkarte von Madeba', *ZDPV* 83: 1–33.

Doron, A. (1965): *Survey of the Development of the Dead Sea Shore*. Tel-Aviv: The Technical Department of HaSomer HaTsair. [H]

Dothan, A. (1986): *The Dead Sea Shore Survey*. The Dead Sea: The Mediterranean Society. [H]

Dothan, M. (1968): 'The Synagogues at Hammath-Tiberias', *Qadmoniot* 4: 116–123. [H]

—— (1981): 'The Synagogue at Hammath-Tiberias', in L.I. Levine (ed.), *Ancient Synagogues Revealed*. Jerusalem: The Israel Exploration Society: 63–69.

—— (1983): *Hammat Tiberias: Early Synagogues and the Hellenistic and Roman Remains*. Jerusalem: The Israel Exploration Society.

—— (1993): 'Hammath-Tiberias', in E. Stern (ed.), *NEAEHL* II, Jerusalem: Israel Exploration Society & Carta: 574–577.

Dothan, M. and Johnson, B.L. (2000): *Hammat Tiberias: Late Synagogues.* Jerusalem: Israel Exploration Society.

Downey, G. (1961): *A History of Antioch in Syria: From Seleucus to the Arab Conquest.* Princeton, New Jersey: Princeton University Press.

—— (1963): *Ancient Antioch.* Princeton, New Jersey: Princeton University Press.

Drimba, O. (1984–1987): *Istoria Culturii şi Civilizaţiei.* I–II, Bucharest: Ştiinţifică şi Enciclopedică.

Drinkwater, J.F. (1983): *Roman Gaul: The Three Provinces, 58 BC–AD 260.* London: Croom Helm.

Dritsas, M. (2002): 'Water, Culture and Leisure: From Spas to Beach Tourism in Greece during the Nineteenth and Twentieth Centuries', in S.C. Anderson and B. Tabb (eds.), *Water, Leisure and Culture: European Historical Perspectives.* Oxford: Berg: 193–208.

Dubnov, S. (1955): *The History of the Jewish People* (4th edn.). I–IV, Tel-Aviv: Dvir. [H]

Dumazedier, J. (1967): *Toward A Society of Leisure* (tr. S.E. McClure). New York: Free Press.

Dunbabin, K.M.D. (1989): 'Baiarum Grata Voluptas: Pleasures and Dangers of the Baths', *PBSR* 57: 6–46.

—— (2003): *The Roman Banquet: Images of Conviviality.* Cambridge: Cambridge University Press.

Dupont, F. (1992): *Daily Life in Ancient Rome* (tr. C. Woodall). Oxford: Blackwell.

Dürr, J. (1881): *Die Reisen des Kaisers Hadrian.* Wien: C. Gerold's Sohn.

Duval, N. (1999): 'Essi sur la signification des vignettes topographiques', in M. Piccirillo and E. Alliata (eds.), *The Madaba Map, Centenary 1897–1997.* Jerusalem: Studium Biblicum Franciscanum: 134–145.

Dvorjetski, E. (1988): *Hammat-Gader during the Hellenistic, Roman and Byzantine Periods: An Historical-Archaeological Analysis,* M.A. thesis, University of Haifa. [H]

—— (1990): 'Women and Coins and Their Connection with Therapeutic Baths', in I. Machtey (ed.), *Progress in Rheumatology: The 5th International Seminar on the Treatment of Rheumatic Diseases.* IV, Petah-Tiqva: Rheumatology Service, Hasharon Hospital: 134–137.

—— (1992a): *Medicinal Hot Springs in Eretz-Israel during the Period of the Second Temple, The Mishnah and the Talmud.* PhD thesis, The Hebrew University of Jerusalem. [H]

—— (1992b): 'Medicinal Hot Springs in Eretz-Israel and in the Decapolis during the Hellenistic, Roman and Byzantine Periods', *ARAM Periodical* 4 (1–2): 425–449.

—— (1993): 'The Coins of Gadara as Historical Documents and Their Affinity to the Baths of Hammat-Gader', *Zion* 58: 387–406. [H]

—— (1994a): 'Medicinal Hot Springs in Eretz-Israel in Antiquity: Sacred Places or Popular Sites of Healing?', *JSJF* 16: 7–27. [H]

—— (1994b): 'The Healing Qualities of the Therapeutic Hot Springs in Eretz-Israel during the Mishnaic and Talmudic Periods', *Proceedings of the Eleventh World Congress of Jewish Studies.* I, Jerusalem: Magness Press, The Hebrew University: 39–46. [H]

—— (1994c): 'Nautical Symbols on the Gadara Coins and Their Link to the *Thermae* of The Three Graces at Hammat-Gader', *MHR* 9: 100–115.

—— (1994d): 'Roman Emperors at the Medicinal Hot Springs in Eretz-Israel', in E. Schiler (ed.) *Studies in the Geography of the Holy Land, Ariel* 105–106: 58–66. [H]

—— (1994e): 'The Theatre in Rabbinic Literature', in A. Segal (ed.), *Aspects of Theatre and Culture in the Graeco-Roman World.* University of Haifa, Faculty of Humanities: 51–68. [H]

—— (1995a): 'On the Use of Smooth Pebbles at the Medicinal Baths of Eretz-Israel in Ancient Times: A Talmudic Analysis', *Koroth* 11: 43–52. [H]

—— (1995b): 'The Medicinal Hot Springs of Kallirrhoe', in G. Barkai, H. Geva and E. Schiler (eds.), *Sites and Places in Jordan.* Jerusalem: Ariel Publishing House: 306–308. [H]

—— (1996a): 'Properties of Therapeutic Baths in Eretz-Israel in Antiquity', in O. Rimon (ed.), *Illness and Healing in Ancient Times*. Hecht Museum, Catalogue No. 13, University of Haifa: Ayalon: 36–42. [H] (English version on pp. 39*–45*).

—— (1996b): 'The Healing Qualities of the Thermo-Mineral Baths in Eretz-Israel and Jordan in Classical Antiquity', *The 35th International Congress on the History of Medicine. Book of Abstracts.* Kos, Greece: 22.

—— (1996c): 'The Thermo-Mineral Springs and the Ships' Load in the Dead Sea according to the Madaba Map', in G. Barkai and E. Schiler (eds.), *Eretz-Israel in the Madaba Map.* Jerusalem: Ariel Publishing House: 82–88. [H]

—— (1997a): 'Medicinal Hot Springs in the Graeco-Roman World', in Y. Hirschfeld (ed.), *The Roman Baths of Hammat Gader, Final Report.* Jerusalem: The Israel Exploration Society: 463–476.

—— (1997b): 'Roman Emperors at the Thermo-Mineral Baths in Eretz-Israel', *Latomus* 56: 567–581.

—— (1999a): 'Social and Cultural Aspects of the Medicinal Baths in Israel according to Rabbinic Sources', in J. DeLaine and D.E. Johnston (eds.), *Roman Baths and Bathing, Proceeding of the First International Conference on Roman Baths held at Bath, 1992. JRA, Supp. Series* 37: 117–129.

—— (1999b): 'Christians at the Thermo-Mineral Baths in the Region of the Kinnert', in G. Barkai and E. Schiler (eds.), *The Kinnert and Its Region in the Christian Tradition, Ariel* 139: 133–141. [H]

—— (1999c): 'Theaters' Culture in the Eastern Mediterranean during the Roman and Byzantine Periods according to the Talmudic literature', in A. Segal, *The History and Architecture of the Theaters in Roman Palestine*, Jerusalem: Mosad Bialik Press: 117–143. [H]

—— (1999d): 'Public Health in Jerusalem during the Second Temple period', in Z. Amar et al. (eds.), *Medicine in Jerusalem through the Ages.* ERETZ—Geographic Research and Publications Project for the Advancement of Knowledge of Eretz-Israel, Tel-Aviv University: 1–32. [H]

—— (2000a): 'The Diseases of Rabbi Judah the Patriarch in Light of Modern Medicine', *HaRefuah* 139 (5–6): 232–236. [H]

—— (2000b): 'The Contribution of the Cairo *Geniza* to the Study of the Medicinal Hot Springs in Eretz-Israel', *Proceedings of the Twelfth World Congress of Jewish Studies.* II, Jerusalem: Magness Press, The Hebrew University: 85–93. [H]

—— (2001a): 'The Maioumas festivals at Ascalon during the Roman-Byzantine Period: "What was perpetrated by the coastal cities was not perpetrated by the generation of the food"', in A. Sasson et al. (eds.), *Ashkelon: A City on the Seashore*, ERETZ—Geographic Research and Publications Project for the Advancement of Knowledge of Eretz-Israel, Tel-Aviv University: 99–118. [H]

—— (2001b): 'A Talmudic Reality in the Erotic Rituals of Dionysiac-Bacchic Cult', in I. Zinguer (ed.), *Dionysos: Origines et Resurgences.* Paris: Librairie Philosophique J. Vrin: 79–93.

—— (2001c): *Ecology and Values: Ecology and Environmental Quality in Jewish Traditional Sources: Selected Sources to the Lectures* (2nd edn.). University of Haifa: Academon Press. [H]

—— (2001–2002): 'Thermo-Mineral Waters in the Eastern Mediterranean Basin: Historical, Archaeological and Medicinal Aspects', *ARAM Periodical* 13–14: 485–512.

—— (2002a): 'The Medical History of Rabbi Judah the Patriarch: A Linguistic Analysis', *Hebrew Studies* 43: 39–55.

—— (2002b): 'The History of Nephrology in the Talmudic Corpus', in G. Eknoyan et al. (eds.), *History of Nephrology, Reports from the 3rd Congress of the International Association for the History of Nephrology.* Freiburg-Paris-London-New York: Karger, Medical and Scientific Publishers: 23–33 [= *AJN* 22 (2002): 119–129].

—— (2002c): 'The Names of Agon Village (Umm Djunni) and Their Geographical-Historical Significance', in A. Demsky (ed.), *These Are The Names: Studies in Jewish Onomastics.* Ramat-Gan: Bar-Ilan University Press: 65–75. [H]

——— (2003): 'The Relations between Jews and Gentiles in Medicinal Hot Springs in Eretz-Israel during the Mishnaic and Talmudic Periods', in A.Oppenheimer et al. (eds.), *Jews and Gentiles in the Holy Land in the Days of the Second Temple, the Mishnah and the Talmud. A Collection of Articles.* Jerusalem: Yad Izhak Ben Zvi Press: 9–39. [H]

——— (2004): 'Healing Waters: The Social World of Hot Springs in Roman Palestine', *BAR* 30 (4): 16–27, 60.

——— (2005): 'Agon Village and Its Affinity to the Leisure Culture in the Land of Israel during the Period of the Second Temple, The Mishnah and the Talmud', in M. Mor et al. (eds.), *For Uriel: Studies in the History of Israel in Antiquity.* The Zalman Shazar Center for Jewish History, Jerusalem: 439–467. [H]

——— (2006–2007): 'Christians at the Thermo-Mineral Baths in Roman-Byzantine Palestine', *ARAM Periodical* 18–19: 13–32.

——— forthcoming [a]: '"Once Happened to Be in a Certain Inn": Aims and Deeds of Our Sages at Hammat-Gader', in Z. Safrai (ed.), *Galilee Studies.* Ramat-Gan: Bar-Ilan University Press. [H]

——— forthcoming [b]: 'Emperor Hadrian at the Thermo-Mineral Baths in The Land of Israel', in P. Zanovello (ed.), *Proceedings of the International Conference on Acque minero-medicinali, terme curative e culti alle acque nel mondo romano.* Padua.

——— forthcoming [c]: 'Maioumas-Shuni and the Maioumas Festivals and Their Affinity to Maioumases and Theatres in the Eastern Mediterranean Basin', in K. Abu-Much (ed.), *Maioumas-Shuni throughout the Ages.* Israel Exploration Society & National Fund of Israel. [H]

——— forthcoming [d]: 'The Dedicatory Inscriptions from the Synagogues at Hammat-Tiberias and at Hammat-Gader and Their Contribution to the Study of the Thermo-Mineral Baths in Byzantine Palestine'. [H]

——— forthcoming [e]: 'Animals As Coin-Type in the Land of Israel in the Roman Period', in B. Arbel, et al. (eds.), *Animals in Historical Prospective. Proceedings of the Conference on Human Beings and Other Animals in Historical Perspective.* The Department of History and the Department of Zoology at Tel-Aviv University and the Department of History at the University of Haifa, 10–11 January 2001: 98–130. [H].

Dvorjetski, E. and Last, R. (1991): 'Gadara: Colony or Colline Tribe: Another Suggested Reading of the Byblos Inscription', *IEJ* 41: 157–162.

Dvorjetski, E. and Segal, A. (1998): 'A Talmudic Reality in Prohibition of Bloodshed in Amusement Places in Eretz-Israel in the Roman and Byzantine Periods', *BAMAH Periodical* 149–150: 83–94. [H]

——— (2001): '"The Kalybē Sanctuaries for the Emperors' Cult in the Hauran and the Trachon: An Historical-Architectonic Analysis', *JHSI* 8: 17–52. [H]

Dyson, S.L. (1991): *Community and Society in Roman Italy.* Baltimore-London: Johns Hopkins University Press.

Eckhardt, K.A. (1933) [repr. 1973]: *Sachsenspiegel, Lehnrecht, Monumenta Germaniae historica. Fontes iuris Germanici Antiqui. Nova Series.* Gottingen: Musterschmidt.

Eckstein, Y. (1975): *The Thermo-Mineral Springs of Israel.* Jerusalem: Geological Institute. [H]

——— (1979a): 'Review of the Heat Flow Data from the Eastern Mediterranean Region', *PAG* 117: 150–179.

——— (1979b): 'Heat Flow and the Hydrologic Cycle: Examples from Israel', in V. Čermák and L. Rybach (eds.), *Terrestrial Heat Flow in Europe.* Berlin-Heidelberg-New York: Springer-Verlag: 88–97.

Eckstein, Y. and Rosental, E. (1965): *Ain Nu'it: Development of Underground Water Sources for Healing.* Jerusalem: The Geological Institute.

Edelstein, L. (2003): 'Soranus', in S. Hornblower and A. Spawforth (eds.), *Oxford Classical Dictionary* (3rd ed. rev.). Oxford: Oxford University Press: 851.

Edwards, P.C., Bourke, S.J., Da Costa, K. et al. (1990): 'Preliminary Report on the University of Sydney's 10th Season of Excavation at Pella (Tabaqat Fahl) in 1988', *ADAJ* 34: 58–93.

Efrati, J.E. (1984): 'Rabbi's Katzra: Thoughts about the Rabbi's Learning', *Shma'atin* 77: 19–20. [H]

Efron, Y. (1988): 'The Deed of Simon Son of Shatah in Ascalon', in A. Kasher, *Canaan, Philistina, Greece and Israel: Realations of the Jews in Eretz-Israel with the Hellenistic Cities (332 BCE–70 CE)*. Jerusaelm: Yad Izhak Ben Zvi: 298–320. [H]

Eftychiadis, A. (1997): 'Diseases in the Byzantine World with Special Emphasis on the Nephropathies', *AJN* 17: 217–221.

—— (2002): 'Renal and Glomerular Circulation according to Oribasius (4th Century)', *AJN* 22: 136–138.

Eggel, W. (1839): *Chemische Untersuchung der heissen Quelle von Ammaus am Galileer Meere.* Tübingen: Ludwig Friedrich Fues.

Ehrlich, M. (1996): 'The Identification of Emmaus with Abū Ġōš in the Crusader Period Reconsidered', *ZDPV* 112: 165–169.

Eisenstein, J.D. (1952): *Ozar Yisrael: An Encyclopedia.* I–X, New York: Pardes. [H]

Elazari-Volcani, B. (1936): 'Life in the Dead Sea', *Nature* 138: 467.

—— (1940): *Studies on the Microflora of the Dead Sea.* PhD thesis, The Hebrew University of Jerusalem. [H]

Eliav, Y.Z. (1993): *Introduction to the Study of Daily Life of the Jews in Roman Baths in Eretz-Israel: History, Halakha and Talmudic Reality.* M.A. thesis, The Hebrew University of Jerusalem. [H]

—— (1995): 'Did the Jews at First Abstain from Using the Roman Bathhouse?', *Cathedra* 75: 3–35. [H]

—— (2000): 'The Roman Bath as a Jewish Institution: Another Look at the Encounter between Judaism and the Greco-Roman Culture', *JSJ* 31: 416–454.

—— (2002): 'Viewing the Sculptural Environment: Shapping the Second Commandment', in P. Schäfer (ed.), *The Talmud Yerushalmi and Graeco-Roman Culture.* III, Tübingen: Mohr-Siebeck: 411–433.

Elitzur, V. (1980): 'Between two Towns', *Eretz-HaGolan* 36: 20–21. [H]

Elmslie, W.A.L. (1967) [repr. 1911]: 'The Mishna on Idolatry "Avoda Zara"', in J.A. Robinson (ed.), *Texts and Studies.* VIII/2, Nendeln: Kraus Reprint.

Engelmann, H., Knibbe, D. and Merkelbach, R. (1980): *Die Inschriften von Ephesos.* III, Bonn: R. Habelt.

Epstein, A. (1957): *From the Antiquity of the Jews.* Jerusalem: Mosad HaRav Kook. [H]

Epstein, J.N. (1930): 'Notes on Talmudic Lexicography', *Tarbiz* 1 (2): 123–127. [H]

—— (1932): 'Emendations on the Yerushalmi', *Tarbiz* 3 (3): 237–248. [H]

—— (1957): *Introduction to the Tannaim Literature.* Jerusalem: Magness Press. [H]

—— (1964): *Introduction to the Mishnah Version* (2nd edn.). Jerusalem: Magness, The Hebrew University. [H]

Escher, B.J. (1899): 'Charites', in *Real-Encyclopädie der classischen Altertumswissenschaft*, in A. Pauly, G. Wissowa and W. Kroll (eds.). VI, München: Druckenmüller: 2150–2167.

Eshel, H. (1992): 'An Inscription Fragment of the Twenty-Four Priestly Courses from Nazareth?', *Tarbiz* 61: 159–161. [H]

—— (1998): 'The History of Research and Survey of the Finds of the Refuge Caves', in H. Eshel and D. Amit (eds.), *Refuge Caves of the Bar Kokhba Revolt.* ERETZ—Geogaphic Research and Publications Project for the Advancement of Knowledge of Eretz-Israel, Tel-Aviv University: 23–68. [H]

Evans, J.K. (1991): *War, Women and Children in Ancient Rome.* London-New York: Routledge.

Even-Shoshan, A. (1969): *The New Dictionary.* I–III, Jerusalem: Kiryat-Sefer. [H]

Eyssenhardt, F.R. (1879): *Epistula Urbica.* Hamburg: [n.s.].

Fagan, G.G. (1999a): *Bathing in Public in the Roman World.* Ann Arbor: The University of Michigan Press.

—— (1999b): 'Interpreting the Evidence: Did Slaves Bathe at the Baths?', in J. DeLaine and D.E. Johnston (eds.), *Roman Baths and Bathing, Proceeding of the First International Conference on Roman Baths held at Bath, 1992. JRA, Supp. Series* 37: 25–34.

Fahd, T. (1958): 'Hubal', in B. Lewis et al. (eds.), *The Encyclopedia of Islam* (new ed.). III, Leiden-London: Brill & Luzac Co.: 536–537.
—— (1971): 'Une pratique cléromantique à la Ka'ba préislamique', *Semitica* 8: 55–79.
Faris, N.A. (tr.) (1952): *The Book of Idols.* Princeton, New Jersey: Princeton University Press.
Feldman, A. (1962): *The Plants of the Mishnah.* Tel-Aviv: Dvir. [H]
Feldman, L.H. and Reinhold, M. (eds.) (1996): *Jewish Life and Thought among Greeks and Romans: Primary Readings.* Edinburgh: T&T Clark.
Feliks, Y. (1994): *Fruit Trees in the Bible and Talmudic Literature.* Jerusalem: R. Mass. [H]
Ferguson, E. (ed.) (1990): 'Didascalia', in *Encyclopedia of Early Christianity.* Chicago-London: St. James.
Ferguson, J. (1970): *The Religions of the Roman Empire.* London: Thames and Hudson.
Ferngren, G.B. (1991): 'Christianity and Healing in the Second Century', in E. Fierens et al. (eds.), *Proceedings of the 32nd International Congress on the History of Medicine.* Bruxelles: Societas Belgica Historiae Medicinae: 131–137.
—— (1992): 'Early Christianity as a Religion of Healing', *BHM* 66: 1–15.
Ferngren, G.B. and Amundsen, D.W. (1996): 'Medicine and Christianity in the Roman Empire: Compatibilities and Tensions', in *ANRW* II.37.3: 2957–2980.
Fiedler, K.G. (1840): *Reise durch alle Theile des Königreiches Griechenland in den Jahren 1834 bis 1837.* I, Leipzig: Leipz.
Figuers, P. (1978): 'Which Way to Emmaus?', *CNI* 3–4: 132–134.
Finkelstein, E.A. (1950): *Introduction to Tractates Avot and Avot de Rabbi Nathan.* New York: Jewish Theological Seminary of America. [H]
Finkelstein, I. (1978): 'Geographical-Historical Remarks for the Description of Eretz-Israel in the Peutinger Map', *Cathedra* 8: 71–79. [H]
—— (197b): 'The Holy Land in the Tabula Peutingeriana: An Historical-Geographical Approach', *PEQ* 111: 27–34.
Finkliesztejn, G. (1986): 'Asklepios Leontonkos et le mythe de la coupe de Césarée Maritime', *RB* 93: 419–428.
Firebaugh, W.C. (1928): *The Inns of Greece and Rome.* Chicago: Norman Lindsay Chicago Pascal Covici, Pub. Inc.
Fischer, H. (1931): *Die verfassungsrechtliche Stellung der Juden in den deutschen Städten während des dreizehnten Jahrhunderts.* Breslau: M. & H. Marcus.
Fisher, C.S. (1938): 'Description of the Site', in C.H. Kraeling (ed.), *Gerasa: City of the Decapolis.* New Haven: American School of Oriental Research: 11–26.
Fisher, M. (1989): 'The Road Jerusalem-Emmaus according to the Excavations in Hurbat Masad', in A. Kasher et al. (eds.), *Greece and Rome in Eretz-Israel: Collected Essays,* Jerusalem: Yad Izhak Ben Zvi: 185–206. [H]
Fischer, M., Issac, B. and Roll, I. (1996): *Roman Roads in Judaea: The Jaffa-Jerusalem Roads.* II, Oxford: Tempus Reparatum.
Fishman-Duker, R. (1984): 'The Bar Kokhva Rebellion in Christian Sources', in A. Oppenheimer and U. Rappaport (eds.), *Bar Kochba Revolt: New Research.* Jerusalem: Yad Izhak Ben Ben Zvi: 233–242. [H]
Fleischer, E. (1986): 'Additions to the Priestly Courses Matter', *Tarbiz* 55: 47–60. [H]
Flexer, A. (1961): 'The Geology of Mount Gilboa', *BRCI* 10: 64–72.
Foerster, G. (1977): 'The Excavations in Tiberias', *Qadmoniot* 10: 87–91. [H]
—— (1983): 'Hammat-Gader: A Synagogue', *HA* 82: 11–12. [H]
—— (1985): 'A Cuirassed Bronze Statue of Hadrian', *'Atiqot EgS* 17: 139–157.
Foerster, G. and Y. Tsafrir, Y. (1992): 'Nysa-Scytopolis in the Roman Period: "A Greek City of Coele Syria", Evidence from the Excavations at Beth-Shean', *ARAM Periodical* 4 (1–2): 117–139.
—— (1993): 'The Beth Shean Excavations Project 1988–91', *ESI* 11: 3–32.
Fontanille, M.T. (1985): 'Les bains dans la médecine Gréco-romaine', in A. Pelletier (ed.), *La Médecine en Gaule: Villes d'eaux sanctuaires des eaux.* Paris: Picard: 15–24.

Forbes, R.J. (1936): *Bitumen and Petroleum in Antiquity.* Leiden: Brill.

Forti, L. (1951): 'Rilievi dedicati alle ninfe Nitrodi', *Rendiconti dell'Accademia di archeologia, Lettere e Belle Arti-Napoli, New Series* 26: 161–191.

Foucault, M. (1990): *The Care of the Self: The History of Sexuality* (tr. R. Hurley). I–III, Harmondsworth: Penguin.

Fowler, W.W. (1969): *The Roman Festivals of the Period of the Republic.* New York: Kennikat Press.

Francus, I. (1988): 'The Halakhic Status of Children Born from Mixed Marriages in Talmudic Literature', *Sidra* 4: 89–110. [H]

Fraschetti, A. (ed.) (2001): *Roman Women* (tr. L. Lappin). Chicago-London: University of Chicago Press.

Frass, O. (1879): 'Der Schwefel im Jordanthal', *ZDPV* 2: 113–119.

Frayn, J.M. (1993): *Markets and Fairs in Roman Italy: Their Social and Economic Importance from the Second Century BC to the Third Century AD.* Oxford: Clarendon Press.

Frazer, J.G. (1951): *The Golden Bough: A Study in Magic and Religion* (3rd edn.). I, New York: The Macmillan Company.

Freeman, P. (2001): 'Roman Jordan', in B. MacDonald, R. Adams and P. Bienkowski (eds.), *The Archaeology of Jordan.* Sheffield: Sheffield Academic Press: 440–452.

French, R. (1994): *Ancient Natural History: Histories of Nature.* London-New York: Routledge.

Frend, W.H.C. (1985): *The Rise of Christianity.* Philadelphia: Fortress Press.

Frere, S.S. and Tomlin, R.S.O. (eds.) (1992): *The Roman Inscriptions of Britain.* II, Oxford: Stroud.

Freund, R., Garfunkel, Z., Zak, I., Goldberg, M., Weissbrod, T. and Derin, B. (1970): 'The Shear Zone along the Dead Sea Rift', *PTRSL* 267A: 107–130.

Freyne, S. (1980): *Galilee from Alexander the Great to Hadrian 323 BCE to 135 CE.* Wilmington: University of Notre Dame Press.

—— (1992): 'Urban-Rural Relations in First-Century Galilee: Some Suggestions from the Literary Sources', in L.I. Levine (ed.), *The Galilee in Late Antiquity.* New York: Jewish Theological Seminary of America: 75–91.

Friedheim, E. (2003): 'Rabban Gamaliel and the Bathhouse of Aphrodite in Akko: A Study of Eretz-Israel Realia in the 2nd and 3rd Centuries CE', *Cathedra* 105: 7–32. [H]

Friedman, S. (1993): 'Historical Aggadah in the Babylonian Talmud', in S. Friedman (ed.), *Jubilee Book for Rabbi Saul Lieberman.* New York: Jewish Theological Seminary of America: 1–46. [H]

—— (1998): 'Recovering the Historical Ben D'rosai', *Sidra* 14: 77–92. [H]

Friedmann, A. (1913a): *Beiträge zur chemischen und physikalischen Untersuchung der Thermen Palästinas.* Berlin: S. Calvary.

—— (1913b): 'Die Thermen von Tiberias und El Hammi in Palästina', *ZBKKH* 6: 429–436.

Friedländer, L. (1922) [repr. 1964]: *Darstellungen aus der Sittengeschichte Roms in der Zeit von August bis zum Ausgang der Antonine* (10th edn.). G. Wissowa (ed.). I–IV, Leipzig: S. Hirzel.

—— (1913) [repr. 1965]: *Roman Life and Manners under the Early Empire.* London-New York: Routledge & Kegan Paul.

Frova, A. (1965): *Scavi di Caesarea Maritima (Israele): Rapporto preliminare della la campagna di scavo della missione archeologica italiano.* Milano: [s.n.].

Fuchs, H. (1964): *Der geistige Widerstand gegen Rom in der antiken Welt* (2nd edn.). Berlin: Walter De Gruyter & Co.

Fuks, G. (1983): *Greece in Eretz-Israel: Beit-She'an in the Hellenistic and Roman Periods.* Jerusalem: Yad Izhak Ben Zvi. [H]

Fulvio, L. (1887): 'Castelforte: Di un edificio termale riconosciuto nel territorio del comune', *Notizie degli Scavi di Antichità* 5: 236–238.

—— (1888): 'Castelforte', *Notizie degli Scavi di Antichità* 2: 460.

Funk, R.W. and Richardson, H.N. (1958): 'The 1958 sounding at Pella', *BA* 21: 82–86.

Funk, S. (1914): 'Die stadt und ihre hochschule', *Festschrift D. Hoffmann*. Berlin: Verlag Hausfreund.

Furrer, K. (1879): 'Die Ortschaften am See Genezareth', *ZDPV* 2: 52–74.

Fytikas, M., Leonidopoulou, G.M. and Cataldi, R. (1999): 'Geothermal Energy in Ancient Greece: From Mythology to Late Antiquity', in R. Cataldi et al. (eds.), *Stories from a Heated Earth—Our Geothermal Heritage*. California: GRC & IGA: 69–101.

Gager, J.G. (ed.) (1992): *Curse Tablets and and Binding Spells from the Ancient World*. Oxford: Oxford University Press.

Galanis, S.-P., Sass, J.H., Munroe, R.J. and Abu Ajamieh, M. (1986): *Heat Flow at Zarqa Ma'in and Zara and A Geothermal Reconnaissance of Jordan*. U.S. Geological Survey. Open File Report.

Garbrecht, G. and Manderscheid, H. (1994): *Die Wasserbewirtschaftung römischer Thermen: Archäologische und Hydrotechnische Untersuchungen*. I–III, Braunschweig: Leichtweiss-Institut für Wasserbau.

Gardiner, E.N. (1930) [repr. 1967]: *Athletics of the Ancient World*. Oxford: Clarendon Press.

Garfunkel, Z. (1997): 'The History and Formation of the Dead Sea Basin', in M. Niemi et al. (eds.), *The Dead Sea: The Lake and Its Setting*. New York-Oxford: Oxford University Press: 36–56.

Garg, S. and Kassoy, D.R. (1981): 'Convective Heat and Mass Transfer in Hydrothermal Systems', in L. Rybach and L.J.P. Muffler (eds.), *Geothermal Systems: Principles and Case Histories*. Chichester-New York-Brisbane-Toronto: Wiley: 37–76.

Garstang, J. (1931): *Joshua-Judges*. London: Constable & Co.

Garzya, A. (1994): 'L'eau dans la littérature médicale de l'antiquité tardive', in R. Ginouvè et al. (eds.), *L'eau, la santé et la maladie dans le monde grec. Actes du colloque organisé à Paris, 1992*. Athènes: Ecole Française d'Athènes & Paris: Diffusion de Boccard: 109–119.

Gask, G. and Todd, J. (1953): 'The Origin of Hospitals', in E.A. Underwood (ed.), *Science, Medicine and History: Essays on the Evolution of Scientific Thought and Medical Practice Written in Honour of Charles Singer*. London-New York-Toronto: Oxford University Press: 122–130.

Gat, J. Mazor, E. and Tsur, Y. (1969): 'The Stable Isotopes Composition of Mineral Waters in the Jordan Rift Valley, Israel', *JH* 7 (3): 334–352.

Gatier, P-L. (1990): 'Un amphithéâtre à Bosra', *Syria* 67: 201–206.

—— (1999): 'The Levant during the Early Byzantine Era: The Continued Survival of Urban Life', in O. Binst (ed.), *The Levant: History and Archaeology in the Eastern Mediterranean*. Cologne: Könemann: 187–240.

Gavrieli, I. and Bein A. (1995): 'Sulphur Iisotopes in the Dead Sea and in Thermal-Saline Springs along the Shores', *Proceeding of the IAEA Meeting on Isotopes in Water Resources Management*. Vienna: 174–176.

Gawlikowski, M. (1990): 'Les dieux des Nabatéens', in *ANRW* II.18.4: 2659–2677.

Geiger, J. (1985): 'Athens in Syria: Greek Intellectuals of Gadara', *Cathedra* 35: 3–16. [H]

—— (1986): 'Eros und Anteros, der blonde und der dunkelhaarige', *Hermes* 114: 375–376.

—— (1994): 'Notes on the Second Sophistic in Palestine', *ICST* 19:221–230.

Gera, D. (1977): *The Rule and the Roman Army from the Destruction of the Second Temple to the Outbreak of Bar-Kokhba Revolt (70–132 CE)*. M.A. thesis, The Hebrew University of Jerusalem. [H]

Geraty, L.T. and Herr, L.G. (eds.) (1986): *The Archaeology of Jordan and Other Studies Presented to Siegfried H. Horn*. Michigan: Andrews University Press.

Germer-Durand, J. (1892): 'Aelia Capitolina', *RB* 1: 369–387.

Gersht, R. (ed.) (1999): *The Sdot-Yam Museum Book of the Antiquities of Caesarea Maritima: In Memory of A. Wegman*. Tel-Aviv: HaKibbutz HaMeuhad. [H]

Gesenius, W. (1899): *Gesenius's Hebrew and Chaldee Lexicon to the Old Testament Scriptures* (rev. & corrected ed.). London: Samuel Bagster & Sons.

Geva, H. (1984): 'The Camp of the Tenth Legion in Jerusalem: An Archaeological Reconsideration', *IEJ* 34: 239–255.

Gibb, H.A.R. and Kramers, J.H. (eds.) (1974): *Shorter Encyclopaedia of Islam*. Leiden: Brill.

Gichon, M. (1978): 'Roman Baths in Eretz-Israel', *Qadmoniot* 11: 37–53. [H]

—— (1979a): 'The Roman Bath at Emmaus: Excavations in 1977', *IEJ* 29: 101–110.

—— (1979b): 'Thermes d'Emmaüs (1977–1978)', *RB* 86: 125–126.

—— (1980): 'Emmaus (Thermen), Emmaus Nicopolis', *ArO* 27: 228–234.

——(1982): 'Military Aspects of the Bar-Kokhba Revolt and the Subterranean Hideaways', *Cathedra* 26: 30–42. [H]

—— (1986–1987): 'The Bath-house at Emmaus', *BAIAS* 6: 54–57.

—— (1993): 'Emmaus', in E. Stern (ed.), *NEAEHL* I, Jerusalem: Israel Exploration Society & Carta: 386–389.

Gichon, M. and Linden, R. (1984): 'Muslim Oil Lamps from Emmaus', *IEJ* 34: 156–169.

Giglioli, G. (1911): 'Note archeologiche sul Latium Novum', *Ausonia* 4: 39–87.

Gil, M. (1981): 'Palestine during the Muslim Period', in Y. Parwer (ed.), *The History of Eretz-Israel: The Muslims and the Crusaders Reigns*. Jerusalem: Keter: 17–160. [H]

—— (1983): *Palestine during the First Muslim Period (634–1099)*. II, Tel-Aviv: Tel-Aviv University Press. [H]

—— (1992): *A History of Palestine 634–1099*. Cambridge: Cambridge University Press.

—— (1994): 'On Sort of Thing of Palestine during the First Muslim Period', *Cathedra* 70: 29–58. [H]

Gilad, D. (1985): *Hydro-Geological Model of the Aquifer of Hammat-Gader*. Hydrological Report, No. 2. Jerusalem: The Hydrological Service, the Governorship of Water and Ministry of Agriculture in Israel. [H]

Gildemeister, J. (1883): 'Beiträge zur Palästinakunde aus arabischen Quellen', *ZDPV* 6: 1–12.

Gilmore, P.M. (1984): 'A Fresh Look at Caracalla's Syrian Silver', *Num. Cir.* 92 (2): 41–42.

—— (1991) 'Palestine in the First Muslim Period (634–1099): Supplement, Remarks and Corrections', *Teuda* 7: 281–345. [H]

Ginouvès, R. (1962): *Balaneutikè: Recherches sur le bain dans l'antiquité grecque*. Paris: De Boccard.

Ginzberg, H.A. (1962): 'Lasha', in *EB*, IV. Jerusalem: Mosad Bialik: 532. [H]

Ginzberg, L. (1909): *Yerushalmi Fragments from the Genizah*. New York: Jewish Theological Seminary of America. [H]

—— (1941–1961): *Explanations and Innovations in the Yerushalmi*. I–IV, New York: Jewish Theological Seminary of America. [H]

Ginzburger, M. (1903): *Pseudo-Jonathan on the Torah*. Berlin: Saluari. [H]

Girdler, R. (1990): 'The Dead Sea Transform Fault System', *Geological and Tectonic Processes of the Dead Sea Rift Zone, Tectonophysics* 180: 1–13.

Gizowska, E. (1998): *Bathing for Health, Beauty and Relaxation*. London: Reader's Digest.

Glaser, F. (2000): 'Fountains and Nymphaea', in Ö. Wikander (ed.), *Handbook of Ancient Water Technology*. Leiden: Brill: 437–449.

Glueck, N. (1943): 'Some Ancient Towns in the Plains of Moab', *BASOR* 91: 7–26.

—— (1951): 'Explorations in Eastern Palestine, Khirbet Fahil', *AASOR* 25–28: 254–257.

Goethert, K.P. (2001): 'Badekultur, Badeorte, Badereisen in den gallischen Provinzen', in M. Matheus (ed.), *Badeorte und Bäderreisen in Antike, Mittelalter und Neuzeit*. Mainzer Vorträge, 5. Stuttgart: Institut für Geschichtliche Landeskunde an der Universität Mainz & Franz Steiner Verlag: 16–33.

Goitein, S.D. (1967): *A Mediterranean Society: The Jewish Communities of the Arab World as Portrayed in the Documents of the Cairo Geniza*. I, Berkeley, California: University of California Press.

—— (1980): *Palestine Jewry in Early Islamic and Crusader Times according to the Geniza Documents*. Jerusalem: Yad Izhak Ben Zvi. [H]

Golan, D. (1989): *Scriptores Historia Augustae, Vita Hadriani*. Jerusalem: Academon. [H]

Golani, U. (1962): *The Geology of Lake Tiberias Region and the Geohydrology of the Saline Springs*. Jerusalem: Report of Tahal, Water Planning for Israel. [H]

Goldin, J. (tr.) (1955): *The Fathers according to Rabbi Nathan*. New Haven: Yale University Press.

—— (1965): 'Something about the House of Study of Rabban Yohanan ben Zakkai', in S. Liberman et al. (eds.), *Jubilee Book for Z. Wolfson*. Jerusalem: The American Academy for Judaic Studies. [H]

Goldstein, A. (1967–1969): 'Medical Nomenclature in Hebrew from Historical Point of View', *Koroth* 4: 452–462, 625–636, 773–786. [H]

Goldstein, A. and Shechter, M. (1956): *The Medicinal and Health Thesaurus*. I–II, Tel-Aviv: Dvir. [H]

Goldsworthy, A. (2003): *The Complete Roman Army*. London: Thames & Hudson.

Golvin, J.C. (1988): *L'amphithéâtre romain: Essai sur la théorisation de sa forme et de ses fonctions*. Paris: Diffusion de Boccard.

Golvin, J.C. and Reddé, M. (1990): 'Naumachies, jeux nautiques et amphithéâtres', in C. Domergue et al. (eds.), *Spectacula*. I, *Gladiateurs et amphithéâtres*: Lattes: Editions Imago: 165–177.

Goodale, T.L. and Godbey, G.C. (1988): *The Evolution of Leisure: Historical and Philosophical Perspectives*. State College, Pennsylvania: Venture Publishing.

Goodenough, E.R. (1953–1968): *Jewish Symbols in the Greco-Roman Period*. I–XIII. [New York]: Pantheon Books.

—— (1958): 'A Jewish-Gnostic Amulet of the Roman Period', *GBS* 1: 71–80.

Goodman, M. (1983): *State and Society in Roman Galilee, AD 132–212*. Totowa, New Jersey: Rowman & Allanheld.

—— (1992): 'The Roman State and the Jewish Patriarch in the Third Century', in L.I. Levine (ed.), *The Galilee in Late Antiquity*. New York: Jewish Theological Seminary of America: 127–139.

—— (1997): *The Roman World 44 BC—AD 180*. London-New York: Routledge.

Gordon, B.L. (1938): 'Ophthalmology in the Bible and the Talmud', *HH* 11: 57–72. [H]

Goshen-Gottstein, A. (1993): 'Rabbi Eleazar ben Arakh: Symbol and Reality', in A. Oppenheimer et al. (eds.), *Jews and Judaism during in the Second Temple Period, the Mishnah and the Talmud, Researches in Honor of S. Safrai*. Jerusalem: Yad Izhak Ben Zvi: 173–197. [H]

Goshen-Gottestein, M. (1965a): 'Borit', in *EB*, II. Jerusalem: Mosad Bialik: 347. [H]

—— (1965b): 'Sulphur', in *EB*, II. Jerusalem: Mosad Bialik: 545–546. [H]

Graf, D.F. (1992): 'Hellenisation and the Decapolis', *ARAM Periodical* 4 (1–2): 1–48.

Grainger, J.D. (1990): *The Cities of Seleukid Syria*. Oxford: Clarendon Press.

Grant, M. (1995): *Art in the Roman Empire*. London-New York: Routledge.

—— (1999): *The Roman Emperor: A Biographical Guide to the Rulers of Imperial Rome 31 BC–AD 476*. London: Phoenix Giant.

—— (2000): *Sick Ceasars: Madness and Malady in Imperial Rome*. New York: Barnes & Noble.

Grätz, H. (1853): 'Palästinenaische Ortsnamen im Talmud: Emmaus or Ammaus', *MGWJ* 2: 112–113.

—— (1897): *Geschiche der Juden von den ältesten Zeiten bis auf die Gegenwart* (4th edn.). IV, Leipzig: O. Leiner.

—— (1908): *Geschichte der Juden* (4th edn.). (tr. S.P. Rabbinovitz). Leipzig: [n.s.].

Graves, R. (1959): *New Larousse Encyclopedia of Mythology.* London-New York: Hamlyn.

—— (tr.) (1986): *Suetonius: The Twelve Caesars: An Illustrated Edition.* London: Penguin Books.

Gray, W.D. (1923): 'The Founding of Aelia Capitolina and the Chronology of the Jewish War under Hadrian', *AJSLL* 39: 248–256.

Green, J. and Tsafrir, Y. (1982): 'Greek Inscriptions from Hammat-Gader: A Poem by the Empress Eudocia and two Building Inscriptions', *IEJ* 32: 77–96.

Green, M. (1995): *Celtic Goddesses: Warriors, Virgins and Mothers.* London: British Museum Press.

Green, V. (1993): *The Madness of Kings: Personal Trauma and the Fate of Nations.* Stroud-New York: Alan Sutton & St. Martin's Press.

Greenvald, Y.Y. (1936): *Eretz-Israel, Babylon and the Diaspora Countries: The Economic Situation of the Sages.* New York: Kampf.

Greitzer, Y. and Levitte, D. (2000): 'Geothermal Update Report from Israel', *Proceeding World Geothermal Congress.* Kyushu-Tohoku, Japan: 209–212.

Grenier, A. (1931–1960): *Manuel d'archéologie gallo-romaine.* I–IV, Paris: A. Picard.

Griffin, M. (1992) [repr. 1976]: *Seneca: A Philosopher in Politics.* Oxford: Clarendon Press.

Grimal, P. (1983): *Roman Cities* (tr. G.M. Woloch). Madison-London: University of Wisconsin Press.

—— (1986): *The Dictionary of Classical Mythology* (tr. A.R. Maxwell-Hyslop). Oxford: Blackwell.

Grossberg, A. (1991): 'A Mikveh in the Bathhouse', *Cathedra* 99: 171–184. [H]

Gsell, S. (1664) [repr. 1963]: 'Gratiae', in C. Daremberg and E. Saglio (eds.), *Dictionnaire des antiquités grecques et romaines.* II, Graz: Akademische Druck-u. Verlagsanstalt: 1658–1664.

Guérin, V. (1868) [repr. 1982]: *Description Géographique, Historique et Archéologique de la Palestine.* I, Paris: Imprimerie imperiale [= idem, *ibid.*, (tr. H. Ben Amram), Jerusalem: Yad Izhak Ben Zvi.

Guhl, E. and Koner, W. (1994): *The Romans: Their Life and Customs.* London: Senate.

Guillemot, J.B. (1882): 'Emmaus-Nicopolis', *LMC* 14: 103–106.

Gur (Garzovski), Y. (1983): *A Hebrew Dictionary.* I–III, Tel-Aviv: Dvir. [H]

Guthrie, D. (1960): *A History of Medicine.* London-Paris-New York: Thomas Nelson.

Guttmann, Y. (1954): 'The Patriarch Judah I: His Birth and His Death', *HUCA* 25: 256–260.

—— (1959): 'Antoninus and Rabbi', *EH*, IV. Jerusalem-Tel-Aviv: Dvir: 422–424. [H]

Habas-Rubin, E. (1996): 'A Poem by the Empress Eudocia: A Note on the Patriarch', *IEJ* 46: 108–119.

Hadidi, A. (1978): 'The Roman Town Planning of Amman', in R. Moorey and P. Parr (eds.), *Archaeology in the Levant: Essays for Kathleen Kenyon.* Warminster: Aris & Phillips: 210–222.

Haffmann, H. (1986): *Itinera Principum: Geschichte und Typologie der Kaiserreisen im Römischen Reich.* Stuttgart: F. Steiner Verlag Wiesbaden.

Hahn, L. (1906): *Rom und Romanismus im griechisch-römischen Osten: Mit besonderer Berücksichtigung der Sprache. Bis auf die Zeit Hadrians: Eine Studie.* Leipzig: Dietrich.

Hakki, W. and Teimeh, M. (1981): *The Geology of Zarqa Ma'in and Zara Areas.* Amman: Natural Resources Authority.

Halbertal, M. (1998): 'Coexisting with the Enemy: Jews and Pagans in the Mishnah', in G. Stanton and G. Stroumsa (eds.), *Tolerance and Intolerance in Early Judaism and Christianity.* Cambridge: Cambridge University Press: 159–172.

Halevi, E.E. (1963): *Numbers Rabbah.* Tel-Aviv: Dvir [H]

Halfmann, H. (1986): *Itinera Principum: Geschichte und Typologie der Kaiserreisen im Römischen Reich.* Stuttgart: F. Steiner Verlag Wiesbaden.

Halov, D. (1838): *The History of Israel Physicians.* Vienna: G. Breg Publishing. [H]

Hammerstaedt, J. (1990): 'Der Kyniker Oenomaus von Gadara', in *ANRW* II.36.4: 2835–2865.

Hammond, N.G.L. and Scullard, H.H. (eds.) (1970): *The Oxford Classical Dictionary*. Oxford: Oxford University Press.

Hangmann, G.M.A. (1968): 'Charites', 'Nymphs', in M. Cary et al. (eds.), *The Oxford Classical Dictionary*. Oxford: Clarendon Press: 227, 615.

Hannestad, N. (2001): 'Castration in the Baths', in N. Birkle et al. (eds.), *Macellum: Culinaria Archaeologica. Festschrift Robert Fleischer zum 60. Geburtstag von Kollegen, Freunden und Schülern*. Mainz: 67–77.

Hanoune, M.R. (1980): 'Thermes romains et Talmud', in R. Chevallier (ed.), *Colloque histoire et historiographie: Clio.Colloquium in honor of L. Foucher. Collection Caesarodunum*. XV, Paris: Société d'édition Les Belles Lettres: 255–262.

Hanson, J.A. (1959): *Roman Theatre-Temples*. Princeton, New Jersey: Princeton University Press.

Harder, G. (1962): 'Herodes-Burgen und Herodes-Städte im Jordangraben', *ZDPV* 78: 49–63.

Harris, H.A. (1967): *Greek Athletes and Athletics*. London: Hutchinson.

—— (1972): *Greek Athletics and the Jews* (eds. and trs. Y. Aluf and M. Bar-Or). Tel-Aviv: AmHaSefer. [H]

Hart, G.D. (2000): *Asclepius: The God of Medicine*. London: Royal Society of Medicine Press.

Hartmann, M. (1973): 'Neue Grabungen in Baden-Aquae Helveticae 1973', *GVJ* 45–51.

Hartmann, R. (1916): 'Politische Geographie des Mamlukenreiches: Kapitel 5 und 6 des Staatshandbuchs Ibn Fadlallâah al Omaris', *ZDMG* 70: 1–40, 477–511.

Harvey, P. (1986) [repr. 1937]: *The Oxford Companion to Classical Literature*. Oxford: Clarendon Press.

Hasson, I. (1982): 'Remarques sur l'inscription de l'époque de Mu'āwiya à Hammat Gader', *IEJ* 32: 97–101.

Hastings, J. (ed.) (1899) [repr. 1958]: *A Dictionary of the Bible*. I–IV, Edinburgh: T.&T. Clark.

Hatcher, R., Zietz, I., Regan, R. and Abu-Ajameh, M. (1981): 'Sinistral Strike-Slip Motion on the Dead Sea Rift: Confirmation from New Magnetic Data', *Geology* 9: 458–462.

Hatt, J.J. (1985): 'Appolon guérisseur en Gaule: ses origines, son caractère, les divinités qui lui sont associées', in A. Pelletier (ed.), *La Médecine en Gaule: Villes d'eaux sanctuaires des eaux*. Paris: Picard: 205–238.

Hayes, C.E. (1997): *Between the Babylonian and Palestinian Talmuds: Accounting for Halakhic Sugyot from Trachtate Avodah Zarah*. New York-Oxford: Oxford University Press.

Haywood, L., Kew, F., Bramham, P., Spink, J., Capenerhurst, J. and Henry, I. (1995): *Understanding Leisure* (2nd edn.) Cheltenham: Stanley Thornes.

Hazel, J. (2001): *Who's Who in the Roman World*. London-New York: Routledge.

Head, B.V. (1963): *Historia Numorum: A Manual Greek Numismatics*. London: Spink.

Healy, J.F. (1986): 'Pliny on Mineralogy and Metals', in R. French and F. Greenaway (eds.), *Science in the Early Roman Empire: Pliny the Elder, His Sources and Influence*. London-Sydney: Croom Helm: 111–146.

Hecker, M. (1961): 'The Roman Road Legio-Sepphoris', *BIES* 25: 175–186. [H]

Heidet, A. (1909): 'Eine Badekur in Kallirrhoë und die Dampfschiffahrt auf dem Toten Meere', *DAH* 53: 121–135.

Heinz, W.H. (1983): *Römische Thermen: Badewesen und Badeluxus im römischen Reich*. München: Hirmer Verlag.

—— (1996): 'Antike Balneologie in späthellenisticher und römischer Zeit: Zur medizinischen Wirkung römischer Bäder', in *ANRW* II.37.3: 2411–2432.

Helck, W. (1972): 'Sarapis', in *Der Kleine Pauly: Lexicon der Antike*. IV, Stuttgart: A. Druckenmüller: 1549.

Henderson, B.W. (1923): *The Life and Principate of the Emperor Hadrian AD 76–138*. London: Methuen.

Hendin, D. (2001): *Guide to Biblical Coins* (4th edn.). New York: Amphora.

Hengel, M. (1974): *Judaism and Hellenism: Studies in their Encounter in Palestine during the Early Hellenistic Period*. Philadelphia: Fortress Press.

Henig, M. (ed.) (1983): *A Handbook of Roman Art: A Survey of the Visual Arts of the Roman World*. Oxford: Phaidon.

—— (1988): 'The Small Objects', in B. Cunliffe (ed.), *The Temple of Sulis Minerva at Bath. The Finds from the Sacred Spring*. II, Oxford: Oxford University Committee for Archaeology. Monograph No. 16: 5–56.

—— (1995) [repr. 1984]: *Religion in Roman Britain*. London: B.T. Batsford.

—— (1999): 'Artistic Patronage and the Roman Military Community in Britain', in A. Goldsworthy and I. Haynes (eds.), *The Roman Army As A Community: Including Papers of A Conference Held at University of London, 1997. JRA, Supp. Series* 34: 151–164.

Henig, M. and Whiting, M. (1987): *Engraved Gems from Gadara in Jordan: The Sa'd Collection of Intaglios and Cameos*. Monograph no. 6. Oxford: Oxford University Committee for Archaeology.

Hennessy, J.B. and Smith, R.H. (1997): 'Pella', in E. Meyers (ed.), *The Oxford Encyclopedia of Archaeology in the Near East*. IV, New York-Oxford: Oxford University Press: 256–259.

Henrichs, A. (1970): 'Zum text einiger zauberpapyri', *ZPE* 6: 204–209.

Hepper, F.N. and Taylor, J.E. (2004): 'Date Palms and Opobalsm in the Madaba Mosaic Map', *PEQ* 136: 35–44.

Herman, D. (1991): 'Directions in Rabbi Yohanan's Decision Making in the Realm of Social and Economic Relations with Gentiles', *SHH* 16–17: 219–241. [H]

Hermansen, G. (1982): *Ostia: Aspects of Roman City Life*. Edmonton: University of Alberta Press.

Herr, M.D. (1970): *The Roman Rule in the Tanaim Literature*. PhD thesis, The Hebrew University of Jerusalem. [H]

—— (1971): 'The Historical Significance of the Dialogues between Sages and Roman Dignitaries', *SH* 22: 123–150.

—— (1977–1978): 'Hellenism and Judaism in Eretz-Israel', *Eshkolot NS* 2–3: 20–27. [H]

—— (1982): 'From the Destruction of the Second Temple to the Ben Kozba War', in M. Stern (ed.), *The History of Eretz-Israel, The Roman-Byzantine Period: The Roman Period from the Conquest to the Ben Kozba War*. IV, Jerusalem: Keter: 301–345. [H]

—— (1985): 'Eretz-Israel from Ben Kozba War to the Distribution of the Roman Empire', in idem, (ed.), *The History of Eretz-Israel, The Roman-Byzantine Period: The Mishna and Talmud Period and the Byzantine Role (70–640)*. V, Jerusalem: Keter: 13–80. [H]

—— (1989): 'External Influences in the World of the Sages in Palestine: Absorption and Rejection', in Y. Kaplan and M. Stern (eds.), *Assimilation, Continuity and Change in the Culture of the Nations and in Israel*. Jerusalem: The Zalman Shazar Center for Jewish History: 83–105. [H]

—— (1994): 'Synagogues and Theatres (Sermons and Satiric Plays)', in S. Elitzur et al. (eds.), *Knesset Ezra: Literature and Life in the Synagogue. Studies Presented to Ezra Fleischer*. Jerusalem: Yad Izhak Ben Zvi and Ben Zvi Institute: 105–119. [H]

Heurgon, J. (1952): 'Le date des gobelets de Vicarello', *RÉA* 54: 39–50.

Heyman, H. (1963): 'Roman Legionary Coins from Phoenicia', *INJ* 3: 47–51.

Hildesheimer, H. (1886): *Beiträge zur Geographie Palästinas*. Berlin: Rosenstein & Hildesheimer.

Hill, G.F. 1914 (repr. 1965): *Catalogue of the Greek Coins in the British Museum: Palestine*. London: Printed by order of the Trustees [of the British Museum].

—— (1922) [repr. 1965]: *Catalogue of the Greek Coins in the British Museum: Arabia, Mesopotamia, and Persia*, London: Printed by order of the Trustees [of the British Museum].

Hill, P. (1989): *The Monuments of Ancient Rome as Coin Types*. London: Seaby.

Hirschberg, A.S. (1920): 'The Therapeutic Sites in Eretz-Israel', *HaTekufah* 6: 215–346. [H]

Hirschfeld, Y. (1976): 'Emmaus: Historical City in View of Orchards', *Papers for the Guides*. Jerusalem: Ministry of Industry, Commerce, and Tourism: 1–12. [H]

—— (1978): 'A Hydraulic Installation in the Water-Supply System of Emmaus-Nicopolis', *IEJ* 28: 86–92.

—— (1987): 'The History and Town-Plan of Ancient Hammat-Gader', *ZDPV* 103: 101–116.

—— (1988): 'Emmaus: "A Nice Water Site and Beautiful Resort": An Historical-Archaeological Survey', *Ariel* 55–56: 9–30. [H]

—— (1989a): 'The Aqueducts of Emmaus-Nicopolis', in D. Amit et al. (eds.), *The Aqueducts of Ancient Palestine*. Jerusalem: Yad Izhak Ben Zvi: 197–204. [H]

—— (1989b): 'Aqueducts in the Graeco-Roman World', in D. Amit et al. (eds.), *The Aqueducts of Ancient Palestine. Collected Essays*. Jerusalem: Yad Izhak Ben-Zvi: 3–27. [H]

—— (1989c): 'Water Supply Networks in the Roman Baths at Hammat-Gader', in D. Amit et al. (eds.), *The Aqueducts of Ancient Palestine*. Jerusalem: Yad Izhak Ben-Zvi: 141–155. [H]

—— (1991a): 'Tiberias, 1990–1991', *HA* 97: 32–35. [H]

—— (1991b): 'The Anchor Church at the Summit of Mt. Berenice, Tiberias', *BA* 54: 122–134.

—— (1991c): *A Guide to Antiquity Sites in Tiberias*. Jerusalem: The Antiquities Authority. [H].

—— (1993): 'Hammat-Gader', in E. Stern (ed.), *NEAEHL* II, Jerusalem: Israel Exploration Society & Carta: 565–573.

—— (1994): *Hammat-Gader and Its Thermae*. Jerusalem: Israel Exploration Society. [H]

—— (1995): 'The Early Bath and Fortress at Ramat Hanadiv near Caesarea', in J.H. Humphrey (ed.), *The Roman and Byzantine Near East: Some Recent Archaeological Research. JRA Supp. Series* 14: 43–44.

—— (ed.) (1997): *The Roman Baths of Hammat Gader, Final Report*. Jerusalem: The Israel Exploration Society.

—— (2002): 'The Aqueducts of Emmaus-Nicopolis', in D. Amit et al. (eds.), *The Aqueducts of Israel*. Portsmoth, Rhode Island: 187–198.

—— (2004): 'Excavations at 'Ein Feshkha, 2001: Final Report', *IEJ* 54: 37–74.

Hirschfeld, Y., Foerster, G. and Vitto, F. (1993): 'Tiberias', in E. Stern (ed.), *NEAEHL* IV, Jerusalem: Israel Exploration Society & Carta: 1464–1473.

Hirschfeld, Y. and Gutfeld, D. (1999): 'Discovery of a Fatimid Bronze Vessels Hoard at Tiberias', *Qadmoniot* 118: 102–107. [H]

Hirschfeld, Y. and Solar, G. (1979): 'Hammat Gader (el-Hamma), Roman Thermae', *IEJ* 9: 230–234.

—— (1981): 'The Roman Thermae at Hammat-Gader: Preliminary Report of Three Seasons of Excavations', *IEJ* 31: 197–219.

—— (1984): 'Sumptuous Roman Baths Uncovered Near Sea of Galilee', *BAR* 10 (6): 22–40.

Hirshman, M. (1988): 'The Stories of the Baths from Tiberias', in Y. Hirschfeld (ed.), *Tiberias: From Beginnings until the Muslim Conquest*. Jerusalem: Yad Izhak Ben Zvi: 119–122. [H]

Hoehner, H.W. (1972): *Herod Antipas*. Cambridge: Cambridge University Press.

Hoffmann, D.Z. (1873): *Mar Samuel*. Leipzig: O. Leiner.

Holden, W. (1970): *Water Treatment and Examination*. Baltimore: Williams and Wilkins.

Holum, K.G., Hohlfelder, R.L., Bull, R.J. and Raban, A. (1988): *King Herod's Dream: Caesarea on the Sea*. New York-London: W.W. Norton & Company.

Horden, F. (2004): 'The Christian Hospital in Late Antiquity: Break or Bridge?', in F. Steger and K.P. Jankrift (eds.), *Gesundheit-Krankheit: Kulturtransfer medizinischen Wissens von der Spätantike bis in die Frühe Neuzeit*. Köln: Böhlau: 77–99.

—— (2005): 'The Earliest Hospitals in Byzantium, Western Europe, and Islam', *JIH* 35 (3): 361–389.

Hornblower, S. and Spawforth, A. (eds.) (2004): *The Oxford Companion to Classical Civilization*. Oxford: Oxford University Press.

Hornum, M.B. (1993): *Nemesis, the Roman State, and the Games*. Leiden: Brill.

Horowitz, A. (2001): *The Jordan Rift Valley*. Lisse-Abingdon-Tokyo: A.A. Balkema.

Horowitz, I.S. (1923): *Eretz-Israel and Its Neibours: Geographical-Historical Encyclopaedia for Eretz-Israel, Syria and Sinai*. Wien: Teitelboim. [H]

Horsley, R.A. (1995): *Galilee: History, Politics, People*. Pennsylvania: Trinity Press International.

Houston, G.W. (1992): 'The Other Spas of Ancient Campania', in R.M. Wilhelm and H. Jones (eds.), *The Two Worlds of the Poet: New Perspective on Virgil*. Detroit: Wayne State University Press: 356–379.

Howell, P.M. (1980): *A Commentary on Book One of the Epigrams of Martial*. London: Athlone.

Hübner, U. (1995): 'Baaras und Zeus Beelbaaros', *BZ* 39: 252–255.

Hugot, L. (1963): 'Die römischen Bücheltermen in Aachen', *BJb* 163: 188–197.

Huizinga, J. (1955): *Homo Ludens: A Study of the Play-Element in Culture*. Boston: Beacon Press.

Hulse, E.V. (1975): 'The Nature of Biblical "Leprosy" and the Use of Alternative Medical Terms in Modern Translations of the Bible', *PEQ* 107: 87–105.

Hull, E. (1889): *Memoir on the Geology and Geography of Arabia, Petraea, Palestine, and Adjoining Districts*. London: P. Watt.

Humphry, J.H. (1986): *Roman Circuses: Arenas for Chariot Racing*. London: Batsford.

—— (1988): 'Roman Games', in M. Grant and R. Kitzinger (eds.), *Civilization of the Ancient Mediterranean: Greece and Rome*. II, New York: Scribner: 1153–1165.

—— (1996): ' "Amphitheater" Hippo-Stadia', in A. Raban and K.G. Holum (eds.), *Caesarea Maritima: A Retrospective after Two Millennia*. Leiden-New York: Brill: 121–129.

Hunger, H. (1980): 'Zum Badewesen in byzantinischen Klöstern', *Klösterliche Sachkultur des Spätmittelalters, Österr. Sitzungsberichte* (Österreichische Akademie der Wissenschaften. Philosophisch-Historische Klasse) 367. Wien: Österreichische Akademie der Wissenschaften: 353–364.

Hunt, E.D. (1982): *Holy Land Pilgrimage in the Later Roman Empire AD 312–460*. Oxford: Clarendon Press.

Hunter, D.G. (1987): 'Resistance to the Virginal Ideal in Late-Fourth Century Rome', *Theatre Survey: JASTR* 48: 45–64.

Hüttenmeister, F. and Reeg, G. (1977): *Die antiken Synagogen in Israel*. I–II, Wiesbaden: Reichert.

Hyman, A.M. (1964): *The History of the Tannaim and Amoraim*. I–III, Jerusalem: Kirya Nemana. [H]

—— (1979): *Torah Haketubah Vehamessurah: A Reference Book of the Scriptural Passages Quoted in Talmudic, Midrashic and Early Rabbinic Literature* (2nd rev. edn.). II, Tel-Aviv: Dvir. [H]

Ilan, Z. (1972): *The Dead Sea and Its Seashores*. Tel-Aviv: Culture & Education. [H]

—— (1974): 'A Broken Slab Containing the Names of the 24 Priestly Courses Discovered in the Vicinity of Kissufim', *Tarbiz* 43: 225–226. [H]

Illani, S. Kronfeld, J. and Flexer, A. (1985): 'Iron-Rich Veins Related to Structural Lineaments and the Search for Base Metals in Israel', *JGE* 24: 197–206.

Ioannou, Th. (ed.) (1884): *Life of Saint Theodore of Sykeon*, Μνημεῖα Ἁγιολογικα. Venetia.

Irby, Ch.L. and Mangles, J. (1823): *Travels in Egypt and Nubia, Syria and Asia Minor during the Years 1817 and 1818*. London: T. White.

Irshai, O. (1984): 'Tiberias during the Mishnah and Talmud Periods', in S. Min HaHar (ed.), *Mitsohar le Tsohar for the Memory of Oron Bergman*. Jerusalem: [n.s.]: 136–153. [H]

Isaac, B. (1978): 'Milestones in Judaea from Vespasian to Constantine', *PEQ* 110: 47–60.

—— (1980): 'Roman Colonies in Judaea: The Foundation of Aelia Capitolina', in

A. Oppenheimer et al. (eds.), *Jerusalem in the Second Temple Period: Abraham Schalit Memorial Volume*. Jerusalem: Yad Ishak Ben Zvi & Ministry of Defence: 340–360. [H]

—— (1980–1981): 'Roman Colonies in Judaea: the Foundation of Aelia Capitolina', *Talanta* 12–13: 31–54.

—— (1981): 'The Decapolis in Syria: A Neglected Inscription', *ZPE* 44: 67–74.

—— (1986): 'The Roman Army in Jerusalem and Its Vicinity', in D. von Planck (ed.), *Studies zu den Militärgrenzen Roms*. III, Stuttgart: Theiss: 635–640.

—— (1988): 'The Roman Administration and the Urbanization', *Cathedra* 48: 9–16. [H]

—— (1993): 'The Essence of the Terms *Burgi* and *Burgarei*', in A. Oppenheimer et al. (eds.), *Jews and Judaism during in the Second Temple Period, the Mishnah and the Talmud. Researches in Honor of S. Safrai*. Jerusalem: Yad Izhak Ben Zvi: 235–242. [H]

—— (2000): *The Limits of Empire: The Roman Army in the East* (rev. edn.). Oxford: Clarendon Press.

Issac, B. and Oppenheimer, A. (1985): 'The Revolt of Bar Kokhba. Scholarship and Ideology', *JJS* 36: 33–60.

Isaac, B. and Roll, I. (1976): 'A Milestone of AD 69 from Judaea: The Elder Trajan and Vespasian', *JRS* 66: 15–19.

—— (1979a): 'Judaea in the Early Years of Hadrian's Regin', *Latomus* 38: 54–66.

—— (1979b): 'Legio II Traiana in Judaea', *ZPE* 33: 149–156.

Isaacs, D. (1994): *Medical and Para-Medical Manuscripts in the Cambridge Geniza Collections*. Cambridge: Cambridge University Press.

Ish-Shalom, M. (1901): 'Assia', in A.M. Luntz (ed.), *Jerusalem*. V, Jerusalem: Darom: 46–51. [H]

Itshaki, A. (ed.) (1978): *Israeli Guide: Useful Encyclopedia for the Geography of the Land*. I–X, Jerusalem: Keter. [H].

Jackson, R. (1988): *Doctors and Diseases in the Roman Empire*. London: British Museum Publications.

—— (1990a): 'Waters and Spas in the Classical World', *MHS* 10: 5–13.

—— (1990b): 'Roman Doctors and Their Instruments: Recent Research into Ancient Practice', *JRA* 3: 5–27.

—— (1993): 'Roman Medicine: The Practitioners and Their Practices', in *ANRW* II.37.1: 79–101.

—— (1994): 'The Surgical Instruments, Appliances and Equipment in Celsus' *De Medicina*', in P. Mudry and G. Sabbah (eds.), *La médecine de Celse. Aspects historiques, scientifiques et littéraires*. Saint-Etienne: Publications de l'Université de Saint-Etienne: 167–209.

—— (1996): 'Eye Medicine in the Roman Empire', in *ANRW* II.37.3: 2228–2251.

—— (1999): 'Spas, Waters and Hydrotherapy', in J. DeLaine and D.E. Johnston (eds.), *Roman Baths and Bathing, Proceeding of the First International Conference on Roman Baths Held at Bath, 1992. JRA, Supp. Series* 37: 107–116.

Jacobs, M. (1995): *Die Institution des jüdischen Patriarchen*. Tübingen: Mohr-Siebeck.

—— (1998a): 'Römische Thermenkultur im Spiegel des Talmud Yerushalmi', in P. Schäfer (ed.), *The Talmud Yerushalmi and Graeco-Roman Culture.* I, Tübingen: Mohr-Siebeck: 219–311.

—— (1998b): 'Theatres and Performances as Reflected in the Talmud Yerushalmi', in P. Schäfer (ed.), *The Talmud Yerusalmi and Graeco-Roman Culture*. I, Tübingen: Mohr Siebeck: 327–347.

Jacobson, D.M. and Wilson-Jones, M. (1999): 'The Annexe of the "Temple of Venus" at Baiae: An Exercise in Roman Geometrical Planning', *JRA* 12: 57–71.

Jaffé, F., Dvorjetski, E., Levitte, D., Massarwah, R. and Swarieh, A. (1999): 'Geothermal Energy Utilisation in the Jordan Valley between Lake Kinneret and the Dead Sea: A View from Antiquity', in R. Cataldi, S.F. Hodgson and J.W. Lund (eds.), *Stories from A Heated Earth: Our Geothermal Heritage*. California: GRC & IGA: 34–49.

Jastrow, M. (1995) [repr. 1950]: *A Dictionary of The Targumim, The Talmud Babli and Yerushalmi, and The Midrashic Literature*. New York: Choreb.
Jayne, W.A. (1925) [repr. 1962]: *The Healing Gods of Ancient Civilizations*. New Haven: Yale University Press.
Jeremias, J. (1932): 'Eine neugefundene Inschrift in Gadara (mkēs)', *ZDPV* 55: 76–80.
Jidejian, N. (1968): *Byblos through The Ages*. Beirut: Dar el-Machreq Publishers.
Joannes Chumnus (1844): Δίαιτα εἰς ποδάγραν. Parisiis: Boissonade JF.
Jobst, W. (1976–1977): 'Das "öffentliche Freudenhaus" in Ephesos', *JÖAI* 51: 61–84.
Johns, C.N. (1950): 'The Citadel, Jerusalem. A Summary of Work Since 1934', *QDAP* 14: 121–190.
Jones, A.H.M. (1940): *The Greek City: From Alexander to Justinian*. Oxford: Clarendon Press.
—— (1964): *The Later Roman Empire, 284–602: A Social Economic and Administrative Survey*. I–III, Oxford: Blackwell.
—— (1971): *Cities of the Eastern Roman Provinces* (2nd edn.). Oxford: Clarendon Press.
Jones, C.P. (1972): 'Aelius Aristides, Eis Basilea', *JRS* 62: 134–152.
Jones, J.M. (1986): *A Dictionary of Ancient Greek Coins*. London: Seaby.
—— (1990): *A Dictionary of Ancient Roman Coins*. London: Seaby.
Jory, E.J. (1986): 'Countinuity and Change in the Roman Theatre', in J.H. Betts et al. (eds.), *Studies in Honour of T.B.L. Webster*. Bristol: Bristol Classical Press: 143–152.
Jost, J.M. (1858): *Geschichte des Judenthumus und seiner Sekten*. Leipzig: Dorffling & Franke.
Jouanna, J. (1994): 'L'eau, la santé et la maladie dans le traité des airs, eaux, lieux', in R. Ginouvè et al. (eds.), *L'eau, la santé et la maladie dans le monde grec. Actes du colloque organisé à Paris, 1992*. Athènes: Ecole Française d'Athènes & Paris: Diffusion de Boccard: 25–40.
Kadman, L. (1956): *The Coins of Aelia Capitolina*. Jerusalem: Universitas-Publishers.
—— (1957): *The Coins of Caesarea Maritima*. Jerusalem: Schocken.
Kadman, L. and Kindler, A. (1963): *The Coin in Israel and Other People*. Tel-Aviv: Dvir. [H]
Kagan, S.R. (1933): 'Hygiene in the Talmud', *HP* 2 (1): 87–93. [H]
—— (1952): *Jewish Medicine*. Boston-Mass.: Medico-Historical Press.
Kahan, D. (1963): *Ecological-Physiological Research of the Hot Springs Fauna in Eretz-Israel*. PhD thesis, The Hebrew University of Jerusalem. [H]
Kahana, A. (2000) [repr. 1937]: *The Apocrypha Books*. Ramat-Gan: Beit-Hillel. [H]
Kahana, T. (1979): 'The Priestly Courses and Their Geographical Settlements', *Tarbiz* 48: 9–29. [H]
Kajanto, I. (1969): 'Balnea, Vina, Venus', in J. Bibauw (ed.), *Hommages à Marcel Renard*. Bruxelles: Latomus: 357–367.
Kallai, Z. (1986): *Historical Geography of the Bible: The Tribal Territories of Israel*. Jerusalem-Leiden: Magness, The Hebrew University & Brill.
Kalner, R.B. (1947): 'The Water Pipe to Beit Yerah and the Date of the Bath', *BJPES* 13: 133–140. [H]
Kampen, N.B. (ed.) (1996): *Sexuality in Acient Art: Near East, Egypt, Greece, and Italy*. New York: Cambridge University Press.
Karcz, I. and Elad, A. (1992): 'The Dating of the "Earthquake of the Sabbatical Year" and its Significance', *Tarbiz* 61: 67–83. [H]
Karcz, I. and Kafri, U. (1978): 'Evaluation of Supposed Archaoseismic Damage in Israel', *JAS* 5: 237–253.
Karcz, I. and Lom, P. (1987): 'Bibliographic Reliability of Catalogues of Historic Earthquakes in and around Israel, I: Methodology and Background', *GSI* 87 (9): 4–17.
Kardos, M.J. (2001): 'l'Vrbs de Martial: Recherches topographiques et littéraires autour des Épigrammes V, 20 et V, 22', *Latomus* 60: 387–413.
Karson, R. (1970): 'El-Hamma', in *The Golan: Anthology of Essays*. Tel-Aviv: The Section of Geography in the Kibbutz Movement: 122–123. [H]

Kasher, A. (1988a): *Canaan, Philistia, Greece and Israel: Relations of the Jews in Eretz-Israel with the Hellenistic Cities (332 BCE–70 CE)*. Jerusaelm: Yad Izhak Ben Zvi. [H]
—— (1988b): 'The Foundation of Tiberias and Its Functioning as the Capital of the Galilee', in Y. Hirschfeld (ed.), *Tiberias: From Beginnings until the Muslim Conquest.* Jerusalem: Yad Izhak Ben Zvi: 3–11. [H]
Kasher, M.M. (1934): *Hammei-Tiberias.* Jerusalem: [n.s.]. [H]
Katzenelson, I.L. (1928): *Talmud and Medicine.* Berlin: Hayim. [H]
Kazhdan, A.P. (1991): 'Baths', in *The Oxford Dictionary of Byzantium*, I. New York-Oxford: Oxford University Press: 271–272.
Kellaway, G.A. (ed.) (1991): *Hot Springs of Bath: Investigations of the Thermal Waters of the Avon Valley.* Bath: Bath City Council.
—— (2001): 'Environment Factors and the Development of Bath Spa, England', in P.E. LaMoreaux and J.T. Tanner (eds.), *Springs and Bottled Waters Bottled Waters of the World: Ancient History, Source, Occurance, Quality, and Use.* Berlin: Springer: 242–256.
Kelley, W.N. Harris, E.D. and Ruddy, E.D. (eds.) (1997): *Textbook of Rheumatology* (2nd edn.). Philadelphia: W.B. Saunders.
Kellogg, J.H. (1918): *Rational Hydrotherapy: A Manual of the Physiological and Therapeutic Effects of Hydriatic Procedures, and the Technique of their Application in the Treatment of Disease* (4th rev. ed.). Battle Creek, Michigan: Modern Medicine.
Keppie, L. (1986): 'Legions in the East from Augustus to Trajan', in P. Freeman and D. Kennedy (eds.), *The Defence of the Roman and Byzantine East. BAR International Series* 297. Oxford: Tempus Reparatum: 411–429.
Kerényi, K. (1951): *The Gods of the Greeks.* London-New York: Thames and Hudson.
—— (1956) [repr. 1960]: *Asklepios: Archetypal Image of the Physician's Existence* (tr. R. Manheim). London: Thames and Hudson.
Kersten, O. (1879): 'Umwanderung des Todten Meeres', *ZDPV* 2: 201–216.
Khouri, R.G. (1986): *Jerash: A Frontier City of the Roman East.* London: Longman.
—— (1988): *The Antiquities of the Jordan Rift Valley.* Amman, Jordan: Al Kutba.
Kiefer, O. (1934) [repr. 1994]: *Sexual Life in Ancient Rome.* London: Constable.
Kiel, G.R. (1982): *Zwei Beiträge zur Geschichte der Balneologie. Die kulturgeschichtlichen und medizinischen Wurzeln des Bäderwesens: 100 Jahre wissenschaftliche Balneologie.* Kassel: Verlag Hans Meister.
Kimelman, R. (1981): 'Birkat HaMinim and the Lack of Evidence for an Anti Christian Jewish Prayer in Late Antiquity', in E.P. Sanders et al. (eds.), *Jewish and Christian Self-Definition.* II, London: SCM Press: 232–236.
—— (1982–1983): 'Rabbi Yohanan and the Rabbinic Authority', *SHH* 9–10: 329–358. [H]
Kimhi, D. (1973): 'Na'aman', in *Encyclopedia of Men and Women in the Bible.* Tel-Aviv: Yavneh: 643–644. [H]
Kindler, A. (1958): 'The Coinage of the Bar Kokhba War', in *The Dating and Meaning of Ancient Jewish Coins and Symbols.* Tel-Aviv-Jerusalem: Schocken Publishing House: 62–80.
—— (1961): *The Coins of Tiberias.* Tiberias: Hammei Tiberia Co.
—— (ed.) (1963): *The Patterns of Monetary Development in Phoenicia and Palestine in Antiquity. Proceedings of International Numismatic Convention.* Tel-Aviv: Schocken.
—— (1973): 'The Coins of Tiberias during the Roman Era', in O. Avissar (ed.), *The Book of Tiberias: The City of Kinnrot and Its Settlement throughout the Ages.* Jerusalem: Keter: 50–59. [H]
—— (1974–1975): 'Numismatic Documentation of Hadrian's Visit to Gaza', *Museum Ha'aretz* 17–18: 61–67. [H]
Kindler, A. and Stein, A. (1987): *A Bibliography of the City Coinage of Palestine from the Second Century BC to the Third Century AD. BAR International Series* 374. Oxford: Tempus Reparatum.
King, A. (1990): *Roman Gaul and Germany.* London: British Museum Publications.

Kisch, G. (1938–1939): 'A Talmudic Legend as the Source for the Josephus Passage in the Sachsenspiegel', *HJ* 1: 105–118.

Klar, B. (1967): 'Tiberias in the Gaonic Period', in H.Z. Hirschberg (ed.), *All the Land of Naphtali. The 24th Archaeological Convvention, 1966.* Jerusalem: Israel Exploration Society: 214–235. [H]

Klausner, J. (1977): 'The Rise of Christianity', in M. Avi-Yonah and Z. Baras (eds.), *The World History of the Jewish People: Society and Religion in the Second Temple Period.* Jerusalem: Am Oved. [H]

—— (1999): *Jesus of Nazareth: His Time, Life and Doctrine.* Jerusalem: Ariel Publishing House. [H]

Kleberg, T. (1957): *Hôtels, restaurants et cabarets dans l'antiquité romaine: études historiques et philologiques.* Uppsala: Almqvist & Wiksells boktr.

Klein, S. (1909): *Briträge zur Geographie und Geschichte Galiläas.* Leipzig: R. Haupt.

—— (1910a): 'Bemerkungen zur Geographie des alten Palästina', *MGWJ* 54: 22–25.

—— (1910b): 'Zur Topographie des alten Palästina', *ZDPV* 33: 26–40.

—— (1910c): 'Rabbi Josué à Emmaüs', *RÉJ* 60: 106–107.

—— (1911–1912): 'The Estates of Rabbi Judah Ha-Nasi and the Jewish Communities in the Trans-Jordanic Region', *JQR* 2: 545–550.

—— (1915): 'Hebräische Ortsnamen bei Josephus', *MGWJ* 59: 156–169.

—— (1920): *Jüdisch-Palästinisches Corpus Inscriptionum.* Wien: Löwit.

—— (1924): *Various Essays on the Study of Eretz-Israel.* Wein: HaMenorah. [H]

—— (1925): *The Jewish Trans-Jordan.* Vienna: HaMenorah.

—— (1929): *Zur Midrasch und Palästinaforschung.* Berlin: HaMenorah.

—— (1930): 'One City Was in Eretz-Israel', *BPSHE* 1 (8–10): 21–24. [H]

—— (1932): 'Kefar Agun', in *EJ*, IX. Berlin: Eschkol Verlag: 1124.

—— (1933): 'The *Nahoti* and Rabba bar Bar Hanna on Matters of Eretz-Israel', *Zion* 5: 1–11. [H]

—— (1934): 'The Cities of the Priests and Levites and the Cities of Refuge', in N. Slousch (ed.), *Collection of the Jewish Palestine Exploration Society Dedicated to the Memory of Dr. A.M. Mazie.* Jerusalem: Rubin Mass: 81–107. [H]

—— (1937): 'Assia-Essia', in *Emet l'Ya'akov: Jubilee Volume for Ya'akov Freimanan.* Berlin: Seminary for Rabbis: 116–127. [H]

—— (ed.) (1939): *Sefer HaYishuv.* Jerusalem: Palestine Historical and Ethnographical Society & Dvir. [H]

—— (1967): *The Land of the Galilee* (2nd edn.). Jerusalem: Mosad HaRav Kook. [H]

Klein, Z. (1968): 'The Dead Sea', in *EH*, XIX. Jerusalem-Tel-Aviv: The Society for Publishing Encyclopaedias: 888–894. [H]

Kleinman, A. (1986): 'Were Fairs in Tannaitic and Amoraic Palestine Artificial and Redundant?', *Zion* 51: 471–484. [H]

Klengel, H. (1971): *Syria Antiqua: Vorislamische Denkmäler der Syrischen Arabischen Republik.* [Leipzig]: Edition Leipzig.

Kliot, N. and Cohen, S.B. (1984): 'The Names of Our Settlements', in E. Schiller (ed.), *Zeev Vilnaey's Jubilee Volume.* I, Jerusalem: Ariel Publishing House: 315–319. [H]

Kloner, A. (1982): 'Judean Subterranean Hideaways from the Time of Bar-Kokhba', *Cathedra* 26: 4–23. [H]

—— (1988): 'The Roman Amphitheatre at Beit Guvrin: Preliminary Report', *IEJ* 38: 15–24.

—— (2001): 'Hippodrum/Amphiteatre in Jerusalem', in A. Faust and E. Baruch (eds.), *New Studies on Jerusalem, Proceedings of the 6th Conference.* Ramat-Gan: Bar Ilan University Press: 75–86. [H]

Kloner, A. and Hübsch, A. (1996): 'The Roman Amphitheatre of Beth Guvrin: A Preliminary Report of the 1992, 1993 and 1994 Seasons', *'Atiqot* 30: 85–106.

Kloner, A. and Tepper, Y. (1987): *The Subterranean Hideaways in the Judean Plain.* Tel-Aviv: HaKibbutz HaMeuhad. [H]

Knapp, A.B. (1993): *Society and Polity at Bronze Age Pella: An Annales Perspective.* Sheffield: JSOT Press.
Kochavi, M. (1989): *Aphek-Antipatris: 5000 Years of History* Tel-Aviv: HaKibbutz HaMeuhad. [H]
Koenen, L. (1962): 'Der brennende Horosknabe: Zu einem Zauberspruch des Philinna-Papyrus', *ChE* 37: 167–174.
Kofsky, A. (1997): 'Peter the Iberian: Pilgrimage, Monasticism and Ecclestical Politics in Byzantine Palestine', *LA* 47: 209–222.
—— (2004): The Byzantine Holy Person: The Case of Barsanuphius and John of Gaza', in M. Poorthuis and J. Schwartz. *Saints and Role Models in Judaism and Christianity.* Leiden-Boston: Brill: 261–285.
Köhler, J. (2002): 'Research on Roman Thermo-Mineral Baths: From Italy to Israel', in C. Ohling et al. (eds.), *Cura Aquarum in Israel. Proceedings of the 11th International Conference on the History of Water Management and Hydraulic Engineering in the Mediterranean Region.* Siegburg: Deutschen Wasserhistorischen Gesellschaft: 295–305.
Köhler, L. and Baumgartner, W. (1967–1984): *Hebräisches und aramäisches Lexicon zum Alten Testament* (2nd edn.). I–III, Leiden: Brill.
Köhne, E. and Ewigleben, C. (eds.) (2000): *Gladiators and Caesars: The Power of Spectacle in Ancient Rome* (tr. R. Jackson). London: British Museum Press.
Kohut, A. (1926): *Aruch Completum* (2nd edn.). I–XII, New York: HaMenorah. [H]
Kokkinos, N. (1998): *The Herodian Dynasty: Origins, Role in Society and Eclipse.* Sheffield: Sheffield Academic Press.
—— (2002): 'Herod's Horrid Death', *BAR* 28 (2): 28–35, 62.
Kolataj, W. (1976): 'La Derniere Période d'utilisation et la destruction des thermes romains Tardifs de Kôm el-Dikka', *ÉT* 9: 218–229.
—— (1983): 'Recherches architectoniques dans les thermes et le théâtre de Kôm el-Dikka à Alexandrie', in G. Grimon et al. (eds.), *Das römisch-byzantinische Ägypten,* Mainz am Rhein: P. von Zabern: 186–194.
Kolton, Y. (1973): 'Springs Alongshore of the Dead Sea', in Z. Ilan (ed.), *Judaen Desert and the Dead Sea. Collection of Essays for the 19th Conference of the Society for the Protection of Nature in Israel.* Tel-Aviv: The Society for the Protection of Nature in Israel in Ein Gedi: 61–67. [H]
Kook, H. (1968): 'The Diseases of Rabbi Yehuda Ha-Nasi', *Koroth* 4: 767–772. [H]
Kottek, S. (1979): 'Du au muguet: a propos de tsafdina', *RHMH* 131: 71–72.
—— (1983): 'The Essenes and Medicine', *Cl. Med.* 18: 81–99.
—— (1994): *Medicine and Hygiene in the Works of Flavius Josephus.* Leiden: E.J. Brill.
—— (1996): 'Selected Elements of Talmudic Medical Terminology with Special Consideration to Graeco-Latin Influences and Sources', in *ANRW* II.37.3: 2912–2932.
—— (1996–1997): Alexandrian Medicine in the Talmudic Corpus', *Koroth* 12: 80–89. [H]
Kraay, C.M. (1980): 'Jewish Friends and Allies of Rome', *ANSM* 25: 53–57.
Kraeling, C.H. (ed.) (1938): *Gerasa: City of the Decapolis.* New Haven: American School of Oriental Research.
—— (1962): *Ptolemais: City of the Libyan Pentapolis.* Chicago: University of Chicago Press.
Krappe, A.H. (1932): 'Les Charites', *RÉG* 45: 155–162.
Krause, J.H. (1841): *Die Gymnastik und Agonistik der Hellenen.* Leipzig: Leipz.
Krauss, S. (1899) [repr. 1964]: *Griechische und Lateinische Lehnwörter im Talmud, Midrasch und Targum.* I–II, Berlin: Berl.
—— (1907–1908): 'Bad und badewesen im Talmud', *HaKedem* 1 (1–4): 87–110; 2 (1–2): 32–50, 171–194.
—— (1909): 'Der Jahrmarkt von Batnam', *ZAW* 29: 294–311.
—— (1910): *Antoninus und Rabbi.* Vienna: Verlag der Israel—Theol. Lehranstalt.
—— (1910–1912): *Talmudische Archäologie.* I–III, Leipzig: G. Fock.
—— (1922) [repr. 1966]: *Synagogale Alertümer.* Berlin: B. Harz.

—— (1929): *Talmudic Antiquities (Qadmoniot HaTalmud)*. I–IV, Berlin: Hertz. [H]
—— (1937): 'From the Romans Rule in Eretz-Israel', *BJPES* 5: 19–21. [H]
—— (1948): *Persia and Rome in the Talmud and Midrashim*. Jerusalem: Mosad HaRav Kook. [H]
—— (1910–1911) [repr. 1966]: *Talmudische Archäologie*. I–II, Hildesheim: [s.n.].
Krencker, D. and Kruger, E. (1929): *Die Trierer Kaiserthermen*. Trier: Augsburg: B. Filser.
Krug, A. (1993): *Heilkunst und Heilkult: Medizin in der Antike* (2nd edn.). München: C.H. Beck.
Kuhnen, H.P. (1990): *Palästina in griechisch-römischer Zeit*. München: Beck.
Künzl, E. (1983): 'Eine Spezialität römischer Chirurgen: die Lithotomie', *AK* 13: 487–493.
—— (1986): 'Operationsräume in römischen Thermen', *BJb* 186: 491–509.
—— (1989–1990): 'Romische Thermen als Spitaler?', *RÖJ* 17–18: 147–152.
—— (1996): 'Forschungsbericht zu den antiken medizinischen Instrumenten', in *ANRW* II.37.3: 2433–2639.
Künzl, E. and Künzl, S. (1992): 'Aquae Apollinares/Vicarello (Italien)', in R. Chevallier (ed.), *Les eaux thermales et les cultes des eaux en Gaul et dans les provinces voisines. Actes du Colloque, Aix-les-Bains 1990*. Turin: Antropologia alpine: 273–296.
Künzl, E. and Weber, Th. (1991): 'Das spätantike grab eines zahnarztes zu Gadara in der Decapolis', *DaM* 5: 81–118.
Kurland, L. (1971a): 'La Radioactivité des eaux thermals en Israël et en particulier à Tibériade (Hamei-Tveria)', *AMIF* 20: 649–655.
—— (1971b): 'The Radioactivity in Hot Springs in Israel, Especially in Hammei-Tiberias', in A. Ya'akov (ed.), *Tiberias Hot Springs. Compilation of Essays in Medicine*. Hammat-Tiberias: Hammei-Tiberias Co.: 44–47. [H]
—— (1976): 'Quelques traits spécifiques des thermes de Tibériade', *AMIF* 24: 21–31. [H]
—— (1977): 'Hammei-Tiberias: A Centre for Reumatic Diseases', *ML* 9: 27–28. [H]
—— (1980): 'Guidance for A Doctor Who Refers to Hammei-Tiberias', *ML* 22: 44–46. [H]
—— (1982): 'The Theory of Baths and the Thermal Centre', *ML* 30: 20–23. [H]
Kutsher, E.Y. (1959): *The Language and the Linguistic Background of Isaiah Scroll from the Dead Sea Scrolls*. Jerusalem: Magness Press, The Hebrew University. [H]
—— (1962): 'The Languages of the Hebrew and Aramaic Documents of Bar Kokhba and His Generation', *Leshonenu* 26: 7–23. [H]
—— (1976): *Studies in Galilean Aramaic*. Ramat-Gan: Bar-Ilan University Press.
Lachmann, S. (1933): 'Die mineralquellen Palästina', *Palästina* 7–9: 221–235.
Ladouceur, D.J. (1981): 'The Death of Herod the Great', *CPh* 76: 25–34.
Lambert, R. (1984) [repr. 1997]: *Beloved and God: The Story of Hadrian and Antinous*. London: Phoenix.
Lämmer, M. (1971): 'The Contribution of King Herod to the Olympic Games', *HaH* 4–5: 10–14. [H]
—— (1972): 'Jason's Gymnasium in Jerusalem', in U. Simri (ed.), *Proceedings of the 1972 Pre-Olympic Seminar on the History of Physical Education and Sport in Asia*. Netanya: Vingate Institute: 51–70.
—— (1976): 'Griechische Wettkämpfe in Galiläa unter der Herrschaft des Herodes Antipas', *KBS* 5: 37–76.
LaMoreaux, P.E. (2001): 'Historical Development', in P.E. LaMoreaux and J.T. Tanner, (eds.), *Springs and Bottled Waters Bottled Waters of the World: Ancient History, Source, Occurance, Quality, and Use*. Berlin: Springer: 16–32.
Landau, G. (1967): 'The Position of Tiberias', in Y. Hirschfeld (ed.), *Tiberias: From Beginnings until the Muslim Conquest*. Jerusalem: Yad Izhak Ben Zvi: 176–177. [H]
Landau, Y.H. (1976): 'Two Inscribed Tombstones', *'Atiqot EgS* 11: 89–91.
Lankester-Harding, G. (1967) [repr. 1990]: *The Antiquities of Jordan*. Cambridge: Lutterworth Press.

Lazarus-Jaffe, H. (1982): 'Between Jewish Religious Laws and Islamic Religious Laws', *Tarbitz* 51: 207–225. [H]

Lazzaro, L. (1981): *Fons Aponi. Abano e Montegrotto nell'antichità*. Abano Terme, Padua: Francisci.

Le Bohec, Y. (1989) [repr. 1994]: *The Imperial Roman Army*. London: B.T. Batsford Ltd.

Le Strange, G. (1890) [repr. 1965]: *Palestine under the Moslems: A Description of Syria and The Holy Land*. Beirut: Khayat.

—— (tr.) (1893): *Palestine Pilgrims' Text Society: Diary of A Journey through Syria and Palestine: Nâsir-I-Khusraw in 1047 AD*. London: Lond.

Lee, G. (2004): *Spa Style Europe*. London: Thames & Hudson.

Lefkowitz, M.R. and Fant, M.B. (1992): *Women's Life in Greece and Rome: A Source Book in Translation* (2nd edn.). Baltimore-London: Johns Hopkins University Press.

Leibner, U. (2003): '"The Carobs of Shikma, the Carobs of Salmona, and the Carobs of Gedora": Geographical or Botanical Names?', *Cathedra* 109: 175–184. [H]

Leibowitz, Y. (1960): 'Hippocrates', in *EH*, XIV. Jerusalem-Tel-Aviv: The Society for Publishing Encyclopaedias: 341–348. [H]

—— (1976a): 'Medicine', in *EB*, VII. Jerusalem: Mosad Bialik: 407–425. [H]

—— (1976b): 'Tsarat', in *EH*, XXVIII. Jerusalem-Tel-Aviv: The Society for Publishing Encyclopaedias: 888. [H]

Leibowitz, Y. and Draifus, P. (1976): 'Ababuot', in *EH*, I. Jerusalem-Tel-Aviv: The Society for Publishing Encyclopaedias: 255–256. [H]

Leibowitz, Y. and Kurland, L. (1972): 'Curative Springs', in *EH*, XXIV. Jerusalem-Tel-Aviv: The Society for Publishing Encyclopaedias: 48–49. [H]

Lemaire, A. (1975): 'Amwâs, vers la solution d'une enigma de l'epigraphie hebraïque', *RB* 82: 15–23.

Lenzen, C.J. and Knauf, E.A. (1987): 'Beit Ras-Capitolias: A Preliminary Evaluation of the Archaeological and Textual Evidence', *Syria* 64: 21–46.

Lester, A. (1997): 'Islamic Glass Finds', in Y. Hirschfeld (ed.), *The Roman Baths of Hammat-Gader, Final Report*. Jerusalem: The Israel Exploration Society: 432–441.

Leutsch, E.L. and Schneidewin, F.G. (eds.) (1965): *Corpus Paroemiographorum Graecorum*. I, Hildesheim: Olm.

Leven, K.H. (1996): 'Attitudes towards Physical Health in Late Antiquity', in J. Woodward and R. Jütte (eds.), *Coping with Sickness: Perspectives on Health Care, Past and Present*. Sheffield: European Association for the History of Medicine and Health Publications: 73–89.

Lévêque, P. (1987): *Aventura Greacă*. Bucharest: Meridiane.

Levick, B. (1999): *Vespasian*. London-New York: Routledge.

Levine, L.I. (1972): 'Coins of Caesarea Maritima', *IEJ* 22: 134–140.

—— (1978): 'Rabbi Simeon b. Yohai and the Purification of Tiberias: History and Tradition', *HUCA* 49: 143–185.

—— (1982): 'On Judah I and the Severan Age', in Z. Baras et al (eds.), *Eretz-Israel from the Destruction of the Second Temple to the Muslim Conquest: Political, Social and Cultural History*. I, Jerusalem: Yad Izhak Ben Zvi: 93–118. [H]

—— (1984): 'Eretz-Israel as a Part of the Roman Empire and the Great Revolt', in M. Stern (ed.), *The History of Eretz-Israel, The Roman-Byzantine Period: The Roman Period from the Conquest to the Ben Kozba War*. IV, Jerusalem: Yad Izhak Ben Zvi & Keter: 11–280. [H]

—— (1985): *The Rabbinic Class in Palestine during the Talmudic Period*. Jerusalem: Yad Izhak Ben Zvi. [H]

—— (1989): *The Rabbinic Class of Roman Palestine in Late Antiquity*. Jerusalem: Yad Izhak Ben Zvi.

—— (1998): *Judaism and Hellenism in Antiquity: Conflict or Confluence*. Seattle University of Washington Press.

—— (2001): 'The Status of the Patriarchate in the Third and Fourth Centuries: Sources and Methodology', in I. Gafni (ed.), *Kehal Yisrael: Jewish Self-Rule through the Ages*. Jerusalem: The Zalman Shazar Center for Jewish History: 103–137. [H]

Levinstam, S.A. (1965a): 'Goni', in *EB*, II. Jerusalem: Mosad Bialik: 458. [H]

—— (1965b): 'Elisha', in *EB*, I. Jerusalem: Mosad Bialik: 355–358. [H]

—— (1965c): 'Hammon', in *EB*, III. Jerusalem: Mosad Bialik: 166. [H]

—— (1965d): 'Hammoth-Dor', in *EB*, III. Jerusalem: Mosad Bialik: 200. [H]

Levitte, D. (1966): *Magmatic Phenomena in the Arava*. MSc thesis, The Hebrew University of Jerusalem. [H]

Levitte, D., and Olshina, A. (1978): *Geothermal Energy Potential of Deep Wells in the Southern Coastal Plain of Israel*. Israel Geology Survey, Report Hydrology.

Levitte, D., Olshina, A. and Wachs, D. (1978): *Geological and Geophysical Investigation in the Hammat Gader Hot Springs Area*. Israel Geology Survey, Report Hydrology.

Levitte, D. and Olshina, A. (1985): *Isotherm and Geothermal Gradient Maps of Israel*. Israel Geology Survey, Report Hydrology.

Levitte, D. and Greitzer, Y. (1997): 'Geothermal Water Potential of Cenomanian-Turonian Aquifer in Central Israel', *IGA News*.

Lévy, J. (1901): 'Cultes et rites Syriens dans le Talmud', *RÉJ* 42: 183–205.

—— (1924) [repr. 1963]: *Wörterbuch über die Talmudim und Midraschim*. I–IV, Berlin: B. Harz.

Levy, J.H. (1969): 'Josephus the Physician', *Studies in Jewish Hellenism*. Jerusalem: Mosad Bialik: 266–293. [H]

Levy, M.A. (1856): *Phönizische Studien*. Breslau: F.E.C. Leuckart.

Lewis, C.T. and Short, C. (1879): *A Latin Dictionary*. Oxford: Oxford Clarendon Press.

Lewy, J. (1943–1944): 'The Old West Semitic Sun-God Hammu', *HUCA* 18: 436–443.

Leyerle, B. (1996): 'Pilgrims to the Land: Early Christians Perceptions of the Galilee', in R.A. Horsley, *Archaeology, History, and Society in Galilee: The Social Context of Jesus and the Rabbis*. Harrisburg, Pennsylvania: Trinity Press International: 345–357.

Licht, C. (1991): *The Legends of the Sages: The Image of the Sage in Rabbinic Literature*. New Jersy: KTAV Publishing House.

Licht, S. (ed.) (1963): *Medical Hydrology*. New Haven: Conn.

Lichtenberger, A. (1999): *Die Baupolitik Herodes des Grossen*. Wiesbaden: Harrassowitz Verlag.

—— (2000–2002): 'Reading a Hitherto Lost Line and the Location of the *Naumachia* at Gadara', *INJ* 14: 191–193.

Liddel H.G. and Scott, R. (1985): *An Intermediate Greek-English Lexicon* (7th edn.). Oxford: Clarendon Press.

Liddell, H.G., Scott, R. and Jones, H.S. (1940): *A Greek-English Lexicon*.Oxford: Clarendon Press.

Lieberman, S. (1931): *The Talmud of Caesarea*. Jerusalem: [n.s.]. [H]

—— (1932a): 'Emendations on the Yerushalmi', *Tarbitz* III/2: 207–209. [H]

—— (1932b): 'Emendations on the Yerushalmi', *Tarbitz* III/4: 452–457. [H]

—— (1935): *HaYerushalmi KiFshuto*. Jerusalem: Darom. [H]

—— (1939a): 'From Legend to Halacha', *Sinai* 4: 54–58. [H]

—— (1939b): *Tosefeth Rishonim*. Jerusalem: *Bamberger & Wahrmann*. [H]

—— (1946): 'Palestine in the Third and Fourth Centuries', *JQR* 36: 329–370.

—— (1950): *Hellenism in Jewish Palestine*. New York: Jewish Theological Seminary of America.

—— (1959): 'Ten Words', *CAC* 3: 73–89. [H]

—— (1955–1988): *Tosefta Ki-Fshutah*. I–X, New York: Jewish Theological Seminary in America. [H]

—— (1963): *Hellenism in Palestine*. Jerusalem: Mosad Bialik. [H]

—— (1968): *Siphre Zutta: The Academy of Ceasarea*. New York: Jewish Theological Seminary of America. [H]

—— (1971): 'Something about the Book of Julianus from Ascalon "Palestine and Its Laws and Customs"', *Tarbiz* 40: 409–417. [H]

—— (1974): *Texts and Studies.* New York: KTAV.

—— (1980): 'That Is How It Was and That Is How It Shall Be: The Jews of Eretz-Israel and World Jewry during Mishnah and Talmud Times', *Cathedra* 17: 3–10. [H]

Lifshitz, B. (1963): 'Inscriptions Latines de Césarée (Caesarea Palaestinae)', *Latomus* 22: 783–784.

—— (1967): *Donateurs et fondateurs dans les synagogues juives.* I, Paris: J. Gabalda.

—— (1977): 'Études sur l'histoire de la province romaine de Syrie', in *ANRW* II.8: 3–30.

Limor, O. (1983): 'Egeria at Mount Nebo', *Cathedra* 27: 49–68. [H]

—— (1998): *Holy Land Travels: Christian Pilgrims in Late Antiquity.* Jerusalem: Yad Izhak Ben Zvi. [H]

—— (1999): 'Christian Pilgrims in the Byzantine Period', in Y. Tsafrir and S. Safrai (eds.), *The History of Jerusalem: The Roman and Byzantine Periods (70–638 CE).* Jerusalem: Yad Izhak Ben Zvi: 391–415. [H]

Lindsey, R.L. (1969): *New Testament: A Hebrew Translation of the Gospel of Mark.* Jerusalem: Dugith Publishers.

Ling, R. (1979): 'The Stanze di Venere at Baiae', *Archeologia* 106: 33–60.

Litchfield, W.R. (1998): 'The Bittersweet Demise of Herod the Great', *JRSM* 91: 283–284.

Louis, A. (1971): 'Hammam', in A. Lewis et al. (eds.), *The Encyclopaedia of Islam* (new ed.), III. Leiden-London: E.J. Brill & Luzac Co.: 139–146.

Löw, I. (1924–1934): *Die Flora der Juden.* I–IV, Wein-Lipzig: R. Löwit.

Luntz, A.M. (ed.) (1904) [repr. 1980]: E. Schiler (com.), *Calender for the Year 1904.* I–III, Jerusalem: Ariel Publishing House. [H]

Luria, B.Z. (1990): 'Mishrephoth Mayim', *Beth Mikra* 105: 187–188. [H]

Luz, M. (1986–1987): 'Abnimos, Nimos and Oenimaus: A Note', *JQR* 2–3: 191–195.

—— (1988): 'Salam, Meleager!', *SIFC* 6 (2): 222–231.

—— (1989): 'A Description of the Greek Cynic in the Jerusalem Talmud', *JSJ* 20: 49–54.

—— (1992): 'Oenomaus and Talmudic Anecdote', *JSJ* 23: 42–80.

—— (2003): 'The Cynics of the Decapolis and Eretz-Israel in the Hellenistic Period', in M. Mor et al. (eds.), *Jews and Gentiles in the Holy Land in the Days of the Second Temple, the Mishnah and the Talmud. A Collection of Articles.* Jerusalem: Yad Izhak Ben Zvi Press: 97–107.

Lynch, W.F. (1854): *Bericht über die expedition der Vereinigten Staaten nach dem Jordan und dem Todten Meere.* Leipzig: Verlag der Dykschen Buchhandlung.

Macchioro, V. (1912): 'Le terme romane di Agnano', *MoA* 21: 224–284.

MacCasland, S.V. (1939): 'The Asklepios Cult in Palestine', *JBL* 58: 221–227.

MacCormack, S. (1972): 'Change and Continuity in Late Antiquity: The Ceremony of Adventus', *Historia* 21: 721–752.

MacDonald, B. (2000): *East of the Jordan: Territories and Sites of the Hebrew Scriptures.* Boston-Mass.: American Schools of Oriental Research.

MacDonald, B. Adams, R. and Bienkowski, P. (eds.) (2001): *The Archaeology of Jordan.* Sheffield: Sheffield Academic Press.

Macdonald, M.C.A. (1995): 'Herodian Echoes in the Syrian Desert', in S. Bourke and J.-P. Descoeudres (eds.), *Trade, Contact and the Movement of Peoples in the Eastern Mediterranean: Studies in Honour of J.B. Hennessy.* Sydney: Meditarch: 285–290.

MacGregor, J. (1869): *The Rob Roy on the Jordan, Nile, Red Sea and Gennesareth.* London: John Murray.

Machtey, I. (1977): 'The Dead Sea as a Curative Region', *ML* 9: 28–29. [H]

—— (1986): 'Sex and Fertility in Rheumatic Diseases', *Eitaniim* 39: 12–13, 115–116. [H]

MacKay, A.G. (1989): 'Pleasure domes at Baiae', in R.I. Curtis (ed.), *Stvdia Pompeiana and Classica in Honor of Wilhelmina F. Jashemski.* II, New Rochelle: 155–172.

Mackillop, J. (1998) [repr. 2004]: *A Dictionary of Celtic Mythology*. Oxford: Oxford University Press.

MacMullen, R. (1967) [repr. 1992]: *Enemies of the Roman Order: Treason, Unrest and Alienation in the Empire*. London-New York: Routledge.

—— (1970): 'Market-Days in the Roman Empire', *Phoenix* 24: 333–341.

—— (1974): *Roman Social Relations 50 BC to AD 284*. New Haven-London: Yale University Press.

—— (1928) [repr. 1981]: *Paganism in the Roman Empire*. New Haven-London: Yale University Press.

Macpherson, J.R. (1896): *Palestine Pilgrims' Text Society: The Pilgrimage of Arculfus*. III, London: Lond.

Macrea, M. (1969): *Viata în Dacia Romană*. Bucharest: Ştiintifică.

Mader, G. (2000): *Josephus and the Politics of Historiography*. Leiden: Brill.

Magen, Y. (1984): 'The Roman Theatre in Shechem', in E. Schiler (ed.), *Zeev Vilnaey's Jubilee Volume*. I, Jerusalem: Ariel Publishing House: 269–277. [H]

—— (2005): *Flavia Neapolis: Shechem in the Roman Period*. Jerusalem: Israel Antiquities Authority.

Magness, J. (2002): 'In the Footsteps of the Tenth Roman Legion in Judaea', in A.M. Berlin and J.A. Overman (eds.), *The First Jewish Revolt: Archaeology, History and Ideology*. London-New York: Routledge: 189–212.

Magoulias, H.J. (1964): 'The Lives of the Saints as Sources of Data for the History of Byzantine Medicine in the Sixth and Seventh Centuries', *ByZ* 57: 127–150.

Maisler, B. and Stekelis, M. (1944–1945): 'Preliminary Report on the Beth Yerah Excavations', *BJPES* 11: 77–84. [H]

Maizler-Mazar, B. (1954): 'Canaan on the Threshold of the Age of the Patriarchs', *Eretz-Israel* 3: 18–32. [H]

Maiuri, A. (1989): *The Phlegraean Fields: From Virgil's Tomb to the Grotto of the Cumaean Sibyl* (5th edn.; tr. and repr. of *I Campi Flegrèi: al sepolcro di Virgilio all'antro di Cuma*. Roma: Libreria dello Stato, 1949). Congleton: Old Vicarage.

Majno, G. (1975) [repr. 1991]: *The Healing Hand: Man and Wound in the Ancient World*. Cambridge, Mass.: Harvard University Press.

Makhouly, N. (1938): 'El-Hamme: Discovery of Stone Seats', *QDAP* 6: 59–62.

Mandelkern, S. (1971): *Veteris Testamenti: Concordantiae Hebraicae Atque Chaldaicae* (3rd edn.). Jerusalem-Tel-Aviv: Schocken. [H]

Manderscheid, H. (1981): *Die Skulpturenausstattung der kaiserzeitlichen Thermenanlagen*. Berlin: Mann.

—— (1988): *Bibliographie zum römischen Badewesen unter besonderer Berücksichtigung der öffentlichen Thermen*. München: In Kommission bei Wasmuth.

—— (2000): 'The Water Management of Greek and Roman Baths', in Ö. Wikander (ed.), *Handbook of Ancient Water Technology*. Leiden: Brill: 467–535.

—— (2004): *Ancient Baths and Bathing: A Bibliography for the Years 1988–2001. JRA, Supp. Series* 55. Portsmouth: Journal of Roman Archaeology.

Manfredi, J. (1903): 'Callirrhoé et Baarou dans la mosaïque géographique de Madaba', *RB* 12: 266–271.

Mann, J. (1922) [repr. 1969]: *The Jews in Egypt and in Palestine under the Fatimid Caliphs*. I–II, New York: KTAV Publishing House.

Manor, Y. (1979): 'Various Traditions on the Location of Emmaus', *Kardom* 6: 21–26. [H]

Maraval, P. (1982): *Égérie: Journal de Voyage (Itinéraire)*. Paris: Éditions du Cerf.

Margalit, D. (1962): *Jewish Sages as Physicians*. Jerusalem: Mosad HaRav Kook. [H]

—— (1970): *The Way of Israel in Medicine*. Jerusalem: The Academy of Medicine. [H]

—— (1976): *The Origins of Health*. Jerusalem: The Academy of Medicine. [H]

Margalioth, M. (1941): 'The Date of the Earthquake at Tiberias', *BJPES* 8: 97–104. [H]

—— (1976): *Encyclopedia of Talmudic and and Geonic Literature*. I–II, Tel-Aviv: Tzetzik. [H].

Margalit, D. (1962): *Jewish Sages as Physicians*. Jerusalem: Mosad HaRav Kook. [H]

—— (1970): *The Way of Israel in Medicine*. Jerusalem: The Academy of Medicine. [H]

—— (1976): *The Origins of Health*. Jerusalem: The Academy of Medicine. [H]

Margulies, R. [n.s.]: *Tal Tehia—Doctors and Medicaments in the Talmud* (2nd edn.). Lwow: Druck Praca. [H]

Mark, S. (2002): 'Alexander the Great, Seafaring, and the Spread of Leprosy', *JHM* 57 (3): 285–311.

Marquardt, J. (1886): *Das Privatleben der Römer*. Leipzig: S. Hirzel.

Marmardji, A.S. (1951): *Textes géographiques arabes sur la Palestine*. Paris: J. Gabalda.

Marmorstein, A. (1977): 'Antoninus', *EH*, II. Jerusalem-Tel-Aviv: The Society for Publishing Encyclopaedias: 1116. [H]

Martin, E.A. (ed.) (1998): *Concise Medical Dictionary*. Oxford: Oxford University Press.

Marwood, M.A. (1988): *The Roman Cult of Salus*. BAR International Series 465. Oxford: Archaeological Reports International Series.

Maas, P. (1942): 'The Philinna Papyrus', *JHS* 62: 33–38.

Masom, S. (2003): *Josephus and the New Testament* (2nd edn). Peabody, Mass.: Hendrickson Publishers.

Massarweh, R. and Swarieh, A. (1995): *Uses of Thermal Water in Jordan*. Amman: The Higher Council for Science and Technology.

Matthews, K. (1994): 'An Archaeology of Homosexuality? Perspectives from the Classical World', *TRAC 94, Proceedings of the Fourth Annual Theoretical Roman Archaeology Conference*. University of Durham, 19–20, March 1994: 118–132.

Mattingly, H. (1936) [repr. 1966]: *Coins of the Roman Empire in the British Museum, Nerva to Hadrian*. III, London: Printed by order of the Trustees [of the British Museum].

Mayer, J. (1910): 'Mar Samuel als arzt', in M. Stern (ed.), *Festschrift Salomon Carlebach*. Berlin: Verlag Hausfreund: 190–195.

Mazar, B. (1954): *Beth Shearim*. I, Jerusalem: The Israel Exploration Society. [H]

—— (1971): *The Excavations in the Old City of Jerusalem, Preliminary Report of the Second and Third Seasons*, Jerusalem: Institute of Archaeology, Hebrew University.

—— (1972): 'Excavations near the Temple Mount', *Qadmoniot* 3–4: 74–90. [H]

Mazar, E. (1999): 'The Camp of the Tenth Roman Legion at the Foot of the South-West Corner of the Temple Mount Enclosure Wall in Jerusalem', in A. Faust and E. Baruch (eds.), *New Studies on Jerusalem, Proceedings of the 5th Conference*. Ramat-Gan: Bar Ilan University Press: 52–67. [H]

—— (2000): 'The Roman-Byzantine Bathhouse at the Foot of the Western Wall of the Temple Mount', in A. Faust and E. Baruch (eds.), *New Studies on Jerusalem, Proceedings of the 6th Conference*. Ramat-Gan: Bar Ilan University Press: 87–102. [H]

—— (2006): 'Hadrian's Legion Encamped on the Temple Mount', *BAR* 32 (6): 53–58, 82–83.

Mazia, A.M. (1926): 'Remarks', in M. Perelman (ed.), *Midrash HaRefuah*. Tel-Aviv: Dvir. [H]

Mazor, E. (1966): 'Geochemical Research on the Origin of Mineral Waters at the Lake Kinneret and the Dead Sea Shores', *Alon Techni (Mekoroth)* 2 (4): 72–81. [H]

—— (1968a): 'Genesis of Mineral Waters in the Tiberias-Dead Sea-Arava Rift Valley, Israel', in M. Malkovsky and J. Petranek (eds.), *Proceedings of Symposium II: Genesis of Mineral and Thermal Waters. Czechoslovakia 1968*. Prague: Academia: 65–80.

—— (1968b): 'On the Radioactivity of the Springs in Jericho Region', *Teva Va'aretz* 10 (6): 387. [H]

—— (1968c): 'The Hot Spring and Cave of Hammam Fhara'on in the Coast of Gulf of Suez', *Teva Va'aretz* 10 (3): 297–299. [H]

—— (1969): 'A Geological View on Sinai, Samaria and the Golan', *Mada* 13 (5): 270–275. [H]

—— (1980) [repr. 1994]: *Geology by Israeli Hammer*. Tel-Aviv: The Open University. [H]

—— (1981a): *Ein Bokek: Development of a Curative and Recreative Site*. Rehovot: Weizmann Institute. [H]

—— (1981b): *Hammei-Zohar: Development of the Baths*. Rehovot: Weizmann Institute. [H]
—— (1997): 'Groundwaters along the Western Dead Sea Shore', in T.M. Niemi et al. (eds.), *The Dead Sea: The Lake and Its Setting*. New York-Oxford: Oxford University Press: 265–276.
Mazor, E. Kaufman, A. and Carmi, I. (1981): 'Hammat-Gader: Geochemistry of Mixed Thermal Spring Complex', *JH* 18: 289–304.
Mazor, E., Levitte, D., Truesdell, A., Healy, J. and Nissenbaum, A. (1980): 'Mixing Models and Ionic Geothermometers Applied to Warm (up to 60°C) Springs: Jordan Rift Valley, Israel', *JH* 45 (1–2): 1–19.
Mazor, E. and Mero, F. (1969): 'Geochemical Tracing of Mineral and Fresh Water Sources in the Lake Tiberias Basin, Israel', *JH* 7: 276–288.
Mazor, E. and Molcho, M. (1970): 'The Springs of Hammat-Gader, Nuqeb and Gophra', *Teva Va'aretz* 11: 260–263. [H]
—— (1972): 'Geochemical Studies on the Feshcha Springs, Dead Sea Basin', *JH* 15: 37–47.
Mazor, E., Nadler, A. and Harpaz, Y. (1973): 'Notes on the Geochemical Tracing of the Kane-Samar Spring Complex, Dead Sea Basin', *IJES* 22: 255–262.
Mazor, E., Nadler, A. and Molcho, M. (1973): 'Mineral Springs in the Suez Rift Valley: Comparison with Waters in the Jordan Rift Valley and Postulation of a Marine Origin', *JH* 20: 289–309.
Mazor, G. (1988): 'The Theatre', *HA* 91: 10–13. [H]
—— (1987–1988): 'The Beit Shean Project', *ESI 1987/88* 6: 7–45.
—— (1999): 'Public Baths in Roman and Byzantine Nysa-Scythopolis (Beth Shean)', in J. De-Laine and D.E. Johnston (eds.), *Roman Baths and Bathing, Proceeding of the First International Conference on Roman Baths held at Bath, 1992. JRA, Supp. Series* 37: 293–302.
Mazor, G. and Bar-Nathan R. (1995): 'Scythopolis: The Capital of Provincia Palestina Secunda', *Qadmoniot* 107–108: 117–137. [H]
McCown, C. (1938): 'The Festival Theater at Birketein', in C. Kraeling (ed.), *Gerasa: City of The Decapolis*. New Haven: American School of Oriental Research: 159–167.
McGinn, T.A.J. (2004): *The Economy of Prostitution in the Roman World: A Study of Social History and the Brothel*. Ann Arbor: University of Michigan Press.
McNamara, M. (1972): *Targum and Testament: Aramaic Paraphrases of the Hebrew Bible. A Light on the New Testament*. Shannon: Irish University Press.
McNicoll, A.W. (1982): *Pella in Jordan*. Canberra: Australian National Gallery.
McNicoll, A.W., Edwards, P.C., Hanbury-Tenison, J., Hennessy, J.B. et al. (1992): *Pella in Jordan*. II, Sydney: Mediterranean Archaeology Supplement.
Medri, M., Soricelli, G. and Benini, A. (1999): 'In Baiano sinu: le Piccole Terme di Baia', in J. DeLaine and D.E. Johnston (eds.), *Roman Baths and Bathing, Proceeding of the First International Conference on Roman Baths held at Bath, 1992. JRA, Supp. Series* 37: 207–219.
Meijer, F. (2004): *Emperors Don't Die in Bed* (tr. S.J. Leinbach). London-New York: Routledge.
Meïmaris, I. (1983): 'Δύο ἐπιγραφὲς τῆς Αὐγούστης Εὐδοκίας (423–460 μ.Χ.) ἀπὸ τῆς Ἐμμάθα παρὰ τὰ Γάδαρα καὶ ἀπὸ τὰ Ἱεροσόλυμα', *Θεολογία* 54: 389–398.
Meir, O. (1990): 'The Story of the Rabbi's Death: A Study of Modes of Traditions' Redaction', *JSHL* 12: 147–177. [H]
—— (1998): *Rabbi Judah Ha-Nasi: A Portrait of a Leader in the Traditions of Eretz-Israel and Babylon*. Tel-Aviv: HaKibbutz HaMeuhad. [H]
Meiri, M. (1973): 'Hammei-Tiberias', in O. Avisar (ed.), *The Book of Tiberias: The City of Kinnrot and Its Settlement throughout the Ages*. Jerusalem: Keter: 29–34. [H]
Melamed, E.Z. (1966): *The Onomastikon of Eusebius*. Jerusalem: The Hebrew University. [H]

Melamed, Y.L. (1971): 'The Chemical Composition of Hammei-Tiberias' Waters', in A. Ya'akov (ed.), *Tiberias Hot Springs. Compilation of Essays in Medicine*. Hammat-Tiberias: Hammei-Tiberias Co.: 13–17. [H]

Mengarelli, R. (1923): 'Civitavecchia. Scavi eseguiti nel 1922 nelle Terme Taurine o Trajane', *NSA* 20: 321–348.

Merrill, R.V. (1944): 'Eros and Anteros', *Speculum* 19 (3): 265–284.

Merrill, S. (1881): *East of the Jordan: A Record of Travel and Observation in the Countries of Moab, Gilead, and Bashan*. London: Bentley.

Mershen, B. and Knauf, E.A. (1988): 'From Gadar to Umm Qais', *ZDPV* 104: 128–145.

Merten, E.W. (1983): *Bäder und Badegepflogenheiten in der Darstellung der Historia Augusta. Antiquitas. Reihe 4, Beiträge zur Historia-Augusta-Forschung*. XVI, Bonn: Habe.

Meshorer, Y. (1966): 'Coins of Gadara City Struck in Commemoration of a Local Naumachy', *Sefunim* 1: 25–27. [H]

—— (1967): *Jewish Coins of the Second Temple Period*. Tel Aviv: Am Hasefer.

—— (1978a): 'Jewish Symbols on Roman Coins Struck in Eretz-Israel', *IMN* 14: 60–63.

—— (1978b): 'The Coins of Sepphoris as Historical Documents', *Zion* 43: 185–200. [H]

—— (1979a): 'Sepphoris and Rome', in O. Mørkholm and N. Waggoner (eds.), *Greek Numismatics and Archaeology: Essays in Honor of Margaret Thompson*. Wetteren: Cultura: 159–171.

—— (1979b): 'A Ring from Gadara', *IEJ* 29: 221–222.

—— (1982): 'Hygieia in Aelia Capitolina', *IEJ* 1: 17–18.

—— (1984): 'Two Finds from the 10th Roman Legion', *IMJ* 3: 41–45.

—— (1985): *City-Coins of Eretz-Israel and the Decapolis in the Roman Period*. Jerusalem: Israel Museum.

—— (1988): 'The Coins of Tiberias', in Y. Hirschfeld (ed.), *Tiberias: From Beginnings until the Muslim Conquest*. Jerusalem: Yad Izhak Ben Zvi: 96–102. [H]

—— (1989): *The Coinage of Aelia Capitolina*. Jerusalem: The Iseael Museum.

—— (2000): *TestiMoney*. Jerusalem: The Iseael Museum.

—— (2004): 'The Three Graces', *Et-Mol* 175: 30. [H]

Meyer, E. (1906): *Die Israeliten und ihre Nachbarstämme: alttestamentliche Untersuchungen*. Halle: Niemeyer.

Meyers, C.M. (1992): 'Roman Sepphoris in Light of New Archaeological Evidence and Recent Research', in L.I. Levine (ed.), *The Galilee in Late Antiquity*. New York Jerusalem: The Jewish Theological Seminary of America & Harvard University Press: 321–338.

Meyers, E.M. (ed.) (1997): *The Oxford Encyclopedia of Archaeology in the Near East. I–V*, New York-Oxford: Oxford University Press.

Meyers, E.M., Netzer, E. and Meyers, C.L. (1992): *Sepphoris*. Winona Lake, Ind.: Eisenbrauns.

Meyshan, J. (1957): 'The Disease of Herod the Great, King of Judaea', *HaRefuah* 53: 154–155. [H]

—— (1973): 'Aeskulapius on Neapolis Coins', *BINS* 5 (1): 9–10. [H]

Michon, M. (1898): 'Inscription d'Amwâs', *RB* 7: 269–271.

Migliolaro, G. (1956): *Montegrotto Terme. Notize Storiche*. Padua.

Miles, G.C. (1960): 'Egyptian Glass Pharmaceutical Measures of the Eighth Century A.D.', *JHM* 15 (4): 384–389.

Milik, J.T. (1954): 'Un contract juif de L'an 134 après J.-C.', *RB* 61: 182–190.

—— (1955): 'Note additionnele sur le contract juif de l'an 134 après J.-C.', *RB* 62: 253–254.

—— (1957): 'Deux documents inédits du Désert de Juda', *Biblica* 38: 245–268.

Millar, F. (1964): *A Study of Cassius Dio*. Oxford: Clarendon Press.

—— (1981) [repr. 2001]: *The Roman Empire and Its Neighbours*. London: Duckworth.

—— (1992): *The Emperor in the Roman World (31 B.C.–A.D. 337)* (2nd edn.). London: Duckworth.

—— (1996): *The Roman Near East 31 BC–AD 337*. Cambridge-Mass.-London: Harvard University Press.

Miller, S.S. (1992): 'Rabbi Hanina bar Hama at Sepphoris', in L.I. Levine (ed.), *The Galilee in Late Antiquity*. New York: Jewish Theological Seminary of America: 175–200.

Miller, T.S. (1985) [repr. 1997]: *The Birth of the Hospital in the Byzantine Empire*. Baltimore: Johns Hopkins University Press.

Milne, J.S. (1907) [repr. 1970]: *Surgical Instruments in Greek and Roman Times*. Oxford: Clarendon Press.

Milson, D. (1987): 'The Late Synagogue at Hammath-Tiberias: A Morphological Study', *LA* 37: 303–310.

—— (2004): 'The Stratum IB Building at Hammat-Tiberias: Synagogue or Church', *PEQ* 136: 45–56.

Mimran, Y. (1984): *The Geology of Wadi al-Malieh*. MSc thesis, The Hebrew University of Jerusalem. [H]

Mitens, K. (1993): 'Theatre Architecture in Central Italy', in P.G. Bilde et al. (eds.), *Aspects of Hellenism in Italy: Towards a Cultural Unity?* Copenhagen: Museum Tusculanum Press, University of Copenhagen: 91–106.

Mittmann, S. (1987): 'Amathous, Essa, Ragaba. Drei hellenistische Festungen im östlichen Randbereich des mittleren Jordangrabens', *ZDPV* 103: 49–63.

Moitreux, G. (1992): 'Hercule et le culte des sources en Lorraine', in R. Chevallier (ed.) *Les eaux thermales et les cultes des eaux en Gaul et dans les provinces voisines. Actes du Colloque, Aix-les-Bains 1990*. Turin: Antropologia alpine: 67–76.

Mommsen, T. (ed.) (1883): *Res Gestae Divi Augusti: Ex Monumentis Ancyrano et Apolloniensi*. Berolini: Apud Weidmannos.

Monteagudo, G.L. (1999): 'The Architecture Models on the Madaba Map', in M. Piccirillo and E. Alliata (eds.), *The Madaba Map, Centenary 1897–1997*. Jerusalem: Studium Biblicum Franciscanum: 256–258.

Mor, M. (1985): 'The Bar-Kokhba Revolt and Non-Jewish Participants', *JJS* 36: 200–209.

—— (1986): 'The Roman Army in Eretz-Israel in the Years AD 70–132', in P. Freeman and D. Kennedy (eds.), *The Defence of the Roman and Byzantine East. BAR International Series* 297. Oxford: Tempus Reparatum: 575–602.

—— (1991): *The Bar-Kokhba Revolt: Its Extent and Effect*. Jerusalem: Yad Izhak Ben Zvi. [H]

—— (2003): *From Samaria to Shechem: The Samaritan Community in Antiquity*. Jerusalem: The Zalman Shazar Center for Jewish History. [H]

Morton, A.H. (1985): *Catalogue of Early Islamic Glass Stamps in the British Museum*. London: British Museum Publications for the Trustees.

Mulas, A. (1978): *Eros in Antiquity*. New York: Erotic Art Book Society.

Münch, G.N. (1893): *Die Zara'ath (Lepra) der Hebraischen Bibel*. Hamburg-Leipzig: [n.s.].

Muntner, Z. (1938): 'On the Terminology of Skin Diseases in the Ancient Hebrew Literature', *HaRefuah* 15: 48–55, 137–144. [H]

—— (1953): 'On the Disease of Herod I', *Koroth* 1: 134–136. [H]

—— (1972): 'Medicine in the Talmud', *Med. Jud.* 2 (1): 4–8.

—— (1983): 'Jews' Gymnastics', in Y. Leibovitz (ed.), *Memorial Book for Prof. Zisman Muntner*. Jerusalem: The Israeli Institute for the History of Medicine: 11–23. [H]

Musil, A. (1907): *Arabia Petraea. Moab*, I. Wien: A. Holder.

Mylius, H. (1936): *Die römischen Heilthermen von Badenweiler, Romisch-germanische Forschungen*. XII, Berlin: W. de Gruyter.

Myslil, V. (1988): *Evaluation of Geothermal Potential of Jordan*. Amman: National Resources Authority.

Naveh, J. (1978): *On Stone and Mosaic: The Aramaic and Hebrew Inscriptions from Ancient Synagogues*. Jerusalem: The Israel Exploration Society. [H]

——— (1991): 'In the Margins of the Bills from Kefar Bero', in M. Goshen-Gottstein et al. (eds.), *Present to Haim Rabin: Essays on Linguistic Studies on His 75 Anniversary*. Jerusalem: Academon. [H].

Naveh, J. and Shaked, S. (1985): *Amulets and Magic Bowels: Aramaic Incantations of Late Antiquity*. Jerusalem: Magness Press, The Hebrew University.

Ne'eman, P. (1971): *Encyclopaedia for Talmudic Geography*. I–II., Tel-Aviv: Tzetzik. [H]

Ne'eman, Y. (1990): 'The Relationship between Jews and non-Jews in the Galilee', *Sinai* 106: 152–166. [H]

——— (1991): 'The Elders of the Galilee', *HaMayan* 31 (2): 21–26. [H]

——— (1993): *Sepphoris in the Second Temple, Mishnah, and Talmud Periods*. PhD thesis, The Hebrew University of Jerusalem. [H]

——— (1996): 'From Beth Shearim to Sepphoris: On Rabbi Judah's Reasons for Moving from Beth Shearim to Sepphoris', *HaMayan* 36 (3): 38–42. [H]

Neev, D. (1965): *The Dead Sea*. PhD thesis, The Hebrew University of Jerusalem. [H]

Neev, D. and Emery, K.O. (1967): 'The Dead Sea: Depositional Processes and Environments of Evaporites', *BGSI* 41: 1–147.

Negev, A. (1972): 'A New Inscription from the High Level Aqueduct at Caesarea', *IEJ* 22: 52–53.

——— (1976): 'Callirrhoe', in R. Stillwell et al. (eds.), *The Princeton Encyclopedia of Classical Sites*. Princeton-New York: Princeton University Press: 187.

Negev, A. and Gibson, S. (2001): *Archaeological Encyclopedia of the Holy Land* (new, rev. and updated ed.), New York-London: Continuum.

Nenova-Merdjanova, R. (1997): 'Roman Precious Bronze Vessels from Moesia and Thracia', *Archaeologia Bulgarica (Sofia)* 1: 30–37.

Nesselhauf, H. and Petrikovits, H. (1967): 'Ein weihaltar fur Appollo aus Aachen-Burtscheid', *BJb* 167: 268–279.

Netzer, E. (1980): 'The Hippodrome that Herod Built at Jericho', *Qadmoniot* 51–52: 104–107. [H]

——— (1995): 'Multi-Purpose Entertainment Structure in Jericho from the Days of Herod', in H. Eshel and H. Erlich (eds.), *Judea and Samaria Research Studies Samaria*. V, Ariel: Research institute: The College of Judea and Samaria & The Center for Judea and Samaria Studies: 135–141. [H]

——— (1999): 'Herodian Bath-houses', in J. DeLaine and D.E. Johnston (eds.), *Roman Baths and Bathing, Proceeding of the First International Conference on Roman Baths held at Bath, 1992. JRA, Supp. Series* 37: 45–55.

——— (2001): *Hasmonean and Herodian Palaces at Jericho: Final Rereports of the 1973–1987 Excavations*. I, Jerusalem: Israel Exploration Society & Institute of Archaeology, The Hebrew University of Jerusalem.

Neubauer, A. (1868) [repr. 1967]: *La Géographie du Talmud*. Paris: Lévy.

Neubauer A. and Cowley, A.E. (1906): *Catalogue of the Hebrew Manuscripts in the Bodleian Library*. II, Oxford: Clarendon Press.

Neuburger, M. (1919): *Die Medizin im Flavius Josephus*. Bad Reichenhall: Buchkunst.

Neuerburg, N. (1965): *L'architettura delle fontane e dei ninfei nell'Italia antica*. Napoli: G. Macchiaroli.

Neumann, C.J.H. and Partsch, J.F.M. (1885): *Physikalische Geographie von Griechenland mit besonderer Rücksicht auf das Alterthum*. Breslau: W. Köbner.

Neusner, J. (1966): *A History of the Jews in Babylonia*. Leiden: Brill.

——— (1970): *A Life of Yohanan ben Zakkai*. Leiden: Brill.

——— (1991): *The Talmud of the Land of Israel, Shabbat*. Atlanta, Ga.: Scholars Press.

Neutsch, K.B. (1949): *Der Sport im Bilde griechischer Kunst*. Willsbach: Scherer.

Neville Havins, P.J. (1976): *The Spas of England*. London: Robert Hale & Co.

Newby, Z. (2002): 'The Heroes of the Baths: Looking at Athletes in the Baths of Caracalla at Rome', *OMNIBVS* 44: 20–21.

Newmyer, S. (1988): 'Antoninus and Rabbi on the Soul: Stoic Elements of a Puzzling Encounter', *Koroth: Special Issue* 9: 108–123.

—— (1996a): 'Talmudic Medicine and Greco-Roman Science: Cross-Currents and Resistance', in *ANRW* II.37.3: 2895–2911.

—— (1996b): 'Public Health in the Holy Land: Classical Influence and Its Legacy', in M. Waserman and S.S. Kottek (eds.) *Health and Disease in the Holy Land: Studies in the History and Sociology of Medicine from Ancient Times to the Present.* Lewiston, N.Y.: Edwin Mellen Press: 67–101.

Newton, A.P. (ed.) (1926): *Travel and Travellers of the Middle Ages.* London-New York: Kegan Paul, Trench, Trübner & Alfred A. Knopf.

Nicolet, H. (1981): 'Une monnaie de bronze frappée à Pella (Décapole) sous Commode', in L. Casson and M. Price (eds.), *Coins, Culture, and History in the Ancient World: Numismatic and Other Studies in Honour of B.L. Trell.* Detroit: Wayne State University Press.

Nielsen, H.S. (1987): 'Alumnus: A Term of Relation Denoting Quasi-Adoption', *Cl. Med.* 38: 141–158.

Nielsen, I. (1985): 'Considerazioni sulle prime fasi dell'evoluzione dell'edificio termale Romane', *ARID* 14: 81–112.

—— (1990): *Thermae et Balnea: The Architecture and Cultural History of Roman Public Baths.* I–II, Aarhus: Aarhus University Press.

—— (1993): 'Det kristne syn pa den romerske badeinstitution', *Religionsvidenskabeligt tidsskrift* 22: 81–96.

—— (1999): 'Early Provincial Baths and Their Relations to Early Italic Baths', in J. DeLaine and D.E. Johnston (eds.), *Roman Baths and Bathing, Proceeding of the First International Conference on Roman Baths held at Bath, 1992. JRA, Supp. Series* 37: 35–43.

Nielsen, I. Andersen, F.G. and Holm-Nielsen, S. (1993): *Gadara-Umm Qes III. Die Byzantinischen Thermen.* Wiesbaden: Harrassowitz.

Niemi, T.M. and Ben-Avraham, Z. (1997): 'Active Tectonics in the Dead Sea Basin', in M. Niemi et al. (eds.), *The Dead Sea: The Lake and Its Setting.* New York-Oxford: Oxford University Press: 73–81.

Nir, D. (1968): *Bibliography on the Dead Sea.* Jerusalem: The Geological Survey of Isreal.

—— (1985): *The Vulcanism in the Golan Hills.* PhD thesis, The Hebrew University of Jerusalem. [H]

Nishri, A. and Stiller, M. (1997): 'Iron, Manganese and Trace Elements in the Dead Sea', in M. Niemi et al. (eds.), *The Dead Sea: The Lake and Its Setting.* New York-Oxford: Oxford University Press: 199–204.

Nissen, H. (1885): *Italische Landeskunde.* Berlin: Weidmannsche Buchhandlung.

Noetling, F. (1886): 'Geologische Skizze der Umgebung des el Hammi', *ZDPV* 9: 58–88.

Nöldeke, Th. (1885): 'Mommsen's Darstellung der römischen Herrschaft und römischen Politik im Orient', *ZDMG* 39: 331–351.

Nolte, A. (2001): *The Ebb and Flow of Hydropathy: The Water-Cure Movement in Europe and America.* PhD thesis. University of Texas at Arlington.

Noth, M. (1928): *Die Israelitischen Personennamen im Rahmen der gemeinsemitischen Namengebung.* Stuttgart: W. Kohlhammer.

—— (1958): *Das Buch Josua* (2nd edn.). Tübingen: J.C.B. Mohr.

Nováček, F. (1966): *Czechoslovak Spas.* Prague: Balnea.

Nriagu, J.O. (1983): 'Saturnine Gout among Roman Aristocrats', *NEJM* 308: 660–663.

Nun, M. (1953): 'Tabgha Valley', *Teva Va'aretz* 10: 389. [H]

—— (1987a): 'Koursi: A Christian Monastery Near Jewish Fish Village', E. Schiler (ed.), *Zeev Vilnay's Jubilee Volume.* II, Jerusalem: Ariel Publishing House: 183–189. [H]

—— (1987b): *Anchorages and Ancient Harbours in the Sea of Galilee.* Jerusalem: Ariel Publishing House. [H]

—— (1996): 'The Fluctuations and Changes in the Kinneret Lake Water Level', *Ariel* 119–120: 267–276. [H]

Nutton, V. (1984): 'Galen in the Eyes of his Contemporaries', *BHM* 58: 315–324.

—— (1995) [repr. 2003]: 'Roman Medicine, 250 BC to AD 200', in L.I. Conard et al. (eds.), *The Western Medical Tradition 800 BC to AD 1800*. Cambridge: Cambridge University Press: 39–70.

—— (2004): *Ancient Medicine*. London-New York: Routledge.

Oded, B. (1971): 'Darb al-Hurana: An Ancient Road', *EI* 10: 192–195. [H]

—— (1972): 'Tseret HaShahar', in *EB*, VI. Jerusalem: Mosad Bialik: 779–780. [H]

Oelmann, F., Bader, W. and Hagen, J. (1932): 'Bericht über die Tätigkeit des Provinzial-museums in Bonn vom 1 April 1930 bis 31 Marz 1931', *BJb* 136–139: 273–278.

Oesterley, W.O.E. (1923): *The Sacred Dance: A Study in Comparative Folklore*. New York: Macmillan.

Olami, J. and Ringel, J. (1975): 'Two New Inscriptions of the Tenth Legion in the Caesarea Aqueduct', *IEJ* 25: 148–150. [H]

Oliphant, L. (1880): *The Land of Gilead with Excursions in Lebanon*. Edinburgh.

Oliver, J.H. (1953): *The Ruling Power: A Study of the Roman Empire in the Second Century AD through the Roman Oration of Aelius Aristides*. Philadelphia: American Philosophical Society.

Olivová, V. (1984): *Sports and Games in the Ancient World*. London: Orbis.

Oppenheimer, A. (1977): 'The Jewish Community in Galilee during the Period of Yavneh and the Bar-Kokhba Revolt', *Cathedra* 4: 51–83. [H]

—— (1978): 'The Academis in Eretz-Israel at the Beginning of the *Amoraim* Period', *Cathedra* 8: 80–89. [H]

—— (1982a): 'Bar-Kokhba Revolt', in Z. Baras et al. (eds.), *Eretz-Israel from the Destruction of the Second Temple to the Muslim Conquest: Political, Social and Cultural History*. I, Jerusalem: 40–74. [H]

—— (1982b): 'Jewish Sources Concerning the Subterranean Hideaways in the Time of Bar-Kokhba', *Cathedra* 26: 24–29. [H]

—— (1983): 'The History of the Sanhedrin in the Galilee', in A. Samueli et al. (eds.), *The Lands of the Galilee*. I, Haifa: University of Haifa Press & Company for Applied Scientific Research: 257–268. [H]

—— (1988): 'Jewish Lydda in the Roman Era', *HUCA* 59: 115–136.

—— (1991): *Galilee in the Mishnaic Period*. Jerusalem: The Zalman Shazar Center for Jewish History. [H]

Oren, E. (1971a): 'Early Islamic Material from Gannai-Hamat (Tiberias)', *Archaeology* 24: 274–277.

—— (1971b): 'Notes and News: Tiberias', *IEJ* 21: 234–235.

—— (1971c): 'Ganei-Hamat (Tibériade)', *RB* 78: 435–437.

Ostrow, S.E. (1979): 'The Topography of Puteoli and Baiae on the Eight Glass Flasks', *Puteoli* 3: 77–140.

Ottosson, M. (1969): *Gilead: Tradition and History* (tr. J. Gray). Lund: Gleerup.

Ousterhout, R. (ed.) (1990): *The Blessing of Pilgrimage*. Urbana-Chicago: University of Illinois Press.

Ovadiah, A. (1972): 'A Jewish Sarcophagus at Tiberias', *IEJ* 22: 229–232.

—— (1997): 'Allegorical Images in Greek Laudatory Inscriptions in Eretz-Israel', *LA* 47: 441–448 [= idem, (1998), ibid., *MOTAR* 6: 15–18. [H]

Ovadiah A. and Gomez-de Silva, C. (1982): 'Supplementum to the Corpus of the Byzantine Churches in the Holy Land', *Levant* 14: 122–170.

Ovadiah A. and Gomez-de Silva, C. and Mucznik, S. (1991a): 'The Mosaic Pavements of Sheikh Zouède in northern Sinai', in E. Dassman and K. Thraede (eds.), *Tesserae: Festschrift für Joseph Engemann. Jahrbuch für Antike und Christentum Ergäzungsband* 18: 181–191.

Ovadiah, A., Mucznik, S. and Gomez-de Silva, C. (1991b): 'A New Look at the Mosaic Floor from Sheikh Zuweid in the Ismailiya Museum', *Qadmoniot* 95–96: 122–126. [H]

Owens, E.J. (1991): *The City in the Greek and Roman World*. London: Routledge.

Ozerman, M. (1980): *Survey of Wadi Malieh*. Tel-Aviv: The National Parks Authority. [H]

—— (1982): 'The Hammam Which Became Dry', *Teva Va'aretz* 24: 72–75. [H]

Özgüler, M.E. and Kasap, A. (1999): 'The Geothermal History of Anatalia, Turkey', in R. Cataldi et al. (eds.), *Stories from A Heated Earth: Our Geothermal Heritage*. California: GRC & IGA: 51–67.

Painter, K.S. (1975): 'Roman Flasks with Scenes of Baiae and Puteoli', *JGS* 17: 54–67.

Palmoni Y. (1969): 'Rabbi Tanhum bar Hiya from Kefar Agin', *Kinnrot* 47 (7): 46–50. [H]

Pantazides, I. (1879): Διόρθωσεις εἰς Μιχαηλ Ψελλοῦ Χρονογράφιαν, Athens.

Paoli, U.E. (1963): *Rome: Its People, Life and Customs* (tr. R.D. Macnaghten). Bristol: Bristol Classical Press.

Parker, D.H. (1970): *Investigation of the Sandstone Aquifer of East Jordan: The Hydrogeology of the Mesozoic-Cenozoic of the Western Highlands and the Plateau of East Jordan*. Rome: FAO.

Parker, H.M.D. (1958): *The Roman Legions* (2nd edn.). Cambridge: Heffer.

Parker, T.S. (1975): 'The Decapolis Reviewed', *JBL* 94: 437–441.

Parness, A. (1965): 'Sulphur', in *EB*, II. Jerusalem: Mosad Bialik: 545–546. [H]

Pasquinucci, M. (ed.) (1987): *Terme romane e vita quotidiana*. Exhibition Catalogue. Modena: Panini.

Patai, R. (1936): *The Water: A Reasearch for the Geography and Folklor of The Land of Israel during the Bible and the Mishnah Periods*. Tel-Aviv: Dvir. [H]

Paton, W.R. (1968): *The Greek Anthology*. London-Cambridge-Mass.: W. Heinemann.

Patrich, J. (2001): 'The *Carceres* of the Herodian Hippodrome/Stadium at Caesarea Maritima and Connections with the Circus Maximus', *JRA* 14: 269–283.

—— (2002): 'On the Lost Circus of Aelia Capitolina', *SCI* 21: 173–188.

Pauly, A., Wissowa, G. and Kroll, W. (eds.) (1919): *Real-Encyclopädie der classischen Altertumswissenschaft*. XX, Stuttgart: J.B. Metzler: 1669.

Payne-Smith, J. (ed.) (1902) [repr. 1957]: *A Compendious Syriac Dictionary*, Oxford: The Clarendon Press.

Pearsall, J. (ed.) (1998): *The New Oxford Dictionary of English*. Oxford: Oxford University Press.

Peck, H.T. (ed.) (1965) [repr. 1897]: *Harper's Dictionary of Classical Literature and Antiquities*. New York: Lond.

Penn, R.G. (1994): *Medicine on Ancient Greek and Roman Coins*. London: Seaby.

Perelman, M. (ed.) (1926): *Midrash HaRefuah*. Tel-Aviv: Dvir. [H]

Perles, J. (1872): 'Miscellen zur rabbinischen sprache und alterthumskunde', *MGWJ* 21: 251–254.

Perowne, S. (1956): *The Life and Times of Herod the Great*. London: Hodder and Stoughton.

—— (1960) [repr. 1986]: *Hadrian*. Dover, N.H.: Croom Helm.

Petrakis, N.L. (1980): 'Diagonal Earlobe Creases, Type a Behavior and the Death of Emperor Hadrian', *WJM* 132: 87–91.

Picard, L. (1932): 'Zur Geologie des Mittleren Jordantales', *ZDPV* 55: 221–225.

Piccirillo, M. (1989): *Chiese e mosaici di Madaba*. Jerusalem: Studium Biblicum Franciscanum.

—— (1993): *The Mosaics of Jordan*. Amman: American Center of Oriental Research.

—— (1995): 'The Mosaics of Trans-Jordan', in G. Barkai, H. Geva and E. Schiler (eds.), *Sites and Places in Jordan*. I, Jerusalem: Ariel Publishing House: 246–262. [H]

Piccirillo M. and Alliata, E. (eds.) (1999): *The Madaba Map, Centenary 1897–1997*. Jerusalem: Studium Biblicum Franciscanum.

Pieper, J. (1963): *Leisure: The Basis of Culture*. New York: Random House.

Pines, K. (1979): 'Thermal Baths at Tiberias', *Mada* 23 (3–4): 181. [H]

Pintsover, P. (1945): 'The Jews—A Swimming Nation', *Atidot* 16: 279–281. [H]

Pleket, H.W. (1975): 'Games, Prizes, Athletes and Ideology', *Stadion* 1: 49–89.

Plommer, H. (1983): 'Scythopolis, Caesarea, and Vitruvius: Sounding Vessels in Ancient Theatres', *Levant* 15: 132–140.

Poldi, R. (1971): 'Instructions Pros and Cons the Treatment in Hammei-Tiberias', in

A. Ya'akov (ed.), *Tiberias Hot Springs. Compilation of Essays in Medicine.* Hammat-Tiberias: Hammei-Tiberias Co.: 60–66. [H]

Pomeroy, S.B. (1975): *Goddesses, Whores, Wives, and Slaves: Women in Classical Antiquity.* London: Robert Hale.

Poole, J.B. and Reed, R. (1961): 'The "Tannery" of Ain Feshkha', *PEQ* 93: 114–123.

Porat, Y. (1995): 'Herod's "Amphitheatre" at Caesarea: A Multipurpose Entertainment', *JRA* 14: 15–27.

Porter, R. (ed.) (1990): *The Medical History of Waters and Spas.* London: Wellcome Institute for the History of Medicine.

—— (1997): *The Greatest Benefit of Mankind: A Medical History of Humanity.* New York: W.W. Norton.

Posner, R., Paul, S. and Stern, E. (eds.) (1987): *The Encyclopedia of the Bible.* I–IV, Tel-Aviv: Miskal. [H]

Potter, D.S. (1999a): 'Roman Religion: Ideas and Actions', in D.S. Potter and D.J. Mattingly (eds.), *Life, Death, and Entertainment in the Roman Empire.* Ann Arbor: University of Michigan Press: 113–167.

—— (1999b): 'Entertainers in the Roman Empire', in D.S. Potter and D.J. Mattingly (eds.), *Life, Death, and Entertainment in the Roman Empire.* Ann Arbor: University of Michigan Press: 256–325.

Potter, T.W. and Johns, C. (2002): *Roman Britain.* London: British Museum Press.

Poulakou-Rebelakou, E. and Marketos, S.G. (1999): 'Kidney Diseases in Byzantine Medical Texts', *AJN* 19: 172–176.

Press, I. (1948–1955): *A Topographical-Historical Encyclopaedia of Palestine.* I–IV, Jerusalem: R. Mass. [H]

Preuss, J. (1978) [repr.1993]: *Biblical and Talmudic Medicine* (tr. and ed. F. Rosner). *Biblisch-Talmudische Medizin.* New York: Sanhedrin.

Price, M.J. and Trell, B.L. (1977): *Coins and Their Cities.* Detroit-London: Vecchi.

Pringle, D. (1993): *The Churches of the Crusader Kingdom of Jerusalem: A Corpus.* I, Cambridge: Cambridge University Press.

Pringsheim, F. (1934): 'The Legal Policy and Reforms of Hadrian', *JRS* 24: 141–153.

Puech, E. (1977–1978): 'L'Acte de vente d'une maison a Kafar Bebayu en 135 de notre ere', *RQ* 9: 213–221.

Purcell, N. (1997): 'The Life of the City', in P. Jones and K. Sidwell (eds.), *The World of Rome: An Introduction to Roman Culture.* Cambridge: Cambridge University Press: 140–180.

Raba, J. (1986): *Russian Travel Accounts on Palestine (12–17 Centuries).* Jerusalem: Yad Izhak Ben Zvi. [H]

Rabani, B. (1953): 'Notes and News', *IEJ* 3: 265.

Rabin, J. (1959): 'Medicinal Folklore in the Beraita and Tosefta', *HH* 32: 149–152. [H]

Rabbinovicz, R.N.N. (1839): *Variae Lectiones in Mischnam et in Talmud Babylonicum.* I–XIV, München: bi-defus H. Rose.

Rabinovitz, Z.M. (1976): *Ginzé Midrash: The Oldest Forms of Rabbinic Midrashim according to Geniza Manuscripts.* Tel-Aviv: Tel-Aviv University Press. [H]

Rajak, T. (1973): 'Justus of Tiberias', *CQ* 23: 345–368.

Rakover, N. (1977): 'On the Protection of Animals', *Koroth* 7: 206–210. [H]

Ramage, N.H. and Ramage, A. (2005): *Roman Art: Romulus to Constantine* (4th edn). London: Laurence King.

Rapoport, S. (1857): *Ereh Millin.* Prague: Landau. [H]

Rappaport U. (1982): 'John of Gischala: From Galilee to Jerusalem', *JJS* 33: 479–493.

—— (1988): 'Tiberias and its Position in the Great Revolt', in Y. Hirschfeld (ed.), *Tiberias: From Beginnings until the Muslim Conquest.* Jerusalem: Yad Izhak Ben Zvi: 12–23. [H]

—— (1992): 'How Anti-Roman Was the Galilee?', in L.I. Levine (ed.), *The Galilee in*

Late Antiquity. New York-Jerusalem: The Jewish Theological Seminary of America & Harvard University Press: 95–102.

Rawson, E.D. (1982): 'The Life and Death of Asclepiades of Bithynia', *CQ* 32: 358–370.

—— (1985): *Intellectual Life in the Late Roman Republic.* London: Duckworth.

Raz, E. (1989): *Review and Analysis of Geothermal Measurments at Ein Gedi Spa (Ein Gedi Borehole 3) during the Period 1962–1983).* Ein Gedi: Kibbutz Ein Gedi.

—— (1993): *The Dead Sea Book.* Tel-Aviv: The National Parks Authority & Tamar Regional Council. [H]

Rebuffat, R. (1991): 'Vocabulaire Thermal', in M. Lenoir (ed.), *Les Thermes romains (Actes de la table ronde organisée par l'Ecole française de Rome, 1988).* Rome: École française de Rome: 1–32.

Reeg, G. (1989): *Die Ortsnamen Israels nach der rabbinischen Literatur.* Wiesbaden: Reichrt.

Re'emi, S.P. (ed.) (1973–1974): *Analitical Concordance to Delitsch Hebrew Translation of the New Testament.* I–III, Jersalem: Nur Press. [H]

Regev, E. (2000a): 'Pure Individualism: The Idea of Non-Priestly Purity in Ancient Judaism', *JSJ* 31: 176–201.

—— (2000b): 'Non-Priestly Purity and its Religious Aspects according to Historical Sources and Archaeological Findings', in M.J.H. Poorthuis and J. Schwartz (eds.), *Purity and Holiness: The Heritage of Leviticus.* Leiden: Brill: 223–244.

Reich, R. (1988): 'The Hot Bath-house (*balneum*), The *Miqweh* and the Jewish Community in the Second Temple Period', *JJS* 39 (1): 102–107.

—— (1995): 'The Synagogue and the *Miqweh* in Eretz-Israel in the Second Temple, Mishnaic and Talmudic Periods', in D. Urman and P.V.M. Flesher (eds.), *Ancient Synagogues: Historical Analysis and Archaeological Discovery.* I, Leiden: Brill: 289–297.

Reich, R. and Biling, J. (2000): 'Theatre's Seats from the Excavation in the Temple Mount', in A. Faust and E. Baruch (eds.), *New Studies on Jerusalem, Proceedings of the 5th Conference.* Ramat-Gan: Bar Ilan University Press: 37–42. [H]

Reland, A. (1714): *Palestina ex Monumentis Veteribus Illustrata.* Utrect: Trajecti Bat.

Renan, E. (1864): *Mission de Phénicie.* Paris: Imprimerie impériale.

Reuling, H. (2004): 'Pious Intrepidness: Egeria and the Ascetic Ideal', in M.J.H. Poorthuis and J. Schwartz (eds.), M. Poorthuis and J. Schwartz. *Saints and Role Models in Judaism and Christianity.* Leiden-Boston: Brill: 243–260.

Richmond, I.A. and Toynbee, J.M.C. (1955): 'The Temple of Sulis-Minerva at Bath', *JRS* 45: 97–120.

Richmond, J. (1934): 'Khirbet Fahil', *PEFQSt*: 18–31.

Ridgway, B.S. (1990): *Hellenistic Sculpture. The Styles of c. 331–200 B.C.* I, Bristol: Bristol Classical Press.

Rimawi, O. and Salameh, E. (1988): 'Hydrochemistry and Ground Water System of Zerka Ma'in-Zara Thermal Field, Jordan', *JH* 98: 147–163.

Ring, J.W. (1996): 'Windows, Baths, and Solar Energy in the Roman Empire', *AJA* 100 (4): 717–724.

Ringwood-Arnold, I. (1960): 'Agonistic Festivals in Italy and Sicily', *AJA* 64: 245–251.

Ritterling, C. (1899): 'Legio X Fretensis', in A. Pauly, G. Wissowa and W. Kroll (eds.) *Real-Encyclopädie der classischen Altertumswissenschaft.* XII/2, München: Druckenmüller: 1071–1077.

Robert, L. (1948): *Recueil d'épigraphie de numismatique et d'antiquités grecques: Épigrammes du Bas-Empire. Hellenica* 4: 1–151.

Robertson, D.S. (1971): *Greek and Roman Architecture* (2nd edn.). Cambridge: Cambridge University Press.

Robertson, M. (1975): *A History of Greek Art.* I–II, London: Cambridge University Press.

Robinson, E. (1865): *Physical Geography of the Holy Land.* London: Lond.

Robinson, E. and Smith, E. (1841) [repr. 1977]: *Biblical Researches in Palestine, Mount Sinai and Arabia Petraea*. III, New York: Arno Press.

Rodnan, G.P. and Benedek, T. (1963): 'Ancient Therapeutic Arts in the Gout', *ArRh* 6: 317–340.

Rogers, J. and Waldron, T. (1995): *A Field Guide to Joint Disease in Archaeology*. Chichester: Wiley.

Roll, I. (1976): 'The Roman Road Network in Eretz-Israel', *Qadmoniot* 9: 38–50. [H]

Roller, D.W. (1998): *The Building Program of Herod the Great*. Berkeley-London: University of California Press.

Romanelli, P. (1959): *Topografia e archeologia dell'Africa romana*. Torino: Società editrice internazionale.

Romanoff, P. (1937): *Onomasticon of Palestine: A New Method in Post Biblical Topography*. New York: Jewish Publication Society.

Roozenbeek, H., Pleket, H.W. and Stroud, R.S. (1990): *Supplementum Epigraphicum Graecum. Consolidated Index for Volumes 26–35 (1976–1985)*. Amsterdam: Gieben.

Rose, H.J. (1968): 'Hygieia', in M. Cary et al. (eds.) *The Oxford Classical Dictionary* (2nd edn.). Oxford: Clarendon Press: 443.

—— (1989): *A Handbook of Greek Mythology* (6th. edn.). London-New York: Routledge.

Rosenberger, M. (1977): *City Coins of Palestine*. Jerusalem: [s.n.].

—— (1978): *The Coinage of Eastern Palestine and Legionary Countermarks. Bar-Kochba Overstruck*. Jerusalem: Rosenberger.

Rosenfeld, B.Z. (1983): 'The Foundation of Tiberias: Changeover in the History of the Jewish Settlement in the Galilee at the end of the Second Temple Period', *Mituv Teveria* 2: 9–20. [H]

—— (1985): 'Tiberias in the Shadows of Wars', *Mituv Teveria* 3: 9–23. [H]

—— (1988): 'The Beginning of Tiberias', *Ariel* 53–54: 23–32. [H]

—— (1997): *Lod and Its Sages in the Days of the Mishnah and the Talmud*. Jerusalem: Yad Izhak Ben Zvi. [H]

—— (1998): 'Innkeeping in Jewish Society in Roman Palestine', *JESHO* 41: 133–158.

Rosenfeld, B.Z. and Menirav, J. (2004): 'Permanent Markets in the Land of Israel during the Periods of the Mishna and Talmud and Their Parallels in the Roman Empire', *Sidra* 19: 161–175. [H]

Rosental, A.S. (1991): 'Baara', *Tarbiz* 60: 325–353. [H]

Rosenthal, D. (1980): *Mishnh Abodah Zarah: A Critical Edition with Introduction*. PhD thesis. The Hebrew University of Jerusalem. [H]

Rosenthal, E. (2001): 'The Roman Springs of Israel', in P.E. LaMoreaux and J.T. Tanner (eds.), *Springs and Bottled Waters Bottled Waters of the World: Ancient History, Source, Occurance, Quality, and Use*. Berlin: Springer: 258–266.

Rosental, R. and Sivan, R. (1978): *Ancient Lamps in the Schloessinger Collection*. Jerusalem: Institute of Archaeology, The Hebrew University of Jerusalem.

Rosner, F. (1977a): *Medicine in the Bible and the Talmud*. New York: KTAV Publishing.

—— (1977b): 'Gout in the Bible and the Talmud', *AIM* 86: 833.

—— (1996): 'Jewish Medicine in the Talmudic Period', in *ANRW* II.37.3: 2866–2894.

—— (2000): *Encyclopedia of Medicine in the Bible and the Talmud*. Northvale-New Jersey-Jerusalem: Jason Aronson Inc.

Rostovtzeff, M. (1957): *The Social and Economic History of the Roman Empire* (2nd edn.). Oxford: Oxford University Press.

Rothstein, J.W. and Hänel, J. (1927): *Das erste Buch der Chronik*. Leipzig: A. Deichert.

Roth-Gerson, L. (1976): 'God Fearers in Jewish Inscription from Sardes', *Eshel Beer-Sheva* 2: 88–93. [H]

—— (1987): *The Greek Inscriptions from the Synagogues in Eretz-Israel*. Jerusalem: Yad Izhak Ben Zvi. [H]

Rouché, C. (1993): *Performers and Partisans at Aphrodisias in the Roman and late Roman Periods*. London: Society for the Promotion of Roman Studies.

Rowland, I.D. (tr.) (1999): *Vitruvius: Ten Books on Architecture.* Cambridge: Cambridge University Press.

Rubin, Z. (1982): 'Joseph the Comes and the Attempts to Convert the Galilee to Christianity in the Fourth Century CE', *Cathedra* 26: 105–116. [H]

Ruoti, R. Morris, D. and Cole, A. (1997): *Aquatic Rehabilitation.* Philadelphia: Lippincott-Raven.

Russell, K.W. (1985): 'The Earthquake Chronology of Palestine and Northwest Arabia from the Second through the Mid-Eighth Century AD', *BASOR* 260: 37–59.

Saarisalo, A. (1927): *The Boundary between Issachar and Naphtali: An Archaeological and Literary Study of Israel's Settlement in Canaan.* Helsinki: Suomalaisen Tiedeakatemian Toimituksia.

Sachs, S. (1914): 'Hammat-Gader', *Kerem Hemed* 8: 16–22. [H]

Safrai, S. (1958): 'Beth Shearim in Talmudic Literature', *EI* 5: 206–212. [H]

—— (1965): *Pilgrimage at the Time of the Second Temple.* Tel-Aviv: Academon. [H]

—— (1969): 'Assia', in A.Z. Melamed (ed.), *Memorial Book for Benjamin De Freis.* Tel-Aviv: Tel-Aviv University: 330. [H]

—— (1971): 'The Relations between the Roman Army and the Jews of Eretz-Israel after the Destruction of the Second Temple', in S. Applebaum (ed.), *Roman Frontier Studies. Proceedings of the 7th International Congress.* Tel-Aviv: Students' Organization of Tel-Aviv University: 124–129. [H]

—— (1975): 'The Chronology of the Nesiim in the Second and Third Century CE', *Proceedings of the Fifth World Congress of Jewish Studies.* II, Jerusalem: Magness Press, The Hebrew University: 51–57. [H]

—— (1982a): 'The Jewish Settlements in the Galilee and the Golan during the Third and Fourth Centuries', in Z. Baras et al. (eds.), *Eretz-Israel from the Destruction of the Second Temple to the Muslim Conquest: Political, Social and Cultural History.* I, Jerusalem: Yad Izhak Ben Zvi: 144–175. [H]

—— (1982b): 'The Recovery of the Jewish Settlement during the Yavneh Period', in Z. Baras et al. (eds.), *Eretz-Israel from the Destruction of the Second Temple to the Muslim Conquest: Political, Social and Cultural History.* I, Jerusalem: Yad Izhak Ben Zvi: 18–39. [H]

—— (1995): 'The Relation of the Aggadah (Tale) to the Halakha (Law)', in A. Oppenheimer and A. Kasher (eds.), *From Generation to Generation: From the End of the Biblical Period to the Sealing of the Talmud. Collection of Researches in Honor of Joshua Ephron.* Jerusalem: Mosad Bialik: 215–234. [H]

Safrai, Z. (1977): 'Samaritan Synagogues in the Roman-Byzantine Period', *Cathedra* 4: 84–112. [H]

—— (1980): *Boundaries and Rule in Eretz-Israel during the Mishnah and the Talmud Periods.* Tel-Aviv: HaKibbutz HaMeuhad. [H]

—— (1984): 'Fairs in the Land of Israel in the Mishnah and Talmud Period', *Zion* 49: 139–158. [H]

—— (1986): 'The Fair as an Economic Institution: Rejoinder', *Zion* 51: 485–486. [H]

—— (1990): 'TheTrade in Roman Palestine', in B. Kedar et al. (eds.), *Chapters in the History of Trade in Palestine. Collections of Essays.* Jerusalem: 108–139. [H]

—— (1992): 'The Roman Army in the Galilee', in L.I. Levine (ed.), *The Galilee in Late Antiquity.* New York-Jerusalem: The Jewish Theological Seminary of America & Harvard University Press: 115–125.

—— (1994): *The Economy of Roman Palestine.* London-New York: Routledge.

—— (1995): *The Jewish Community in Eretz-Israel during the Mishnah and the Talmud Periods.* Jerusalem: The Zalman Shazar Center for Jewish History. [H]

Salameh, E. (1990): *A Study of Spas in Jordan.* Amman: University of Jordan. [A]

Salameh, E. and Bannayan, H. (1993): *Water Resources of Jordan, Present Status and Future Potential.* Amman: Friedrich Ebert Stiftung.

Salameh, E. and Udluft, P. (1985): 'The Hydrodynamic Pattern of the Central Part of Jordan', *GJ* 38: 39–53.

Salarneh E., Rimawi, O. and Hamed, K.H. (1991): *Curative Thermal and Mineral Water in Jordan*. Water Resources Center, Issue. No. 15. Amman : University of Jordan.

Saldarini, A.J. (1975): 'Johanan ben Zaccai's Escape from Jerusalem', *JSJ* 6: 189–204.

Sanders, E.P. (1992) [repr. 1994]: *Judaism: Practice and Belief, 63 BCE–66 CE*. London-Philadelphia: SCM Press & Trinity Press International.

Sandison, A.T. (1967): 'The Last Illness of Herod the Great, King of Judaea', *Med. Hist.* 11: 381–388.

Sapir, J. (1970): *Even Sapir Book*. Jerusalem: Mekorot Library. [H]

Sarfatti, G.B. (1975): 'A Fragmentary Roman Inscription in the Turkish Wall of Jerusalem', *IEJ* 25: 151.

Sartre, M. (1992): 'Les Cités de la Décapole septentrional: Canatha, Raphana, Dion et Adraha', *ARAM Periodical* 4 (1–2): 139–156.

Satlow, M.L. (1995): *Tasting the Dish: Rabbinic Rhetorics of Sexuality*. Atlanta: Scholars Press.

Sauer, B. (1996): 'An Inscription from Northern Italy, The Roman Temple Complex in Bath and Minerva as a Healing Goddess in Gallo-Roman Religion', *OJA* 15 (1): 63–93.

—— (1999): 'The Augustan Army Spa at Bourbonne-les-Bains', in A. Goldsworthy and I. Haynes (eds.), *The Roman Army As A Community: Including Papers of A Conference Held at University of London, 1997. JRA, Supp. Series* 34: 52–79.

Sawyer, D.F. (1996): *Women and Religion in the First Christian Centuries*. London-New York: Routledge.

Scarborough, J. (1969): *Roman Medicine*. London: Thames and Hudson.

Scarre, C. (1995): *Chronicle of the Roman Emperors*. London: Thames and Hudson.

Schäfer, P. (1979): 'Die Flucht Johanan b. Zakkais aus Jerusalem und die Gründung des "Lehrhauses" in Jabne', in *ANRW* II.19.2: 43–101.

—— (1990): 'Hadrian's Policy in Judaea and the Bar Kokhba Revolt: A Reassessment', P.R. Davies and R.T. White (eds.), *A Tribute to Geza Vermes: Essays on Jewish and Christian Literature and History*. Sheffield: JSOT Press: 281–303.

Schalit, A. (1951): 'Alexander Yannai's Conquests in Moab', *EI* 1: 104–121. [H]

—— (1968): *Namenwörterbuch zu Flavius Josephus*. Leiden: Brill.

—— (1973): *Flavii Josephi: Anquitates Judaicae*. Jerusalem: Mosad Bialik. [H]

—— (1975): 'Die Erhebung Vespasians nach Flavius Josephus, Talmud and Midrasch. Zur Geschichte einer messianischen Prophetie', in *ANRW* II.2: 208–327.

—— (1978): *King Herod: The Man and His Activities*. Jerusalem: Mosad Bialik. [H]

Schapiro, D. (1901): 'Les Connaissances médicales de Mar Samuel', *RÉJ* 42: 14–26.

Scharf, J., Nahir, M. and Rubilovitch, M. (1975): 'Scleritis Associated with Hyperuricaemia', *RhRe* 14 (4): 251–252.

Schattner, I. (1962): 'The Lower Jordan Valley: A Study in the Fluviomorphology of an Arid Region', *SH* 9: 59–66.

Scherrer, A. (1936): 'Die Thermen von Tiberias', *IMZ* 55: 5–8.

Schick, C. (1898): 'Birket es Sultan, Jerusalem', *PEFQSt* 224–229.

Schlatter, A. (1893): *Zur Topographie und Geschichte Palästinas*. Calw-Stuttgart: Calw &c.

Schlatter, T. (1918): 'Des Gelaiet der Zehnstadte', *Palästinajahrbuch* 14: 90–110.

Schmitt, G. (1975): 'Topographische Probleme bei Josephus', *ZDPV* 91: 50–68.

Schmitt, L. and Prieur, M. (2004): *Les Monnaies Romaines*. Paris: Les Chevau-légers.

Schmitz, L. (1870) [repr. 1967]: 'Charis', in W. Smith (ed.), *A Dictionary of Greek and Roman Biography and Mithology*. London: J. Murray.

Schocett, R. (1933): 'The Treatment of Diseases as Found in the Talmud', *HP* 2 (1): 77–86. [H]

—— (1936): 'Hammei-Tiberias in the Past', *HP* 9: 164–168. [H]

Schochat, A. (1960): 'On the Ambiguous Oracle in the Works of Josephus', in M. Haendel (ed.), *Studies in Memory of Joseph Shilo*. Tel-Aviv: Department of Education and Culture at Tel-Aviv City Council: 163–165. [H]

Schrötter, H. (1924): *Das Tote Meer: Beitrag zur physikalischen Geographie und Balneologie mit Bemerkungen zur Flora der Ufergelände*. Wien-Leipzig: Moritz Perles.
Schulman, N. (1959): 'The Geology of the Central Jordan Valley', *BRCI* 8: 63–90.
—— (1968): 'Geological Survey on the Golan', *Teva Va'aretz* 10: 179–181. [H]
Schulman, N. and Bartov, Y. (1978): 'Tectonics and Sedimentation along the Rift Valley, in Sedimentology in Israel, Cyprus and Turkey', *The 10th International Congress on Sedimentology. Guidebook*. II, Jerusalem: 37–94.
Schult, H. (1966): 'Zwei Häfen aus römischer Zeit am Toten Meer, rugm el-bahr und el-beled (ez-zâra)', *ZDPV* 82: 139–148.
Schumacher, G. (1886a): *Across the Jordan*. London: Lond.
—— (1886b): 'Beschreibung des Dscholan', *ZDPV* 9: 294–301.
—— (1888a): *The Jaulân: Surveyed for the German Society for the Exploration of the Holy Land*. London: Richard Bentley.
—— (1888b): *Pella*. London: The Society's office.
—— (1890): *Northern 'Ajlûn*. London: A.P. Watt.
Schürer, E. (1907) [repr. 1964]: *Geschichte des judischen Volks im Zeitalter Jesu Christi*. (4th edn.). I–III, Hildesheim: G. Olms.
—— (1991) [repr. 1979]: *The History of the Jewish People in the Age of Jesus Christ (175 BC–AD 135)*. G.Vermes, F. Millar and M. Black (rev. and eds.). I–IV, Edinburgh: T. & T. Clark.
Schwabe, M. (1912): 'Les Manuscrits du Consistoire Israélite de Paris provenant de la Gueniza du Caire', *RÉJ* 64: 100–196.
—— (1949): 'The History of Tiberias: An Epigraphical Research', in M. Shwabe and Y. Guttmann (eds.), *Studies in Jewish Hellenism*. Jerusalem: Magness Press, The Hebrew University: 200–251. [H]
—— (1957): 'Documents of a Journey through Palestine in the Years 317–323 CE', *Eretz-Israel* 3: 181–185. [H]
—— (1968): 'Tiberias Revealed through Inscriptions', in H.Z. Hirschberg (ed.), *All the Land of Naphtali. The 24th Archaeological Convention, 1966*. Jerusalem: Israel Exploration Society: 180–191. [H]
Schwabe M. and B. Lifshitz, B. (1967): *Beth Shearim*. II, Jerusalem: The Israel Exploration Society.
Schwartz, J.J. (1982): 'The Settlement in Judaea Region during the Third and the Fourth Centuries', in Z. Baras et al. (eds.), *Eretz-Israel from the Destruction of the Second Temple to the Muslim Conquest: Political, Social and Cultural History*. I, Jerusalem: Yad Izhak Ben Zvi: 180–201. [H]
—— (1983): 'The Tension Between the Southern Sages and the Galilean Sages during the Mishnah and Talmud Periods', *Sinai* 93: 102–109. [H]
—— (1986): *Jewish Settlement in Judaea from the Bar-Kokhba Revolt to the Muslim Conquest*. Jerusalem: Magness. [H]
—— (1988): 'Everyday Life in Tiberias in the Mishnah and Talmud Periods', in Y. Hirschfeld (ed.), *Tiberias: From Beginnings until the Muslim Conquest*. Jerusalem: Yad Izhak Ben Zvi: 103–110. [H]
—— (1990): 'Once More on the "Boundary of Gezer" Inscriptions and the History of Gezer and Lydda at the End of the Second Temple Period', *IEJ* 40: 47–57.
—— (1991): *Lod (Lydda), Israel: From Its Origins through the Byzantine Period*. BAR International Series 571. Oxford: Tempus Reparatum.
—— (1998a): 'Aspects of Leisure-Time Activities in Roman Period Palestine', in P. Schäfer (ed.), *The Talmud Yerushalmi and Graeco-Roman Culture*.I, Tübingen: Mohr-Siebeck: 313–325.
—— (1998b): 'Archaeology and the City', in D. Sperber, *The City in Roman Palestine*. New York-Oxford: Oxford University Press: 149–187.
—— (2003): 'The Relations between Jews and Gentiles during the Mishnah and the Talmud Periods according to their Attitude to Game Culture and Leisure-Time Activities', in A. Oppenheimer et al. (eds.), *Jews and Gentiles in the Holy Land in the*

Days of the Second Temple, the Mishnah and the Talmud. A Collection of Articles. Jerusalem: Yad Izhak Ben Zvi Press: 132–141. [H]

Schwartz, S. (1998): 'Gamaliel in Aphrodite's Bath: Palestinian Judaism and Urban Culture in the Third and Fourth Centuries', in P. Schäfer (ed.), *The Talmud Yerushalmi and Graeco-Roman Culture.* I, Tübingen: Mohr-Siebeck: 203–217.

—— (2001): *Imperialism and Jewish Society 200 BCE to 640 CE.* Princeton-Oxford: Princeton University Press.

Scott, J.T. (1988): 'Gout in Antiquity', *The Arthritis and Rheumatism, Council for Research: The Antiquity of the Erosive Arthropathies, Conference Proceedings.* Bath: 25–29.

Scullard, H.H. (1981): *Festivals and Cermonies of the Roman Republic.* London: Thames and Hudson.

Sear, F.B. (1990): 'The Theatre at Leptis Magna and the Development of Roman Theatre Design', *JRA* 3: 376–383.

—— (1982) [repr. 1998]: *Roman Architecture.* London-New York: Routledge.

Seetzen, U.J. (1854): *Ulrich Jasper Seetzen's Reisen durch Syrien, Palästina, Phönicien, die Transjordan-Länder, Arabia Petraea und Unter-Aegypten.* Berlin: Verlegt Bei G. Reimer.

Segal, A. (1988): *Town Planning and Architecture in Provincia Arabia: The Cities along the Via Traiana Nova in the 1st–3rd Centuries CE. BAR International Series*, 419. Oxford: Tempus Reparatum.

—— (1995a): *Theatres in Roman Palestine and Provincia Arabia.* Leiden: Brill.

—— (1995b): *Monumental Architecture in Roman Palestine and Provincia Arabia.* Haifa: University of Haifa Press. [H]

—— (1997): *From Function to Monument: Urban Landscapes of Roman Palestine, Syria and Provincia Arabia.* Oxford: Oxbow Books.

Segert, S. (1976): *A Grammar of Phoenician and Punic.* München: Beck.

Segev, G. (1989): 'Hammei-Tiberias in the Past and Present: Balneological Treatments', in I. Goldrat (ed.), *Hot Springs and Curative Baths in the Kinnert Lake.* Tel-Aviv: Open University: 149–153. [H]

Sepp, N. (1863): *Jerusalem und das Heilige Land: Pilgerbuch nach Palastine, Syrien und Aegypten.* Schaffhausen: Fr. Hurter.

Serruya, C. (ed.) (1978): *Lake Kinneret,* Boston: W. Junk.

Settis, S. (1974): '"Esedra" e "ninfeo" nella terminologia architettonica del mondo romano. Dall'età repubblicana alla tarda antichità', in *ANRW I.4:* 661–745.

Seyffert, A.O. (1891): *A Dictionary of Classical Antiquities: Mythology, Religion, Literature and Art* (2nd edn.): Lond.

Seyrig, H. (1959): 'Temples, cults et souvernirs historiques de la Décapole', *Syria* 36: 60–73.

Shaked, S. (1964): *A Tentative Bibliography of Geniza Documents.* Paris: Mouton.

Shalem, N. (1941): 'On the Dating of the "Earthquake of the Sabbatical Year"', *BJPES* 8: 117. [H]

—— (1953): 'Jerusaem and Its Desert', in M. Ish-Shalom et al. (eds.), *Yerushalayim: Review for Eretz-Israel Research.* I, Jerusalem: Mosad HaRav Kook: 300–326. [H]

—— (1956): 'Seismic Tidal Waves (Tsunamies) in the Eastern Mediterranean', *BIES* 20: 159–170. [H]

Shapira, A. (1997): 'On the Seismicity of the Dead Sea Basin', in M. Niemi et al. (eds.), *The Dead Sea: The Lake and Its Setting.* New York-Oxford: Oxford University Press: 82–88.

Shapira, N. (1962): 'The Wine Industry Concerning the Ancient Hebrew Sources', *Koroth* 3 (1–2): 40–72. [H]

Shatzman, I. (1983): 'Security Problems in Southern Judaea Following the First Revolt', *Cathedra* 30: 3–32. [H]

Shaw, B.D. (1995): 'Rural Markets in North Africa and the Political Economy of the Roman Empire', in B.D. Shaw (ed.), *Rulers, Nomads, and Christians in Roman North Africa.* Aldershot: Variorum: 37–73.

Shaw, T. (1738): *Travels, or Observations Relating to Several Parts of Barbary and the Levant.* Oxford: Printed at the Theatre.

Sheedy, K., Carson, R.A.G. and Walmsley, A.G. (2001) *Pella in Jordan 1979–1990: The Coins.* Sydney: Adapa.

Shelomi-Friedmann, M. (1936): 'The Chemical Analysis of the Springs in Eretz-Israel', *HH* 9: 169–178. [H]

Shelton, J.-A. (1988): *As The Romans Did: A Source Book in Roman Social History.* New York-Oxford: Oxford University Press.

Shenhav, E. (1997): 'The Maioumas Cult in Light of the Excavations at Shuni', E. Regev (ed.), *New Studies on the Coastal Plain, Proceedings of the 17th Conference of the Dept. of the Land of Eretz-Israel Studies in Honour of Prof. Y. Feliks.* Ramat-Gan: Bar-Ilan University Press: 56–70. [H]

Shew, I. (1845): *Hydropathy or The Water-Cure: Its Principles, Modes of Treatment* (2nd edn.), New York: Wiley and Putnam.

Shiponi, A. (1962): *Hammei-Tiberias in the Halakha and the Aggadah.* Hammat-Tiberias: Hammat-Tiberias Co. [H]

Shorek, Y. (1981): 'Jason's Gymnastics and Agonistic Contribution (168–175 BCE)', *HaH* 3: 8–10. [H]

—— (1977): *Cultural Physical Training in Eretz-Israel during the Mishnah and the Talmud Periods.* Tel-Aviv: Vingate Institute for Sport and Phisical Education. [H]

Shoshan, A. (1977): 'The Illness of Rabbi Judah the Patriarch', *Koroth* 7: 521–524. [H]

Sijpesteijn, P.J. (1969): 'A New Document Concerning Hadrian's Visit to Egypt', *Historia* 18: 109–118.

Simchoni, I.N. (1968): *The History of the Jewish War Against the Romans.* Givatiim-Ramat-Gan: Masada. [H]

Simon, I. (1978a): 'Bains, ablutions et cures thermales dans l'antiquité hebraïque', *RHMH* 125: 7–10, 33–38.

—— (1978b): 'Bains, ablutions et cures thermales dans l'antiquité hebraïque', *RHMH* 126: 57–62.

Simons, J. (1959): *The Geographical and Topographical Texts of the Old Testament: A Concise Commentary in XXXII Chapters.* Leiden: Brill.

Skinner, J. (1963): *The International Critical Commentary: A Critical and Exegetical Commentary on Genesis* (2nd edn.). Edinburgh: T. & T. Clark.

Slousch, N. (1921): 'Excavations of the Israel Antiquities Society in Hammat of Tiberias', *BJPES* 1/1: 5–39. [H]

—— (1925): 'Addition to the Excavations at Hammat of Tiberias', *BJPES* 1/2: 49–52. [H]

Slouschz, Z.A. (1993): 'The Priestly Courses in the Temple', *Shmatin* 113: 65–77. [H]

Small (1987): 'Late Hellenistic Baths in Palestine', *BASOR* 266: 59–74.

Smallwood, E.M. (1981): *The Jews under Roman Rule from Pompey to Diocletian* (2nd edn.). Leiden: Brill.

Smith, G.A. (1920): *The Historical Geography of The Holy Land* (21st edn.). London: Hodder & Stoughton.

Smith, J.R. (1922): *Springs and Wells in Greek and Roman Literature: Their Legends and Locations.* New York: G.P. Putnam's sons.

Smith, M. (1956): 'Palestinian Judaism in the First Century', in M. Davis (ed.), *Israel: Its Role in Civilization.* New York: Jewish Theological Seminary of America: 67–81.

Smith, P. and G. Kahila (1991): 'Bones of a Hundred Infants Found in Ashkelon Sewer', *BAR* 17 (4): 47.

Smith, R.A.L. (1944): *Bath.* London: B.T. Batsford.

Smith, R.H. (1968): 'Pella of the Decapolis, 1967', *Archaeology* 21: 134–137.

—— (1973a): *Pella of the Decapolis.* I, Wooster, Ohio: College of Wooster.

—— (1973b): 'A Sarcophagus from Pella: New Light on the Earliest Christianity', *Archaeology* 26: 250–256.

—— (1992): 'Some Pre-Christian Religions at Pella of the Decapolis', *ARAM* 4: 1–2: 197– 214.
—— (1993): 'Pella', in E. Stern (ed.), *NEAEHL* III, Jerusalem: Israel Exploration Society & Carta: 1174–1180.
Smith, R.H. and Day, L.P. (1989): *Pella of the Decapolis.* II, Ohio: College of Wooster.
Smith, R.H., McNicoll, A.W. and Hennessey, J.B. (1982): *Pella in Jordan 1979–1981.* Canberra-Wooster: College of Wooster.
Smith, W. (1904): *A Classical Dictionary.* London: T. Allman.
Smith, W. and Lockwood, J. (1988): *Chambers Murry: Latin-English Dictionary.* Cambridge: Cambridge University Press.
Sobel, H. (1990): *Hygieia: Die Göttin der Gesundheit.* Darmstadt: Wissenschaftliche Buch-gesellschaft.
Sokoloff, M. (1990): *A Dictionary of Jewish Palestinian Aramaic of the Byzantine Period.* Ramat-Gan: Bar-Ilan University Press.
Sourdel, D. (1952): *Les cultes du Hauran à l'époque romaine. Bibliothèque archéologique et his-torique.* LIII, Paris: Imprimerie nationale & Paul Geuthner.
Sowers, S. (1970): 'The Circumstances and Recollection of the Pella Fight', *TZ* 26: 305–320.
Speller, E. (2002): *Following Hadrian, A Second-Century Journey through the Roman Empire.* London: REVIEW.
Sperber, D. (1971): 'Oenomaos of Gadara', in *EJ*, XII. Jerusalem: Keter Books: 1331–1332. [H]
—— (1982): *Essays on Greek and Latin in the Mishna, Talmud and Midrashic Literature.* Jerusalem: Makor.
—— (1986): *Nautica Talmudica.* Ramat-Gan: Bar-Ilan University Press.
—— (1998): *The City in Roman Palestine.* New York-Oxford: Oxford University Press.
Spijkerman, A. (1978): *The Coins of the Decapolis and Provincia Arabia.* (ed. M. Piccirillo), Jerusalem: Studium Biblicum Franciscanum.
Stacey, D.A. (1995): *The Archaeology of Early Islamic Tiberias.* PhD thesis, University of London.
Staehelin, F. (1948): *Die Schweiz in römischer Zeit.* Basel: Schwabe.
Stager, L.E. (1991): 'Eroticism and Infanticide at Ashkelon', *BAR* 17 (4): 34–53, 72.
Stahl, Z. (1986): *The Coins in Palestine during the Roman Period.* Tel-Aviv: Liderman. [H]
Starinski, A., Katz, A. and Levitte, D. (1979): 'Temperature-Composition-Depth Relationship in Rift Valley Hot Springs: Hammat Gader, Northern Israel', *CG* 27: 233–244.
Starowieyski, M. (1979) 'Bibliografia Egeriana', *Augustinianum* 19: 297–318.
Starr, J. (1935): 'Byzantine Jewry on the Eve of the Arab Conquest (565–638)', *JPOS* 15: 280–293.
Stein, M. (tr.) (1968): *The Life of Josephus.* Ramat-Gan: Masada. [H]
Steinberg. J. (1960): *Dictionary of the Bible: Mishpat HaUrim.* Tel-Aviv: Yisraeel. [H]
Steinespring, W.F. (1939): 'Hadrian in Palestine A.D. 129/130', *JAOS* 59: 360–365.
Steinfeld, Z.A. (1986): 'The Prohibition on Gentile Dish', *Sidra* 2: 125–143. [H]
Stern, E. (1968): 'Natrium', in *EB*, V. Jerusalem: Mosad Bialik: 989–990. [H]
Stern, M. (1964): 'Sympathy for Judaism in Roman Senatorial Circles in the Early Empire', *Zion* 29: 155–167. [H]
—— (ed.) (1974–1980): *Greek and Roman Latin Authors on Jews and Judaism.* I–III, Jerusa-lem: Israel Academy of Sciences and Humanities.
—— (1981): 'The Hellenism of Eretz-Israel and the Hasmonean Revolt', in M. Stern (ed.), *The History of Eretz-Israel: The Hellenistic Period and the Hasmonean State (332–37 BCE).* III, Jerusalem: Yad Izhak Ben Zvi & Keter: 11–190. [H]
—— (1982): 'The Roman Regime in Provincia Judaea from the Destruction to the Bar-Kokhba Revolt', in Z. Baras et al. (eds.), *Eretz-Israel from the Destruction of the Second Temple to the Muslim Conquest: Political, Social and Cultural History.* I, Jerusalem: Yad Izhak Ben Zvi & Keter: 1–11. [H]

—— (1983a): 'Herod's Kingship', in M. Avi-Yonah (ed.), *The World History of the Jewish People: The Herodian Period.* Jerusalem: Am Oved: 53–90. [H]

—— (1983b): 'The Sicarii and the Zealots', in M. Avi-Yonah and Z. Baras (eds.), *The World History of the Jewish People: The Herodian Period.* Jerusalem: Am Oved: 167–196. [H]

Steuernagel, C. (1927): *Der 'Adschlūn.* Leipzig: [n.s.].

Stevenson, S.W. (1889): *A Dictionary of Roman Coins, Republican and Imperial.* London: G. Bell and sons.

Stewart, A. (1896): *Palestine Pilgrims' Text Society of the Holy Places Visited by Antoninus Martyr.* II, London: Lond.

Stiebel, G.D. (1999): 'The Whereabouts of the Xth Legion and the Boundaries of Aelia Capitolina', in A. Faust and E. Baruch (eds.), *New Studies on Jerusalem, Proceedings of the 5th Conference.* Ramat Gan: Bar Ilan University Press: 68–103. [H]

Stobbe, J.E.O. (1866): *Die Juden in Deutschland während des Mittelalters in politischer, Socialer und rechtlicher Beziehung.* Braunschweig.

Strack, P.L. (1933): *Untersuchungen zur römischen Reichsprägung des zweiten Jahrhunderts.* Stuttgart: W. Kohlhammer.

Strobel, A. (1966): 'Zur Ortslage von Kallirrohë', *ZDPV* 82: 149–162.

—— (1989): 'Zar'ah (el) / Kallirrhoe', in D. Homès-Frederiq and J.B. Hennessy (eds.), *Archaeology of Jordan.* II/2: *Field Reports: Sites L-Z.* Leuven: Peeters.

—— (1990): 'Ez-Zara: Mukawer Survey', in S. Kerner (ed.), *The Near East in Antiquity: Archaeological Work of National and International Institutions in Jordan.* IV, Amman: German Protestant Institute for Archaeology: 81–85.

—— (1997): 'Ancient Roads in the Roman District of South Peraea: Routes of Communication in the Eastern Area of the Dead Sea', in G. Bisheh et al. (eds.), *Studies in the History and Archaeology of Jordan.* VI, Amman: Department of Antiquities: 271–280.

Strobel, A. and Clamer, C. (1986): 'Excavations at Ez-Zāra', *ADAJ* 30: 381–384.

Sukenik, E.L. (1926): 'Three Ancient Jewish Inscriptions from Palestine', *Supp. Zion* 1: 16–17. [H]

—— (1930): 'Cathedra of Moses', *Tarbiz* 1: 145–151. [H]

—— (1935a): *The Ancient Synagogue of El-Ḥammeh (Hammat by Gadara).* Jerusalem: R. Mass. [= idem, *ibid.*, (1935b): *JPOS* 15: 101–180].

—— (1935b): 'The Ancient Synagogue in Hammat-Gader (A Primarily Survey)', in N. Slousch (ed.), *Collection of the Jewish Palestine Exploration Society Dedicated to the Memory of Dr. A.M. Mazie.* Jerusalem: Rubin Mass: 41–61. [H]

Swaddling, J. (1980) [repr. 1999]: *The Ancient Olympic Games.* London: Published for the Trustees of the British Museum by British Museum.

Swarieh, A. (1990): *Hydrogeology of the Wadi Wala Sub Basin and Zarka Ma'in Hot Springs.* MSc thesis, University of London.

—— (2000): 'Geothermal Energy Resources in Jordan: Country Update Report', *Proceeding World Geothermal Congress.* Kyushu-Tohoku, Japan: 469–472.

Swarieh, A. and Massarweh, R. (1993): *Thermal Springs in Wadi Ibn Hainmad.* Amman: Natural Resources Authority.

—— (1995): *Geothermal Water in Zara and Zarqa Ma'in Area.* Report No. 8. Amman: Natural Resources Authority.

—— (1997): *Geothermal Water in Mukhiebeh and North Shuneh Areas.* Report No. 9. Amman: Natural Resources Authority.

Syme, R. (1991): 'Journeys of Hadrian', *RP* 6: 347–357 [= idem, (1988) *ZPE* 73: 159–170].

Szabó, A. (1978): *Ape și Gaze Radioactive în R.S. România.* Cluj-Napoca: Dacia.

Tal, A. (1991): 'Etelin', *Teuda* 7: 155–159. [H]

Talmon, S. (1958): '"These are the Ken'ites Who Came from Hammath, the Father of the House of Rechab" (*Chronicles* 2, 55)', *EI* 5: 111–113. [H]

Tameanko, M. (1999): *Monumental Coins: Buildings and Structures in Ancient Coinage.* Iola, WI: Krause Publications.

Tannahill, R. (1980): *Sex in History.* London: Hamish Hamilton.

Ta-Shma, I.M (1971): 'Judah (Nesiah)', in *EJ*, X. Jerusalem: Keter Books: 333. [H]

Taylor, J.E. (ed.) (2003): *Palestine in the Fourth Century AD: The Onomasticon by Eusebius of Caesarea*. Jerusalem: Carta.

Teixidor, J. (1977): *The Pagan God: Popular Religion in the Greco-Roman near East.* Princeton, New Jersey: Princeton University Press.

Thomas, D.W. (1933): 'En-Dor: A Sacred Spring?', *PEFQSt*: 205–206.

—— (1934): 'The Meaning of the Name Hammoth-Dor', *PEFQSt*: 147–148.

Thomsen, P. (1907): *Loca Sancta: Verzeichnis der im 1. bis 6. Jahrhundert n. Chr. erwähnten Ortschaften Palästinas.* Halle: a.S.

Thomson, W.A.R. (1978): *Spas That Heal.* London: Adam and Charles Black.

Thornton, M.K. (1975): 'Hadrian and His Reign', in *ANRW* II.2: 432–476.

Thrämer, E. (1951): 'Health and Gods of Healing', in J. Hastings (ed.), *Encyclopædia of Religion and Ethics.* V, New York: Charles Scribner's Sons: 540–556.

Timbalist-Zori, N. (1943–1944): 'Umm Juni', *BJPES* 10: 119–122. [H]

Timm, S. (1989): *Moab zwischen den Mächten: Studien zu historischen Denkmälern und Texten.* Wiesbaden: Otto Harrassowitz.

Tokatzinski, N.A. (1970): *The Land to Its Boundaries.* Jerusalem: [n.s.]. [H]

Tomlin, R.S.O. (1988): 'The Curse Tablets', in B. Cunliffe (ed.), *The Temple of Sulis Minerva at Bath. The Finds from the Sacred Spring.* II, Oxford: Oxford University Committee for Archaeology. Monograph No. 16: 59–277.

Toner, J.P. (1995): *Leisue and Ancient Rome.* Cambridge: Polity Press.

Tournaye, D. (1990): *Etude du potentiel et des utilisations des ressources géothermales de Jordanie.* Companie Française de Géothermie, Orléans, France.

—— (1992): *Etude de l'utilisation des ressources géothermiques pour le chauffage des serres, zone sud d'Amman.* Companie franrtaise de géothermie, Orléans, France.

Trall, R.T. (1869) [repr. 1877]: *The Hydropathic Encyclopedia: A System of Hydropathy and Hygiene.* New York: Samuel R. Wells.

Traversari, G. (1960): Gli spettacoli in Acqua nel Teatro tardo-antico. Roma: L'Erma di Bretschneider.

Tristram, H.B. (1866): *The Land of Israel: A Journal of Travels in Palestine Undertaken with Special Reference to its Physical Character* (2nd edn.). London: Society for Promoting Christian Knowledge.

—— (1871): *The Topography of the Holy Land.* London: Society for Promoting Christian Knowledge.

—— (1873): *The Land of Moab: Travels and Discoveries on the East Side of the Dead Sea and the Jordan.* London: Lond.

Tsafrir, Y. (1968): 'The Conflict between the Christians and Jews in the Tiberias Region in the Byzantine Period', in H.Z. Hirschberg (ed.), *All the Land of Naphtali. The 24th Archaeological Convention, 1966.* Jerusalem: Israel Exploration Society: 79–90. [H]

—— (1984): *Eretz-Israel from the Destruction of the Second Temple to the Muslim Conquest, Archaeology and Art.* II, Jerusalem: Yad Izhak Ben Zvi. [H]

Tsafrir, Y. and Foerster, G. (1989): 'The Dating of the "Earthquake of the Sabbatical Year" of 749 CE in Palestine', *Tarbiz* 58: 357–362. [H]

—— (1992): 'The Dating of the Earthquake of the Sabbatical Year in 749 C.E.', *BSOAS* 55: 231–235.

—— (1995): 'On the *Earthquake of the Sabbatical Year* in 749 C.E.', *Cathedra* 74: 179–180. [H]

Turner, V.W. (1987): 'Pilgrimage', in M. Eliade et al. (eds.), *The Encyclopedia of Religion.* X, New York: Macmillan & London: Collier Macmillan: 327–338.

Turner, V.W. and Turner, E. (1978): *Image and Pilgrimage in Christian Culture: Anthropological Perspectives.* Oxford: Blackwell.

Tur-Sinai, N.H. (1956): 'Following the Language and the Book', *Leshonenu* 20: 1–10. [H]

—— (1965): 'Yemim, HaYemim', in *EB*, III. Jerusalem: Mosad Bialik: 702–703. [H]

Tweig, S. (1979): 'Thrapeutic Baths in Israel', *Kardom* 1 (6): 27–28. [H]

Tzaferis, V. (1983): 'The Excavations of Kursi-Gergesa', *'Atiqot EgS* 16: 1–51.
—— (1993): 'Kursi', in E. Stern (ed.), *NEAEHL* III, Jerusalem: Israel Exploration Society & Carta: 893–896.
Tzondak, B. (1938): 'The Estrous Hormone and Coloured Material Similat to Vitamin B$_2$ in the Dead Sea', in J.N. Epstein et al. (eds.), *Magness Book. Collection of Essays.* Jerusalem: Society for Publishing Books by The Hebrew University: 428–432. [H]
Ullman, M. (1970): *Die Medizin im Islam.* Leiden-Köln: Brill.
Ulmann, S.B. (1950): 'Medical Plants in the Bible', *Sinai* 26: 134–205. [H]
Unz, C. (1971): 'Römische Militärfunde aus Baden-Aquae Helveticae', *GVJ:* 41–45.
Urman, D. (1995): 'Hammat Gader', in D. Urman and P.V.M. Flesher (eds.), *Ancient Synagogues: Historical Analysis and Archaeological Discovery.* II, Leiden: Brill: 595– 605.
Urbach, E.E. (1953): 'The Jews in Their Land during the *Tannaim* Period', *Behinot* 4: 61–72. [= M.D. Herr and J. Frankel (eds.) (1988): ibid., *Researches in Judaic Studies.* II, Jerusalem: Magness Press, The Hebrew University: 687–700. [H]
—— (1968): 'Rabbi Judah the Patriarch', *EH,* XIX. Jerusalem-Tel-Aviv: Dvir: 208. [H]
—— (1971) *The Sages: Their Concepts and Beliefs* (2nd edn.). Jerusalem: Magness Press, The Hebrew University. [H]
—— (1973): 'Mishmarot U'Ma'amadot', *Tarbiz* 42: 304–327. [H]
—— (1976): 'Halakhah and History', in R.H. Hamerton-Kelly and R. Scroggs (eds.), *Jews, Greeks and Christians: Religious Cultures in Late Antiquity. Essays in Honor of W.D. Davies.* Leiden: Brill:
—— (1984): *The Halakha: Its Origins and Development.* Givatayim: Yad LaTalmud. [H]
—— (1988): 'The Laws of Idolatry in the Light of Historical and Archaeological Facts in the Third Century', *From the World of the Sages: Research Essays* (2nd edn.). Jerusalem: Magness Press, The Hebrew University: 125–178. [= ibid., *Eretz-Israel* 5 (1958): 189–205]. [H]
Vallance, J.T. (1990): *The Lost Theory of Asclepiades of Bithynia.* Oxford: Clarendon Press.
—— (1993): 'The Medical System of Asclepiades of Bithynia', in *ANRW* II.37.1: 693–727.
van der Vliet, N. (1950): *Monnaies inédites ou très rares du medaillier de sainte Anne de Jérusalem.* Paris: Lecoffre, J. Gabalda et Cie.
van Kasteren, J.P. (1892): 'Emmaus-Nicopolis et les auteurs arabes', *RB* 1: 80–99.
van Nijf, O.M. (1997): *The Civic World of Professional Associations in the Roman East.* Amsterdam: J.C. Gieben, Publisher.
van Rose, S. and Mercer, E. (1999): *Volcanoes.* London: The National History Museum.
Van Zyl, A.H. (1960): *The Moabites. Pretoria Oriental Series,* 3. Leiden: Brill.
Vann, R.L. (1989): *The Unexcavated Buildings of Sardis. BAR International Series* 538. Oxford: Archaeological Reports International Series.
Varhaftig, S. (1987): 'Marketing Merchandises in the Talmud', *Sinai* 100 (1): 429–451. [H]
Vengosh, A., Starinksy, A., Kolodny, Y. and Chivas, A. (1994): 'Boron Isotope Geochemistry of Thermal Springs from the Northern Rift Valley, Israel', *JH* 162: 165–169.
Villard, L. (1994): 'Le bain dans la médicine hippocratique', in R. Ginouvè et al. (eds.), *L'eau, la santé et la maladie dans le monde grec. Actes du colloque organisé à Paris, 1992.* Athènes: Ecole Française d'Athènes & Paris: Diffusion de Boccard: 41–60.
Vilnaey, Z. (1970–1985): *Ariel: Encyclopaedia for the Geography of Eretz-Israel.* I–IX, Sifriyat HaSade. [H]
Vincent, L.H. (1902): 'Inscription Romaine d'Abou Ghôch', *RB* 11: 428–433.
—— (1908): 'Amulette Judeo-Araméenne', *RB* 17: 382–394.
—— (1921–1922): 'Les fouilles juives d'El-Hammam, a Tibériade', *RB* 30: 438–442. *Ibid.,* 31: 115–122.
—— (1936): 'Chronique: Autour du groupe monumental d'Amwas', *RB* 45: 403–415.

—— (1948): 'La chronólogie du groupe monumental d'Amwas', *RB* 55: 348–375.

Vincent, L.H. and Abel, F.M. (1912–1914): *Jerusalem: Recherches de Topographie, d'Archéologie, et d'Histoire.* I–III, Paris: J. Gabalda.

—— (1932): *Emmaüs: Sa basilique et son histoire.* Paris: E. Leroux.

Vogel, E.K. (1971): 'Bibliography of Holy Land Sites', *HUCA* 42: 1–96.

Vogel, E.K. and Holtzclaw, B. (1981): 'Bibliography of Holy Land Sites', *HUCA* 52: 1–92.

Vohalman, M. (1939): *Studies of the Land.* Tel-Aviv: Stibel. [H]

von Bergmann, A. (1897): *Die Lepra.* Stuttgart: F. Enke.

Wacher, J. (1998): *Roman Britain.* London: Sutton Publishing.

—— (ed.) (2002): *The Roman World.* I–II, London-New York: Routledge.

Wagner-Lux, U., Vriezen, K.J.H. et al. (1993): 'Vorläufiger Bericht über die Ausgrabungs- und Vermessungsarbeiten in Gadara (Umm Qes) in Jordanien im Jahre 1992', *ZDPV* 109: 64–72.

Walbank, F.W. (1981) [repr. 1992]: *The Hellenistic World.* [London]: Fontana Paperbacks.

Walford, E. (1855): *Sozomen's Ecclesiastical History.* London: Henry G. Bohn.

Walker, P.W.L. (1990) *Holy City, Holy Places? Christian Attitudes to Jerusalem and the Holy Land in the Fourth Century.* Oxford: Clarendon Press.

Walker, S. (1987): 'Roman Nymphaea in the Greek World', in S. Macready and F.H. Thompson (eds.), *Roman Architecture in the Greek World.* London: Burlington House, Picadilly: 60–71.

Wallack-Samuels, C., Rynearson, P. and Meshorer, Y. (2000): *The Numismatic Legacy of the Jews.* New York: Stack's Publications Numismatic Review.

Walmsley, A.G. (1988): 'Pella/Fihl after the Islamic Conquest: A Convergence of Literary and Archaeological Evidence', *Med. Arch.* 1: 142–159.

—— (1992): 'Archaeology in Jordan: Pella', *AJA* 96: 539–541.

—— (1995): 'Christians and Christianity at Early Islamic Pella (Fihl)', in S. Bourke and J.-P. Descoeudres (eds.), *Trade, Contact, and the Movement of Peoples in the Eastern Mediterranean: Studies in Honour of J. Basil Hennessy.* Med. Arch. Supp. 3: 321–324.

—— (2002): 'Die Dekapolis-Städte nach dem Ende des römischen Reiches. Kontinuiat und Wandel', in A. Hoffman and S. Kerner (eds.), *Gadara, Gerasa und die Dekapolis.* Mainz: Zaberns Bildbänd zur Archäologie: 137–145.

Walmsley, A.G., Macumber, P.G., Edwards, P.C. et al. (1993): 'The Eleventh and Twelfth Seasons of Excavation at Pella (Tabaqat Fahl) 1989–1990', *ADAJ* 37: 165–231.

Walner, A. (2000): 'The Twenty-Four Priestly Courses in Eretz-Israel', in Y. Alfasi (ed.), *Searei-Shmuel: Memorial Book for Shmuel Klughaft.* Bat-Yam: Family Klughaft 125–141. [H]

Walters, H.B. (1921): *Catalogue of the Silver Plates. Greek, Etruscan and Roman in the British Museum.* London: British Museum Press.

Ward, R.B. (1992): 'Women in Roman Baths', *HTR* 85 (2): 125–147.

Ward-Perkins, J.B. (1981): *Roman Imperial Architecture* (2nd edn.). New Haven-London: Yale University Press.

Waterhouse, S.D. and Ibach, R. (1975): 'Heshbon 1973: The Topographical Survey', *AUSS* 13: 217–233.

Waterman, L. (1937) [repr. 1980]: *Preliminary Report of the University of Michigan, Excavations at Sepphoris, Palestine in 1931.* Ann Arbor: University Microfilms International.

Watson, P. and Tidmarsh, J. (1996): 'Pella/Tall al-Husn Excavations 1993. The University of Sydney: 15th Season', *ADAJ* 40: 293–313.

Weber, M. (1996): *Antike Badekultur.* München: C.H. Beck.

Weber, T. (1988): 'Gadara of the Decapolis: A Summary of the 1988 Season at Umm-Qeis', *ADAJ* 32: 349–352.

—— (1989): 'Umm-Qeis (Gadara)', in D. Homes-Fredericq and J.B. Hennessy (eds.), *Archaeology of Jordan, Field Reports.* II/2, *Akkadica, Supplementum* 8: 606–611.

—— (1991): 'Gadara of the Decapolis. Preliminary Report on the 1990 Season at Umm Qeis', *ADAJ* 35: 223–235.

—— (1992): 'Ein frühchristliches Grab mit Glockenketten zu Gadara in der syrischen Dekapolis', *JÖB* 42: 249–286.

—— (1993): *Pella Decapolitana: Studien zur geschichte, architektur und bildenden kunst einer hellenisierten Stadt des nordlichen Ostjordanlandes*. Wiesbaden.

—— (1997): 'Thermal Springs, Medical Supply and Healing Cults in Roman-Byzantine Jordan', in G. Bisheh et al. (eds.), *Studies in the History and Archaeology of Jordan*. VI, Amman: Department of Antiquities: 331–338.

—— (2002): *Gadara: Umm Qes. Gadara Decapolitana. Untersuchungen zur Topographie, Geschichte, Architektur und der Bildenden Kunst einer 'Polis Hellenis' im Ostjordanland*. I, Wiesbaden: Harrassowitz.

Weber, W. (1907): *Untersuchungen zur Geschichte des Kaisers Hadrianus*. Leipzig: Teubner.

Weeber, K.W. (1999): *Panem et Circenses: Massenunterhaltung als Politik im antiken Rom*. Mainz am Rhein: Philipp von Zabern.

Weinfeld, M. (1982): *Genesis*, in M. Haran et al. (eds.), *Encyclpaedia of the World of the Bible*. I–XXIV, Tel-Aviv: Revivim. [H]

Weiss, H.B. and Kemble, H.R. (1962): *They Took to the Waters*. Trenton, New Jersey: Past Times Press.

—— (1967): *The Great American Water-Cure Craze: A History of Hydropathy in the United States*. Trenton, New Jersey: The Past Times Press.

Weiss, Z. (1988): 'The Ancient Synagogues at Tiberias and Hammat', in Y. Hirschfeld (ed.), *Tiberias: From Beginnings until the Muslim Conquest*. Jerusalem: Yad Izhak Ben Zvi: 35–46. [H]

—— (1992): 'Social Aspects of Burial in Beth Shearim', in L.I. Levine (ed.), *The Galilee in Late Antiquity*. New York: Jewish Theological Seminary of America: 357–371.

—— (1994): *Zippori*. Jerusalem: Israel Exploration Society.

—— (1995): 'Roman Leisure Culture and Its Influence upon the Jewish Population in the Land of Israel', *Qadmoniot* 109: 2–19. [H]

—— (1998): 'Buildings for Entertainment', in D. Sperber, *The City in Roman Palestine*. New York-Oxford: Oxford University Press: 77–102.

—— (2001): 'The Jews of Ancient Palestine and the Roman Games: Rabbinic Dicta vs. Communal Practice', *Zion* 66: 427–450. [H]

Weiss, Z. and Netzer, E. (1996): *Promise and Redemption: The Synagogue Mosaic of Sepphoris*. Jerusalem: Israel Museum.

—— (1997): 'The Hebrew University Excavations at Sepphoris', *Qadmoniot* 113: 3–21. [H]

Welch, K. (1991): 'Roman Amphitheatres Revived', *JRA* 4: 272–281.

Weller, C.H. (1903): 'The Cave at Vari', *AJA* 7: 263–288.

Welles, C.B. (1938): 'The Inscriptions in Gerasa', in C.H. Kraeling (ed.), *Gerasa: City of the Decapolis*. New Haven: American School of Oriental Research: 355–494.

Wellhausen, J. (1876): *Die Composition des Hexateuchs* (1885; from essays: 1876–1877).

Wells, C.M. (1992) [repr. 1984]: *The Roman Empire* (2nd ed.). London: Fontana.

Westermann, C. (1984): *Genesis 1–11: A Commentary* (tr. J.J. Scullion). London-Minneapolis: S.P.C.K. & Augsburg.

White, D. (1985): 'Roman Athletics', *Expedition* 27 (2): 30–40.

Wiedemer, H.R. (1967): 'Die Entdeckung der romischen Heilthermen von Baden: Aquae Helveticae 1967', *GVJ*: 83–93.

Wiedermann, T. (1992) [repr. 2001]: *Emperors and Gladiators*. London-New York: Routledge.

Wilkinson, J. (1977): *Jerusalem Pilgrims before the Crusades*. Warminster: Aris & Phillips.

—— (1981): *Egeria's Travels* (rev. edn.). Warminster: Aris & Phillips.

Wilkinson, L.P. (1981): *The Roman Experience*. Lanham, MD: University Press of America.

Williams, C.A. (1999): *Roman Homosexuality: Ideologies of Masculinity in Classical Antiquity.* New York-Oxford: Oxford University Press.

Williams, F. (tr.) (1987): *The Panarion of Epiphanius of Salamis.* Book I (Sects 1–46). Leiden: Brill.

Willis, B. (1928): 'Earthquaqe in the Holy Land', *BSSA* 18: 73–103.

Wilmanns, G. (ed.) (1873): *Exempla inscriptionum latinarum in usum praecipue academicum.* Berolini: Apud Weidmannos.

Wilson, C.W. (tr.) (1888): *Palestine Pilgrims' Text Society: The Pilgrimage of the Russian Abbot Daniel in The Holy Land, 1106–1107 A.D.* IV: Lond.

Wilson, J.F. (2004): *Caesarea Philippi: Banias, The Lost City of Pan.* London: I.B. Tauris.

Winogradov, Z. (1988): 'Berenice Aqueduct: The Ancient Aqueduct of Tiberias', in Y. Hirschfeld (ed.), *Tiberias: From Beginnings until the Muslim Conquest.* Jerusalem: Yad Izhak Ben Zvi: 151–165. [H]

—— (2002): 'The Aqueduct of Tiberias', in D. Amit et al. (eds.), *The Aqueducts of Israel.* Portsmoth, Rhode Island: 295–304.

Witt, R.E. (1971): *Isis in the Graeco-Roman World.* Ithaca, N.Y.: Cornell University Press.

—— (1997): *Isis in the Ancient World.* Baltimore-London: Johns Hopkins University Press.

Wohnlich, S. (2001): 'The Spa of Baden-Baden, Germany', in P.E. LaMoreaux and J.T. Tanner (eds.), *Springs and Bottled Waters Bottled Waters of the World: Ancient History, Source, Occurance, Quality, and Use.* Berlin: Springer: 164–165.

Wood, K.E. (2004): *Spa Culture and the Social History of Medicine in Germany.* PhD thesis, University of Illinois at Chicago.

Worschech, U. (1992): 'Der gott Kemosch versuch einer charakterisierung', *UF* 24: 393–401.

Wright, C. (1988): *Guide to Health Spas around the World.* Chester: Globe Pequot Press.

Wroth, W. (1885): 'Hygieia', *JHS* 5: 82–101.

Wunderbar, R.J. (1850): *Biblish-talmudische Medicin oder pragmatische Darstellung der Arzneikunde der alten Israeliten.* Riga-Leipzig: [n.s.].

Yakobovitz, M. (1981): *Lexicon of Waters.* I–II, Tel-Aviv: Sifriyat Maariv. [H]

Yankelvitz, R. (1988): 'Hammei-Tiberias Baths in Antiquity', *Ma-Tov Tiberias* 6: 15–21. [H]

Yaretzky, A. (1982): 'Hereditary Factors in Rheumatic Diseases', *FPMJ* 10: 427–432. [H].

Yaron, F. (1952): 'The Springs of Lake Kinnereth and Their Relationship to the Dead Sea', *BRCI* 2: 121–128. [H]

Yaron, H. (2001): *Health Tourism and Ecological Desert Tourism: Perceived Density and Willingness to Pay.* MSc. Thesis. The Technion, Israel Institute of Technology. [H]

Yavetz, Z. (1974): 'The Position of the Physician in the Ancient Roman Society', *HaRefuah* 86 (7): 373–377. [H]

Yechieli, Y. and Gat, J.R. (1997): 'Geochemical and Hydrological Processes in the Coastal Environment of the Dead Sea', in M. Niemi et al. (eds.), *The Dead Sea: The Lake and Its Setting.* New York-Oxford: Oxford University: 252–264.

Yegül, F. (1988): 'The Function of the Thermo-Mineral Bathing Complex at Baiae', (Abstract), *AJA* 92: 282.

—— (1992): *Baths and Bathing in Classical Antiquity.* New York-Cambridge-Mass.: The MIT Press.

—— (1996): 'The Thermo-Mineral Complex at Baiae and *De Balneis Puteolanis*', *The Art Bulletin* 78 (1): 137–161.

Yeivin, S. (1956): 'The Extent of Egyptian Domination in Hither Asia under the Middle Kingdom', *EI* 4: 37–40. [H]

Yudelevitz, M.D. (1950): *Tiberias: The Jewish Life during the Talmudic Era.* Tel-Aviv: Mosad HaRav Kook. [H]

Zanovello, P. and Basso, P. (2004): *Montegrotto Terme: Via Neroniana: gli scavi 1989–1992*. Padova: Il poligrafo.

Zajac, N. (1999): 'Thermae: A Policy of Public Health or Personal Legitimation?', in J. DeLaine and D.E. Johnston (eds.), *Roman Baths and Bathing, Proceeding of the First International Conference on Roman Baths held at Bath, 1992. JRA Supp. Series* 37: 99–105.

Zayadine, F. (1966): 'Samaria-Sebaste, Le Theatre', *RB* 72: 576–580.

Zeide, J. (1954): *History of Medicine*. Tel-Aviv: Neuman. [H]

Zeuner, P.A. (1960): 'Notes on Qumran', *PEQ* 92: 33–36.

Zevin, S.Y. (1980): 'Hammet-Tiberias', *Talmudic Encyclopedia for Halakhic Issues*. XVI, Jerusalem: *Talmudic Encyclopedia* Publication & Mosad HaRav Kook: 44–52. [H]

Zeyadeh, A. (1992): 'Urban Transformation in the Decapolis Cities of Jordan', *ARAM Periodical* 4 (1–2): 101–115.

—— (1994): 'Settlement Patterns, An Archaeological Prespective: Case Studies from Northern Palestine and Jordan', in G.R.D. King and A. Cameron (eds.) *The Byzantine and Early Islamic Near East*. II, Princeton, N.J.: Darwin Press: 117–131.

Zellinger, J. (1928): *Bad und Bäder in der altchristlichen Kirche: eine Studie über Christentum und Antike*. München: Hueber.

Zias, J. (1989): 'Lust and Leprosy: Confusion or Correlation?', *BASOR* 275: 27–31.

—— (1997): 'Disease and Healing Methods in Ancient Land of Israel in Paleo-Pathological Research', *Qadmoniot* 113: 54–59. [H]

Ziegenaus, O. (1981): *Altertümer von Pergamon: Das Asklepieion*. III, Berlin: W. de Gruyter.

Ziegler, K. (1919): 'Thermai Himeraiai', in A. Pauly, G. Wissowa and W. Kroll (eds.) *Real-Encyclopädie der classischen Altertumswissenschaft*. München: Druckenmüller: 2385.

Zielinski, T. (1924): 'Charis and Charites', *CQ* 18: 158–163.

Zipor, M.A. (2005): *The Septuagint Vrsion of the Book of Genesis*. Ramat-Gan: Bar-Ilan University Press. [H]

Zlotnick, D. (1993): 'Proklos ben Plslws', in S. Friedman (ed.), *Saul Liberman Memorial Volume*. New York: The Jewish Theological Seminary of America: 49–52.

Zorell, F. (ed.) (1984): *Lexicon Hebraicum et Aramaicum Veteris Testamenti*. Roma: Pontificium Institutum Biblicum.

Zulay, M. (1937): 'Poetry for the Memorial of Various Events: The Earthquake in Tiberias and in Other Parts of the Country', *BIHPR* 3: 151–162. [= ibid., (1995) in E. Hazan (ed.). *Eretz-Israel and Its Poetry: Studies in the Piyyutim from the Cairo Geniza*. Jerusalem: The Magness Press, The Hebrew University]. [H]

Zuri, I.S. (1924): *The Southerners' Culture*. Warsow: Merkaz. [H]

—— (1931–1933): *The History of the Public Jewish Law, The Reign of the Presidency and The Committee*. I–III, Paris [s.n.]. [H]

GENERAL INDEX

Hammat-Selim, 59
Hammat-Tiberias, 3, 8, 125, 138, 253, 255, 311, 312, 421
Hammatu, 163
hamme, 59
hammei, 11, 127
Hammei-Ba'arah, xxxi, 92, 99, 144, 169, 180, 189, 192, 195, 196, 199, 227, 228, 239, 259, 278, 282, 402, 418, 425, 428
Hammei-Livias, xxxi, 92, 196, 197, 199, 223, 401, 417, 425
hammei-marpeh, 11
Hammei-Mazor, 63, 66
Hammei-Shalem, 63
Hammei-Tiberias, xxxi, xxxii, 1, 2, 4, 6, 12, 14, 15, 20, 24, 54, 56, 57, 58, 59, 60, 64, 68, 71, 72, 75, 76, 77, 78, 79, 81, 92. 125, 126, 127, 128, 129, 130, 131, 132, 134, 135, 136, 138, 139, 140, 142, 143, 168, 169, 180, 187, 192, 195, 231, 232, 233, 234, 235, 236, 239, 242, 247, 248, 253, 259, 269, 270, 274, 276, 277, 278, 280, 281, 282, 291, 301, 313, 324, 332, 338, 348, 351, 352, 395, 396, 397, 417, 421, 425, 427
Hammei-Yesha, 63, 64
Hammei-Yoav, 69
Hammei-Zohar, 63, 65, 66, 81
Hammim, 11, 15
Hammon, 13, 14
Hammoth, 167, 425
Hammoth-Dor, 13, 14
Hammt, 14
Hammta, 14, *See Hammtha*
Hammtha, xxx, 14, 30, 69, 164, 165, 210, 213, 215, 223, 301, 302, 317, 318, 330, 426, *See Hammta*
Hammtha de Gader, 11
Hammtha de Peḥal, 14, 30, 164, 165, 166, 167, 237
Hammthan, 11, 15, 30, 31, 165, 166, 203, 207, 278, 281, 292, 302, 317
Hamuel, 14
Hana bar Ketina, Rav, 277
Hanania ben Akavia, 187
Hanina, Rabbi, 144, 241, 262, 297, 299, 303, 304, 307, 308
Hanina bar Hama, Rabbi, 299, 303
Hanina bar Joseph
Hanina bar Pappa, Rabbi, 375
Hanina of Ein Te'enah, 296
Hansen disease, 244

HaRambam, 8, 142, *See* Maimonides
HaRamban, 8, 143, 235, 248
harara, 35
haruspex, 101
Hasmonean, 47, 150, 172, 210, 291
Hauran, 12, 60, 126, 192, 372
HaYamim, 16, 17, 183
Hazor, 126, 182
headaches, 74, 87, 267, 336
healing cults, xxix, xxx, xxxi, 4, 88, 125, 169, 201, 226, 232, 237, 252, 278, 285, 287, 306, 313, 318, 335, 354, 358, 359, 397, 400
healing qualities, xxxi, 2, 9, 80, 83, 88, 143, 171, 220, 223, 228, 236, 241, 242, 248, 313, 349, 352, 403, 423, 428, 431
health ailments, 9, 223, 241, 403, 423
health resorts, xxxi, 9, 425
Hebron, 387
hegemon, 156, 318, 325
Hellenistic, xxix, 1, 3, 7, 40, 65, 85, 94, 110, 125, 127, 143, 163, 165, 211, 282, 325, 347, 348, 350, 353, 357, 363, 375, 378, 426
Hellenistic-Roman, 40, 127, 163, 324, 370
Hemam, 18
hemar, 24
hemmet, 13
Hephaestus, 93, 95
Heptapegon, 57
Heracles, 89, 92, 93, 94, 105, 148, 285, 288, 338, 343, 344, 355, 399, *See* Hercules
Herculanum, 123
Hercules, 97, 99, 250, 338, 355, *See* Heracles
Hercules Bibax, 104
Hermes, 96, 97
Hermon, 182, 374
Herod Antipas, 127, 128, 130, 198, 401
Herod Archelaus, 360
Herod the Great, 2, 38, 40, 170, 171, 174, 178, 189, 198, 232, 254, 360
Herodium, 173, 329
Herodotus, 93, 378
Heshbon, 166, 173, 182, 197, 198, *See* Hisban, Esbus
Hezekiah, 276, 277, 298, 308
hibil, 196
Hierapolis (Pamukkale), 93, 203
Hierocles, 7, 198, 401
Hieromices, 363, 371, 387, *See* Yarmuk
Hieronymus, 7, 16, 17, 25, 31, 148,

GREEK WORDS

ILLUSTRATIONS

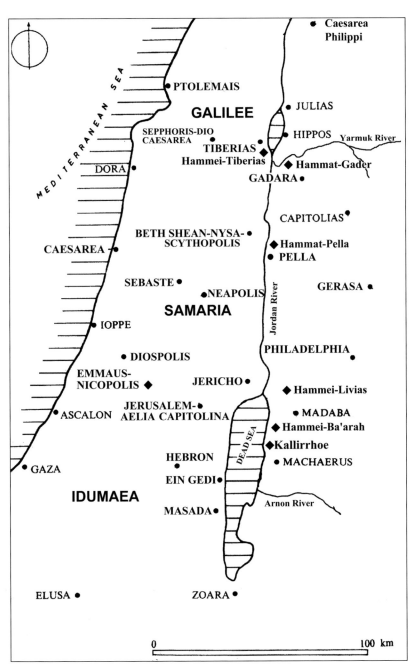

Map 1 Location of the thermo-mineral baths in Roman Palestine and
Provincia Arabia
(Drawing by Meiri Dvorjetski)

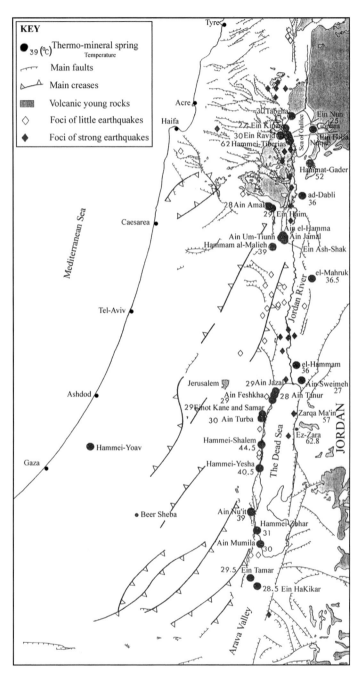

Map 2   Location of the thermo-mineral springs in Israel and Jordan
(After Eckstein [1975]: *The Thermo-Mineral Springs of Israel*, with additions).
(Drawing by Meiri Dvorjetski)

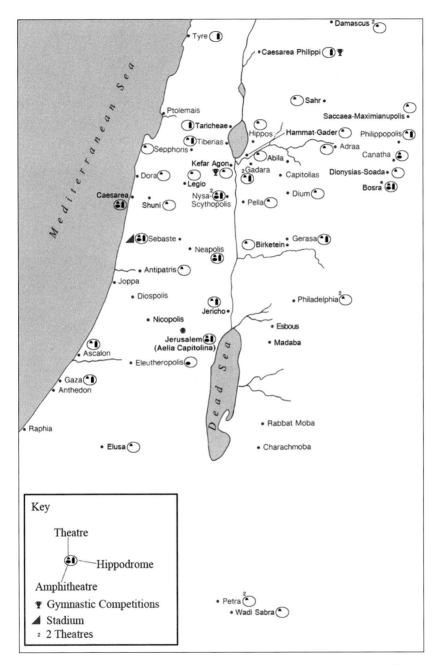

Map 3   Distribution of leisure and pleasure sites in the eastern Mediterranean according to historical evidences and archaeological remains
(Drawing by Meiri Dvorjetski)

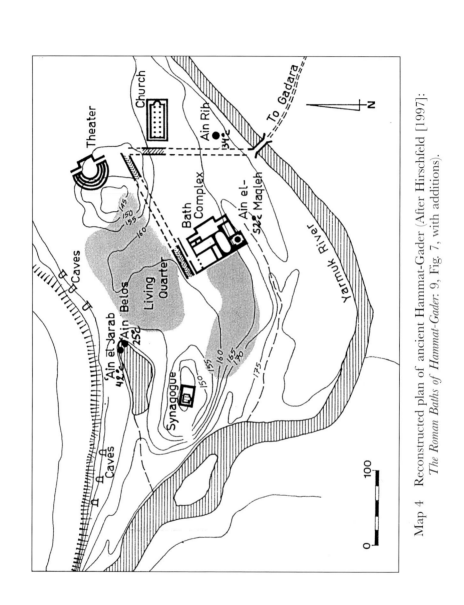

Map 4 Reconstructed plan of ancient Hammat-Gader (After Hirschfeld [1997]:
The Roman Baths of Hammat-Gader: 9, Fig. 7, with additions).

Tab. 1   Sample of Temperature and Chemical Composition of hot springs in Israel and the Dead Sea
(Concentrations are given in milligram/liter)

The Spring	Location	HCO$_3^-$	SO$_4^{-2}$	Cl$^-$	Br$^-$	Ca^{-2}	Mg^{+2}	Na$^+$	K$^+$	°C	°F
Hammei-Tiberias	2017 / 2414	150	770	17,800	228	3,340	682	6,590	380	62	143.6
Hammat-Gader 1	2126 / 2320	330	177	506	5.4	152	39.8	24.5	21.8	52	125.6
Hammat-Gader 2	2124 / 2322	344	121	300	3.7	105	44.5	140	13.1	42	107.6
Hammat-Gader 3	2128 / 2321	361	100	218		124	37.5	120	10.5	37	98.6
Hammat-Gader 4	2310 / 2327	381	58	87	2	89	32.7	55	3.9	29	84.2
Ein Nuqeb	2106 / 2462	263	356	1,663	16.1	156	105	925	51.0	30	86.0
Ein Gophra	2105 / 2457	322	205	2,430	27.5	265	172	1,100	68.5	33	91.4
Al-Malieh (upper)	1952 / 1928	137	333	1,625	19.4	335	89	720	50.0	36	96.8
Al-Malieh (lower)	1952 / 1928	251	263	1,245	12.1	263	76	565	37.4	38	100.4
Einot Tsukim (Feshkha) 3	1927 / 1246	275	45	1,740	29	228	263	495	57.0	26	78.8
Einot Tsukim (Feshkha) 11	1927 / 1240	281	84	3,241	83	410	484	805	224	28	82.4
Einot Tzukim (Feshkha) 14	1925 / 1233	298	225	40,180	886	3,546	6,895	8,560	1,350	31	87.8
Ein Kane 6	1880 / 1142	294	116	1,390	26	175	290	350	76	26	78.8
Ein Samar 12	1885 / 1122	276	125	2,970	63	300	562	780	120	26	78.8
Hammei-Yesha	1859 / 0920	86	1,030	121,680	825	10,180	19,520	28,650	3,660	40	104.0
Hammei-Zohar	1848 / 0640	177	704	41,840	815	3,497	6,580	10,395	1,030	28	82.4
Hammam Fhara'on	951 / 848	179	725	7,620	49	1,118	151	3,525	126	72	161.6
The Dead Sea		230	600	218,130	4,650	15,150	39,600	38,000	6,600		

Key: HCO$_3$ - Bicarbonate; SO$_4$ - Sulphate; Cl - Chlorine; Br - Bromine; Ca - Calcium; Mg - Magnesium; Na - Sodium; K - Potassium
(After Mazor [1980]: *Geology*: 303, Tab. 18, with addition).

Tab. 2   Thermo-mineral springs and diseases According to Ancient and Modern Sources (Author Original)

DISEASES / SPRINGS	Gyneco-logical	Neuro-pathies	Rheumatisms Arthrities	Gastro-intestinal	Debili-tation	Urinary	Dermato-pathies	Endo-crinology	Respiratory
Hammei-Tiberias	▲		▲	▲	▲	▲	▲		▲
Hammat-Gader			▲	▲		▲	▲	▲	
Hammat-Pella		▲	▲	▲			▲		
Kallirrhoe			▲	▲	▲	▲			
Hammei-Baʾarah	▲	▲	▲	▲	▲	▲	▲		
Hammei-Livias		▲	▲				▲		
Emmaus-Nicopolis			▲	▲					

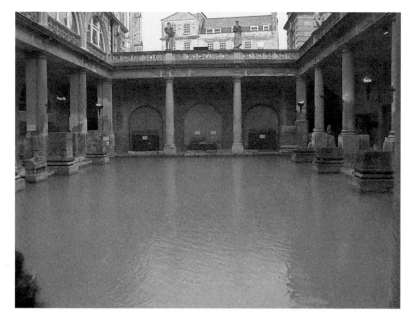

Fig. 1 The great bath at Bath Spa, England (Author original)

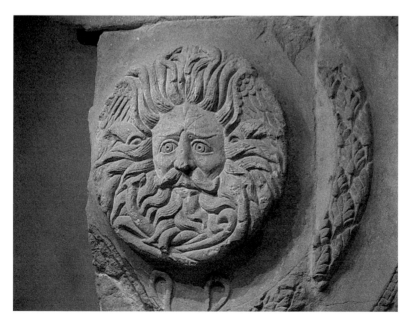

Fig. 2 The Gorgon's head pediment from the front of the temple of
Sulis-Minerva, Bath Spa, England
(Author original)

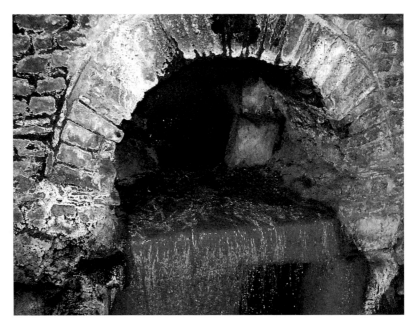

Fig. 3   The sacred spring of Bath Spa, England (Author original)

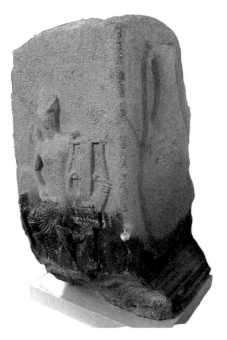

Fig. 4   Alter found in Aachen depicting the image of Apollo-Grannus
(Author original)

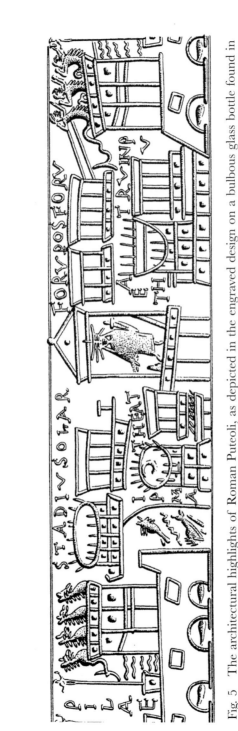

Fig. 5   The architectural highlights of Roman Puteoli, as depicted in the engraved design on a bulbous glass bottle found in North Africa (From Jackson [1999]: 'Spas, Waters and Hydrotherapy', *JRA Supp.* 37 [1]: 115, Fig. 4). (Drawing by Philip Compton, British Museum, by courtesy of Dr. Ralph Jackson)

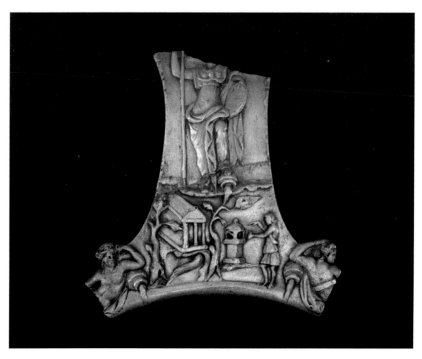

Fig. 6   Silver and gilt patera handle from Capheaton, Northumberland, showing the goddess Minerva presiding over a sacred spring, possibly Bath (From Jackson [1988]: *Doctors and Diseases*: 165, no. 44).

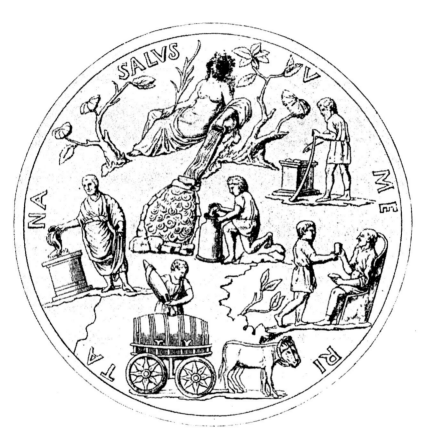

Fig. 7 Scenes of the Spanish spa of Salus Umeritana on a silver and gilt
bowl from Otañes, Castro Urdiales, Northern Spain. (From Jackson [1999]:
    'Spas, Waters and Hydrotherapy', *JRA Supp.* 37 [1]: 116, Fig. 5).

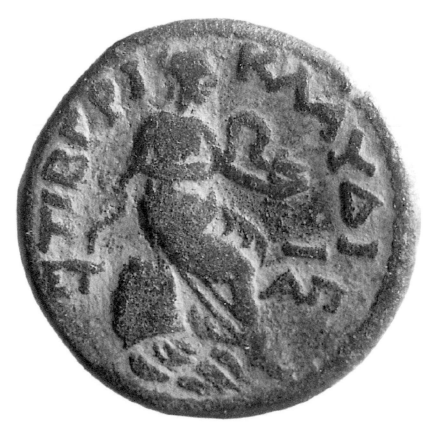

Fig. 8   Hygieia, goddess of health seated on a rock from which gushes a spring and feeding a serpent from a bowl. A coin of Tiberias (Trajan, 99/100 CE) (From Meshorer [2000]: *TestiMoney*: 50, Fig. 1).

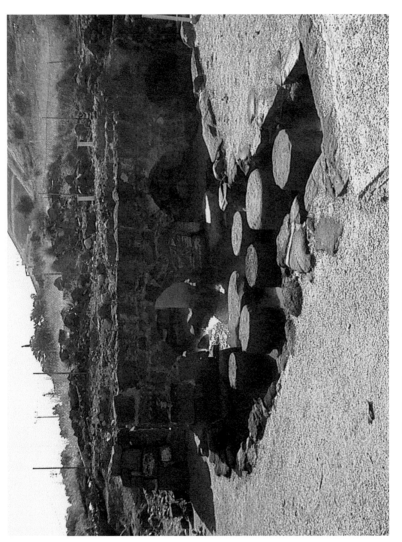

Fig. 9   The remains of Hammei-Tiberias (Author original)

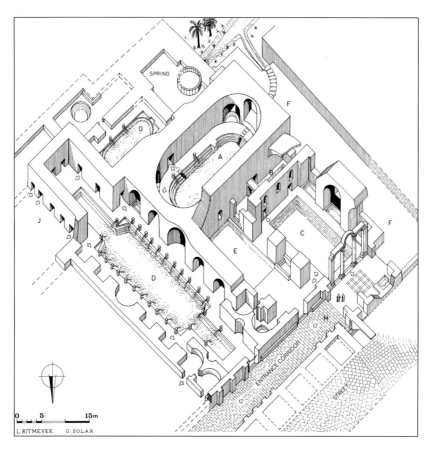

Fig. 10 Partial reconstruction of the baths complex at Hammat-Gader, with identification of the excavations areas and the conjectured bathing route [marked by arrows] (From Hirschfeld [1997]: *The Roman Baths of Hammat-Gader*: 55, Fig. 51).

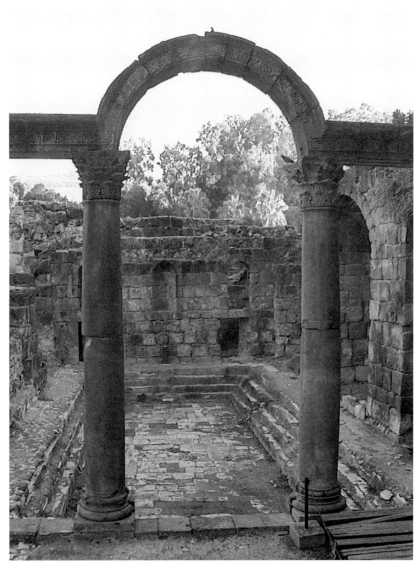

Fig. 11 Hammat-Gader, Beyond the columned portal; The Hall of Piers
and the wall with niches, looking southwest
(Author original)

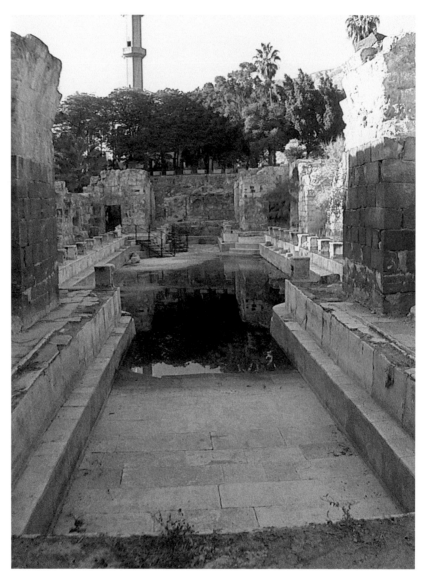

Fig. 12 Hammat-Gader, view of the central bathing pool of the Hall of
Fountains, looking south
(Author original)

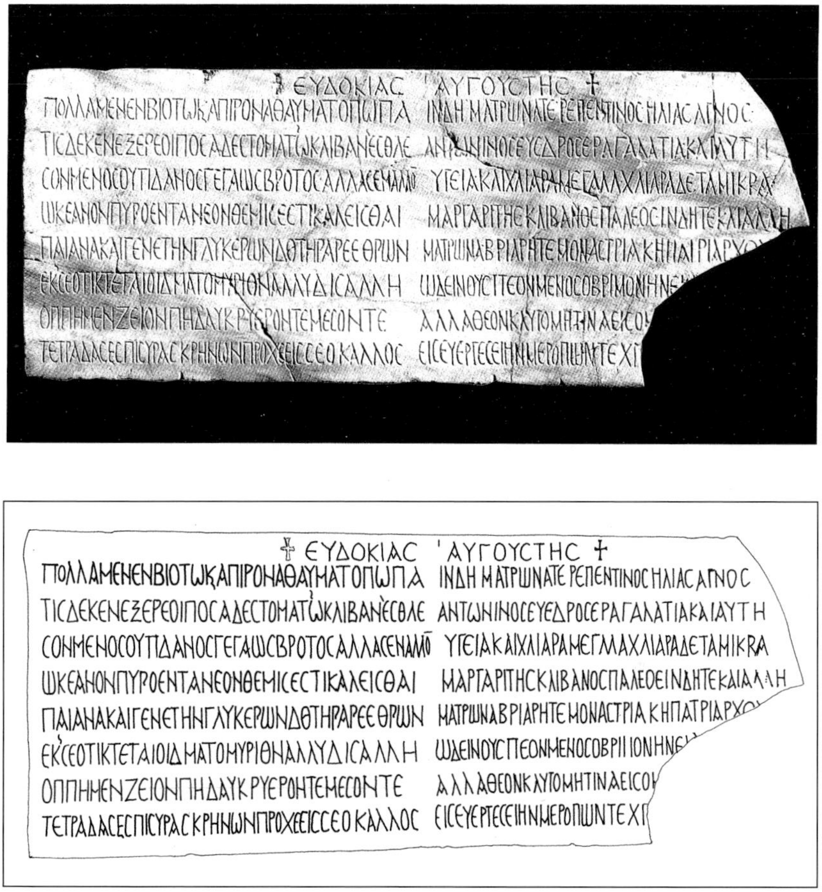

Fig. 13   Empress Eudocia's inscription from Hammat-Gader (From Di Segni [1997]: 'The Greek Inscriptions of Hammat Gader', in Hirschfeld, *The Roman Baths of Hammat-Gader*: 231, Fig. 45).

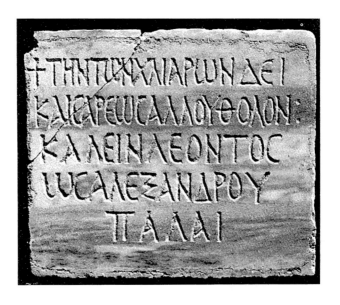

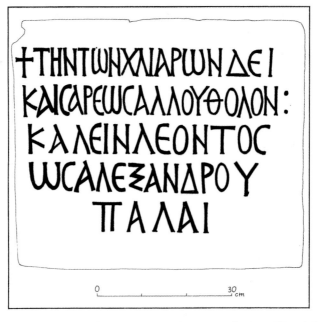

Fig. 14   The *tholos* of the lukewarm pool at Hammat-Gader: 'The *tholos* of the lukewarm pool should be named after another Caesarean, Leo, as it once (used to be named) after Alexander' (From Di Segni [1997]: 'The Greek Inscriptions', in Hirschfeld, *The Roman Baths of Hammat-Gader*: 237, Fig. 49).

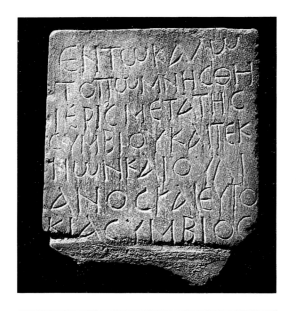

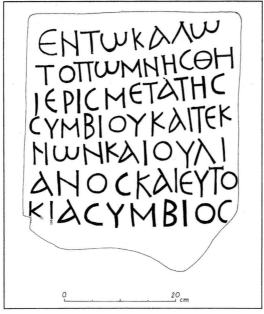

ΕΝΤωΚΑΛω
ΤΟΠΤωΜΝΗϹΘΗ
ΙΕΡΙϹΜΕΤΑΤΗϹ
ϹΥΜΒΙΟΥΚΑΙΤΕΚ
ΝωΝΚΑΙΟΥΛΙ
ΑΝΟϹΚΑΙΕΥΤΟ
ΚΙΑϹΥΜΒΙΟϹ

Fig. 15   A Greek inscription from Hammat-Gader, 'this beautiful place': 'In this beautiful place may Hierius be remembered, with (his) wife and children, and Julian and (his) wife Eutocia'. (From Di Segni [1997]: 'The Greek Inscriptions', in Hirschfeld, *The Roman Baths of Hammat-Gader*: 241, Fig. 51).

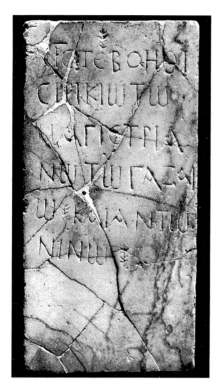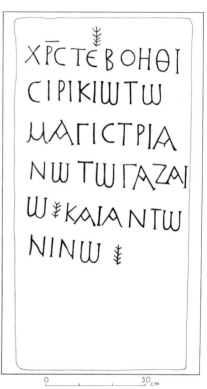

Fig. 16   A Greek inscription from Hammat-Gader, 'Christ, help!': 'Christ, help
Siricius the Gazean *in rebus*, and Antoninus' (From Di Segni [1997]: 'The Greek
Inscriptions', in Hirschfeld, *The Roman Baths of Hammat-Gader*: 210, Fig. 26).

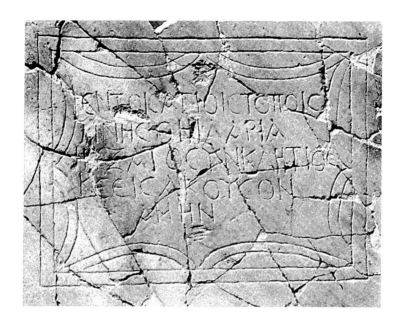

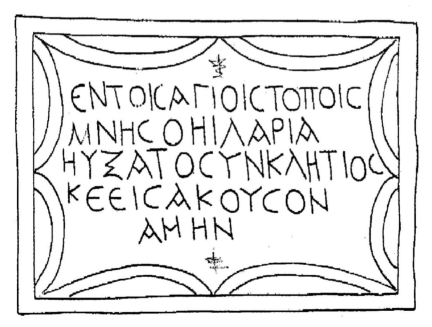

Fig. 17   A Greek inscription from Hammat-Gader, 'These holy places': 'In these holy places may Hilaria be remembered. Syncletius uttered this prayer: hearken, O Lord! Amen' (From Di Segni [1997]: 'The Greek Inscriptions', in Hirschfeld, *The Roman Baths of Hammat-Gader*: 219, Fig. 33).

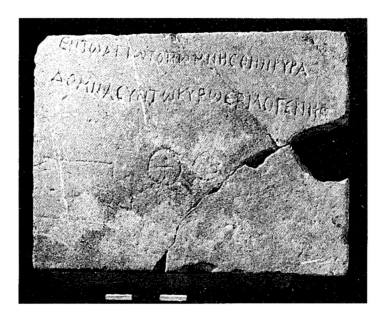

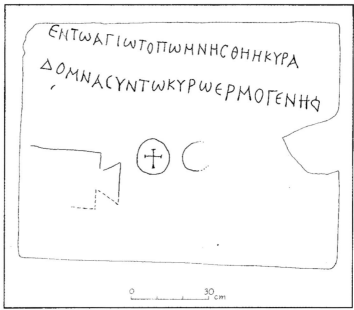

Fig. 18   A Greek inscription from Hammat-Gader, 'This holy place': In this holy place may the lady Domna be remembered, with the lord Hermogenes' (From Di Segni [1997]: 'The Greek Inscriptions', in Hirschfeld, *The Roman Baths of Hammat-Gader*: 244, Fig. 54).

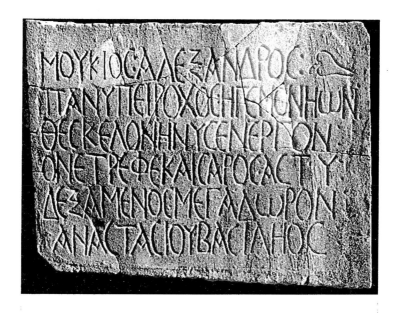

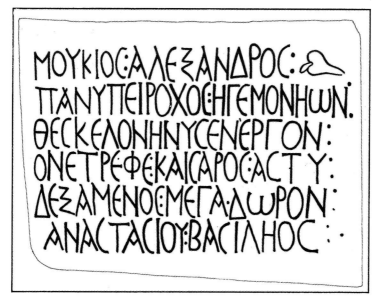

Fig. 19   A Greek inscription of the supreme governor from Hammat-
Gader: 'Mucius Alexander, supreme governor (or: the greatest of governors),
accomplished this wondrous work, (he) whom the city of Caesar nourished,
having received a great gift from Emperor Anastasius' (From Di Segni [1997]:
'The Greek Inscriptions', in Hirschfeld, *The Roman Baths of Hammat-Gader*:
235, Fig. 47).

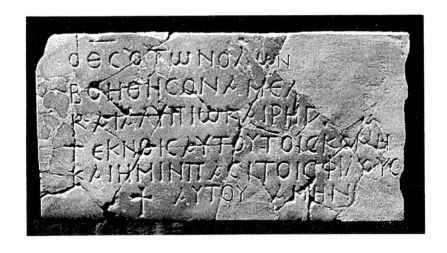

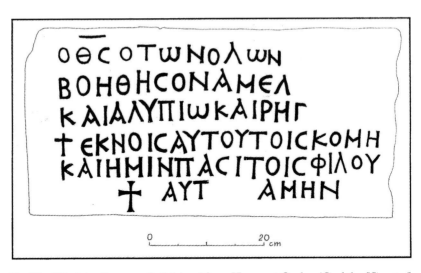

ΟΘϹ Ο Τῶ ΝΟλῶΝ
ΒΟΗΘΗϹΟΝΑΜΕλ
ΚΑΙΑλΥΠΙῶΚΑΙΡΗΓ
✝ΕΚΝΟΙϹΑΥΤΟΥΤΟΙϹΚΟΜΗ
ΚΑΙΗΜΙΝΠΑϹΙΤΟΙϹΦΙλΟΥ
✝ ΑΥΤ   ΑΜΗΝ

0   20 cm

Fig. 20   'God the Creator of all things' from Hammat-Gader: 'God the [Creator] of all things, help Ameli[anus], and Alypius and Reginus [?] his children, the counts, and us all who love them. Amen'. (From Di Segni [1997]: 'The Greek Inscriptions', in Hirschfeld, *The Roman Baths of Hammat-Gader*: 200, Fig. 16).

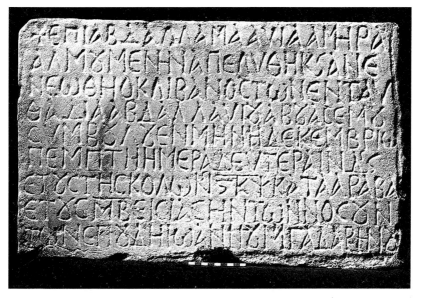

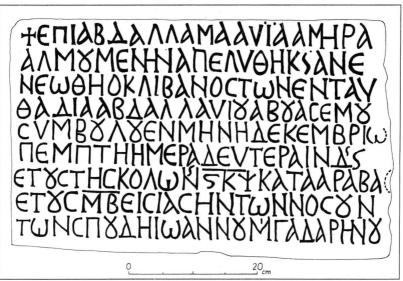

Fig. 21   Caliph Abdallah Muʾāwiya's inscription from Hammat-Gader (From Di Segni [1997]: 'The Greek Inscriptions of Hammat Gader', in Hirschfeld, *The Roman Baths of Hammat-Gader*: 238, Fig. 50).

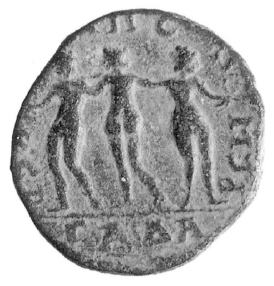

Fig. 22   The Three Graces. A coin of Gadara (Elagabal, 218 CE). (From
Meshorer [2000]: *TestiMoney*: 52, Fig. 1).

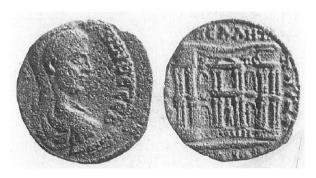

Fig. 23   The Nymphaeum. A coin of Pella (Elagabal, 220 CE) (From
Meshorer [1985]: *City-Coins*: 92, Fig. 251).

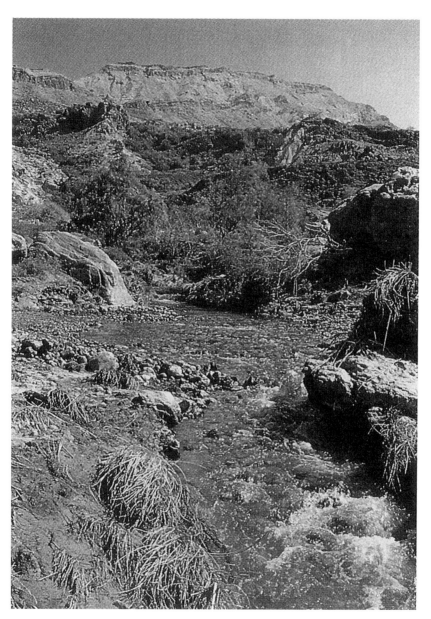

Fig. 24   Hot springs at Ez-Zara-Kallirrhoe (From Piccirillo and Alliata [1999]: *The Madaba Map*: 206).

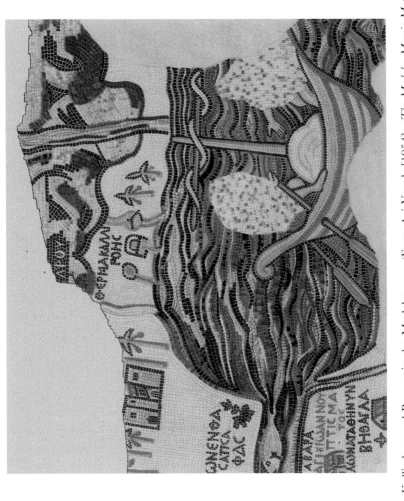

Fig. 25   Kallirrhoe and Baarou in the Madaba map (From Avi-Yonah [1954]: *The Madaba Mosaic Map*: Pl. 2).

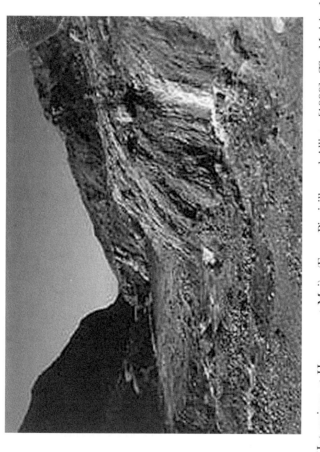

Fig. 26 Hot springs at Hammamat Maiʾn (From Piccirillo and Alliata [1999]: *The Madaba Map*: 206).

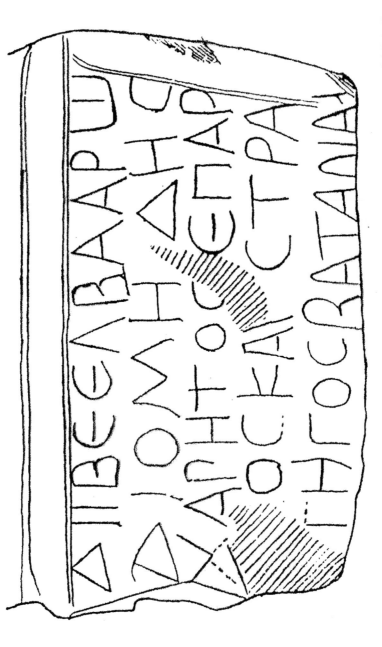

Fig. 27 A votive inscription from southern Syria to Zeus Beelbaaros of Hammei-Baʾarah (From Sourdel [1952]: *Les cultes du Hauran à l'époque romaine*: 45–46, Pl. 4:1).

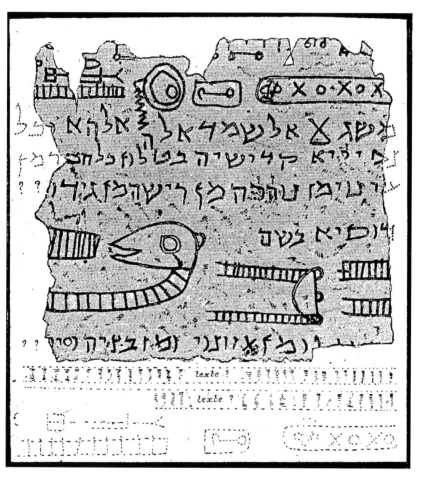

Fig. 28   Amulet from Emmaus-Nicopolis (From Vincent [1908]: 'Amulette
Judeo-Araméenne', *RB* 17: 382).

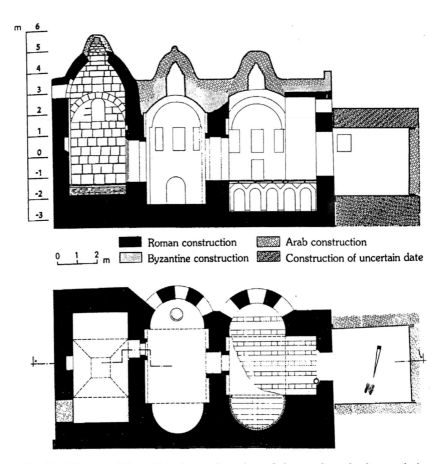

m
6
5
4
3
2
1
0
-1
-2
-3

■ Roman construction   ▨ Arab construction
0 1 2 m ▨ Byzantine construction ▨ Construction of uncertain date

Fig. 29 Emmaus-Nicopolis, plan and section of the southern baths, on their reduced scale (From Gichon [1993]: 'Emmaus', in Stern *NEAEHL* I: 387).

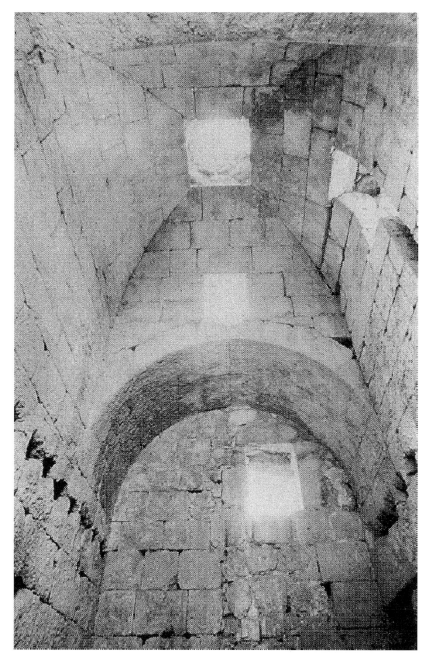

Fig. 30   Emmaus-Nicopolis, Room 4, cupola and north wall (From Gichon
(1979a): 'The Roman Bath at Emmaus', *IEJ* 29: Pl. 12A).

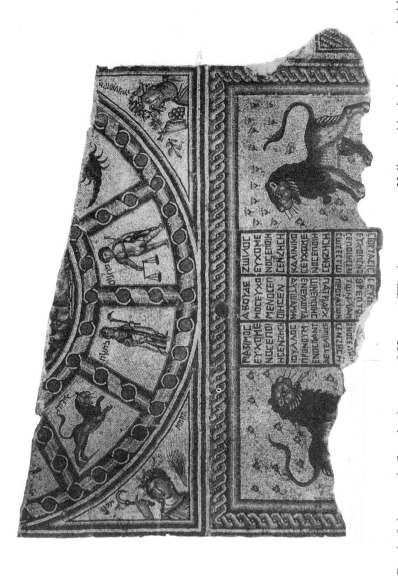

Fig. 31 Panel of the mosaic floor in the nave of Hammat-Tiberias synagogue. Helios on his chariot surrounded by a zodiac and a dedicatory Greek inscription (From Dothan [1993]: 'Hammat-Tiberias', in Stern *NEAEHL* II: 576).

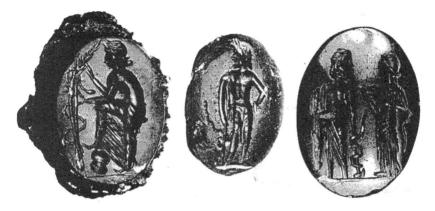

Hygieia and Aesculapius

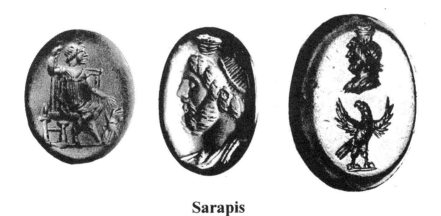

Sarapis

Fig. 32   Engraved gems of Hygieia, Aesculapius and Sarapis from Gadara
(From Henig and Whiting [1997]: *Engraved Gems from Gadara*: Figs. 26, 30, 38,
185, 190, 191).

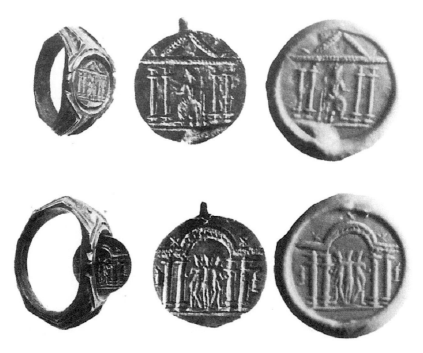

Fig. 33   A ring from Gadara; Disk revolving on two pivots (From Meshorer
[1979]: 'A Ring from Gadara', *IEJ* 29: Pl. 25 C & D).

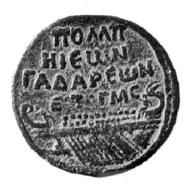
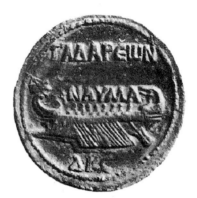
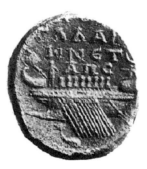

Fig. 34   Nautical symbols on the Gadara coins; Right: Galley with ramming prow, rudder, and oarsmen. Greek inscription 'the people of Gadara city and the *naumachia*. Year 224'. (Medallion, Marcus Aurelius, 161 CE); Left: Greek inscription 'of the people of Pompeian Gadara. Year 243' (Medallion, Commodus, 180 CE); Bottom: Galley with details clearly visible and two dolphins below. Greek inscription Year 283' (Elagabal, 220 CE). (From Meshorer [1985]: *City Coins*: 80–82: Figs. 218, 219, 224).